EVALUATION,
DIAGNOSIS, AND
TREATMENT OF
OCCLUSAL PROBLEMS

EVALUATION, DIAGNOSIS, AND TREATMENT OF OCCLUSAL PROBLEMS

PETER E. DAWSON, D.D.S.

SECOND EDITION
with 879 illustrations, including 19 in color

The C. V. Mosby Company

ST. LOUIS • BALTIMORE • TORONTO   1989

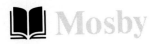

Editor: Robert W. Reinhardt
Assistant editor: Maureen Slaten
Project manager: Kathleen L. Teal
Production editor: Carl Masthay
Design: John Rokusek
Production: Ginny Douglas, Teresa Breckwoldt

SECOND EDITION

Copyright © 1989 by The C.V. Mosby Company

Previous edition copyrighted 1974

Printed in the United States of America

The C.V. Mosby Company
11830 Westline Industrial Drive, St. Louis, Missouri   63146

Library of Congress Cataloging in Publication Data

Dawson, Peter E., 1930-
Evaluation, diagnosis, and treatment of occlusal
problems.

   Includes bibliographies and index.
   1. Malocclusion.   2. Temporomandibular joint—
Diseases.   3. Orthodontics, Corrective.   I. Title.
II. Title: Occlusal problems. [DNLM: 1. Malocclusion—
diagnosis. 2. Malocclusion—therapy.   3. Orthodontics,
Corrective.   WU 440 D272e]
RK523.D38   1989   617.6'43   88-8346
ISBN 0-8016-2788-5

C/MV/MV   9   8   7   6   5

This book is dedicated
to the great incentives in my life

To my God . . .
the architect of the masticatory system. The more I understand the logic behind
its beautifully integrated design, the more I realize its every element was planned
by a loving creator. The words of affection that we speak, the smiles we share,
the songs we sing, and the kisses we give to our loved ones are possible only
because an element of love was integrated into this design.

To my family . . .
especially to Jodie, my best friend, helper, and supporter. In her special way, a
real contributor to this endeavor. And to Mark, Anne, Kelly, and Cary, who have
made being parents a wonderful and joyous experience.

To my profession . . .
especially to those in it who make really *caring* for each patient their top
priority. It's for those true professionals that this book was written.

Foreword
to the second edition

When I wrote the foreword for the first edition, there was no way to know how applicable those comments would be 15 years later. During those years dentists have had the benefit of excellent research, which has led to improved diagnostic capabilities. Concepts and methods for providing complete dentistry have continued to improve and have certainly received growing acceptance from a better educated public. Even severely complex problems can be treated now with more predictability than ever. There is enough information available today for the general practitioner to become as competent as he or she chooses if the commitment to excellence is strong enough.

Some things do not seem to change, however, and there is still a very small percentage of practitioners who are willing to step up and pay the price required to become a true master. The need and the opportunity are greater than ever, but the percentages regarding the index of competency do not seem to change. I have requested that the original foreword be reprinted because the message I tried to convey in it is just as applicable today as it was when it was written. I hope it may stimulate some to achieve a higher level of competence in this wonderful profession of ours.

The practitioner who chooses excellence as his or her goal will find in this expanded text the fundamentals for diagnosing, planning, and executing complete dentistry. Dr. Dawson has taken a sound approach by starting with a basic explanation of how the masticatory system functions before progressing to more and more complex problems. He has emphasized the importance of conservative treatment and pointed out the need for more complete diagnosis based on a better understanding of causes and effects.

The importance of conservative treatment cannot be overstressed and you should understand that the use of complex approaches is considered only after an orderly analysis of simpler methods fails to provide the answers. It should be remembered that the majority of patients can be treated very successfully with basic time-tested procedures as long as each step is done with great care.

On the other hand, if you learn the basics well and practice them carefully, you had better be prepared to recognize the more complex problems because people with those special problems will seek you out if you are successful.

Lindsey D. Pankey, Sr.

Foreword
to the first edition

Possibly a Foreword should not be a testimonial, but after reading and studying the well-arranged and valuable material in manuscript form, I am reminded of the statement regarding the different kinds of dentists, namely:

Those who can talk about it,

Those who can write about it,

Those who can do it.

Occasionally, there is one who can do two of the above, but it is a rare individual who can do all three. From my many years of contact with the author, I knew he was master of two, and now I find in his well-organized and logical arrangement of the various facets of complete dental care, as presented in this book, he is the rare individual who can do all three. I commend this treatise to the general practitioner and the specialist alike. It may not be amiss to form a lending library in your office and let your dentally deteriorating patients read it, especially the first chapter. This is suggested after you are sure you know the theory and have attained technical competency at a fairly high level.

To master technical skills by actual doing, the general practitioner must organize and execute the complex subject matter of "complete dentistry" in such a way as to give optimal dental health to patients.

It has been said, and I think with generosity, that the general practitioners' index of competency is as follows: 2% are masters, 8% are adept, 36% are students, and 54% are indifferent.

The masters can interview, diagnose, plan treatment, educate, motivate, and do case explanation. More importantly, they can technically execute the dental services they render on a very high level. The adept are well versed, are proficient and skilled, and can render high level physiological dental services. The student may need help in various areas, but, with time, he will progress to a higher level. All must know their limitations and use the services of the specialist in dentistry as needed for the case to give optimum dental health care to the patient. It is the responsibility of the profession (and the public too if they have a high dental I.Q. and can do it) to bring the indifferent, and the whole profession, to a concept of attainment for "complete dentistry." During my five decades in dentistry, and especially the last two, I have seen unbelievable progress in this direction. The higher level of attainment in the specialized fields has been a great factor in this progress. However, they too can upgrade their services.

The author has presented such a concept in a step by step outline, and he has discussed it in an understandable way for the master and the adept. The serious student should grasp its meaning and with further collateral, meaningful study, he should bring it to fruition in his practice for the welfare of his patients. In a great country like ours, there will always be room for the serious students, the adept, and the masters even though the indifferent will probably always be with us. All should be goal oriented to optimum dental health care for their patients in order to earn the spiritual (through self-fulfillment) and material rewards for superior service.

Much confusion has been brought about by men listening to clinicians or to essayists through colored slides on some given technique rather than the basic principles. This is especially true in panel discussions where three or four men with a moderator are allowed to discuss various techniques that in reality agree 90% or more, with very little, if any, disagreement except through so-called techniques and instrumentation. To the student, to some of the adept, and to the indifferent ones, it is all very confusing. Many times it is discouraging to the point that the student could very well become indifferent. The indifferent justifies his position by saying: "If they cannot agree, why should I bother?"

In work of this nature, or any other, one should stick to basic fundamental principles, understand occlusion in depth, know what he is actually trying to obtain as a goal, and avoid becoming sidetracked through what appears to be different opinions.

Dr. Dawson has given a realistic outline and discussion of the subject of completed dentistry. In order for the professional student to bring it to practical significance, he should carry it further to a learning experience through actual "doing" in group participation.

Lindsey D. Pankey, Sr.

Preface

In the 15 years since the first edition of this text was published, interest in occlusion and the temporomandibular joint has expanded in many directions and from many sources. Although there is obviously a higher level of awareness about the importance of occlusion than before, there is also a high level of confusion about diagnosis and treatment of occlusal problems, especially regarding the relationship between occlusion and the temporomandibular joints.

TMJ therapies that violate basic principles of occlusion are still in use. And we commonly see occlusal treatment, including orthodontics, prosthodontics, and maxillofacial surgery performed independently of any regard for the physiologic function of the jaw joints. Attempts to isolate temporomandibular joint problems as unrelated to the teeth have missed the fundamental fact that the condyles and the lower teeth have a fixed relationship to each other. Short of surgery, it is simply not possible to alter jaw-to-jaw relationships at the occlusal interface without affecting the position of the joints, and it is equally impossible to alter the alignment of the articular components without affecting the occlusion. Thus one cannot master the subject of occlusion without also being a student of the temporomandibular joint. And certainly the complexities of temporomandibular joint disorders cannot be grasped as a separate issue. The teeth and the joints are part of a functional unit that must be understood in its entirety. All the parts of the masticatory system are interrelated and must work in anatomic and functional harmony or disequilibrium results. Only when we know how the system was designed to work will we know what's wrong with it when it isn't working correctly.

In developing the format for this text, my principle purpose was to simplify a very complex subject by attempting to explain how the masticatory system functions. I have tried to make this learning process easier by using numerous illustrations so that each of the important concepts can be clearly visualized in a logical sequence. I am convinced that most of the confusion about diagnosis and treatment could be cleared up for anyone who understands the logic that went into the design of the masticatory system.

In my working with dentists for many years in seminars and study groups it is more apparent than ever that the best way to understand occlusion is to divide it into parts. That is the way this text has been organized. I would strongly recommend that each chapter should be read and understood before you move on to the next chapter because a definite *sequence* of understanding is essential. As an example centric relation must be understood before a discussion of "long centric" makes sense. Anterior guidance must be understood before posterior occlusion can be discussed logically. And requirements for occlusal stability must be digested before the causes of instability can be analyzed. Several new chapters have been added to ensure that all the necessary interrelationships are clarified. A wide variety of diagnostic methods are discussed and controversial views are evaluated pro and con.

Problems of occlusion are organized by type, and so those chapters can be used as a reference for specific kinds of malocclusion. Guidelines for diagnosis and treatment of every type of occlusal problem are explained.

There are many treatment regimens still in use today that do not serve the patient's best interest, but they prevail because of the failure of adequate scientific examination of them.

Bites are still being raised because of the erroneous idea that lost vertical dimension is the cause of TMJ disorders. Pivot appliances are still being placed in the molar region "to take pressure off the condyles." Expensive and useless devices for TMJ diagnosis are being used because dentists are misled by unsubstantiated claims. Such methods or devices would never be accepted by anyone with a basic knowledge of the requirements for anatomic and functional harmony. The sad consequence is that such methods lead so often to unconscionable overtreatment of the patient without solving the problem.

Dentists are often surprised to find that every decision regarding treatment can be made on a scientific basis, and this even includes esthetic determinations. This is so only if the *why* is understood as a predecessor of the *how*. There is a *reason* behind every incisal edge position, every labial contour, every lingual contour, and every cusp-tip position. There is a *reason* why some teeth get loose, and others wear away. There is a *reason* why some temporomandibular joints hurt or click, why muscles become tender, and why teeth get sensitive. There is a *reason* why some occlusions remain stable and others do not.

In this text, I have tried to approach every diagnostic or treatment decision on the basis of understanding the reasons for the problem and the reasons for the treatment. The reasons will generally relate in one way or another to some form of disequilibrium in the masticatory system, which can be readily determined if the determinants of functional harmony are understood.

A more complete understanding of the masticatory system is important for another reason. Dentists today are expected to be the physician of the masticatory system. It is a role for which no other medical specialist has adequate training. Equilibrium in the system cannot be achieved separate from the dentition, nor can stability of the dental arches be achieved in a disharmonious relationship with the joints, the muscles, or the skeletal base.

Through the years new scientific data have strengthened some of our viewpoints and completely changed others. Some old definitions had to be changed, and some earlier concepts had to be discarded. When we rely on a scientific attitude, we realize that true scientific criticism never stops. No question is ever completely closed. As new facts appear or a new way of understanding old facts is shown, the scientific mind is willing to reexamine, to modify, or even to overthrow its own theories if the facts do not fully support the concept. In so doing we should also realize, however, that careful clinical observation is often the stimulator of meaningful research.

It is also very easy though to misinterpret clinical results alone because relief of symptoms may not mean a problem has been corrected. We have learned through long-term observation that symptoms may be relieved at the expense of causing later problems, which may be more severe.

I have tried to expose my own clinical observations and ideas to the test of time as well as to the invited scrutiny of a wide variety of special expertise. I'm grateful that there have been so many great minds in our profession who were willing to share so generously.

On the importance of occlusion, my eyes were opened by Dr. Sigurd Ramfjord, and because of his help early in my practice years, my entire concept of clinical dentistry was changed. He has continued to be a source of information as well as a valued friend.

Soon after I became aware of the importance of occlusion, I had the great good fortune of attending the first of many seminars by Dr. L.D. Pankey. Since that time his friendship and his guidance have had a profound influence on my practice and my life. His contributions to our profession cannot be measured. As I look back, I marvel at the insight he had in such a wide range of clinical dentistry, including diagnosis, restorative principles, occlusal concepts, and a phenomenal understanding of people. The L.D. Pankey Institute for Advanced Dental Education stands as tangible proof that many others feel the same gratitude as I do.

So many people have done so much to increase my understanding, it would be impossible to name them all, but I'm particularly appreciative of the many evenings that Dr. Vincent Trapozzano spent with me and a small study group. He encouraged in us an appreciation of the literature while insisting on critical evaluation of all that we heard or read. His contribution to my education was enormous.

Dr. Clyde Schuyler gave dentistry the first sound principles of occlusion, and many of the thoughts in this book started with seeds that were sown by Dr. Clyde. I was privileged to have him as a friend, and his visits to my office that extended into long evenings of discussion are treasured memories.

One of my closest friends in dentistry was also one of my greatest sources of motivation. Dr. James Cosper was a constant sounding board for ideas and a continuous voice of encouragement.

Dr. Alvin Fillastre, Jr., continues to be one of my most favorite stimulators of new ideas. He's an innovator and a scientific thinker as well as a superb clinician. Our time together during "Dawson-Fillastre Week" at the Pankey Institute is one of my most treasured weeks of the year. I've learned a lot of dentistry from Alvin, and I appreciate his help and analysis of my own thinking.

In orthodontics, I was blessed with a marvelous educator in my early years. Dr. Clare McCreary helped me gel most of my thinking about orthodontic diagnosis and minor tooth movement. Dr. Walt Sheffield has also helped my education by introducing me to a variety of conceptual approaches to treatment. Dr. Gerry Francatti has been a constant source of information, and I have benefited greatly from the work of Dr. Rudolph Slavicek and Dr. Robert Ricketts.

Dr. Sidney Frederick has spent a lifetime of study on the importance of muscle influence on the dentition. His clinical observations and research have been generously shared and form the major foundation for an understanding of the neutral zone. I thank him for his generous contributions to this text.

One of the brightest stars to come along in dentistry is Dr. Mark Piper, a brilliant surgeon and an exceptional diagnostician and innovator. Through an exciting synergy between our different disciplines in dentistry, we have been able to combine concepts of occlusal diagnosis with a unique opportunity to see into the temporomandibular joint from the surgeon's perspective. Mark is the developer of Doppler auscultation for the TMJ, differential arthrography, microsurgical techniques for TMJ reparative surgery, new methods for reshaping and repairing disks, and numerous other notable improvements in diagnosis and treatment. The opportunity to work with Mark and his partners Dr. Bob Chong and Dr. Tom Boland has been a great experience for me and the other doctors in our group.

Dr. Parker Mahan deserves special acknowledgment. He continues to be a seemingly unlimited source of special knowledge. His understanding of anatomy, physiology, neurology, pharmacology, and so on is always generously shared. It is a special privilege to share his friendship.

Many other generous people have added to my understanding. As I look back, I appreciate the stimulating challenges I received from Dr. Charles Stewart and Dr. Peter K. Thomas. I'm grateful for the strong friendship and exchange of ideas from Dr. Niles Guichet. Dr. Arne Lauritzen had a great influence on my thinking, and Dr. Harry Sicher, more than any other, turned me on to become a student of TMJ anatomy. Drs. J. Hart Long and Billy Buhner provided the means for evaluating our concepts of centric relation. Dr. Eugene Williamson has been a major source of information, stimulation, and some of the most useful research that has been related to our field. Dr. Terry Tanaka has also been a scientifically minded treasure chest of information. Mariano Rocabado has shared generously his knowledge as a physical therapist regarding the importance of coordinated muscle function and the role of connective tissue in joint disorders.

I owe a special debt of appreciation to my partners in practice: Dr. Pete Roach, Dr. Glenn DuPont, and Dr. Witt Wilkerson. They are all constant sources of new ideas and information. Without their support and unselfish dedication, I could not have taken the time needed to complete this text. My long-time technicians, Paul Muia, Lee Foreman, and Ben Crocker have made restorative dentistry a pleasure, and I thank them also.

What started out to be a revision turned into a 5-year rewrite of the first edition. I guess no one can know how much time and effort is required to put together a text of this scope except the ones involved. Special thanks must go to my artist, Nancy Howcroft-Therrien, for her talent in preparing hundreds of new illustrations.

A special bouquet goes to my daughter, Anne Dawson, who typed the final manuscript and coordinated all the pieces for the publisher. It was really a joy to have such a dedicated helper.

Finally, I want to thank the wonderful staff at Mosby. Their professionalism and helpfulness is greatly appreciated.

This book has been a labor of love. If it serves the purpose intended for it, it will be well worth all the effort that has gone into it.

Peter E. Dawson

Contents

1

The concept of complete dentistry

A dental examination is complete if it allows identification of all active factors that are capable of causing or contributing to the deterioration of oral health or function. It is *in*complete if it does not provide enough information to develop a total treatment plan aimed at optimum *maintainability* of the teeth and their supporting structures.

Since there is no effective way to achieve maintainable oral health without a harmony of all parts of the masticatory system, the total system must be evaluated. What affects one part of the system will eventually affect the other parts. The alteration of form or function of teeth, muscle, joints, bone, or ligaments is interrelated and must be understood before any part of the system can be properly analyzed or predictably treated.

Deterioration or malfunction of any part should be viewed as an *effect* that is the direct or indirect result of one or more identifiable *causes*. The careful diagnostician must first be a careful examiner who observes every deleterious effect in the form of signs or symptoms and then looks for every possible cause for each observed effect. Both causes and effects must be analyzed carefully so that they can be related to specific goals of treatment.

The establishment of definitive goals is the foundation for complete dentistry. If a goal is clear enough, it can be visualized and in fact *must* be visualized. A good rule is to avoid starting any treatment until the result can be clearly visualized. The ultimate goal of all dental treatment is optimum oral health, but until the practitioner can visualize how each type of tissue looks and acts when healthy, there will be no point of reference for knowing whether treatment is needed or if it is successful when rendered. Clearly defined goals give purpose to treatment planning and make it possible to be highly objective.

Complete dentistry has four comprehensive goals:
1. Optimum oral health
2. Anatomic harmony
3. Functional harmony
4. Occlusal stability

If each of these goals is achieved, treatment success is assured. When the entire gnathostomatic system is healthy, and there is a harmony of form and function, and the relationships are stable, the treatment can be considered "complete." Furthermore, esthetic requirements will also be fulfilled, since the appearance of the smile is dependent on the same harmony of form that is necessary for harmony of function.

In the analysis of any oral diagnosis problem, each of the above goals should be evaluated for fulfillment. This is practical only if the *reasons* for form and function relationships are understood, along with the cause-and-effect nature of health versus disease. This type of analysis also eliminates dependency on empiric treatment or making patients fit averages. There are many stable, healthy dentitions that do not fit the averages, are not Class I occlusion, and seemingly violate all the customary guidelines. Attempts to "correct" these dentitions often end in failure because the existing harmony of form and function is disturbed by the treatment. Such mistakes can be prevented, and a high degree of predictability can be developed if the goals of treatment are based on a foundation of why rather than how. There is a reason for every position, contour, and alignment of every part of the gnathostomatic system. There is a reason for every incisal edge position, every labial contour, every lingual contour, or every cusp tip position. There is a reason why some teeth get loose and others wear away. There is a reason why temporomandibular joints get sore, why muscles become tender, and teeth get sensitive. There is a reason why certain occlusions remain stable and others do not. Treating the effect without correcting the cause is rarely successful.

Every diagnostic or treatment decision should be made on the basis of understanding the reasons for the problem and the reasons for the treatment. Planning must then be directed at definitive goals by therapeutic use of cause-and-effect relationships. Let us explore each of the four basic goals in detail to show how effectively they can be used to help solve problems of oral diagnosis and treatment.

OPTIMUM ORAL HEALTH

All treatment should be consistent with the goal of providing *and maintaining* the highest degree of oral health possible for each patient. In this regard, diagnosis and treatment planning can be condensed into two fundamental objectives:

1. Finding all factors that contribute in any way to deterioration of oral health
2. Determining the best method of eliminating each factor of deterioration

Total elimination of all causative factors to the point of complete reversal of deterioration is not always possible. The problems of some patients are too severe or have gone on too long to expect a complete return to ideal health. But the degree to which we can elimi-

nate the *causes* will directly relate to our degree of success in changing unhealthy mouths to healthy ones.

Causes of deterioration

Dental disease rarely results from a single entity. It is almost always the result of a combination of factors. The same causative insult can produce a variety of responses because of differences in host resistance. The response can also be altered by variations in intensity or duration of the insult, sometimes to such an extent that a completely different set of symptoms may result from increased intensity of the same causative factor.

Because similar symptoms may result from completely different causes and a variety of symptoms may result from the same causative factor, treating symptoms is generally short sighted therapy. It is always advantageous to determine the specific *cause* of both signs and symptoms. If the causative insult can be completely eliminated, the normal adaptive response of the body should activate a return to normalcy. Of course, it may still be necessary to repair damaged tissues, but this can then be done with a greater chance of a long-term successful prognosis.

Much of the confusion about cause-and-effect relationships results from failure to differentiate between *causative* factors and *contributing* factors.

A contributing factor does not by itself cause disease. Rather, it lowers the resistance of the host to the causative factor. Host resistance may be lowered biochemically or biomechanically, and resistance may be lowered in a specific tissue or in an entire system. Generally, the weakest link breaks down. Contributing factors may also work by increasing the intensity of function or tension. The greatest susceptibility to disease occurs when a causative factor is present in a host with increased stress and lowered resistance. Both causative and contributing factors must be considered when one is deciding on a course of treatment, but the most direct approach is to give the highest priority to *direct* causative factors. Attempts at increasing host resistance and decreasing stress levels should be kept in proper perspective as adjunctive therapy.

Let us use a simple illustration to show how a single direct causative factor can produce a variety of signs and symptoms depending on variations in how different patients respond.

In a healthy patient with a perfect dentition, let us explore the variety of responses that can occur if a high crown with incline interferences is placed on a second molar. There are at least 15 different ways that patients might respond to this specific insult.

1. The tooth may become sensitive to hot or cold, or it may ache.
2. The tooth may become tender to touch.
3. The tooth may become loose.
4. The tooth may become worn.
5. The mandible may deviate around the interference, causing the other teeth to be worn down.
6. The deviated jaw function may cause other teeth to be loosened.
7. The deviated jaw function may cause the masticatory muscles to become hyperactive, or become spastic.
8. Trismus may result from the muscle spasticity.
9. Muscle tension headaches may develop.
10. The combination of sore teeth, sore muscles, and headaches may cause tension and stress.
11. Tension and stress may lead to depression.
12. The combination of the deviated mandible and the spastic musculature may cause a condyle-disk derangement.
13. The combination of the disk derangement and the elevator muscle spasm may initiate degenerative arthritic changes in the temporomandibular joint.
14. All of the above.
15. None of the above.

All the signs and symptoms listed above are a direct result of the same causative factor, the occlusal interference from the high crown. None of the contributing factors that altered the response actually *caused* the problems. If the causative insult had been corrected before irreversible damage, all symptoms would have disappeared without any changes having to be made in host resistance.

Host resistance is not the only variable. Variations in intensity of function can alter response to the same potentially damaging causative factor. The same type of occlusal interference mentioned above may go completely un-

noticed by the very relaxed patient who has no tendency to clench or brux. The mouth breather or the person who sleeps with the mouth open will have fewer if any symptoms because no stress results in the absence of tooth contact. The same patient under duress may begin to clench or brux, activating the trigger that programs the muscles into an avoidance pattern, further complicating the symptoms in the teeth, the muscles, and possibly the joints.

Diagnosis and treatment planning

Despite the complexity of the multicausality concept, it is still possible to simplify our approach to diagnosis and treatment planning. The law of cause and effect is so seldom repudiated that from a practical standpoint if we find an effect there will always be a cause. Good patient management requires the recognition of all causative factors along with an understanding of how and why each factor affects the health or function of any part of the system. The first step then in achieving complete dentistry is careful diagnosis to observe both causes and effects of disharmony, instabilty, or disease.

The method of diagnosis and treatment planning consists in the following:

1. A careful examination to isolate and analyze every factor that is capable of causing disease, disharmony, or instability, in other words, finding each *detrimental causative factor.*
2. An analysis of *host resistance* and an evaluation of any other contributing factors.
3. An evaluation of the *effects* of causative factors. Effects should be related to time, intensity, and host resistance. When you see an effect, search until you find the cause. Is the causative factor still active, or has it already run its course in producing its effect?
4. An *analysis of all possible methods* that could be used to eliminate detrimental causative factors or neutralize their harmful effects.
5. Selection of the *best* treatment approach.

Finding the causative factors

Patients lose their teeth in two ways: either the teeth break down, or the supporting structures break down. As simplistic as it may sound, if we exclude neoplastic disorders or injury, almost every deteriorating effect on the teeth or supporting structures is a direct result of one or both of two causative factors:

1. Microorganisms
2. Stress

If the intensity of the causative factors is constant, the degree or rapidity of deterioration is dependent on the contributing factor of host resistance. Patients should understand the role each factor plays, since they must share the responsibility for keeping each factor under control.

Causative factor 1—microorganisms. There seems to be no doubt that the elimination of bacterial plaque and the thorough cleaning of gingival sulci are essential to oral health. The acid microbial waste products not only cause caries through decalcification of the tooth surfaces, but they are also highly inflammatory to soft tissues and destructive to the bony support.

Any condition that prevents thorough cleaning of any tooth surface or any portion of the sulcus should be considered a causative factor that can lead to loss of teeth. There is no such thing as a "healthy" mouth that has long-standing deposits of bacterial plaque. As long as organized masses of microorganisms are present, progressive breakdown of the supporting tissues will occur. The only variable is the *rate* of deterioration, which may vary from patient to patient and even from tooth to tooth in the same mouth. The tissue response to the noxious products of the microbial colonies depends both on the general resistance of the host and on the resistance of the specific areas that are being subjected to the microbial toxins.

Even in a dentition that is uniformly coated with plaque, the destructive effects are not uniform. Periodontal destruction around some teeth may be severe, whereas other teeth may retain all or most of their bony support. Since the intensity of the microbial attack is about the same around all the teeth, there must be a tooth-by-tooth difference in resistance to the microbial toxins. The differences in resistance from one tooth to the next most often is directly related to differences in intensity of occlusal stress. It is a common clinical finding that the degree of bone breakdown is in direct

proportion to the occlusal stress exerted on each tooth.

Although there does appear to be a clinical relationship between the amount of microbial damage and the amount of occlusal stress, occlusal stress is not a *necessary* factor. Severe periodontal disease can occur in an environment of occlusal perfection. It is important to understand that the best occlusal treatment cannot prevent deterioration of the supporting structures if inflammation is present. Occlusal therapy without control of plaque is incomplete dentistry. On the other hand, soft-tissue management, even with exceptional control of plaque, falls short of the long-term maintainability that can be achieved when excessive occlusal stresses are also reduced.

The short-term improvement that can be accomplished by *either* occlusal therapy *or* plaque elimination can be impressive, but judging results too soon can be misleading.

A concentrated mouth hygiene program may transform bleeding, edematous gingivae into healthy-appearing tissue. In addition, occlusal correction may dramatically improve the comfort of the teeth and eliminate hypermobility. But even such noticeable improvement can be misleading if underneath the healthy-looking tissue an untreated pocket remains. No matter how healthy the gingiva appears, deterioration of the alveolar bone will continue if the entire sulcus is not cleanable. The healthy appearance on the outside merely produces a false sense of security while deterioration continues in the depth of the pocket.

No matter how thorough the plaque control program, even if combined with occlusal therapy, it is incomplete dentistry if there remain deep lesions that are capable of producing continued deterioration of the periodontal support.

Causative factor 2—stress. Hyperfunction and misdirected occlusal forces can cause or contribute to any or all of the following effects:

1. Hypermobility of teeth
2. Excessive wear
3. Hypersensitivity
4. Masticatory muscle imbalance
5. Temporomandibular disorders
6. Periodontal breakdown
7. Formation of noxious oral habits
8. Fracture of cusps or split teeth

Since the teeth, their supporting structures, and the entire masticatory apparatus are adversely affected by excessive stress, a major goal of treatment is always the reduction of stress to a point that is not destructive. The amount of stress exerted against the dentition is always related in some way to whether the teeth are in harmony with the mechanical movements of the mandible. Because the mandible is a lever arm with a fulcrum and a power source of strong muscles, it is axiomatic that the teeth must not interfere with its powerful functional movements. The patterns of mandibular function are definite and are dependent on two determinants:

1. The anatomic limits of movement that are imposed on the temporomandibular joints by their articulating surfaces and their ligaments
2. The physiologic action of the muscles as they move the mandible within or up to its border limitations

If the teeth interfere with the physiologic harmony of muscle-and-joint function, the conflict produces stress. The stress may result in harm to any or all parts of the mechanism. The damaging effects of such stress can be obscured by the adaptive responses in the system, but there is usually a price to pay for adaptation. The adaptive response may be to wear away the tooth interferences in an attempt to regain structural balance between the teeth, the joints, and the musculature. Often, it is easier to loosen the teeth than to wear the hard enamel, whereas in other cases the teeth are just forced out of alignment.

Muscle activity is almost always affected by occlusal interferences because when the physiologic position of the joint is not compatible with the intercuspation of the teeth, muscle will be directed to move the jaw to make the teeth fit even if it requires displacement of the joints. The exquisitely sensitive proprioceptive innervation around the roots directs the muscles, which can then easily become hyperactive by the constant demand to function in the displaced jaw position.

If there have been any major shortcomings in the understanding of occlusal diagnosis, the first has been failure to understand how little it takes to throw the system out of balance. The second problem of communication has been disagreement on what constitutes correct position and alignment of the condyle-disk assembly. Both points must be clarified because when we talk about an occlusal interference we mean that one or more tooth surfaces interfere with the physiologic functional pattern of the condyle-disk assembly. The result is stress in the mechanism. The proprioceptive nerve endings around the teeth are so exquisitely sensitive to even minute variations of pressure that the slightest interference by a single tooth is sufficient to change the whole pattern of muscle function. The nature of the myoneural mechanism is to protect the teeth. If the teeth are not in harmony with the joints, the muscles must not only move the mandible into the convenient position, but they are also given the job of bracing the condyles on the slopes of the eminences against the force of antagonistic elevator muscle contraction. In other words muscles are forced into the long-term bracing role that is properly the job of bone and ligaments. Although bone and ligaments in normal function do not become fatigued, muscles in abnormal function do. Muscle fatigue can produce a variety of problems and symptoms. Prolonged contraction of a fatigued muscle may produce painful spasm of the muscle itself, or it may do the same to its antagonistic muscle by forcing it into an incoordinated stretch-reflex contraction.

The imbalanced masticatory muscles may affect the postural muscles of the head, neck, and eventually the shoulders, as one system out of harmony disrupts other functional units. All these disruptions produce stress, and stress takes its toll in many different ways from simple acceleration of wear to complex excruciating pain. The pain may masquerade as an earache, a toothache, or quite often a headache. It is a common occurrence for long-standing headache problems to disappear when muscle harmony is reestablished. A high percentage of headaches are the result of muscle tension. Very often, the trigger for the whole chain of head and neck muscle hyperactivity is from a minute occlusal interference.

Despite the extreme mobility patterns that can be caused by traumatogenic occlusion, there is no evidence to show that occlusal trauma can cause an increase in pocket depth unless inflammation is present in the region of the gingival attachment. If the gingival attachment is intact and there is a sufficient level of supporting bone remaining, even severely mobile teeth can be returned to normal firmness and health by correcting the occlusion. With meticulous hygiene to keep the sulci completely free of plaque, inflammation can be prevented, even in extremely loose teeth. In the absence of inflammation we do not expect pocket depth to increase, and this is probably so whether the occlusion is correct or faulty. Lindhe and Nyman[1] have shown rather conclusively that occlusal trauma of the jiggling type, even with greatly reduced periodontal support, will not cause further destruction of the attachment apparatus, once the plaque-induced periodontal disease has been cured. However, the combination of plaque-induced periodontitis and occlusal trauma causes a more progressive loss of connective tissue attachment than in nontraumatized teeth.

Some authorities have argued that occlusal factors play *no* role in periodontal breakdown because inflammation is the essential causative factor for increased pocket depth. This opinion presents a limited viewpoint of what constitutes periodontal disease. A total picture of periodontal health should include the health of *all* the structures that support the teeth, not just the gingival attachment. The way in which bone is destroyed can be learned from careful clinical observation. The reason why teeth in hyperfunction become loose is that the bone around the roots breaks down. The bone breakdown follows a specific pattern because the bone resorption is a direct result of pressure stimulation, which causes thrombosis, hemorrhage, and destruction of collagen. The fibroblasts that are put under excessive pressure convert into osteoclasts, which in turn destroy bone in direct proportion to the intensity and direction of the pressures exerted. This means then that intra-alveolar bone breakdown follows a pattern that is definitively related to occlusal stress patterns. Careful clinical observation repeatedly confirms this relationship. If the occlusion is corrected *before* inflammation or injury deepens the sulcus to communicate with the area of bone resorption, osteoblastic activity will replace the osteoclastic destruction and bone will complete fill back in to its original levels. The loose tooth will tighten and can return to normal health and function.

If the occlusal correction is delayed, our clinical experience has consistently shown that it will eventually communicate with a deepened sulcus or pocket. Understand that the increase in pocket depth requires bacterial inflammation or injury and so it theoretically can be prevented. It has in fact been prevented on selective patients who are willing and able to follow extraordinary hygiene procedures under increased professional supervision. Although theoretically possible, it is not generally practical or consistently predictable. Bone resorption often occurs worse in furcation areas that are hardest to clean and where communication with the pocket is most likely to occur. Once there is any breakthrough between the sulcus and the area of bone breakdown, the pocket is immediately deepened to the extent of the intra-alveolar defect and a major periodontal lesion results. It is now too late for occlusal correction to resolve the bony defect. Major periodontal therapy will be required, and even then the bone level will not be returned to its original contour. That opportunity is lost whenever occlusal correction is delayed too long.

The repair of intraosseous defects is more predictable when the teeth are firm. From almost every viewpoint of treatment it is more difficult to keep the supporting tissues healthy around a loose tooth than it is around a firm one. Occlusal stress must be considered as a primary cause of supporting structure breakdown around the teeth. Correction of misdirected or excessive forces against the teeth is one of the essential considerations in achieving optimum maintainability of any dentition.

How stress affects the teeth

Tooth enamel is the hardest structure in the body. It was designed to last a lifetime of normal function. Even the contour of each crown is designed to maximize the amount of wear it can withstand without harm to its functional capabilities. Electromyographic research has also shown the presence of an energy conservation system for the masticatory muscles so that contraction of all three pairs of elevator muscles is reserved by pressure sensors around the roots for when there is a bolus of food between the teeth. The system is designed to use minimal muscle contraction when there is no food to penetrate, thereby saving wear and tear on the teeth.

The system works well as is evidenced by the number of elderly patients we see with intact dentitions that still have enamel surfaces in good function. Whenever you observe such a patient with no excessive wear or hypermobility in their later years, you will find consistently that there is a harmony of the occlusal surfaces with the functional movements of the mandible.

Whenever the intercuspation is not in harmony with the physiologic function of the temporomandibular joints, you will find almost without exception either excessive wear, hypermobility, or adaptive realignment of the teeth. When a tooth interferes with correct joint position, the pressure sensors around the roots of the prematurely contacting tooth misinterpret the pressure as a bolus and thus activate all the elevator muscles to contract with excessive force against the teeth when it is not needed. The result is acceleration of wear and tear on the dentition.

ANATOMIC HARMONY

No system works well if its parts are not in their proper place. The masticatory system is no exception. If any part of it becomes misaligned, the entire system must adapt. Adaptation to misalignment creates stress and accelerates wear.

Anatomic harmony is permissive harmony. It is the starting point from which function occurs. Whether all parts of the system are in a balanced static relationship determines whether there will be a peaceful neuromuscular system. This is so because muscle controls all function, and muscle must have a static resting relationship from which functional activity begins and to which it returns when functional demands are completed. Anything that interfers with static harmony of any part alters normal muscle function into an unbalanced relationship of constant demand. Muscle has an optimum length of contraction and an optimum length at rest, and correct anatomic harmony depends on allowing muscle to function to its normal limits without interference.

The most common shortcoming in analyzing or treating occlusal relationships is failure to consider *all* the parts of the masticatory system. We are prone to many mistakes if our understanding of occlusion is limited to occlusal contacts alone. The teeth are merely a *part* of the total system, and frankly there is no way to evaluate occlusal relationships until we have first ascertained that the temporomandibular articulation is in harmony. There is no such

thing as a perfected occlusion with a misaligned temporomandibular articulation. There can be no occlusal harmony when any part of the masticatory apparatus is at war with muscle. That includes the lips, tongue, and cheek musculature.

A harmony of form is a prerequisite for harmony of function, and it is necessart to have a working knowledge of how the two interrelate. Every aspect of each tooth's position and contour can be determined on the basis of its harmony with functional requirements. As examples, the upper anterior teeth must relate to the closing path of the lips as they seal for swallowing; the incisal edges must relate to the lower lip contour for proper phonetics and the lingual contours must relate to the tongue in swallowing. Many other functional relationships are discussed in other chapters, but the important thing to understand at this point is that every part of the system has an understandable reason for its position, contour, and alignment. If any anatomic component is not in harmony, the entire system must adapt. Adaptive changes should always be evaluated as responses to imbalance. Whether the body's attempts at correcting imbalance are beneficial or destructive is dependent on the resistance or response of the altered tissue or part. Astute diagnosticians must know the norm and must be able to determine when an imbalance exists and whether the tissue or parts have successfully adapted to the altered imbalance.

If we can achieve anatomic harmony of all parts of the system, we are assured of the best possible esthetics as well as the comfort of a peaceful neuromuscular system. The best esthetic result is a natural appearance. Having all parts properly shaped and positioned in total harmony is the formula for a pretty smile and an attractive face, according to the best plan in nature.

FUNCTIONAL HARMONY

Because it is a dynamic system, organized for performing a variety of functions, each part of the masticatory apparatus has several different functions. Besides mastication, the same system is also designed to be used for drinking, sucking, swallowing, and breathing, not to mention smiling, kissing, licking, and spitting. The same parts also serve simultaneously as the organ of speech. The total gnathostomatic system is truly a remarkable example of multiple-use bioengineering. To perform such a variety of functions, it is obvious that the lips, tongue, cheeks, bone, joints, and muscles must have a highly organized relationship to each other and to the teeth, which must fit into the system without disturbing any of the other functional demands, or vice versa.

I cannot overstress the importance of understanding the functional interrelationships involved in the masticatory system. It is impossible to adequately evaluate cause-and-effect influences in the dentition or the joints without knowledge of functional interdependencies. If we do not know what *causes* a malrelationship, we will probably fail in our treatment. We may subject our patients to unnecessary treatment or inadquate treatment if we are forced to treat the symptoms without understanding the causes.

Functional disharmony usually provokes a chain reaction of responses. A child with enlarged adenoids has difficulty breathing unless he thrusts his tongue forward to increase the size of the airway. The forward tongue thrust overpowers the normal pressure of the lips, and the anterior teeth adapt to the outward pressure by moving forward until they reach the new position of balance between the tongue and lips. The lower lip may now find it is easier to fit behind the upper anterior teeth than to stretch over the protruded arrangement.

The lower lip thus may force the upper anterior teeth into a more severe protrusion while crowding the lower incisors lingually. If attempts are made to correct the alignment of the teeth, without correcting the cause of the tongue thrust, the treatment will fail.

Teeth simply do not move out of alignment, do not get loose, or do not wear away without a specific underlying cause. As already shown, the cause may be at the beginning of a chain reaction, but regardless of when and how the process was initiated, treatment will not be successful unless all currently active causes for disharmony are corrected.

An acceptable analysis of occlusal disharmony cannot be made from examination of *unmounted* diagnostic casts. For an examination to be considered complete, all functional relationships must be evaluated to determine how the dentition relates to all the other structures that influence anatomic or functional har-

mony. This requires a facebow orientation of the casts to the condylar axis.

The goal of functional harmony is a peaceful neuromuscular system. The masticatory system is capable of high-capacity demands. The system must be free to function to its anatomic limit without mechanical interference but must not be restricted to function solely at that limit. It must function to the limit when needed. It must be at peace when functional demands are reduced.

OCCLUSAL STABILITY

The essence of both anatomic and functional harmony is *balance*. Every system in the body (as well as the entire universe) relies on a centered relationship between equal and opposite forces. Every cell wall is balanced between the osmotic pressure of intracellular fluids and that of extracellular fluids.

The sympathetic nervous sytem is balanced by the parasympathetic system. Every chemical, thermal, or mechanical function in the body responds to antagonistic forces until the opposing forces are equalized. Recognition of this basic law of nature serves as a framework for recognizing when, how, and why each part of the masticatory system is either in peaceful balance or stressful disharmony.

A Class I relationship is not in itself indicative of occlusal stability. Orthodontic guidelines and other textbook norms for analyzing occlusal relationships are unquestionably beneficial, but there are no rigid standards of tooth alignment that of themselves guarantee stability or instability. Some of the most perfect Class I occlusions break down, whereas some of the most obvious malocclusions remain stable. There is a reason, and the reason is clinically determinable. The teeth are the most adaptably movable part of the masticatory system. Their position is rather easily altered, either vertically or horizontally by the forces exerted against them. For any tooth position to be stable it must be in balanced harmony with all forces, both vertical and horizontal, and so it is just as important to have a knowledge of the forces that exert pressures against the teeth as it is to understand classic occlusal relationships. A general knowledge of the forces that are critical to occlusal stability will illustrate the natural law of balance between equal and opposite forces.

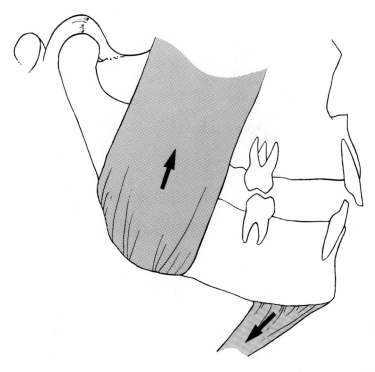

Fig. 1-1. The mandible is balanced at a position of equilibrium between the opposing pull of the elevator versus the depressor muscles. When the opposing nuscles are in a normal state of resting tonicity, the mandible is at its postural rest position. At the rest position, the teeth should be separated.

The resting position of the mandible is the result of balance between the resting length of the elevator muscles and the resting length of the depressor muscles (Fig. 1-1).

If either the elevator muscles or the depressor muscles contract, the mandible will be moved toward the more powerful contraction. If both the elevator and depressor muscles contract simultaneously, the stronger elevator muscles will usually overpower the depressor muscles and the "resting" position of the mandible will be more elevated, thus reducing the freeway space. Both sets of antagonistic muscles will be stressed by the isometric hyperactivity, if the contraction is prolonged.

The anteroposterior position of the mandible is determined by the harmonious function of the lateral pterygoid muscles versus the fibers of the temporalis (Fig. 1-2). Each condyle is positioned on the slope of the eminence and moved up or down its convex incline by the balanced contraction versus release of these two antagonistic muscles.

When the mandible is at rest, the condyle-disk assemblies are centered against bone and

ligament stops so that the positioner muscles can be at peace.

The disk itself is balanced between the opposing forces of the elastic fibers behind the disk and the superior belly of the lateral pterygoid muscle in front (Fig. 1-3).

Because the disk is attached to points on the medial and lateral poles of the condyle, it is free to rotate around those points of attachment. Its position on the condyle is thus controlled by whether the pull of the retrodiskal elastic fibers is stronger, weaker, or the same as the muscle contraction in front.

The vertical positioning of the mandible *in function* is controlled by a dynamic balance of muscle that requires coordinated contraction and release of antagonistic muscles. As the elevator muscles contract, the depressor muscles must release allowing the mandible to be hinged closed around its condylar axis. The habitual closed position of the mandible is a highly repetitive position in relation to the maxilla. The consistency of the mandible-to-maxilla relationship is the result of a physiologic optimum length of contraction of the el-

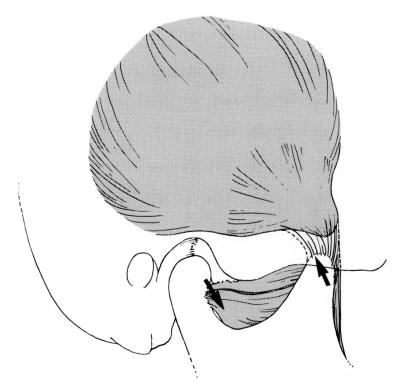

Fig. 1-2. The position of the condyles is dependent on a balanced relationship between the protruding muscles (lateral pyerygoids) versus the retrusive muscles (temporalis). In normal function, contraction of one muscle is coordinated with the release of the opposing muscle to allow the condyle to move forward and back.

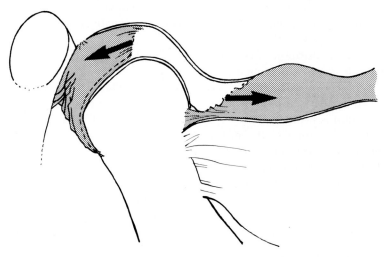

Fig. 1-3. The position of the disk is determined by a balance between the elastic fibers pulling back versus the superior lateral pterygoid muscle pulling forward. The disk rotates on the condyle to a point of neutrality between the opposing forces.

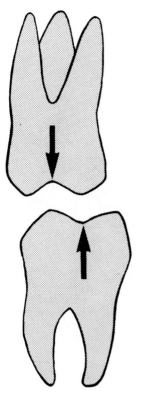

Fig. 1-4. Teeth erupt toward each other as the result of an ever-present eruptive force that stays active throughout life. When the eruptive force of the lower tooth meets an equal opposite force from the upper tooth, the eruptive forces are balanced.

evator muscles balanced to an optimum length of the released stretch of the depressor muscles. It is this consistent point of dynamic balance that determines the vertical dimension of the mandible to the maxilla. The vertical dimension of occlusion is quite naturally determined by this relationship because of the natural law of balance applied to the *eruption* of the teeth.

The law of balanced, equal-and-opposite force consistently applies to the eruption of teeth. Each tooth has an ever-present eruptive force that causes it to continue to erupt until it is met by an opposite force that equals the eruptive force (Fig. 1-4).

The ideal stops for eruption are the teeth in the opposing arch. If the opposing force is greater than the eruptive force, the tooth will be intruded. If the resistance is less than the eruptive force, the tooth will continue to erupt until the forces are equal. What determines the precise point of balance? It is the repetitious closed position of the mandible that is determined by the optimum length of *contraction* of the elevator muscles (Fig. 1-5). Any interference to this balance of eruptive force versus optimally contracted length of muscle will dis-

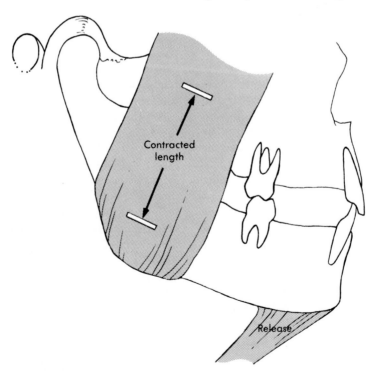

Fig. 1-5. The eruptive forces of the upper and lower teeth meet at the repetitive jaw-to-jaw dimension that is determined by the repetitive contracted length of the elevator muscles. Thus there is a balanced equilibrium between the eruptive force of the teeth versus the *contracted* length of the elevator muscles.

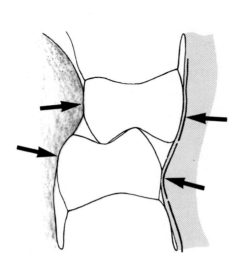

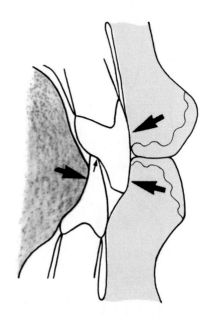

Fig. 1-6. The horizontal position of the posterior teeth is determined by the neutral zone, which is the point of balance between the outward force of the tongue versus the inward force of the buccinator bands of muscle.

Fig. 1-7. The anterior teeth erupt into a balance between the forward pressure from the tongue versus the inward pressure from the lips. The point at which the opposing forces are balanced is called the *neutral zone.*

rupt the optimum vertical dimension of occlusion. Indiscriminate use of bite planes is one of the most common causes of long-term occlusal disharmony because of the chain of damaging events that are initiated by the disruption of the naturally existing harmony. Chapter 5 explains the details of vertical dimension.

Horizontal stability of the posterior teeth results from a position of balance between the outward force of the tongue and the inward force of the buccinator muscle (Fig. 1-6). The centerpoint of balance forms the posterior neutral zone, which will be moved by whichever force is stronger. See Chapter 6 regarding the neutral zone.

To have long-term stability of the anterior teeth, one must position them in a balanced relationship between the forward pressure of the tongue and the inward pressure of the lips. As teeth erupt, they are guided into this balanced position of neutrality between opposing forces (Fig. 1-7). The precise location of this anterior neutral zone is one of the most critical determinations that must be made as it affects the entire pattern of masticatory function (see Chapter 16, Anterior Guidance).

The interrelationships previously described are just a few examples of the balance that must exist between all functional components of the entire gnathostomatic system if we are to achieve long-term stability of the system. There are many other less obvious examples that could be used to illustrate this basic law of nature. Even the quality of speech requires a balance between oral and nasal resonance that can be disturbed by improper positioning of teeth because of the forced alteration of tongue position.

When the need for balance in all aspects of the masticatory system is understood, it will be obvious that knowledge of the anatomy and physiology of the system is also a requirement for proficiency in diagnosis and treatment planning. Without this knowledge, the practitioner will be prone to accept far too many of the empiric approaches, including harmful procedures, gimmickry, and a general tendency to overtreat. But if the interrelationships and interdependencies of the parts of the system are understood, along with knowledge of physiologic principles, diagnosis becomes a logical routine of finding a cause for every deleterious effect. Treatment then evolves from the determination of what is the best way to restore the system to functional harmony and optimum, maintainable health. That is the concept of complete dentistry.

EXPLAINING THE TREATMENT RATIONALE TO THE PATIENT

An oversimplified but effective way to relate the treatment requirements to patients is to explain, as follows:

If we are to make your mouth healthy and keep it that way, we must accomplish two things:
1. We must leave no place in your mouth that is not completely cleanable.
2. We must reduce all the stresses in your mouth to a point where they are not destructive.

These two are *my* responsibility. Your responsibility is to keep your mouth spotlessly clean and to report any uneven stresses that may occur so that they can be corrected. It is also your responsibility to maintain your best level of general health through proper diet and exercise. If we *both* do a complete job of fulfilling our responsibilities, you should have your teeth as long as you need them.

Hygiene appointments should be scheduled *after* diagnosis and treatment planning. It should be part of the treatment prescribed by the dentist to help each patient learn the proper way to care for the mouth. Mouth hygiene is a very important part of the preliminary mouth preparation, which is usually necessary before one starts restorative procedures.

It is also ideal for the hygienist to record dietary habits and to counsel patients on proper nutrition for prevention of future dental disease.

REFERENCE

1. Lindhe, J., and Nyman, S.: The role of occlusion in periodontal disease and the biological rationale for splinting in treatment of periodontitis, Oral Sciences Rev. **10**:11, 1977.

SUGGESTED READINGS

Arnim, S.S.: The connective tissue fibers of the marginal gingiva, J. Am. Dent. Assoc. **47**:271, 1953.

Arnim, S.S.: Microcosms of the mouth—role in periodontal disease, Texas Dent. J. **82**:4, March 1964.

Cheraskin, E., Ringsdorf, W.M., Jr., and Clark, J.W.: Diet and disease, Emmaus, Pa., 1977, Rodale Books.

Lindhe, J., and Svanberg, G.: Influence of trauma from occlusion on progression of experimental periodontitis in the beagle dog, J. Clin. Periodontol. **1**:3, 1974.

Ramfjord, S., and Ash, M.M.: Occlusion, ed. 3, 1983, W.B. Saunders Co.

Rocabado, M.: Biomechanical relationship of the cranial, cervical, and hyoid regions, J. Craniomandibular Pract. **1**:3, 1983.

Rudd, K.D., O'Leary, T.J., and Stumpf, A.J., Jr.: Horizontal tooth mobility in carefully screened subjects, Periodontics **2**:65, March 1964.

Sicher, H.: Functional anatomy of the temporomandibular joint. In Sarnat, B., editor: The temporomandibular joint, ed. 2, Springfield, Ill., 1964, Charles C Thomas, Publisher.

2

Occlusal therapy

Because of the earlier tendencies to evaluate occlusal relationships solely on the basis of how the teeth intercuspate, any occlusion that had the appearance of "proper" intercuspation was considered correct, and any tooth arrangement that did not have the textbook version of correct intercuspation was considered a *mal-*occlusion. Consequently most treatment of occlusion was designed to make the teeth *look like* the "correct" version of proper intercuspation. The results were inconsistent, were often unstable, and had an unpredictable effect on problems of muscle dysfunction, tooth hypermobility, abrasion, and temporomandibular disorders. Many clinicians reasoned that if a "properly" intercuspated occlusion did not solve problems predictably the problems were unrelated to occlusion. This viewpoint led to a downplay of the role of occlusion and an upsurge of a wide variety of empiric treatment techniques. The indiscriminate use of drugs to treat the *symptoms* of the disorders has probably been the most damaging approach, though many attempts at so-called occlusal therapy were also harmful, even though they may have achieved a tentative relief of symptoms. The improper use of bite planes, bite-raising appliances, pivots, and mutilative occlusal grinding are common examples of "therapies" that have been advocated because of claimed successes in relieving symptoms. The claims however could often be disputed under scientific conditions, and careful observers often pointed out that it was common for the "successful" results to degenerate into disharmonies that were fre-

quently worse than the original problem. Because of the high percentage of bad results from occlusal treatment, many clinicians decided it had no value at all. Although some authorities were decrying the total concept of occlusal therapy, many practicing clinicians were finding that proper intercuspation was only part of the picture. Ramfjord and Ash[1] showed that an occlusion should be evaluated more by the way it influenced the function of the stomatognathic system than by the way the teeth intercuspate. Frederick[2] showed that teeth that were not in harmony with the musculature would be moved regardless of how they intercuspated.

As more clinical observations were made and more research was done, it became obvious that successful occlusal therapy is not possible if occlusal contacts are not directly related to the temporomandibular articulation. The teeth function in direct biomechanical relationship with the temporomandibular joints and the muscles. Storey[3] showed that the *occlusal interface* is not determined by occlusal contacts alone, but also involves the anatomy of the joints, the limiting influence of the ligaments, and the shape and orientation of the occlusal plane. These he characterizes as the passive factors. The active parts of the system include not only the muscles themselves but also the reflex responses that arise in and around the teeth, the joints, the muscles, and the mucosa and probably in the periosteum and the skin. Storey has suggested that these neuromuscular reflex responses appear to protect the teeth and their supporting structures against damage but when they become continuously active they lead to pathogenesis.

Because of these reflex responses and the intricate interdependencies of the stomatognathic system, the alteration of even one tooth incline has the potential for disrupting the balance and thus the stability of the entire system. Such minute incline interferences often occur in occclusions that appear to have ideal intercuspation.

Our clinical experience has repeatedly demonstrated the effect of minute occlusal interferences on muscle harmony and temporomandibular function. We have found that even the slight depression of a prematurely contacting tooth is sufficient to activate muscle incoordination and can result in symptoms of a wide range of severity. It is not necessary for the occlusal interference to cause an actual slide or horizontal deviation. The slight vertical overloading of a single tooth can be the trigger that keeps the muscles in an incoordinated state of hypercontraction.

The detection of such minute interferences requires very careful technique, but it is a practical clinical procedure. Occlusal contacts are marked with two colors of very thin articulating ribbon—one color for very light closing contact color, the other for firmer closing contact. If both color marks are not in the same location, it indicates tooth movement on closure. Failure to refine an occlusion so that both the light contacts and the firm contacts are identical can often lead to failure in eliminating muscle incoordination and the symptoms that go with it. Many occlusal treatments stop short of achieving equalized axial pressures even though the slide is eliminated. When symptoms remain, the therapist then often rules out occlusal factors when in fact the occlusal triggers are still active.

In the past few years, a considerable amount of excellent research data has confirmed the cause-and-effect relationship between occlusal interferences and muscle incoordination. Recent studies have further confirmed the importance of *minute* occlusal interferences and the positive results achieved by their correction.

Riise[4,5] has shown through the use of quantitative electromyography that a single, minor occlusal interference, experimentally induced in the intercuspal position, may change not only the postural muscle activity, but also the

activity during submaximal and maximal bite. This change in muscle activity also occurs in mastication. Perhaps of most importance is the finding that when the interference is removed, the muscular coordination improves.

Bakke and Møller[6] have documented significant changes in muscular activity from induced interferences as thin as 50 µm. Several other research studies have also shown the negative influence on the function of the stomatognathic system from various types of occlusal interferences.

It is apparent that the periodontal receptors are exquisitely sensitive to slight variations in pressure. It is also apparent and has been documented by several investigators that disturbances of harmonious input to the periodontal receptors caused by occlusal interference can result in functional disorders of the stomatognathic system. It has been verified that the correction of the occlusal interferences results in a return to normal function and harmony of muscle activity.

Ramfjord and several other investigators have documented the relief of pain and related its timing with the return to symmetric muscle activity when occlusal interferences were removed in patients with pain and muscle dysfunction. Krogh-Poulsen[7] has shown the relationship between specific interferences and functional muscle abnormalities. Beyron[8] has shown the relationship of occlusal interferences to asymmetric abrasion of the tooth surfaces. Graf[9] showed the relationship of occlusal interferences to alterations in the deglutition reflex and also concluded that a stable occlusal contact relationship in maximum intercuspation seems to be essential for adequate masticatory function. The ample evidence proves rather conclusively the following:

1. Minute occlusal interferences can trigger muscle into hyperactivity, incoordination, and dysfunction.
2. The correction of the interferences eliminates the muscle dysfunction, relieves the pain, and allows the muscles to return to normal balanced activity.

Why there is lack of agreement regarding the importance of occlusal disharmony as a cause of muscle pain and dysfunction

Many authorities have minimized the importance of occlusion as a factor in temporomandibular dysfunction and muscle pain. I have observed repeatedly that the less importance a clinician puts on occlusal factors the more he will advocate the use of drugs or psychologic approaches. The less that occlusal factors are understood, the more there will be the tendency to resort to gimmickry, kinesiology, bite raising, and other procedures with questionable scientific rationale. Unfortunately, many of the most common treatments are actually harmful, even though they may provide momentary relief. Since many well intentioned dentists have resorted to these empiric procedures because of failure to get results through occlusal treatment, the reason for their disregard for occlusal therapy should be explained.

Three statements could sum up the reasons:

1. Dentists *distrust* occlusal therapy if they fail to get predictive results from its use.
2. Dentists *oppose* occlusal therapy if they have caused their patients to get worse off from its use.
3. Predictive occlusal therapy requires more preciseness than most dentists are aware of. If occlusal therapy is not done carefully enough, it will not help, and the altered occlusion may actually intensify the problem or cause new problems of discomfort.

There are two extremely important aspects of occlusal treatment that demand preciseness if predictability is to be achieved:

1. Precise position and alignment of the condyle-disk assembly in a physiologically correct relationship to the fossa. The condyles need not *stay* in the centrically related position, *but they must have access to it without interference from the teeth.*
2. *Preciseness* in the elimination of all interferences to the centric relation position of the condyles.

Some observations that we (Dawson and Arcan[10]) have made through using precise measuring techniques for quantifying occlusal interferences (photocclusion) have shown that the proprioceptive sensitivity is greater than is generally realized and the muscle response to minute discrepancies varies from patient to patient but can reach an exquisite sensitivity in some patients.

Some other observations from our photocclusion studies follow:

1. From the standpoint of establishing muscle harmony, the *number* of tooth contacts is less important than the complete elimination of deviating inclines or premature contacts.
2. Two contacts (one on each side) in complete harmony with the uppermost condyle-disk position can produce muscle harmony in some patients. Generally this occurs in combination with tongue-biting habits.
3. The absence of a slide does not in itself indicate complete symmetry, since uneven pressure may result in the movement of a tooth or teeth without producing a discernible slide. Such asymmetric pressure is difficult to discern, but it can constitute a potent trigger that activates muscle hyperactivity. Photocclusion methods have enabled us to record not only pressure against deviating inclines, but also variations of intensity of axial nondeviating pressure.
4. It is not uncommon for the symptoms of occluso-muscle disharmony (such as pain and limitation of function) to remain even in the absence of a slide, but such symptoms are frequently eliminated only when the axial pressures are equalized.
5. *The goal is to obtain the maximum number of axially directed contacts that are equal in intensity.* The pressure of even one tooth contact with greater intensity is sufficient to destroy the muscle harmony and activate a hyperactivity of the unbalanced muscles.
6. Although it is often necessary to precisely equalize all occlusal contacts to eliminate muscle pain and dysfunction, it is not usually necessary to *maintain* the same degree of occlusal perfection once the muscle activity is normalized. This varies from patient to patient depending on tension levels and some psychologic factors that reduce the normal adaptive capacity of the body.
7. Teeth that have had excessive axial pressures will almost always rebound after occlusal correction. They may require repeated adjustments before they stabilize.

REQUIREMENTS FOR SUCCESSFUL OCCLUSAL THERAPY

There is, at this time, enough scientific evidence to logically assume that occlusal treatment must be related to both the active and passive elements of the entire stomatognathic system. The goal of occlusal therapy is to reduce stresses to a point that is not destructive to any part of the system. This can be accomplished when one follows a logical sequence for evaluation or treatment of any occlusal problem. The sequence parallels the requirements for successful treatment.

There are three requirements for success when treating problems of occlusal stress or instability, as follows:

1. *Comfortable condyles.* The temporomandibular articulation must be able to function and resist pressure with no discomfort. This is the essential *starting point* for any dental treatment that involves the occlusal surfaces of the teeth. When we speak of an "occlusal interference," we are referring to an interference to comfortable mandibular function. Until we have determined the comfortable, physiologically correct relationship of the condyle-disk assemblies we cannot know the functional mandible-to-maxilla relationship to which the occlusion must be related.

2. *Anterior teeth in harmony with the envelope of function.* Just as the condylar paths determine how the back end of the mandible moves in function, the anterior teeth determine how the front end moves. There are many factors that dictate correct position and contour of the anterior teeth and that in turn cause the development of the *functional* pathways that the mandible travels in mastication, speech, swallowing and other functions. The lips, tongue, occlusal plane, and optimum contracted muscle lengths are some of the determining factors. The anterior guidance is one of the most important relationships that determines the character of the entire occlusal arrangement.

3. *Noninterfering posterior teeth.* As already stated, we want to develop the maximum number of axially directed contacts that are equal in intensity, but we do not want any posterior contact to interfere with either the comfortable condyles in the back or the anterior guidance in front.

The complexities of occlusion can be simplified if each of the above requirements is understood, along with its relationship to the other requirements. Each requirement is discussed separately. The essential starting point for any understanding of occlusion is a thorough knowledge of the anatomy, physiology, and biomechanics of the temporomandibular joints and their relationship to the stomatognathic system.

REFERENCES

1. Ramfjord, S., and Ash, M.M.: Occlusion, ed. 3, Philadelphia, 1983, W.B. Saunders Co.
2. Frederick, S.: The buccinator, orbicularis complex, Manual prepared for the Florida Prosthodontic Seminar, 1987.
3. Storey, A.T.: Controversies related to temporomandibular joint function and dysfunction. In Zarb, G.A., and Carlsson, G.E.: Temporomandibular joint function and dysfunction, St. Louis, 1979, The C.V. Mosby Co.
4. Riise, C., and Sheikholeslam, A.: Influence of experimental interfering occlusal contacts on the activity of the anterior temporal and masseter muscles during mastication, J. Oral Rehabil. **11**:325, 1984.
5. Sheikholeslam, A., and Riise, C.: Influence of experimental interfering cuspal contacts on the activity of the anterior temporal and masseter muscles during submaximal and maximal bite in intercuspal position, J. Oral Rehabil. **10**:207, 1983.
6. Bakke, M., and Møller, E.: Distortion of maximal elevator activity by unilateral premature tooth contact, Scand. J. Dent. Res. **88**:67, 1980.
7. Krough-Poulson, W.G., and Olsson, A.: Management of the occlusion of the teeth: background, definitions, rationale. In Schwartz, L., and Chayes, C., editors: Facial pain and mandibular dysfunction, Philadelphia, 1968, W.B. Saunders Co.
8. Beyron, H.: Occlusal changes in adult dentition, J. Am. Dent. Assoc, **48**:674, 1954.
9. Graf, H.: Occlusal forces during function. In Rowe, N.H., editor: Occlusion: research in form and function, Ann Arbor, Mich., 1975, University of Michigan Press.
10. Dawson, P.E., and Arcan, M., Attaining harmonic occlusion through visualized strain analysis, J. Prosthet. Dent. **46**:615, 1981.

3

The stomatognathic system

Before we can evaluate dysfunction and disease, we must have a clear picture of normal function and health. The basis for cause-and-effect diagnosis is an understanding of normal form and its relation to function. The anatomist Moffett has observed that "we will not find much of a disturbance in function without having a corresponding degree of alteration in structure." The healthy interrelationship between form and function provides us with a base line that can be used in distinguishing normal function from pathofunction.

Most of the diagnostic procedures described in this text are designed to *test* the various components of the system to determine whether each part is healthy and then to decide if that part is in correct position and alignment to function normally.

A basic knowledge of the stomatognathic system starts with the temporomandibular joint, since it is the center of structural and functional interrelationships.

Some of the most obvious aspects of the temporomandibular joint are often missed, even though they are extremely important. In fact some of the most popular techniques for treating temporomandibular disorders are based on misconceptions of how the joint functions, and many of the procedures that are advocated for restorative or orthodontic treatment are either unnecessary or detrimental to long-term stability. To relate each aspect of form to function, it is helpful to separate the various components of the joint into understandable segments, starting with the passive structures of articulation and then progressing to an understanding of how the active elements make the system function.

THE ARTICULATING SURFACES

If we examine a dry skull, it is apparent that the articulating surfaces of the condyle and its reciprocal socket merely *allow* movement to occur. The joint is often described as a universal joint, but that description does not apply because each condyle imposes limitations of movement on the other. One condyle cannot move in any manner without reciprocal movement on the opposite side. In opening-closing movements, the two condyles form a common axis and so, in effect, act as one hinge joint. Despite the fact that the condyles are rarely symmetric, the axial rotation occurs around a true hinge that is on a fixed axis when the condyles are fully seated. Rotation around a *fixed* horizontal axis seems improbable because of the angulation of the condyles in relation to the horizontal axis. Each condyle is normally at about a 90-degree angulation with the plane of the mandibular ramus, which places their axes at an obtuse angle to each other. To understand how the condyles with different axes can rotate around a fixed common axis, we must look to the contour of the *medial poles* and their relation to the articular fossae. Because of the different angles and the

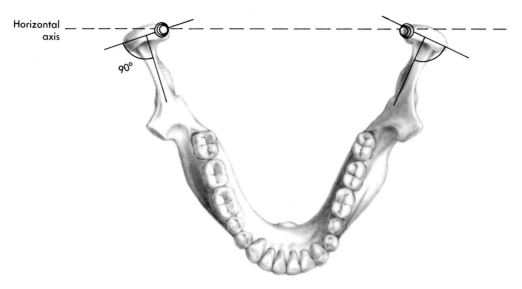

Horizontal
axis

90°

Fig. 3-1. The medial poles of the condyles are the only rotation points that would permit a fixed axis of rotation because the condyles are not parallel to the horizontal axis. This means that the lateral poles of the condyles must translate, even if the medial poles are rotating around a fixed axis (as occurs in centric relation).

asymmetry of the condyles, the medial pole appears to be the only logical common rotation point that would permit a true rotation to occur on a fixed axis (Fig. 3-1).

For the medial pole to serve as a point of rotation, the articular fossa must be contoured to receive it. Its triangular shape (Fig. 3-2) serves this mechanical function very well, and in addition the medial part of the fossa is reinforced with thick bone and so it can also serve as a stop for the upward force of the elevator muscles and the inward force of the medial pterygoid muscles (Fig. 3-3).

Other than the strongly braced medial portion, the roof of the fossa is always quite thin. Hold a skull up to the light and you will see that the bone in the roof is quite translucent, but notice the density of the medial portion and relate that difference to the relation of form to function. The temporomandibular joint is designed to bear stress and must be capable of resisting forces that measure into hundreds of pounds. The condyles serve as a bilateral fulcrum for the mandible, and so the joints are always subjected to stress whenever the powerful elevator muscles contract. The spe-

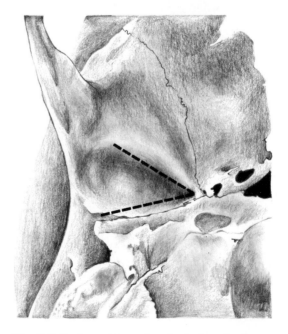

Fig. 3-2. Further evidence that the horizontal axis runs through the medial poles of the condyles is found in the triangular fossae with the apex related to the medial pole. A horizontal axis through any part of the condyle other than the medial pole would result in translatory movements of the medial pole during a fixed rotational axis, and this would be incompatible with the V shape of the fossa.

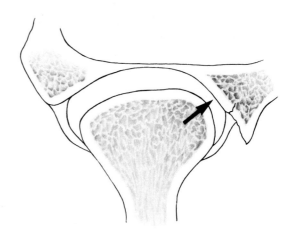

Fig. 3-3. The condyle-disk assemblies are braced at the midmost, uppermost position by compression of the medial poles against the medial apex of each triangular fossa. To resist the inward, upward pressure from the internal pterygoid muscles, the fossae are heavily buttressed with bone in line with the direction of load. The anterior surface of each condyle is simultaneously compressed against the posterior slope of the eminentia.

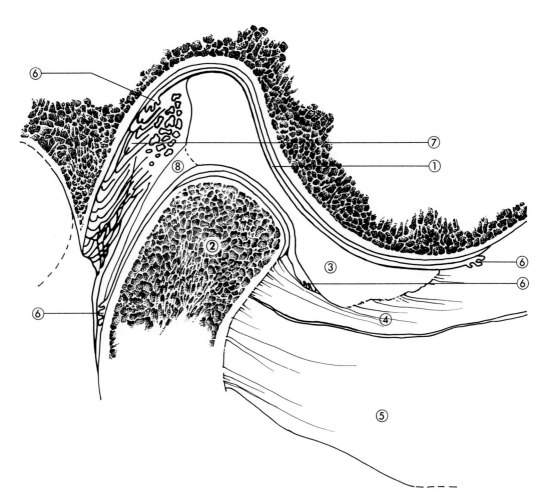

Fig. 3-4. Lateral view of cross section through the temporomandibular joint. *1,* Posterior slope of the eminentia (notice typical convex contour); *2,* condyle; *3,* disk (notice biconcave shape to fit both convex condyle and convex eminentia); *4,* superior lateral ptergoid muscle; *5,* inferior lateral pterygoid muscle; *6,* synovial tissue; *7,* retrodiskal tissue including posterior attachment of disk to temporal bone; *8,* posterior ligamentous attachment of disk to the condyle.

cific areas of reinforcement of the fossa conform with the bearing areas for the upward, forward, and inward forces of the musculature.

The *articular eminence* forms the anterior part of the articular fossa (Fig. 3-4). Because of the slightly forward pull of the elevator muscles, the condyles are always held firmly against the eminence (with the disk interposed). Of great importance is the strongly *convex* contour of the eminence. Since the anterior aspect of the condyle is also convex, one can see the purpose and the importance of the biconcave *articular disk* that fits between the two convex surfaces. Because of its position between the condyle and the temporal bones, the disk divides the joint into an upper and a lower compartment. The lower compartment serves as the socket in which the condyle rotates, whereas the upper compartment allows the socket to slide up and down the eminence. Thus the mandible can hinge freely as either one or both condyles translate forward.

Since each condyle serves as a fulcrum and is subjected to a predominantly upward force from the elevator muscles, it is provided with a definite stop to resist those forces. The condyle-disk assembly is able to slide up the eminence until the medial pole is stopped by the reinforced medial part of the fossa. This occurs at the highest point to which the properly aligned condyle-disk assembly can move. It occurs simultaneously with contact still maintained against the eminence. The uppermost position is also the position at which the medial pole is braced against the medial articular lip (with disk interposed). This relationship stabilizes the *midmost* position of the mandible in centric relation and prevents any lateral translation from occurring while the condyle-disk assembly is in the uppermost position (Fig. 3-5). Sicher[1] has stated that "only the fracture of the internal lip or its destruction could permit a medial displacement of the condyle. The presence of the medial articular lip also prevents a lateral displacement of the

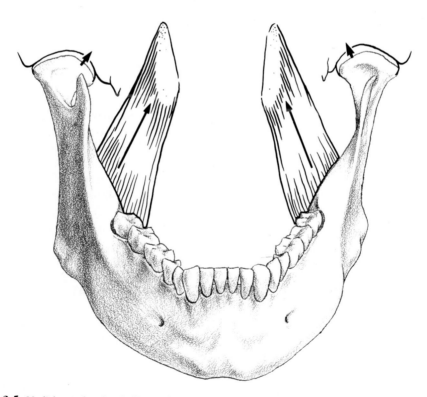

Fig. 3-5. Medial pole bracing in line with internal pterygoid muscle contraction establishes the midmost position at centric relation. This braced position is consistently simultaneous with the uppermost position. This medial pole stop also prevents the lower posterior teeth from moving horizontally toward the midline, an essential anatomic design that makes a normal curve of occlusion possible. It also explains why an immediate side shift is not possible from the fully seated position of the condyles (centric relation).

condyle, since this could occur only under simultaneous medial displacement of the other condyle."

As further evidence that this is a stress bearing joint, all the articular surfaces of the condyle, the fossa, and the eminence are covered with avascular layers of dense fibrous connective tissue. The absence of blood vessels is a sure sign that those specific areas are designed to receive considerable pressure. The avascular areas are also devoid of innervation, and this includes the bearing areas of the disk; so if the condyle and the disk are in proper alignment in the fossa they can receive great pressure with no sign of discomfort, since there are no sensory nerves in the bearing areas to report discomfort.

The disk itself is a classic example of design for function. It is composed of layers of collagen fibers oriented in different directions to resist the shearing effect that might occur in a sliding joint. The bearing area is avascular, and so it is nourished by synovial fluids that also lubricate the joint for smooth gliding function. The reason for using collagen fibers instead of hyaline cartilage in the temporomandibular joint is that the stiffer cartilage that works well in most other joints would not be pliable enough to change shape as it conforms to the contours of the convex eminence in the sliding movements.

The disk is firmly attached to the medial and lateral poles of the condyle, and such attachment is the reason it moves in unison with the condyle. The diskal ligaments, which bind the disk to the poles, allow it to rotate from the front of the condyle to the top and vice versa. In normal function the disk is always positioned so that pressure from the condyle is directed through its central bearing area. Positioning of the disk is controlled by the combination of elastic fibers attached to the back of the disk, which keep it under tension against the action of the superior lateral pterygoid muscle that is attached to the front of the disk. So while the diskal ligaments pull the disk along as the condyle moves, its rotation on the condyle is determined by the degree of contraction or release of the superior lateral pterygoid muscle.

Many of the misconceptions about the disk have resulted from its depiction in illustrations as a little round cap that sits on top of the condyle. It actually wraps around the condyle

to the points of attachment medially and laterally, and its posterior border is quite thick. The steeper the slope of the eminentia, the thicker the distal lip of the disk becomes, a feature that seems to indicate the importance of the disk as one of the structures that combine to determine the uppermost position of the condyle. The functional positioning of the disk is a critical factor in mandibular movements, and several disorders can result from its discoordination.

Although the articulating surfaces *allow* movement by providing the mechanical framework for the sliding hinge, the function of the *ligaments* is to *limit* the movements of the mandible. The capsular ligament is not attached medially or laterally to the disk, but it is attached to the neck of the condyle below the attachments of the disk. The capsule that appears thin and loose is strongly reinforced laterally as the temporomandibular ligament. This has the effect of limiting retrusive and lateral movement of the condyle without preventing its rotation.

Some confusion exists regarding how the temporomandibular ligaments can brace the condyle without restricting its function, since in most two-dimensional drawings of the joint it would appear that the ligaments are placed in a position that would simply stop the opening of the jaw. This is the function of only one part of the ligament. Its fan shape permits different bundles of the ligament to function in different movements of the jaw. The nearly horizontal fibers of the temporomandibular ligaments limit posterior movement in a manner that permits a pure rotation at the terminal hinge position. This pure rotation is usually limited to a jaw opening of about 15 mm before the opening is stopped by the ligaments at the neck of the condyle. At that point the condyle-disk assembly pivots against the ligament and must translate forward to permit further opening (Fig. 3-6). This is a very ingenious design that moves the mandible forward as it opens, to keep the floor of the mouth from hinging back into an interference with the airway.

The strength of the ligaments that limit the rearward movement of the condyles is sufficient to protect the thin tympanic plate and the soft tissues behind the condyle. The combination of the ligaments, the thick distal lip of the disks, and the reinforced areas of the fossae

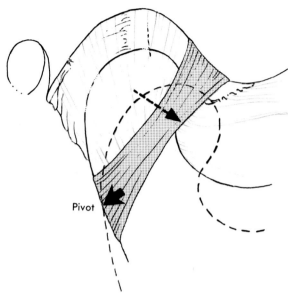

Pivot

Fig. 3-6. Positioning of part of the temporomandibular ligament is designed to prevent the mandible from opening too far on a pure hinge rotation at the uppermost position. As the jaw opens on a fixed axis, the floor of the mouth is directed back into the airway. To prevent this, the ligament reaches its full length at about 15 to 20 mm of jaw opening, at which point it becomes a pivot that initiates a forward translation of the rotating condyle. This requires the mandible to move forward away from any airway obstruction during full opening.

are so protective that even a hard direct blow to the jaw will fracture the mandible rather than drive the condyle back into the tympanic plate or up through the thin roof of the fossa.

If one studies the structure and arrangement of the temporomandibular articulation, it should become apparent that the joint should be able to hinge freely and resist very strong pressure with complete comfort *if all the parts are healthy and are in correct alignment*. This is so because all the bearing areas are reinforced for strength and receive all functional pressures on avascular, noninnervated surfaces. But this occurs only if all the passive parts are in balance with the active forces of the musculature. It has been my consistent clinical finding that whenever I find discomfort or dysfunction, I will also find muscle incoordination. Since muscle incoordination can so easily start a chain reaction of structural misalignment, it is necessary to determine whether muscle incoordination is the cause or the result of the structural malrelationship. To do this, we must understand how the muscles function harmoniously.

THE MASTICATORY MUSCLES

It is helpful to divide the muscles of mastication into the positioner muscles and the elevator muscles. The *positioner muscles* are responsible for the horizontal position of the mandible. This relationship is determined by the inferior lateral pterygoid muscles that pull

the condyles forward, and the fibers of the temporal muscles that pull the mandible back. The superior lateral pterygoid muscle is responsible for keeping the disk properly aligned with the condyle during function.

The *elevator muscles* are all positioned distally to the teeth so that they elevate the condyles and hold them firmly against the eminence while hinging the jaw. The masseter, internal pterygoid, and the major part of the temporal muscle are responsible for elevation.

In the normal resting position of the mandible, the elevator muscles and their antagonistic depressor muscles are in a resting state of postural contraction. The mandible is balanced between. To open the jaw from the resting position requires the contraction of the depressor muscles and the simultaneous release of the elevator muscles. As the jaw continues to open, the temporomandibular ligament reaches its restricting length at the neck of the condyle to stop the pure hinge rotation of the condyle. At this point, the condyle must translate forward. As the inferior belly of the lateral pterygoid muscle contracts, it pulls the condyle forward down the convex eminentia, and the disk is pulled along with the condyle. As the condyle-disk assembly moves down the steep incline and onto the crest of the eminence, the elastic fibers behind the disk keep tension on it to rotate it onto the top of the condyle so that the disk will be maintained in line with the direction of force. To permit the retrodiskal elastic fibers to rotate the disk to the top of the condyle, the muscle attached to the front of the disk must remain passive, and so the superior belly of the lateral pterygoid does not contract on opening or protrusive movements of the mandible (Fig. 3-7).

The superior stratum of the bilaminar zone is responsible for the positioning of the disk in protrusive movements. The inferior stratum is attached to the condyle, and so as the disk rotates back, tension is reduced in those fibers. Increasing tension in the superior stratum occurs as the condyle moves *forward.*

As the mandible starts its closure, the middle and posterior fibers of the temporal muscle contract to pull the mandible back while the inferior lateral pterygoid releases its protrusive action. The depressor muscles also release as the elevator muscles start their contraction. The combined contraction of the elevator muscles pulls the condyle up the lubricated incline until it is stopped by the bracing of the medial pole and the restraining ligaments. The forwardly directed muscle contraction holds the condyle against the eminence.

The disk, being firmly attached to the poles of the condyle, is pulled up the incline with the condyle, but during that movement it must be rotated from the top of the condyle back to the more anterior relationship; so on closure the superior pterygoid becomes active to counteract the pull of the retrodiskal elastic fibers and, through controlled contraction, holds the disk so that it is rotated to the front of the condyle as it moves back up the incline (Fig. 3-8).

When the condyle-disk assembly moves down the eminence, the vacated space above and behind the condyle must be filled rapidly, since the closed system could not tolerate a vacuum. The area must be emptied just as rapidly when the condyle returns. To accomplish this, a glomus cell arteriovenous shunting system shunts blood in and out of the area to replace the volume of the condyle as rapidly as it moves forward and to empty the space as rapidly as the condyle moves back. This shunting system is called the *vascular knee* (Fig. 3-9). In order for such rapid reversals in hydraulic pressure to occur, the medium around the area is composed of loose areolar connective tissue, which can more readily conform to the unique effects of compression and tension.

It is obvious that much of the structural complexity of the temporomandibular joint is necessary to maintain coordinated function between the condyle and the disk. The past few years has brought new insight into condyle-disk function and pathofunction. It has become apparent that condyle-disk discoordination does not occur without the involvement of muscle. One must determine whether incoordination of muscle is the cause of the disk misalignment and, if so, he must follow the chain of muscle responses back until the originating stimulus for the muscle disharmony is determined. If structural alterations have occurred in the joint, he must determine whether correction of the alignment will allow healing of the affected part, or whether the patient can function at a tolerable comfort level with the damaged part. If the damage is too severe and reparative surgery is the choice, it must be accompanied by a return to structural and functional balance of the entire system or the surgery will probably fail. The severing of sensory nerves during surgery may produce a tentative relief of pain, but if balanced function is not achieved, the symptoms will probably reoccur when the sensory nerves regenerate.

IMPORTANCE OF OCCLUSAL HARMONY

Ideal mandibular function results from a harmonious interrelationship of all the muscles that move the jaw. Muscle becomes fatigued if it is not allowed to rest. Muscle should not be forced into prolonged activity with no chance to rest. When teeth are added to the stomatognathic system, they can exert a unique influence on the entire interbalance of the system because if the intercuspation of the teeth is not in harmony with the joint-ligament-muscle balance a stressful and tiresome protective role is forced onto the muscles. When the muscles elevate the mandible *in the absence of any deviating interferences,* the closing muscles pull the condyle-disk assembly up until it is stopped by bone at the medial pole. If tooth inclines interfere with this uppermost position, the lateral pterygoid muscle is forced into positioning the mandible to accommodate to the teeth. The mandible is thus realigned to make the teeth intercuspate even though to do so requires the lateral pterygoid muscles to take over the bracing function normally assigned to the bone and ligaments.

The lateral pterygoid muscles are capable of holding the condyles during protrusive func-

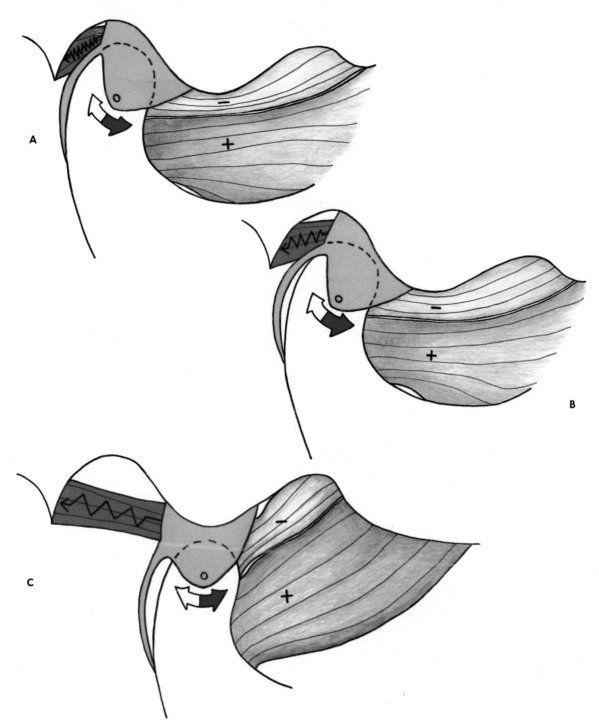

Fig. 3-7. A, When the condyle is at its uppermost position against the steepest part of the posterior slope of the eminentia, the disk is positioned on the front of the condyle in line with the forward direction of force. As the condyle is pulled forward by contraction of the inferior lateral pterygoid muscle (+), the superior lateral pterygoid (−) releases contraction. This allows the elastic fibers attached to the back of the disk to rotate it to the top of the condyle as it moves down the slope. **B,** As the condyle is pulled down the slope, tension from the retrodiskal elastic fibers increases to rotate the disk toward the top of the condyle and keep it aligned with the changing direction of force. The superior lateral pterygoid must stay released (−) to permit the elastic fibers to pull the disk back. Notice the progressive slackening of the posterior ligamentous attachment of the disk *(PL)* to the condyle. **C,** When the condyle reaches the crest of the eminentia, the direction of force from the elevator muscles is up through the top of the condyle, against the more horizontal surface of the eminentia. The superior lateral pterygoid stays passive through the full protrusive movement to allow the retrodiskal elastic fibers to control the alignment of the disk on opening. Notice that the superior lateral pterygoid muscle attaches to the condyle as well as the disk, thus preventing the disk from being pulled too far distally.

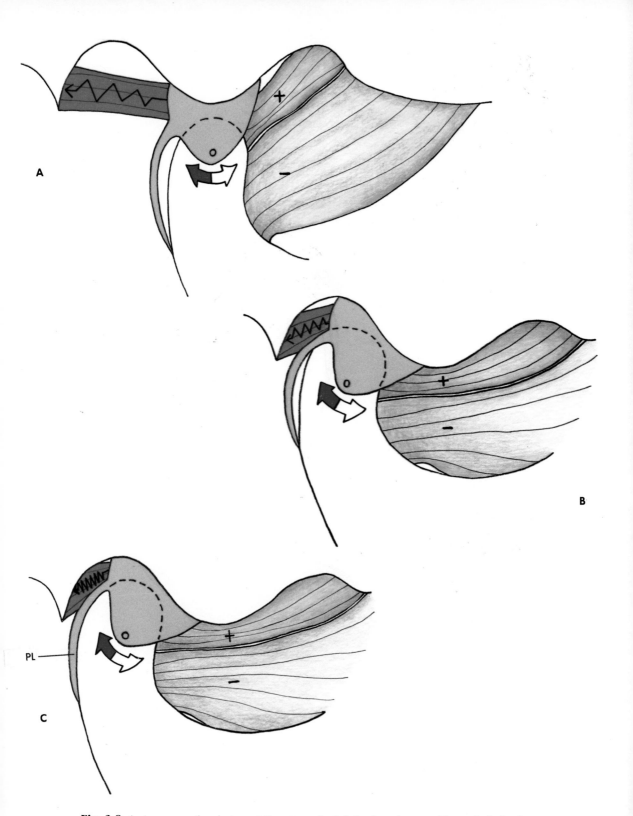

Fig. 3-8. A, As soon as the closing rotation starts, the inferior lateral pterygoid muscle ($-$) releases contraction to allow the condyle to be pulled back and up the slope by the elevator muscles. Simultaneously, the superior lateral pterygoid muscle ($+$) activates its contraction to hold the disk forward, in opposition to the pull of the elastic fibers as the condyle starts to move distally. **B,** As the condyle returns up the slope, the contraction of the superior lateral pterygoid muscle ($+$) controls the alignment of the disk, rotating it around the lateral and medial diskal ligaments back to the front of the condyle. The retrodiskal elastic fibers maintain constant tension against the forward pull of the muscle on the disk. **C,** The inferior lateral pterygoid ($-$) stays passive through the full range of closure to allow the condyle to slide up the slope of the eminentia. The superior lateral pterygoid maintains a controlled contraction ($+$) to hold the disk forward so that it is automatically rotated back to the front of the condyle as the condyle moves back to centric relation. At this point the posterior ligament *(PL)* is taut, preventing the disk from being rotated too far forward.

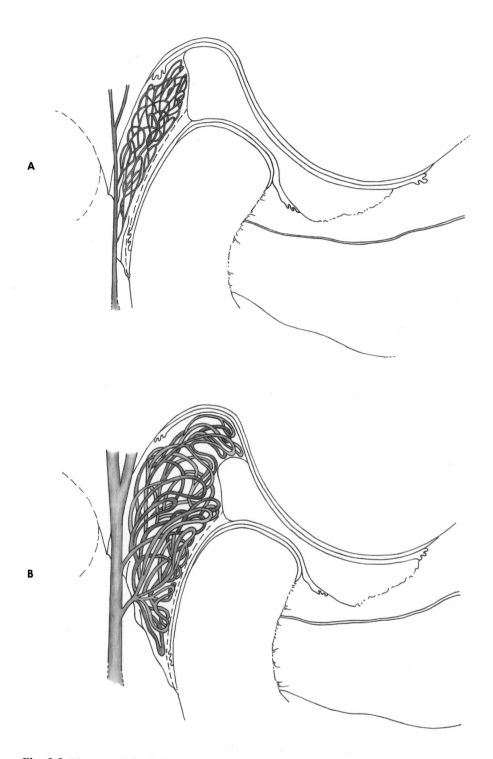

Fig. 3-9. The space behind the condyle changes rapidly as the condyle moves forward and back. A network of blood vessels, **A,** with elastic walls allows blood to rush in as the condyle moves forward to fill the space with the expanded vessels, **B.** As the condyle moves back, the blood is shunted out the vessels. This shunting system is called the *vascular knee.*

tion, *but in the presence of an occlusal interference they can never be relieved of this function without allowing the malaligned teeth to be stressed.*

The mechanism that forces this prolonged contraction onto the lateral pterygoid muscles is the exquisitely sensitive protective reflex system that guards the teeth and their supporting structures against excessive stress. Proprioceptive nerve endings scattered through the periodontal ligaments are sensitive to even minute pressures on individual teeth. The proprioceptive system is designed like a glove of periodontal receptors capable of evaluating the direction and intensity of stresses on the teeth and designed to program the lateral pterygoid muscles to position the jaw so that the elevator muscles can close directly into maximum occlusal contact. If tooth interferences cause the mandible to move left, the right lateral pterygoid must contract to pull that condyle forward. Contraction of the left pterygoid moves the jaw to the right. Contraction of both pterygoids moves the jaw forward. There are unlimited variations of timing and degree of muscle contraction to precisely position the mandible for maximum intercuspation of the teeth, but the lateral pterygoid muscles are always involved in any deviation from centric relation.

This unique relationship between the lateral pterygoid muscles and the proprioceptive periodontal receptors is so definite that it even overrides the normal tendency of the muscle to rest when it becomes fatigued. The muscles cannot relax the protective bracing contraction as long as the occlusal interference is present.

The pattern of deviation is reinforced every time contact is made, and it is retained in the brain's memory bank so that muscular closure into the deviated jaw relationship becomes automatic. One important facet of the proprioceptive memory, however, is that it fades rapidly if continual reinforcement of the pattern ceases. Elimination of interfering contacts permits an almost immediate return to normal muscle function. The deviation pattern is forgotten as soon as it is no longer needed.

In the past few years, new research has shown that the effect of occlusal harmony or disharmony is more definitive than had been realized. Many investigators have documented the cause-and-effect relationship between oc-

clusal interferences and muscle incoordination, but the work of Williamson[2] has given a new perspective to the importance of *precise* occlusal harmony and its relationship to physiologic condyle positioning.

Williamson has demonstrated the precise effect of occlusal interferences on muscle coordination and normal muscle activity. Using electromyographic procedures, he showed that interfering contacts on posterior teeth in any eccentric postion caused hyperactivity of the elevator muscles. But if the anterior guidance was allowed to disclude all posterior teeth from any contact other than centric relation, the elevator muscles either stopped active contraction or noticeably reduced it the moment the posterior teeth were discluded.

If heavy contact on any posterior tooth in any eccentric position causes a response of muscle hyperactivity, it has the effect of loading the tooth or teeth with the occlusal interferences, but the elevator muscle hypercontraction also loads the joint with the same hyperactivity.

Williamson's research has particular meaning to the principles of occlusion outlined in this text because of his agreement with the description of centric relation and his meticulous attention to its precise recording. This is the type of research that has been needed because it relates electromyographic results to a specifically described centric relation position that was verified and documented.

The noticeable reduction in elevator muscle activity at the precise moment of disclusion is one of the most important and clinically useful findings in many years.

An incoordinated musculature rarely exists without some form of adaptive structural change. Because of their tendency to wear, become loose, or move, the teeth are the usual site for structural alteration. The temporomandibular joint has generally been regarded as the most stable component of the masticatory system, but remodeling can change the shape of the disk or the condyles. Mongini[3] has shown that a direct relationship exists between the shape of the condyle after remodeling and the abrasion patterns on the teeth. His findings give strong support to the concept that remodeling of the joint can be considered, to a certain extent, a functional adaptation to a new occlusal situation.

The apex of force positioning of the

condyle seems to relate rather consistently with Mongini's findings regarding the relationship between the type of displacement and condylar shape caused by remodeling. He showed that flattening and flaring of the anterior surface are the most common changes in condylar shape and are accompanied in most cases by anterior condylar displacement. Remodeling of the posterior surface of the condyle, leading to flattening or concavities, is frequent in posterior displacement.

When all the notable, related research of the past few years is analyzed, it is apparent that the occlusal interface must involve the articulating surfaces of the temporomandibular joints with equal importance to the occlusal surfaces of the teeth. All the active and passive elements of this interrelationship must be carefully evaluated to make certain that a harmony of parts exists. Signs and symptoms of temporomandibular disorders are the effects that occur when some part of this interrelationship goes awry.

Healing is part of the body's adaptive response, but for healing to achieve proper repair, it must occur in a friendly environment of balance. Mongini has shown that if the parts of the stomatognathic system can be restored to a balanced relationship even a flattened condyle may regain a normal contour. Occlusal therapy and consequent condylar repositioning led to improved contour of a previous flattened condyle in 7 out of 11 patients, and in 3 of the patients in whom degenerative lesions were also present the lesions were healed.

The new insights that so much of the recent research has given us has confirmed what many other clinicians and I have observed clinically: successful occlusal treatment is dependent on complete harmony of all the passive and active components of a very precise and complex *system*. It is not possible to have an adequate understanding of occlusion outside of the framework of the total stomatognathic system.

Although the problem posed to the occlusal therapist or the restorative dentist is to organize the dentition in harmony with the musculature, it must first be determined that it is a *peaceful* neuromuscular system. It is imperative to ascertain that the muscles are not being stimulated into stressful patterns of function that would simply be perpetuated.

The muscles must have complete freedom to function with no *extended* demands on any muscle or group of muscles. Ligaments must be permitted to assume their bracing roles to permit muscles to rest. All tooth inclines should fall outside of nonfunctional jaw movements but should be easily reached when functional contact is desired.

Limiting jaw movements to a terminal hinge arc of closure is tolerated by some patients but is restrictive to most because it imposes limitations on muscle function that can stimulate an erasure attempt to brux away the interference or move it out of its restricting position. Limiting jaw movements to a protruded closure is worse because it places continuous demands on the lateral pterygoid muscles by preventing condylar access to the bony stop at centric relation.

Limiting jaw movements to a distalized joint position is worse yet because it forces the condyle onto a vascular innervated area that is not designed to resist pressure and encourages damage and displacement of the disk. The resulting inflammatory response incites muscle spasm and eventual degenerative changes.

A minimal stress occlusion is *permissive*. It never forces muscles into protective contraction or incites nonfunctional hyperactivity. It permits the entire range of the stomatognathic system to function harmoniously with no excessive demands placed on the joints, the ligaments, the neuromuscular system, or the teeth.

REFERENCES

1. Sicher, H.: The temporomandibular joint. In Sarnat, B., editor: The temporomandibular joint, ed. 2, Springfield, Ill., 1964, Charles C Thomas, Publisher.
2. Williamson, E.H., and Lundquist, D.O.: Anterior guidance: its effect on electromyographic activity of the temporal and masseter muscles, J. Prosthet. Dent. 49(6):816-823, 1983.
3. Mongini, F.: Influence of function on temporomandibular joint remodeling and degenerative disease, Dent. Clin. North Am. 27(3):479, 1983.

SUGGESTED READINGS

Gibbs, C.H., Messerman, T., Reswick, J.B., et al.: Functional movements of the mandible, J. Prosthet. Dent. 26:604, 1971.
Mahan, P.E.: The temporomandibular joint in function and pathofunction, U.C.L.A. Symposium on temporomandibular Function and Pathofunction, Chicago, 1980, Quintessence Publishing Co., Inc., pp. 33-47.
Mahan, P.E., Gibbs, C.H., and Mauderli, A.: Superior and inferior lateral pterygoid EMG activity, J. Dent. Res. 61:272, 1982. (Abstract.)
Mahan, P.E.: Anatomic, histologic, and physiologic features of TMJ. Chapter 1 in Irby, W.B., editor: Current advances in oral surgery, vol. 3, St. Louis, 1980, The C.V. Mosby Co.
Posselt, V.: Range of movement of the mandible, J. Am. Dent. Assoc. 56:10-13, 1958.
Ramfjord, S., and Ash, M.M.: Occlusion, ed. 3, Philadelphia, 1983, W.B. Saunders Co.
Sarnat, B., editor: The temporomandibular joint, ed. 2, Springfield, Ill., 1964, Charles C Thomas, Publisher.
Sessle, B.J., and Hannam, A.G., editors: Mastication and swallowing, Toronto, 1976, University of Toronto Press.
Sicher, H., and DeBrul, E.L.: Oral anatomy, ed. 5, St. Louis, 1970, The C.V. Mosby Co.
Zola, A.: Morphologic limiting factors in the temporomandibular joint, J. Prosthet. Dent. 13:732-740, 1963.

4

Centric relation

An understanding of occlusion starts with centric relation. Fail to have a clear grasp of its meaning, and confusion about occlusion is assured. Fail to develop the skills required for locating, verifying, and recording centric relation, and clinical results will be compromised.

The differential diagnosis of temporomandibular disorders requires accuracy in determining centric relation. The predictability of all types of occlusal treatment is directly related to the ability of the dentist to precisely record centric relation. If one were asked to select the one arch-to-arch relationship that is most important to the comfort, function, and health of the stomatognathic system, one would have to say, without reservation, *centric relation.*

It is impossible for one to develop a harmonious occlusal relationship without *first* determining that each condyle is properly aligned with its disk and the condyle-disk assembly is properly positioned in its fossa in centric relation. This is the starting point of occlusion. If the condyles are not in correct position when the occlusion is altered, the occlusion will be harmonized to malrelated condyle position. Thus the correctness of any occlusal treatment is dependent on where the temporomandibular joints are positioned when the occlusion is "corrected."

There are many misconceptions about the term "centric relation." It has been defined in so many different ways that the word "centric"

has all but lost its importance. A main point of confusion arises from failure to differentiate between the two terms *centric relation* and *centric occlusion.* Furthermore, the standard definition of centric relation as being "most retruded" is not correct from the standpoint of anatomic harmony, and most methods for recording centric relation do not position the mandible in a physiologically correct relationship with the fossae.

Practice of the definition of "most retruded" not only is unphysiologic, but also can actually be harmful to the condyle-disk alignment and can result in serious problems to the joints, the muscles, and the teeth. Attempting to shove the mandible *back* into centric relation is quite possibly the most erroneous procedure in dentistry. Unfortunately, it is also one of the most commonly used.

Further confusion results from describing centric relation as "unstrained" in the most often quoted definition. When the condyles are pulled up into the terminal hinge position by forceable contraction of the elevator muscles, it would appear that the terminal hinge position is a *strained* relationship.

Let's define centric relation to conform with anatomic and functional harmony. Remember that centric relation refers to a positional relationship of the *temporomandibular joints.* As such, it is a mandible-to-maxilla relationship. It is an axial position, meaning the joints can rotate to open or close the jaw without moving

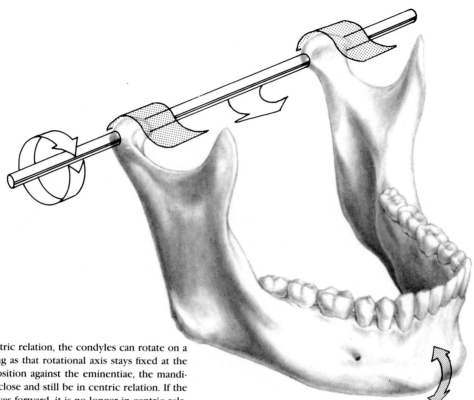

Fig. 4-1. In centric relation, the condyles can rotate on a fixed axis. As long as that rotational axis stays fixed at the most superior position against the eminentiae, the mandible can open or close and still be in centric relation. If the condyle axis moves forward, it is no longer in centric relation.

off the centric relation position and so the mandible can be in centric relation even when the teeth are separated (Fig. 4-1). Remember too that the hinge axis can move down and up the eminentia permitting the jaw to open or close at any position from centric relation to most protruded, but only in centric relation can the jaw hinge on a fixed axis without requiring the lateral pterygoid muscles to brace against the closing muscles. With the requirements for physiologic harmony in mind, a redefinition of centric relation is needed:

Centric relation may be defined as the relationship of the mandible to the maxilla when the properly aligned condyle-disk assemblies are in the most superior position against the eminentia, irrespective of tooth position or vertical dimension.

Centric occlusion refers to the relationship of the mandible to the maxilla when the teeth are in maximum occlusal contact, irrespective of the position or alignment of the condyle-disk assemblies. This is also referred to as the *acquired position* of the mandible or the *maximum interocclusal position* (MIOP).

When the intercuspation of the teeth is in harmony with both correctly positioned and aligned condyle-disk assemblies, centric relation and centric occlusion are the same. This is the goal of occlusal treatment.

APEX-OF-FORCE POSITION OF THE CONDYLES

The apex-of-force position is the position a healthy condyle assumes if its disk is properly aligned and there is no muscle bracing to prevent it from going to the most superior position against the eminentia.

At this position the anterior surface of the condyle-disk assembly rests firmly against the convex eminentia, and so the condyle obviously cannot move forward without being guided downward.

Because the medial pole of each condyle is braced at the uppermost medial part of its reciprocal fossa contour, the condyle-disk assembly cannot move backward from that position without moving downward. The thick distal lip of the disk that extends over the contour of the condyle can also direct the condyle down-

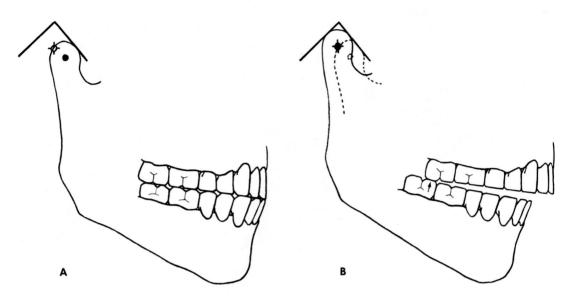

Fig. 4-2. If the occlusion is harmonized at a protruded-jaw relationship, the forward position of the condyle requires downward movement, **A.** When the elevator muscles contract behind the teeth, the condyles are elevated into the more superiorly seated position at centric relation, **B.** This causes the most posterior teeth to become the occlusal pivot and puts the entire load onto these teeth until the jaw shifts forward.

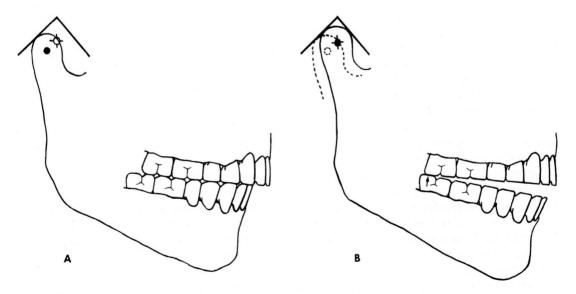

Fig. 4-3. If the occlusion is harmonized to a distalized condyle position, **A,** the full occlusal load shifts to the most posterior teeth when the condyles are elevated into the seated position at the centric relation, **B.**

ward if it moves distally from its centralized position in the disk.

When the mandible is forced distally, the arrangement of the restraining ligaments can also be a factor in directing the condyles downward according to some authorities. However, if the intact condyle-disk assembly is observed carefully, it appears that the medial pole relationship is the dominant factor in guiding the condyle downward from the apex position.

If the disk is properly related to the condyle, the position at the apex of force relates to the most superior position against the eminentia. This position can be recorded with extremely accurate repeatability and is the position I have described as centric relation. There are both physiologic and mechanical reasons for advocating this uppermost position.

From a mechanical standpoint, the condyle cannot move forward or backward from centric relation without moving downward, and so any error of recording centric relation results in a downwardly displaced condyle. If the occlusion is harmonized to a downwardly displaced condyle, whether it is anterior or posterior to centric relation, the greatest stress will be placed on the most posterior teeth when the elevator muscles contract. (Figs. 4-2 and 4-3). Remember that the elevator muscles are all behind the teeth and so contraction during closure has the tendency to seat the condylar axis up.

From a physiologic standpoint an occlusion harmonized to a downwardly displaced condyle forces a protective hypercontraction of the lateral pterygoid muscles and activates the medial pterygoid and masseter muscles into unnecessary contraction during swallowing thus creating excessive forces on the interfering teeth.

If there are no tooth interferences to centric relation, the condyle-disk assemblies are free to slide all the way up the eminentia until the medial poles are stopped by bone. So the lateral pterygoid muscles can release contraction and do not have to remain as the sole counteractant to the strong elevator muscles. There is thus no stimulus for antagonistic muscle hyperactivity at a bone-braced centric relation.

There has been a considerable amount of debate regarding both the position of the condyles in centric relation and the need for

precision in recording it. The confusion is understandable to anyone who has observed the variety of joint positions that are commonly recorded as centric relation. For many years, I have used the Buhnergraph and the Verichek instruments to compare the joint positions achieved by hundreds of different dentists. When several bite records are made on the same patient, it is very unusual to find two dentists who locate the same condyle position, and it is also unusual for the same dentist to precisely duplicate his own recording. Because of this, many dentists have assumed that centric relation is not a precise position and that the condyles really seat into a fairly broad area with no particular specificity needed. We are often admonished that the patient is not a machine and that the body does not function with precision. The term "long centric" has frequently been misinterpreted as referring to an *area* of centric.

Such assumptions are misleading. The articulating surfaces do have *very precise limitations* of movement, and the sensory nerves and reflex organs are exquisitely sensitive. The sensory receptors and the reflex responses they initiate in muscle are unbelievably precise and extremely rapid in response. There are many functional mechanisms in the body that work with microscopic detail at lightning-fast response times (such as the eye, the parts of the ear, and the complex patterns of speech). The integration of so many functional responsibilities into one system requires precision in the stomatognathic system. The need for precise recording of centric relation must not be confused with a *restriction* of function to a precise position, but rather a *permissive* freedom to move in and out of that border position with no interferences.

The reason for advocating the *uppermost* position of the condyle-disk assembly is that it is the physiologic position of the condyles when the mandible is elevated firmly by normal muscle function. Normal muscle function, however, is dependent on the absence of interferences from the teeth.

When there are tooth interferences that prevent either condyle from going to its uppermost hinge position during intercuspation, the pattern of muscle function changes to pull the condyle down the slope and into the position that aligns the mandible with the maximum intercuspation position. The positioner muscle (lateral pterygoid) must then hold the condyle down the slippery incline while the elevator muscles contract.

The reason muscle changes jaw position in the presence of interferences is to protect the interfering tooth or teeth from absorbing the entire force of the closing musculature. The deviation is initiated by the exquisitely sensitive periodontal receptors around the roots of the interfering teeth. Remember that these pressure-sensitive receptors are the protectors of the teeth and if they do not program the muscles to deviate the mandible a tooth that interferes with centric relation would be subjected to the entire closing muscle force. To accommodate to all types of interferences, the periodontal receptors can trigger the lateral pterygoid muscles to pull one or both condyles forward. The mandible can thus be deviated by the muscles to accommodate to almost any occlusion. Because of constant repetition of the proprioceptive trigger to the muscles, they become patterned to the devious closure. Such memorized patterns of muscle activity are called "engrams." The physiology of muscle engrams has been described by Sicher, Ramfjord, and others, and no study of occlusion is complete without a thorough understanding of the role engrams play.

The proprioceptive-engram system works so effectively to guide the mandible around interferences and into the "acquired position" that it is easy to be fooled into believing that the deviated jaw position is correct. Some clinicians even advocate the muscle-positioned relationship as inviolate and attempt to perpetuate it as the correct jaw-to-jaw relationship regardless of the position of the joints. To accept this physiologic disharmony between the teeth and the joints, one would have to be unaware of the destructive effects of such disharmony. Although the harmful effects vary as the adaptive capacity of individuals varies, the patient who has interferences to centric relation and no problems is extremely rare. Our experience is that in most instances, patients with "no problems" have just not been examined carefully. Experience has also shown that patients are more comfortable if they have the freedom to close their teeth together in centric relation. Furthermore, it is impossible to harm a patient by allowing him the freedom to close into centric relation.

If freedom to close into centric relation cannot hurt anyone and it predictably produces the most comfortable, physiologically sound occlusion, a logical question would be, Why doesn't everyone accept it? If it is so clinically superior to other concepts, it should be easy to convince anyone of its value. During the past few years, there has been enough related research evidence to convince a growing number of clinicians that the centric relation position is precise and that muscle incoordination can occur when there are even minute interferences to it. There are however many authorities who still do not subscribe to the importance of joint positioning before analysis or treatment of an occlusion. The reason for this divergence of opinion should be explained.

If centric relation interferences are not eliminated *completely,* the patient may actually be *less* comfortable than he was with his acquired occlusion. To achieve predictable success with equilibration or restorative procedures, the arch-to-arch relationship must be perfectly located. When interocclusal bite records are used, they must be made with meticulous attention to accuracy and transfers to an articulator must be done with extreme precision. Failure either to record or transfer with precision accuracy will produce unpredictable results. Although extreme care with each procedure is essential, the most careful operator will still achieve unpredictable results if the method is wrong. Unfortunately, most of the methods used for recording centric relation do not achieve the precision required for predictable success. Furthermore, even a skilled therapist cannot be certain of the correctness of a jaw relationship unless that position is tested for verification. Because of engram effects on the musculature, it is very easy to be fooled by a freely hinging jaw that appears to be in a correct centric relation but is actually braced by muscle, or is not correctly aligned on its disk.

Most of the current techniques for recording centric relation are still based on the erroneous concept of the "most retruded" condyle position, and so they tend to force the condyle *back* off the eminentia and fail also to get the condyles *up* far enough to achieve the essential combination of bracing from the medial pole, the ligaments, and the eminentia.

One-handed chin-point guidance techniques rarely ever record an accurate centric relation.

If the operator is skillful enough to "romance" (ease) the jaw into a neuromuscular release so that the jaw hinges freely, the condyles will almost always be forced *back and down* by the distalizing pressure. If the operator is not skillful and tends to push back before the muscular release, the lateral pterygoid muscles will resist the tension applied against them with a stretch-reflex contraction that will actually hold the condyles *forward* of centric relation and down the eminentia. This is a very common problem with *all* techniques for recording centric relation unless the operator has learned the combination of delicacy and timing when manipulating the mandible so that muscles are not triggered into contraction by applying pressure at the wrong time or in the wrong direction.

Based on more than 30 years of clinical practice and the carefully *measured* comparison of the centric relation attempts by hundreds of dentists and the careful observation of comparative results achieved by different dentists in a clinical environment for treating temporomandibular disorders, two statements can be made relative to centric relation if the general quality of care is similar:

1. Dentists who learn to position the joints in a precisely correct centric relation are generally highly successful in diagnosing and treating occlusal problems and temporomandibular disorders.
2. Very few dentists record centric relation accurately and probably still fewer achieve accuracy in mounting casts on the articulator. Dentists who do not learn and practice these skills require more time, more adjustments, and use of more bite planes, more drugs, and more gimmickery and do not achieve the level of predictability that is possible.

The above comments are not mere opinions. They are made on the basis of a continuing long-term study that has enabled our group to compare with needlepoint accuracy the condyle positions that result from every method known to us for recording centric relation. Recording materials and devices have been compared as well as positioning techniques. For several years the study has utilized the research technique and instrumentation developed by Long and Buhner[1] (Fig. 4-4). Results from the study have had added meaning because they have been carried out with the

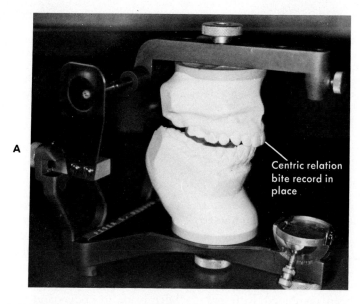

Fig. 4-4. A, Buhnergraph conversion of a Hanau University Model 130-22 Articulator. Models have been mounted with centric bite record and facebow before replacing condyle assemblies with needle point axis and graph paper plate for marking condyle axis location. Upper half of articulator just rests on centric bite record.
Continued.

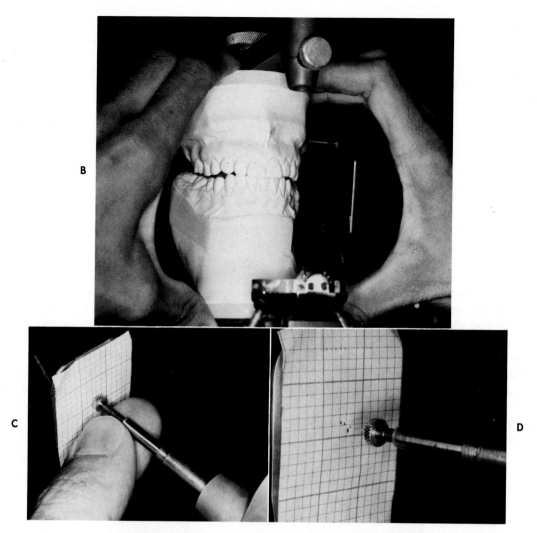

Fig. 4-4, cont'd. B, When condyle axis location is being recorded, models should be firmly seated and held in place against the bite record. **C,** While an assistant holds the models in precise relationship to the centric bite record, the needle point is slid out to penetrate the graph. This notes condyle location for this particular bite record. A new bite record can then be placed between the models, and condyle location can be compared from one bite to another. **D,** Comparative condyle location for several different bite records. Needle holes are made extra large for photographic purposes, but normally only the very fine tip of the needle is used for extremely precise comparison.

diagnosis and treatment of several thousand patients with occlusal or temporomandibular disorders, or both, so that a comparison of condyle positioning can be matched with a comparison of clinical results over a long period of time. The study of comparative condyle positions has also been combined with precisely quantified recording of occlusal interferences (photocclusion) so that both the accuracy of the condyle position and the accuracy

of the occlusal correction can be analyzed and related to relief of signs and symptoms.

All clinical impressions that have resulted from the studies just described have been analyzed as carefully as possible from an anatomic and physiologic perspective. An attempt has been made to understand the cause-and-effect pattern of all signs and symptoms, and there appears to be a recognizable relationship between each type of occlusal disorder and the specific effects that occur in the stomato-gnathic system.

One must be careful not to misinterpret the role of occlusion and centric relation. The term "occlusionist" has been used to describe the dentist who treats *all* temporomandibular disorders with varying types of occlusal procedures. It is critically important to understand that occlusal therapy must be reserved for specific, definitive problems that relate to occlusal disharmony. There is a wide variety of causes for temporomandibular disorders and a still wider variety of causes for craniofacial pain. A differential diagnosis must always allow determination of the cause of the problem before any treatment is selected. If expertise in evaluating joint position and occlusal factors is not developed however, the therapist has no basis for knowing whether they are or are not a factor to contend with. Knowledge regarding the role of centric relation is as important to making a negative diagnosis as it is in isolating it as a direct causative factor.

There are two aspects of recording centric relation. The first consideration is proper manipulation of the mandible such as that necessary for equilibration procedures or examining for premature contacts. The second consideration is concerned with the manner of making interocclusal bite records for correct articulation of mounted casts. Each is discussed separately.

METHODS OF MANIPULATION FOR CENTRIC RELATION

In evaluating the many techniques for positioning the mandible in centric relation, several important observations have been consistently noted.

1. One-handed techniques almost never achieve correct centric relation positioning. Chin-point guidance tends to push the condyles down and back.
2. The mandible cannot be *forced* into centric relation. The uppermost terminal axis must be *delicately* located in an open position *without pressure* on the mandible, and *then* it must be firmly held on that axis while the jaw is closed to the first point of contact. Pressure applied before the joints are in centric relation activates muscle contraction.
3. It is difficult to record centric relation when the patient is upright. Manipulation of the mandible is simpler and far more consistent if the patient is supine.
4. If upward pressure toward the condyles causes any sign of discomfort or tension, the position cannot be accpeted as centric relation. A differential diagnosis must be made to determine the cause of the discomfort before one proceeds (see Chapter 8).
5. The most commonly found cause for discomfort from upward pressure is related to tension of hypercontracted muscle. Muscle spasm can affect both the position of the condyle and the alignment of the disk. In most instances, delicate manipulative techniques can be used to release the spasm and ease the condyles into the correct position.
6. Once a correct method of manipulation is learned, patients will not resist the operator. Drugs, injections, or appliances are rarely needed if the mandible is manipulated properly. This is true even in patients with acute trismus in all but the rarest cases unless an intra-articular problem is present.

The techniques of manipulation must be learned and perfected as one learns any skill requiring dexterity. Because effective manipulation requires a combination of delicacy and firmness used with a keen sense of timing, the operator should have a clear visualization of what is occurring in the joints and how the muscles are affected by various movements and pressures. Whenever a patient tenses up and does not cooperate, it is almost always because force is applied to the mandible *before* it is gently positioned into its uppermost position with the teeth separated. Patients nearly always resist sudden movements, rapid jiggling, or terse commands. The essential first step of finding centric relation is to deprogram muscle contraction. This is achieved best with a gentleness that I must admit I rarely see in the usual attempts of most dentists. But if you observe some of the masters who are extremely successful such as Ramfjord, Fillastre, and Mahan, you will notice a special gentleness that is not generally observed, but you will also notice that it is combined with firm control as the muscles release. Although all use different methods to position the jaw, they are

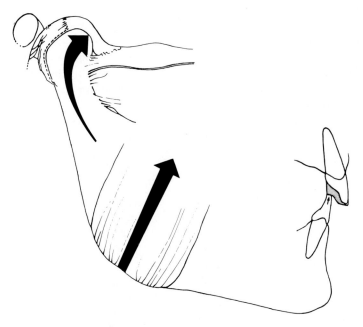

Fig. 4-5. The Lucia jig provides a flat anterior stop that separates all posterior teeth. This allows the elevator muscles to seat the condyles in the correct direction with no chance of posterior occlusal interference.

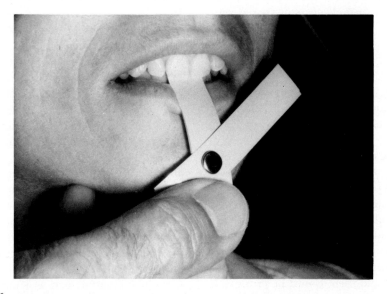

Fig. 4-6. The leaf gage provides a variable thickness anterior stop that separates the posterior teeth, allowing the condyles to seat without interference.

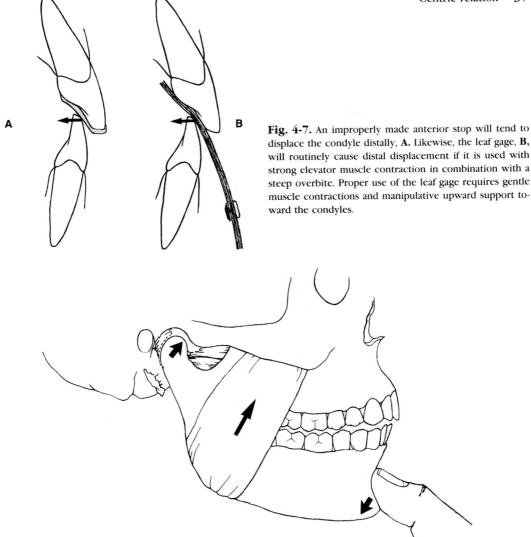

Fig. 4-7. An improperly made anterior stop will tend to displace the condyle distally, **A.** Likewise, the leaf gage, **B,** will routinely cause distal displacement if it is used with strong elevator muscle contraction in combination with a steep overbite. Proper use of the leaf gage requires gentle muscle contractions and manipulative upward support toward the condyles.

Fig. 4-8. Keeping the teeth separated by downward chin-point pressure allows the elevator muscles to seat the condyles into centric relation. This is a useful procedure, but it does not provide the level of verification that can be achieved by firmer load testing of the joints.

highly successful in achieving superlative results. The bruised or sore chin is an absolute sign of improper manipulation.

There is no one specific way that must be used to record centric relation correctly, but there are important similarities that are common in all the techniques that consistently achieve it. Besides the gentleness timed with firmness already described, a common procedure that we have consistently noted among successful occlusal therapists is firmness of upwardly directed pressure at or near the angle of the mandible to ensure that the condyles are seated superiorly against the eminentiae. Some very successful operators utilize anterior stops to separate the posterior teeth so that the muscles can fully seat the condyles with no possibility of tooth interferences. The anterior stop advocated by Lucia[2] (Fig. 4-5) and the leaf gage advocated by Long (Fig. 4-6) are good examples. As with all techniques, both the anterior stop and the leaf gage have the potential for deviating the mandible if not used properly (Fig. 4-7). Anderson and Tanner successfully used a one-handed manipulation but relied on downward pressure applied at the symphysis with the teeth separated, so that contraction of the elevator muscles against the chin point could seat the condyles up (Fig. 4-8).

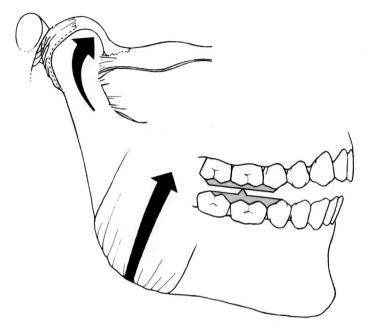

Fig. 4-9. Central bearing point techniques are excellent muscle deprogrammers because they allow full movement of the mandible in any direction. Elevator muscle contraction can seat the condyles with no chance of occlusal interference.

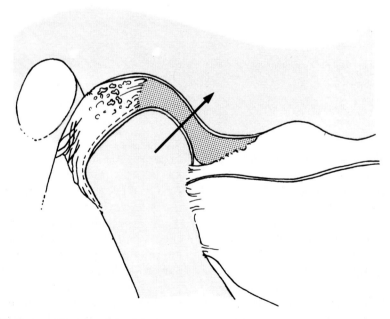

Fig. 4-10. Correct alignment of the disk is a critical requirement of centric relation. At that alignment, all loading forces are directed through avascular, noninnervated tissues that are designed to be stress bearing without discomfort.

A central bearing point, as used in pantographic or stereographic techniques is an excellent muscle-deprogramming device that allows the elevator muscles to seat the condyles in the proper direction (Fig. 4-9). It also prevents any chance of mandibular displacement from occlusal contacts. But as with any technique, the arrived-at condyle positions should still be load tested for verification of centric relation before they are accepted.

In the analysis of any manipulative techniques for recording centric relation, the rationale for the position is far more important than the method used to record it, but because there is such importance in the preciseness of the recording, I analyzed not only the results achieved, but also the degree of difficulty in learning the various procedures. My findings using Buhnergraph or Verichek analysis have consistently shown the bilateral manipulative technique (Dawson technique) to be not only the most consistently repeatable, but also the most easily learned. Several university studies[3-5] have verified that bilateral manipulation is the most repeatable and achieves the most superior position of the condyles. But by far the most important reason for using bilateral manipulation is that it provides a method of *verification* of the following:

1. Correctness of the condyle position
2. Alignment of the condyle-disk assembly
3. Integrity of the articular surfaces

This is unquestionably the most important difference between bilateral manipulation and other manipulative techniques. The ability to exert firm upward pressure toward the condyles while the teeth are separated is the key to verifying the acceptability of the centric relation position.

The reason why healthy condyles in centric relation must be completely comfortable even when firmly loaded can be explained. Only in centric relation are both condyles:

1. Correctly aligned with their disks and
2. Stopped by a bony stop.

Correct condyle-disk alignment ensures that all forces are loaded through avascular, noninnervated tissues (Fig. 4-10).

A bony stop for the condyle-disk assemblies ensures that the lateral pterygoid muscles do not have to resist the upward loading forces.

Complete comfort when there is loading also indicates that there is no active inflammation or pathosis on any of the bearing surfaces of the articulation.

HOW VERIFICATION WORKS

If the first requirement for successful occlusal treatment is *comfortable condyles,* one needs to know what causes *dis*comfort. The condyles should be able to resist even very firm pressure with no sign of tenderness or tension, and that is the reason we apply pressure as a test.

There are three basic causes of temporomandibular discomfort that respond to the test of upward pressure:

1. Improper position of the condyle
2. Improper alignment of the disk
3. Pathosis of the articulating surfaces

To test the joints for these problems, one must exert *firm* pressure and in the right direction to elicit a specific response that has diagnostic significance. Correct bilateral manipulation is essential.

The verification of the centric relation position is dependent on complete comfort during the application of the firm pressure, with simultaneous slow hinging of the mandible to test all the bearing surfaces of the condyles. The presence of *any* discomfort or tension under pressure must be analyzed further to determine what must be done to achieve a correct centric relation.

DIAGNOSING IMPROPER CONDYLE POSITION

If the condyle-disk assembly is forward of centric relation, it was pulled there by the contraction of the lateral pterygoid muscle. If the muscle does not release its contraction, pressure upward will have to be resisted by the muscle (Fig. 4-11) rather than by bone and ligament. Pressure up should be firm enough to stretch the shortened muscle so that it will respond with a feeling of tenderness or tension. A *spastic* muscle will generally respond more painfully to forced stretching. If the condyle-disk assembly is braced against bone and ligament in centric relation, it is not possible to stretch the lateral pterygoid muscle because the condyle is already stopped from going higher.

If upward pressure causes tenderness in either TMJ area, it has been our consistent experience that in more than 95% of the patients so tested the tenderness has been in muscle. If the condyle-disk assembly is allowed to go further up the eminentia to its bone-braced stop at the medial pole, the need for muscle contraction is eliminated and upward pressure will

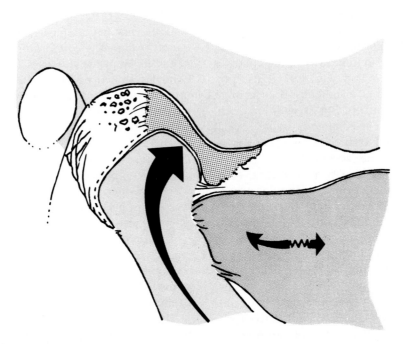

Fig. 4-11. Upward pressure, through a condyle that is held down the eminence by muscle, will exert a stretching effect on the contracted muscle. This will elicit some response of tension or tenderness. If the condyle is fully seated, it is impossible to stretch the muscle because it is impossible to move the condyle-disk assemblies higher.

then produce no tenderness or tension. The relief should be an immediate response when the condyle reaches centric relation.

If gentle manipulation does not work to ease the condyle up, release of lateral pterygoid muscle contraction can be aided by any procedure that disengages the occlusal deviation. This takes away the proprioceptive trigger that activates positioner muscle contraction. A cotton roll between the teeth generally works quite well in 5 to 20 minutes to release muscle contraction or spasm and permits easier manipulation to centric relation.

Bite planes permit a release of muscle spasm by providing a smooth surface to replace the deviating inclines. This gives the condyles the freedom to go to their physiologic position rather than forcing the muscles to relate them to the malrelated occlusion.

DIAGNOSING MISALIGNMENT OF THE DISK

The stress-bearing area of the disk is dense fibrous connective tissue. It is avascular and has no sensory nerve endings, so that when the condyle is properly aligned with the disk it can resist great pressure with no discomfort.

The tissues around the periphery of the support area of the disk, however, are vascular and are innervated with sensory nerve endings. Pressure on these tissues stimulates a response of discomfort or pain. So upward pressure exerted on the condyle will produce discomfort if the disk is not properly aligned (Fig. 4-12).

If it is not possible to manipulate the condyles into a position that can resist pressure comfortably and separation of the teeth with a cotton roll gives no relief, we *suspect* a condyle-disk derangement or a pathologic intra-articular problem.

If a click or pop accompanies jaw opening or closing, this is further evidence of condyle-disk discoordination. Transcranial radiographs will generally (but not always) show the condyle to be against the distal wall of the fossa if the disk is displaced anteriorly.

If the condyle and the disk are not properly aligned, the mandible is not in centric relation. The misalignment must be corrected before the occlusion can be properly harmonized to the TMJ, or the condyle-disk discoordination will be perpetuated.

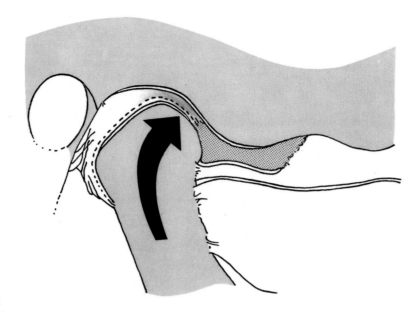

Fig. 4-12. If the condyle is off the disk, upward pressure loads the condyle directly onto the vascular, innervated tissue and causes a response of tenderness or pain. The degree of discomfort may be extreme in early displacements. Any discomfort, however, during loading indicates the possibility of a disk derangement and signifies that centric relation is not being achieved.

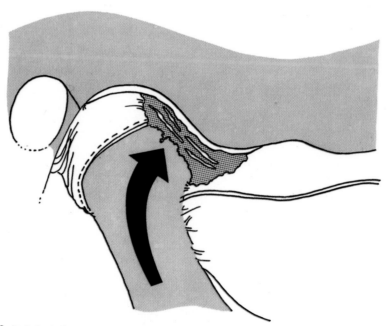

Fig. 4-13. Pathologic breakdown of the articulating surfaces is often accompanied by an invasion of blood vessels and nerves. Loss of the articular cartilage may also expose vascular, innervated surfaces that are sensitive when loaded. Any destruction of the avascular bearing surfaces is likely to result in some discomfort when the condyles are load tested.

DIAGNOSING PATHOSES OF THE ARTICULATING SURFACES

The third possibility to evaluate when upward pressure causes discomfort in the joint area is the chance that the pain is the result of pressure on the bony articulating surfaces. This is possible only if there is some degeneration of the bony surface that involves vascularization with resultant exposed innervation of the bearing area of the condyle or the fossa (Fig. 4-13). Such is the case in arthritic deformity of the joint surface. It may also be the result of tumors, cysts, developmental anomalies, or injury.

Radiographic analysis is most often the differentiating method for determining which type of intra-articular problem is causing the discomfort. However, exploratory surgery is sometimes required before a final diagnosis can be made. Doppler auscultation has eliminated much of the need however for invasive methods of differential diagnosis.

Each of the preceding problems is discussed in greater detail in Chapter 8. It should be obvious however that if any such disorders exist it will not be possible to locate a precise centric relation position, and so the *verification* of centric relation is an essential procedure that should be routinely utilized before initiation of any occlusal treatment.

THE METHOD FOR BILATERAL MANIPULATION

Correct manipulation requires *delicacy first* to encourage neuromuscular release and *then* firmness to verify the position and hold the condyle-disk assemblies in the uppermost hinge axis position while the relationship is being recorded. Several points are important to assure consistency in the manipulation of the mandible to its precise centric relation axis.

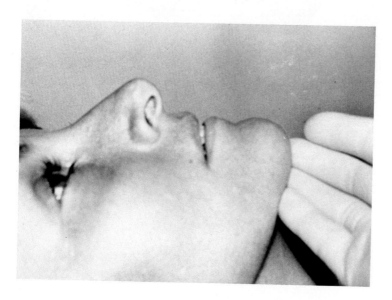

Step one

Recline the patient all the way back; point the chin up. When the patient is supine, it is comfortable for the operator to work in a seated position and it is easy for the patient to relax. Pointing the chin up makes it easier to position the fingers on the mandible and prevents the tendency of some patients to protrude the jaw.

Step two

Working from a seated position behind the patient, firmly stabilize the head. I prefer to stabilize the head between my forearm and rib cage as shown. Some dentists find it is more comfortable to position the top of the patient's head in the center of their abdomen. Whatever method is used, it is essential that the head be stabilized in a firm grip so that it will not move when the mandible is being manipulated. Failure to do this is one of the most common mistakes.

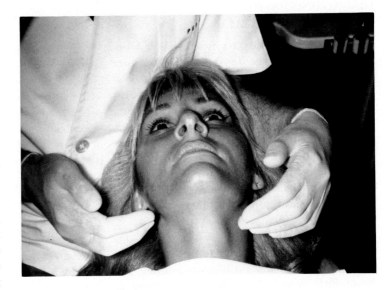

Step three

With the head firmly stabilized, position the four fingers of each hand on the lower border of the mandible. The little fingers should be even with the angle of the mandible or even slightly behind it. Position the fingers as if you were going to lift the head.

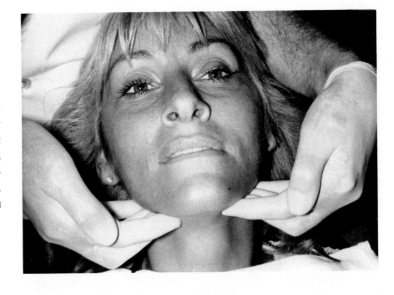

Step four

Bring thumbs together to form a C with each hand. The thumbs should fit in the notch above the symphysis. No pressure is applied at this time. The hand position should be comfortable to both the patient and the dentist.

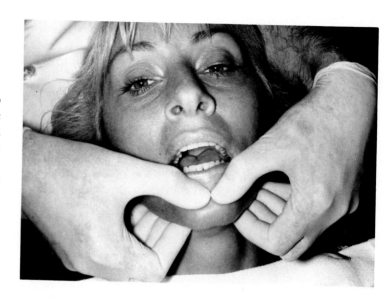

Step five

Now, *with a very gentle touch,* the jaw is manipulated so that it slowly hinges open and closed. As it hinges, the mandible will usually slip up into centric relation automatically *if no pressure is applied.* Any pressure applied before the condyles are completely seated will be resisted by the lateral pterygoid muscles. The contracted muscles will be stretched by the pressure and will respond with greater muscle contraction (stretch-reflex reaction). Once these positioner muscles have been stimulated to contraction, it is extremely difficult to seat the condyles into centric relation.

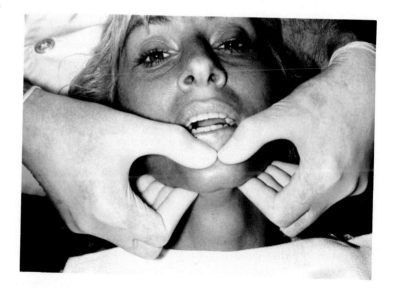

The key at this point is delicacy. *No pressure.* No jiggling, because this also activates muscle response. Use slow hinging movements so that the muscles are not triggered into contraction.

The whole purpose of this step is to deactivate the muscles. We often describe this procedure as "romancing the mandible." Remember we are really just *letting* the condyles go where they physiologically want to be—properly seated in their respective fossae. When the jaw is being hinged in this position, it is not necessary to open wide. An arc of 1 to 2 mm is acceptable. When arcing, do not let the teeth touch.

If the patient resists even gentle manipulation by holding the jaw in protrusion, position the hands *gently* and then *ask the patient* to hinge open and closed. At the point that closing action starts to occur, the mandible will usually retrude automatically. If the hands simply ride along with the patient's own jaw movement, you will feel the jaw go back. *Then* hold it firmly on that hinge position in preparation for the next step.

Step six

After the mandible feels as though it were hinging freely and the condyles seem to be fully seated up in their fossae, most experienced operators will assume that the mandible is in centric relation. But no matter how solidly the condyles seat or how freely the mandible hinges, you *cannot* be certain the position is correct by feel alone. *The centric relation position must be verified.* Both the position of each condyle and its proper alignment with the disk must be tested by application of very firm pressure *upward* with the fingers while the teeth are kept firmly apart with *downward* thumb pressure in the notch above the symphysis (Fig. 4-14). With proper hand position, very firm upward pressure can be maintained while a free axial rotation of the condyles on the terminal axis is still allowed.

The instructions to the patient at this point must be very specific. Ask the patient, Do you feel *any sign* of *tenderness* or *tension in the area of either joint* when I apply pressure? It is a good idea to rub your finger lightly on the skin over the joint area so that the patient knows exactly where the joints are before pressure is applied. If there is *any* sign of tenderness or even tension in either joint area when pressure is applied upwardly toward the fossa seat, you *cannot* accept that position as centric relation. If the articulating surfaces of the TMJ are healthy and in proper alignment with the disk and the condyle-disk assembly is in the uppermost position without muscle bracing, there will be no tenderness or tension of any kind, even with very firm pressure.

If the patient feels *any* degree of tenderness or tension in either condyle area, the pressure should be released and gentle arcing resumed. With experience, the dentist will be able to lightly manipulate the mandible *toward* the tender side. The relationship of the lower midline to the upper midline should be watched. As one works through the muscle contraction and the muscle releases the condyle-disk assembly to its bony stop, the lower midline will move toward the tender side. (It is not necessary for midlines to be in line with each other. They are used for reference points only.)

When the shift toward the tender side is noticed, the position should again be tested by resumption of upward pressure to load the joints. There will be no tenderness if the condyle has reached its centric relation—stopping place. If tenderness increases as the condyle is moved distally, the possibility of pathosis or derangement should be considered.

The ability to manipulate the mandible through the release of a contracted muscle comes only with practice and understanding. Until that ability is developed to produce consistent results, it may be necessary to use some other methods to get the condyles into centric relation. The simplest aid is also one of the most effective, that is, to place a cotton roll across the first premolar area so that the posterior teeth cannot touch (Fig. 4-15). If the cotton roll is held in place for several minutes, the proprioceptive input from interfering teeth to the muscles will be lost and the mandible can then be easily manipulated into position unless there is pathosis or a nonreducible disk displacement.

It should be noted again that free rotation around the condylar axis is not a guarantee that the axis is a superiorly placed one. The condyle can rotate freely in its disk at any position from terminal hinge to extreme protrusion. Even experienced operators can be fooled unless the load test is used as a confirmation of centric relation.

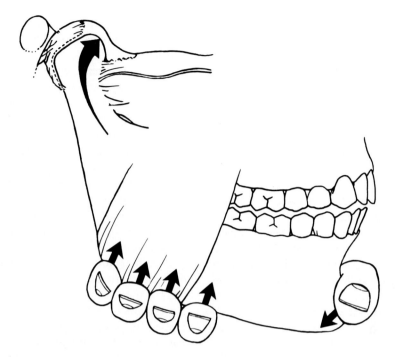

Fig. 4-14. Proper hand position for bilateral manipulation uses *downward* pressure from the thumbs to keep the teeth separated whereas *upward, slightly forward* pressure from the fingers loads the condyles against the posterior wall of the eminentiae. This hand position can then be used to help slide the condyles up the slopes but still maintain loaded pressure against the eminentiae.

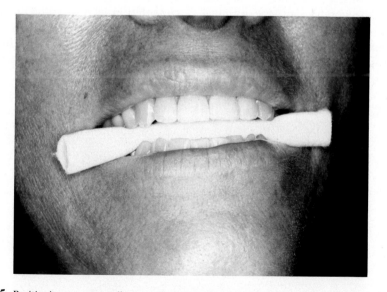

Fig. 4-15. Positioning a cotton roll across the bicuspids prevents occlusal interferences from contacting. It is a very effective way to deprogram hyperactive masticatory muscles. Muscle contraction will usually start to release in a few minutes though in some patients more time may be required.

Step seven

When it is possible to freely and painlessly arc the mandible while exerting firm pressure up toward the condyles, the dentist is then ready to close the mandible to the first point of contact.

The mandible should not be forced closed in one motion, rather it is held firmly on its terminal axis and arcing begun in small opening-closing arcs. Each closing arc should be progressively closer to tooth contact.

As the closing mandible brings the interfering teeth closer together, resistance to closure will progressively increase. Because of muscle memory engrams developed from long-standing patterns of avoiding the premature contact, it will be difficult to close the mandible the last millimeter or so in many instances. *The mandible should not translate off its terminal axis,* but it should be held firmly at the point of resistance to closure or a millimeter or two open. If the mandible is held there for a few moments, the proprioceptive influence will be lessened and the arcing closure may be resumed. It may be necessary to close in increments of a fraction of a millimeter at a time, but with careful manipulation the dentist will be able to close to the first point of contact without letting the condyles off the terminal hinge.

It is frequently helpful to tell the patient, "Just let your jaw close now until the first tooth touches." But if the patient is allowed to help, the condyles should be held on their terminal axis.

There are many ways of encouraging patients to relax and cooperate with the manipulative efforts. Asking the patient to "let the jaw hang loosely" will frequently help. Sometimes having the patient relax the shoulders helps diminish resistance to manipulation, but usually the resistance is caused by exertion of pressure on the jaw too soon, *before* the condyles are in the terminal axis position. The axis *must be gently located in the open position before pressure is applied. The patient should be lying flat with the chin pointed up.*

7. When initial tooth-to-tooth contact is made, the first interference to centric relation has been located. With the mandible held on its terminal axis, the interfering teeth are tapped together two or three times so that the patient can feel the prematurities. The jaw is closed to this premature contact. The patient is asked to help hold that position for a second and then the teeth are squeezed together.

The direction in which the mandible deviates from its first tooth contact to its maximum occlusal contact should be noted. This is commonly called a "slide in centric," but the connotation is misleading since it is really a slide *from* centric relation. Such a slide indicates that the teeth are not in harmony with centric relation. When such a slide is present,

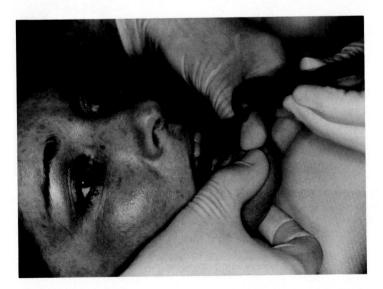

Fig. 4-16. To mark centric relation interferences, arc the mandible on a firmly held terminal axis while the assistant holds the ribbon.

the condyle-disk assembly is not permitted to go to its physiologic position of bracing against bone when the teeth are together. The result of such a relationship is stress.

The purpose of equilibration is to eliminate such stress by eliminating the interferences that cause the mandible to deviate off its terminal arc of closure. The procedures for equilibration are described in Chapter 24, but it should be noted here that the effectiveness of the equilibration procedures will depend on the dentist's ability to properly manipulate the mandible as described.

To mark the interfering contact that has been located by manipulation, it is necessary to have help. Either the chairside assistant or the patient must hold the marking ribbon while the mandible is manipulated with both hands (Fig. 4-16).

If mounted models are to be used, a record will have to be made so that the casts will be related to each other on the articulator exactly as the mandible is related to the maxilla in centric relation. To record this jaw relationshp at the first point of contact, an interocclusal bite record must be made. There is no one method of taking centric relation bite records that will work on all patients. Both the technique and the materials used must be changed to accommodate varying conditions. An understanding of the various problems will enable the dentist to select the best method for each particular situation.

METHODS FOR TAKING CENTRIC BITE RECORDS

The purpose of a centric bite record is to capture, in some stable material, the relationship of the mandible to the maxilla when the condyles are in their terminal axis position. The record should be made at a vertical opening that does not permit the first interfering tooth to contact. The record must fit the models as perfectly as it fits the mouth.

In selecting the technique and the material to be used for making an interocclusal record, several factors should be considered.

1. *The ability of the operator to manipulate the mandible.* If the dentist has perfected manipulative techniques so that he can quickly position the jaw into centric relation and close it without deviation into the bite material, he may use wax effectively in selected cases. If too much time is required

to manipulate the mandible, the wax will cool and become too hard. Unless the wax is very soft when the bite is taken, there is a danger of depressing the teeth or moving them laterally.

2. *The ability of the patient to cooperate.* Once manipulative techniques have been perfected, patient cooperation will cease to be a problem except for unusual cases.

3. *Tooth mobility.* The teeth should not be moved by the bite material. Very loose teeth may even require stabilization before a correct bite can be taken. Soft materials that do not depress the teeth should be used with special techniques when hypermobility is a problem.

4. *Edentulous areas.* When the bite material is being indented by edentulous areas, extreme care must be taken not to distort the soft tissues. A model made from nondistorting impression material will not fit into an interocclusal record that has compressed soft tissue.

5. *Condylectomy.* The procedure for taking bite records on patients who have lost one or both condyles is entirely different from the methods used for recording terminal hinge position of the condyles.

6. *Occlusal interferences.* The method for taking a centric bite record on a patient with gross interferences will be different from the method used for the patient who can close without deviation to the correct vertical dimension. If interfering teeth contact, the mandible will deviate and the bite record will be in error. It may be necessary to record centric relation at a very open vertical to avoid contacting the interference. If so, special precautions should be taken to make sure the terminal hinge axis is correctly recorded along with the interocclusal bite record.

There are four basic techniques from a practical clinical standpoint for making a centric relation interocclusal record:

1. Wax bite procedures
2. Anterior stop techniques
3. Use of preadapted bases
4. Central bearing point techniques

Each of these techniques has advantages and disadvantages that should be understood if they are to be used effectively. It would be unrealistic to single out any one of these or any other technique as being practical for all cases because no one technique lends itself to all the different conditions that the restorative dentist faces. The ideal technique for any given case is the method that enables the dentist to accurately record centric relation in the simplest way. Complicated procedures are used only if accuracy cannot be achieved with a simpler technique.

There are four criteria for accuracy in making an interocclusal centric bite record:

1. The bite record must not cause any movement of teeth or displacement of soft tissue.
2. It must be possible to check the accuracy of the bite record in the mouth.
3. The bite record must fit the models as accurately as it fits the mouth.
4. It must be possible to check the accuracy of the bite record on the models.

It will usually be possible to fulfill all four requirements for accuracy by proper selection of one of the techniques to be described. However, it may be necessary to combine techniques or to improvise in very clever ways to ensure that all four criteria for accuracy are fulfilled with absolute preciseness. Such flexibility of combining or improvising should be kept in mind when you are studying the following details of the four basic techniques.

Wax bite

The use of wax for making interocclusal records is by far the most popular method. The main reason for its popularity lies in its simplicity. Simplicity is not a valid reason for using a technique unless it also fulfills all criteria for accuracy.

Perhaps we tend to underrate the wax bite because we see it used so commonly in such inaccurate ways, but along with its simplicity, the wax bite rates with the best techniques in regard to accuracy *if it is properly used.*

If direct wax bite procedures are to be used, it is important to select the right type of wax. If the wax record can bend and mold itself to fit the models, errors can be masked. Therefore the wax must be brittle hard when it is cooled but must be soft enough not to cause movement of teeth when it is warm. Extra-hard base plate wax is an excellent bite material. The correct choice of wax will not bend at normal room temperature without snapping.

The following procedures are basic for making a direct wax interocclusal record (wax bite).

The surfaces of a sheet of extra-hard base plate wax are heated over a bunsen burner and the end thirds folded onto the middle third. While the wax is still warm, it is pressed very lightly against the upper arch either in the mouth or against a model. The indentations are noted, and with a warm knife, the wafer is trimmed to just fit the arch. If enough posterior teeth are present to get a firm index for the models, the wax is trimmed so that the anterior teeth are not included in the bite.

Only the outer edge of the wax is softened over the flame where the teeth will be indenting it. The upper teeth are dried and the wax is pressed against them, making sure to get a good indentation against each tooth.

With the patient lying back flat, the mandible is manipulated to guide it into the wax without allowing it to deviate off its terminal axis. With use of the procedure described in this chapter for manipulation of the mandible, the jaw is closed almost to the point of first tooth contact. If the upper teeth are dry and the lower teeth are wet with saliva, the wax will usually stick firmly to the upper teeth and enable the dentist to tap into the wax without dislodging it. The wax must have been softened enough at the edges so that it will not cause movement of the teeth when they close into it.

The bite is cooled slightly with air and removed. It is checked to make sure there are no penetrations. Then with a very sharp knife, the indentations made by the buccal cusp tips of both upper and lower teeth are trimmed. This will enable the dentist to check the accuracy of the bite record in the mouth.

Now the wax record is returned to the upper arch and the mandible is guided into it, making sure there is no deviation during closure. The mouth is closed firmly against the wax, which is still slightly warm, and perfect adaptation of the wax to the teeth is checked. There should be a tooth-wax-tooth relationship with no cracks between the wax and any tooth (Fig. 4-17). This will be easy to check because the wax has been trimmed back to the upper and lower buccal cusp tips.

The wax is again removed and any wax that contacts soft tissue is trimmed. It is then rechecked for accuracy in the mouth to make sure the record has not been distorted by the trimming. If it is necessary to resoften the wax to correct for a slight distortion, it is best to soften only the edge of the wafer where the teeth indent it. The wax is placed back against

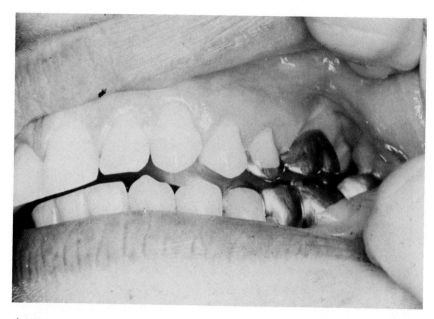

Fig. 4-17. A correctly made wax bite record. There are no cracks between the teeth and the wax when the jaw is manipulated into centric relation. Wax should be brittle hard so that it cannot be distorted when the models are placed in the bite record.

the upper teeth and the mandible closed into it to readapt it. The wax wafer should extend directly across the arch without touching palatal tissue (Fig. 4-18).

When it is fairly certain that the record is correct, it is checked again for perfect tooth-wax-tooth adaptation and to be certain that there is no impingement of soft tissue. Now the dentist is ready to verify the accuracy of the record in the mouth. One of the biggest advantages of the wax record is that it can be checked out so precisely in the mouth as well as on the models.

The wax is chilled in ice water. If the correct type of extra-hard base plate wax is being used, it will become extremely hard when it is chilled in this manner. Now the record is placed against the upper teeth and the mandible manipulated to check for occlusal interferences. Any errors in the wax record will show up as interferences. Using extremely careful manipulation (as outlined), check all teeth to be sure that they touch the bite record at the same time. The patient should be asked, Which side touches first? He must not be able to discern any difference.

If any teeth had been depressed or moved laterally in taking the bite, careful manipulation at this check point will show it. Any devi-

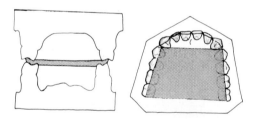

Fig. 4-18. Correctly made wax wafer for recording centric relation. Wax should be sufficiently thick (two or three thicknesses) so that it does not bend, and it should avoid all soft tissue whenever possible. *One-piece* wafer is easy to control and helps to stabilize teeth during centric record making. Individual quadrant bites are easily dislodged and are difficult to adapt to the model accurately.

ation when closing into the bite record can be observed. There is no time problem in checking the chilled record. All the time needed should be taken to make sure the record is perfect before it is accepted. It is sometimes possible to correct minor discrepancies by resoftening the lower side only and then repeating the closure in centric relation.

Wax bite records can be stored safely when they are floated in water. Plastic denture containers that have a tight-fitting lid are ideal for safe keeping of the records until they are

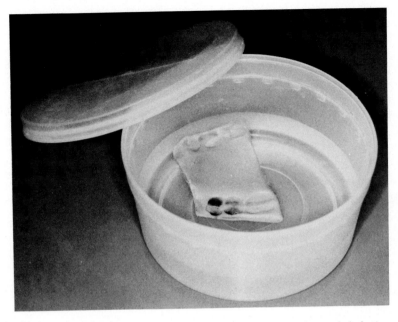

Fig. 4-19. Store wax bite records until needed by floating them in water in a sealed plastic container. Careless handling of bite records is responsible for many mounting errors.

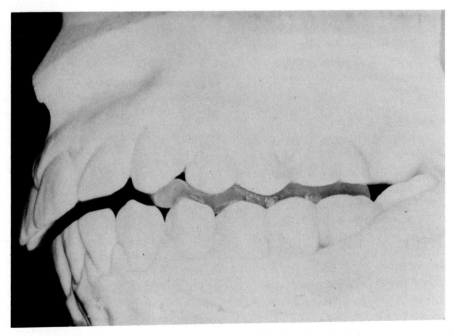

Fig. 4-20. The bite record should fit the model as accurately as it fits the mouth. There should be no cracks showing between stone-wax-stone.

needed. Enough water to float the bite will eliminate distortion in the container (Fig. 4-19).

A wax bite made in the manner just described permits very accurate mounting and checking of the mounting of the stone models. When the models have been mounted, they should fit the bite record just as perfectly as the record fits the mouth. It is easy to check for stone-wax-stone adaptation in the same manner that tooth-wax-tooth adaptation was checked intraorally (Fig. 4-20). If there is so much as a crack between the wax and the stone, the mounting should be rejected.

Failure of the models to adapt perfectly to the bite may be the result of several possible errors. It could be caused by peduncles on the models or by using too much stone in one mix for mounting the models to the instrument. A large mix of stone produces considerable distortion upon setting, and so it is always better to build up with smaller mixes. A model made from a distorted impression will not fit the bite accurately; neither will a bite record that has been distorted by improper handling fit correctly made models.

Regardless of the cause of the discrepancy, properly made wax bite records will show it up if the stone-wax-stone adaptation is carefully noted.

It should be rather obvious that the technique just described depends on proper manipulation of the mandible. It is not suitable for patients who have extremely loose teeth or large edentulous areas. However, when conditions lend themselves to the use of this technique, it can be relied upon with confidence as a simple but extremely accurate procedure for recording centric relation.

Anterior stop techniques

Of all the techniques for carefully recording centric relation, methods using some form of anterior stop are the easiest to learn and offer the greatest flexibility. Anterior stop techniques may be modified and adapted to almost any clinical situation in which anterior teeth are present. It is an extremely accurate technique, and the accuracy can even be achieved with very loose teeth, posterior edentulous ridges, and patients with temporomandibular joint problems.

The term "anterior stop" as it is used here refers to contact in the incisor area *only.*

When the mandible is closed, the lower incisors strike against a "stop" that is precisely adapted to fit against the upper incisors. The stop should be thin enough so that the first point of posterior tooth contact just barely misses, but under no circumstances should any posterior tooth be allowed to touch when the anterior stop is in place.

The great advantage of using an anterior stop is that it allows the condyles to seat *up* without any possible deviation or restriction from the posterior teeth. If the anterior stop is correctly made, there is no tendency for the patient to shift the jaw in any direction while a soft material such as plaster can set up to form the bite record between the posterior teeth. Neither is there any problem of compression of hypermobile posterior teeth by the soft bite material.

If the manipulation of the mandible is made difficult by muscle spasm, the pain-dysfunction syndrome can be relieved when one allows the patient to rest the mandible for a few minutes with the anterior stop in place. Since deviating interferences cannot be reached when the anterior stop is in place, the proprioceptive trigger to the muscles is lost and the mandible can be freely manipulated into its terminal hinge position.

Variations in the technique are mostly variations of materials used. As an example, the anterior stop may be made from acrylic resin or from hard compound. It may be processed on previously mounted models, or it may be adapted directly in the mouth. The anterior teeth themselves may serve as the anterior stop if they contact perfectly in centric relation and if the posterior teeth are missing or have been taken out of contact through preparation for crowns or onlays.

The choice of a bite material for the posterior teeth has great flexibility. Since the anterior stop enables the mandible to be held in a very stable position for several minutes, the choice of materials is almost unlimited. Plaster is used effectively, since it sets quickly and is easy to use. Zinc oxide impression pastes are frequently used and can be very effective.

Self-curing acrylic resin has been used though it requires special attention because of its tendency to generate heat while setting. Distortion might also be a problem with many types of acrylic resins, and acrylic bite records are very hard on dies.

Wax may be used very effectively on posterior teeth with anterior stop techniques if the wax is heated to a dead-soft consistency. It can then be checked out after it has hardened in the same manner that has already been described for checking the accuracy of a conventional wax bite.

Firm-setting silicone impression material makes an excellent posterior bite material for edentulous ridges because of its accuracy after it sets and because of its nondistorting flow before it sets. A stable anterior stop enables the patient to hold the jaw in centric relation for the relatively long setting required by many silicone products.

A bite record made from firm-setting silicone adapts easily and accurately to the stone model and can be checked on the model for accuracy in the same manner that is used for checking a wax bite.

The flexibility of anterior stop techniques is limited only by the imagination of the operator. The choice of materials can be made according to the varied needs of the patient. The more mobile the teeth, the softer the posterior bite material must be to keep from moving them until it sets firm. Bite materials that do not set firm cannot be checked for accuracy on the mounted models. Consequently they should not be used.

The following step-by-step procedures should serve to illustrate the basic techniques of utilizing anterior stop techniques for recording centric relation.

1. A little ball of red compound is softened and adapted to the upper central incisors so that their lingual surfaces are completely covered. It is extended over the incisal edges for stability.

2. With the patient in a supine position, the mandible is manipulated into centric relation and closed until the lower incisors indent the softened compound. The patient closes into the compound until the posterior teeth just barely miss contacting. The mandible is arced on its terminal axis to see whether there is any deviation off the axis as the lower incisors fit into the depressions in the compound. If there is any deviation off the arc of centric closure, the compound is resoftened and the procedure begun again.

The anterior stop shoud always be checked meticulously for accuracy before one proceeds with the bite record on the posterior teeth.

This is done by checking against the hardened anterior stop. The centric relation axis of closure should be verified by checking for any tenderness in the joint areas while applying pressure on the mandible toward the condyles. If pressure produces tenderness in either joint area, the axis of closure is not correct.

When it is certain that the axis of closure is correct, the patient should close into the indentations in the compound. The lower incisors should go directly into the indentations with no movement of the teeth or deviation off the axis.

3. When the accuracy of the anterior stop has been verified, the material for the bite record is mixed and a roll of it placed on the lower teeth. The patient closes into the stop position and holds his jaws together with firm pressure. The firm pressure will seat the condyles up. The anterior stop will keep the patient from deviating off that position.

4. When the bite material has set, it is removed and trimmed back to the tips of the lower buccal cusps and the central grooves of the upper teeth. (This can vary with malposed or prepared teeth so long as the fit of the teeth against the bite material can be checked.) Now the bite record is trimmed back wherever it touched soft tissue.

5. The bite record is placed back on the upper teeth. It will usually fit snugly enough so that it will stay in place. The jaw is manipulated very carefully into a terminal axis closure, and any discrepancies between the teeth and the bite material are noted. If the record checks out as correct in the mouth, it can then be accepted for mounting. It should be rechecked on the models to make sure it fits them as well as it fits in the mouth.

Posterior teeth opposed by edentulous ridge

If posterior teeth are opposed by an edentulous ridge, certain types of heavy-bodied silicone can be used to make a preliminary bite record with an anterior stop. Two balls of putty-like silicone base material of sufficient size to fill the space between the teeth and the ridges should be mixed. They should be adapted to the occlusal surfaces of the teeth and part of the material folded around the teeth and into some of the undercut areas of each tooth. The mandible is manipulated into the previously perfect anterior stop, making sure the ridges are in contact with the silicone. When the silicone has completely set, it should be removed and the edentulous side trimmed back slightly so that it does not contact the ridge. The tooth side should be trimmed back so that it does not contact soft tissue.

A wash of light-bodied impression material is added to the base material on the edentulous side only. The bite record is reinserted by being snapped back in over the teeth and the jaw is closed into the anterior stop. If there are no posterior teeth in contact in centric relation, the anterior teeth may serve as the anterior stop, provided that they cause no deviation and the patient can hold perfectly still against them.

The light-bodied material adapts nicely to the edentulous ridge without distorting it. The heavier-bodied mix keeps a snug grip on the opposing teeth for easy manipulation without loosening the bite material.

When set and removed, the bite record can then be trimmed and checked for adaptation to the teeth the same as other bite records. There should be no space between the bite record and any of the posterior teeth. In most cases the silicone can be trimmed back to check the adaptation to the rest of the ridge also.

When this procedure is followed, the silicone material used for the preliminary bite should be the type that can be worked with like putty. Materials that flow too easily will not hold their shape in the fairly large mass that is usually required for edentulous areas. When set, the material must be firm enough to ensure positive seating of the models without permitting distortion of the bite record.

Several usable silicone materials are available. If the technique is fully understood, a careful operator can accurately evaluate any number of materials and use the ones that suit him best.

Making centric bite records on preformed bases

Whenever there is a danger that teeth will be moved or soft tissue compressed by an intraorally made bite record, the use of a preformed base is indicated.

A bite record that moves teeth or compresses or distorts soft tissue will not accurately fit a stone model made from a soft, nondistorting impression material. The problem is especially evident when one is trying to record centric relation in a mouth with hypermobile teeth or with opposing edentulous ridges. The problem is amplified if hypermobile teeth are spaced far apart or if the edentulous ridge areas are flabby and mobile.

Accuracy demands that the bite record must fit the models as perfectly as it fits the mouth. If the base for the bite record is made on the model that it must fit, the criteria for accuracy can be served quite well.

The possible variations in the use of premade bases are endless. Although we tend to think of the procedure as being limited to bases that rest on soft tissue, one of the most important advantages of a premade base is its capacity for stabilizing hypermobile teeth in their correct position while the bite record is being made.

One of the most effective ways of using a premade base is also one of the simplest. A triple-layered wafer of extra-hard base plate wax is adapted to an accurate model that has been dampened so that the warm wax will not stick to it. The wafer should extend across from one side of the arch to the other in order to provide cross-arch stabilization for the teeth. The wax should be pressed firmly around the teeth on the model in a manner that not only will hold the teeth in the mouth firmly but will also stabilize the base (Fig. 4-21). Whenever practical, the base should be adapted to the upper arch where it is not so easily dislodged by the tongue. It should be trimmed back to within a millimeter of the buccal surface of the teeth so that the cheeks do not push it loose when it is in place.

Wax over any occluding surfaces should be thinned to allow maximum closure without tooth-to-tooth contact. If the posterior teeth have been prepared for restorations and the anterior centric contacts have been perfected, the wax base should be limited to posterior teeth and it should not touch opposing teeth when the anterior teeth are in contact.

If there are large edentulous areas that must support the base, the wax should be meticulously adapted so as not to impinge on any muscle attachments that could dislodge the base. The wax should be at least three thicknesses for strength and should be extra hard and brittle enough to break rather than bend when it is cool.

When the stability of the premade base is

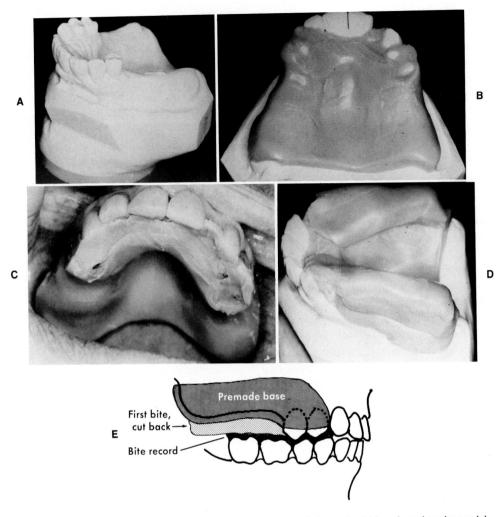

Fig. 4-21. When large edentulous areas are present, a premade base should be adapted to the model and the interocclusal record made on the fitted base. **A,** The upper model is mounted on the articulator with a facebow registration. **B,** *Extra-hard* base plate wax is adapted to the models. Three thicknesses should be used on the palate to prevent distortion. Wax can be wrapped around some teeth for stabilization of the base or the teeth themselves. If base is made sturdy enough, it will fit precisely back on the model after the bite record is made. **C,** The base is tried in the mouth and relieved of any deviating contacts. It should be adjusted so that the bite can be taken at or near the correct vertical dimension. **D,** Softer wax is added on the model and returned to the mouth for a preliminary bite record. The wax is then cut back to just miss tooth contact, and the final bite record is made using dead-soft wax *that turns hard when chilled.* **E,** Diagram showing layers of bite record. Ideally, final bite record is made with front teeth in contact at correct vertical dimension. The final bite record should be made with the minimum amount of wax required to just barely indent the teeth in the opposing arch.

perfected and it has been cleared of any occlusal interferences, it should be put back on the model and rechecked to make sure it still fits the cast perfectly. It should be chilled to prevent it from distorting, and then, where the opposing teeth will touch it, a small strip of base plate wax that has been heated to dead-soft consistency should be added. The base should be reinserted into the mouth and the mandible manipulated into a terminal axis clo-

sure to indent the dead-soft wax strip with the lower posterior teeth.

The most common mistake in using wax for the bite record is using too much wax. Only enough should be added to the base to provide an index of the tips of the opposing teeth. Another frequent source of error is using wax that is too flexible. The wax should be dead soft when heated but should be brittle hard when cooled. Extra-hard waxes can be checked for accuracy both in the mouth and on the models. Soft waxes can be adapted incorrectly after the bite record is made without showing any evidence of the error either in the mouth or on the models.

The manipulative technique described in this chapter must be practiced until it can be achieved with precise accuracy and repeatability. In my many years of teaching the procedures, it has become obvious that although some learn the method quite easily most dentists must work very diligently before mastering the technique. Some dentists never achieve acceptable accuracy though, thankfully, they are in the minority. Most dentists can learn to position the mandible in a very precise centric relation and repeat the same recording with needlepoint accuracy.

The procedure is well worth learning. Although centric relation records can be accurately made using other methods, there is no good substitute for correct manipulation when it comes to equilibration procedures. For differential diagnoses of TMJ disorders, the ability to test the joints is essential. Bilateral manipulation provides the most practical, direct method for verifying centric relation and ruling out intra-articular problems.

The one best method for learning the procedures is to practice by taking several bite records on the same patient and comparing the positions on a Verichek instrument or Buhnergraph. If two or three dentists can work together on the same patient, valuable input can be gleaned from a comparison of subtle differences in technique. The procedures should be refined until all recordings are identical.

Any dentist who is willing to spend the time and energy to master the technique of recording and verifying precisely correct centric relation will benefit in untold ways. There is no procedure in dentistry that can produce as many tangible benefits to both the doctor and the patient as the routine correct recording of centric relation, verified for accuracy.

REFERENCES

1. Long, J.H., Jr.: Location of the terminal hinge axis by intraoral means, J. Prosthet. Dent. **23**:11, 1970.
2. Lucia, V.O.: A technique for recording centric relation, J. Prosthet. Dent. **14**:492, 1964.
3. Kantor, M.E., Silverman, S.I., and Garfinkel, L.: Centric-relation recording techniques: a comparative investigation, J. Prosthet. Dent. **28**:593, 1972.
4. Lundeen, H.: Centric relation records, the effect of muscle action, J. Prosthet. Dent. **31**(3):244-251, 1974.
5. Hobo, S., and Iwata, T.: Reproducibility of mandibular centricity in three dimensions, J. Prosthet. Dent. **53**:649, 1985.

SUGGESTED READINGS

Beyron, H.: Optimal occlusion, Dent. Clin. North Am. **13**:537, 1969.

Celenza, F.V.: The centric position: replacement and character, J. Prosthet. Dent. **30**:591, 1973.

Celenza, F.V., and Nasedkin, J.N.: Occlusion: the state of the art, Chicago, 1978, Quintessence Publishing Co., Inc.

Dawson, P.E.: Optimum TMJ condyle position in clinical practice, Int. J. Periodontics Restorative Dent. **5**(3):10, 1985.

Frederick, D.R., Pameyer, D.H., and Stallard, R.E.: A correlation between force and distalization of the mandible in obtaining centric relation, J. Periodontol. **45**:70, 1974.

Gilboe, D.: Centric relation as the treatment position, J. Prosthet. Dent. **50**(5):685, 1983.

Ingervall, B., Helkimo, M., and Carlsson, G.E.: Recording of the retrusive position of the mandible with application of varying external pressure to the lower jaw in man, Arch. Oral Biol. **16**:1165, 1971.

Mohl, N.: Comments in Solberg, W.K., and Clark, G.T.: Abnormal jaw mechanics, Chicago, 1984, Quintessence Publishing Co., Inc., p. 46.

Palla, S.: Condyle positioning and radiological analysis. In Solberg, W.K., and Clark, G.T.: Abnormal jaw mechanics, Chicago, 1984, Quintessence Publishing Co., Inc., pp. 51-53.

Stuart, C.E.: Good occlusion for natural teeth, J. Prosthet. Dent. **14**:716, 1964.

Williamson, E.H.: Laminographic study of mandibular condyle position when recording centric relation, J. Prosthet. Dent. **39**:561, 1978.

Zola, A.: Morphologic limiting factors in the temporomandibular joint, J. Prosthet. Dent. **13**:732-740, 1963.

5

Vertical dimension

The *vertical dimension of occlusion* refers to the vertical position of the mandible in relation to the maxilla when the upper and lower teeth are intercuspated at the most closed position.

Even though the vertical dimension of occlusion occurs when the teeth are fully articulated, the teeth are not the determinants of vertical dimension. Rather their position is determined *by* the vertical dimension of the space available between the fixed maxilla and the muscle-positioned mandible.

The most important thing to understand about vertical dimension is that the mandible goes repetitiously to the position dictated by the *contracted* elevator muscles (Fig. 5-1). The upper and lower teeth erupt into the space until they meet at that jaw-to-jaw relationship (Fig. 5-2). Thus the elevator muscle–contracted length during the power cycle of the elevator muscles sets the limits of jaw separation to which the teeth erupt.

The second important aspect of vertical dimension that must be understood is that the vertical position of each tooth is adaptable to the space provided, not vice versa, and that the capacity of the teeth to erupt or intrude is present throughout life. There is an ever-present eruptive force that causes teeth to erupt until they meet an equal, opposite force. If the opposing force is greater than the eruptive force, the teeth are intruded until the eruptive force equals the resistive force against them. If the resistive force is less than the

eruptive force, the teeth will continue to erupt.

All resistive forces are solely the result of pressure exerted by the *musculature-controlled* elevation of the mandible toward the maxilla. The neutral point to which the teeth erupt is the optimum point at which the muscle contraction is completed in its repetitive power cycle. It is possible to contract the muscles further by conscious demand, but the habitual pattern of closure is amazingly constant and is the controlling factor of vertical dimension. In fact, the dimension of this jaw-to-jaw relationship is so constant that even severe bruxing, clenching, and abrading parafunction do not alter the jaw-to-jaw dimension between bony landmarks in each jaw (Fig. 5-3). This is evidenced by the consistent observation that eruption keeps pace with wear. Because of elongation of the alveolar process, even severe abrasion of teeth does not cause a loss of vertical dimension. The only explanation for this phenomenon is the constancy of the mandible-to-maxilla dimension at the completion of the elevator-muscle contraction cycle.

VERTICAL DIMENSION AT REST

When a muscle is neither hypotonic nor hypertonic, it is said to be "at rest." Even resting muscle is in a mild state of contraction. This mild contraction of antagonistic muscles is necessary to maintain the posture and alignment of the skeletal parts. Contraction of one muscle beyond its resting length affects its an-

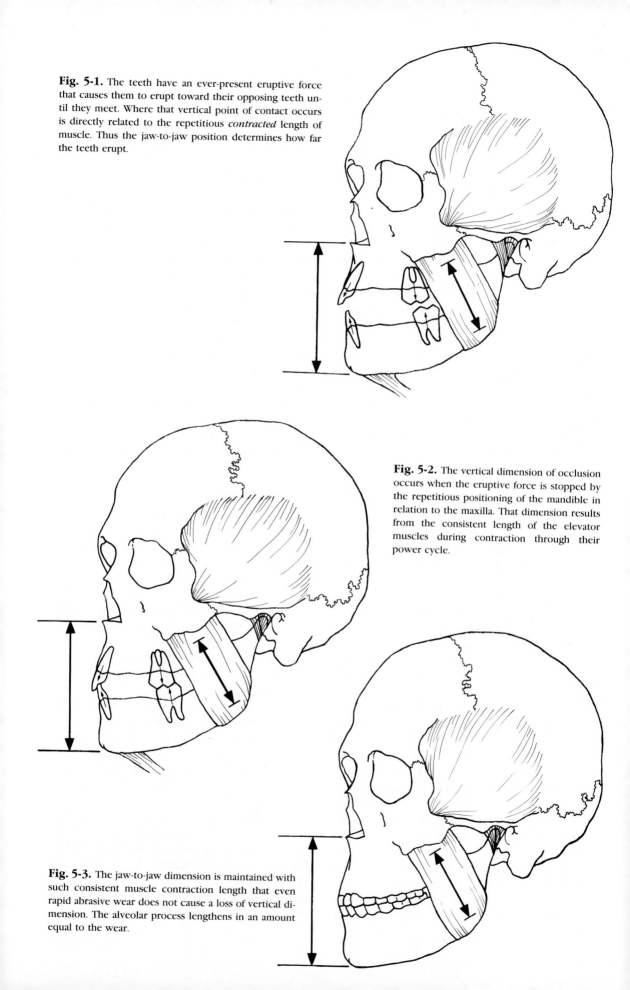

Fig. 5-1. The teeth have an ever-present eruptive force that causes them to erupt toward their opposing teeth until they meet. Where that vertical point of contact occurs is directly related to the repetitious *contracted* length of muscle. Thus the jaw-to-jaw position determines how far the teeth erupt.

Fig. 5-2. The vertical dimension of occlusion occurs when the eruptive force is stopped by the repetitious positioning of the mandible in relation to the maxilla. That dimension results from the consistent length of the elevator muscles during contraction through their power cycle.

Fig. 5-3. The jaw-to-jaw dimension is maintained with such consistent muscle contraction length that even rapid abrasive wear does not cause a loss of vertical dimension. The alveolar process lengthens in an amount equal to the wear.

tagonistic muscle to some degree. The antagonist must release and give the contracting muscle its way, or it must respond by isometrically contracting more forcefully itself to counterbalance the effect of the antagonist. Either way, the harmony of resting muscle is disturbed by any factor that interferes with its resting length.

From Niswonger's[1] early postulations that the rest position was constant and inviolate, numerous proponents of this concept have generated a variety of methods using the rest position for determining the vertical dimension of occlusion. Despite the popularity of using rest position as a starting point for determining occlusal vertical dimension, it is an unreliable approach because the dimension between the teeth at the rest position is not consistent for different patients. The rest position is not consistent even in the same patient. Atwood[2] found variations as great as 4 mm at the same sitting and even greater variations at different sittings. Finding the vertical dimension of rest position and then arbitrarily closing a specific amount is an unsatisfactory approach.

Recent research efforts have also shown that the rest position is anything but constant. The jaw position at rest not only is highly variable, but it also changes noticeably in the same patient in response to a variety of factors including how much stress the patient is subjected to. The rest position is also altered by the presence of any noxious stimuli from occlusal interferences that can cause varying degrees of muscle incoordination. The effects of masticatory muscle incoordination can range from slight hypercontraction to severe trismus, all of which can have a profound effect on the postural position of the mandible at rest.

Although the length of the elevator muscles varies through a wide range of contraction in the so-called resting position, the contracted length in the power cycle appears constant.[3] That consistency results from the "all-or-none" contraction of a sufficiently constant number of muscle fibers to establish an unvarying dimension during the repetitious swallowing pattern.

To simplify the concept, the contracted length of the elevator muscles during the repetitive power cycle used in swallowing is constant (at least within the range of clinical

importance). The length of muscle at rest position is not constant, nor is the rest position consistently related to the vertical dimension of occlusion. Some muscles may contract to half of their resting length, whereas others shorten very little. The variations of muscle contraction are as great as the differences in people themselves.

Gibbs and Mahan[4] have pointed out that the maximum force with which muscle resists elongation is applied when it is completely committed to contraction. If teeth erupt until they reach a resistance that equals their eruptive force, it is logical that the muscular placement of the mandible in relationship to the maxilla would determine the point at which that resistance is met. It is also apparent that an increase in the vertical dimension of the teeth would interfere with the optimum length of muscle in its power-stroke contraction cycle.

If the vertical dimension can be established in harmony with the optimum repetitive length of the contracted elevator muscles, the muscles will be free to rest at whatever length is comfortable. The practical approach therefore is to concentrate on accurately recording the *vertical dimension of occlusion* and allowing the dimensions of the freeway space to be the natural result of the difference between the optimum length of contracted muscles and the length of the muscles at rest.

The concept of using the rest position as a starting point for finding the vertical dimension of occlusion is unreliable for two reasons:

1. The rest position is not constant and continuously changes, and so it is not a logical base line from which to measure the fixed dimension at maximum intercuspation.
2. The interocclusal freeway space is highly variable from one patient to another, and so there are no set dimensional relationships that could be used to find the occlusal vertical dimension even if the rest position could be determined with consistent accuracy.

Nevertheless, attempts to determine a consistent rest position have been pursued using transcutaneous electrical neural stimulation (TENS). The use of the Myomonitor to accomplish a TENS-induced relaxation of the masticatory muscles has become a popular procedure that allegedly leads to determination of the correct vertical dimension of occlusion. Williamson,[5] however, showed that the TENS-induced rest position differs significantly from the clinical rest position, and other researchers[6] have reported similar discrepancies, along with a frequent inability to duplicate the dimensions recorded. Williamson also showed that even after 1 hour of muscle pulsation to ensure adequate muscle relaxation, the vertical dimension at rest changed significantly on the same patient even while the Myomonitor was being used continuously. When the patient was subjected to varying levels of stress, from playing a competitive electronic game, with electrical stimulation via surface electrodes from the Myomonitor continuing, the vertical dimension of rest decreased significantly.

Even if a transcutaneous electrical neural type of stimulation could be used with consistent results to determine the vertical dimension of rest, it would still not be an acceptable method for determining the vertical dimension of occlusion. The muscle-*contracted* position is unrelated to any consistent comparison with the resting musculature, regardless of how resting length is determined. The finding that stress affects the resting posture of the mandible, even while the Myomonitor is being used, just adds another variable to an already questionable modality.

The safest rule for determining the vertical dimension of occlusion on patients with teeth is, *Do not change the vertical dimension of occlusion that occurs when the teeth are intercuspated in maximum contact.* In patients with occluding natural teeth this means, *Do not open the bite.*

The reason for giving two similar rules is to try to overcome some of the misleading but popular concepts regarding *bite raising.* There was a time when bite raising was almost synonymous with oral rehabilitation. Even the finest dentists used bite-raising techniques with little or no concern for the consequences. The detrimental effects of bite raising are insidious, however, so it took years of practicing the procedure to learn that it was not a wise approach.

There are definite exceptions to the rules against bite raising. It is sometimes necessary, and with the better understanding we now have regarding the potential for vertical change within the alveolar process we can of-

ten take advantage of alterations of vertical during the treatment stage, knowing that the muscular control over jaw relationships will, in time, return the vertical dimension to its pretreatment measurement.

Although there are valid reasons for increasing the vertical dimension, most bite raising has been traditionally done for one of the following reasons:

1. To relieve a temporomandibular disorder.
2. To "unload" the temporomandibular joints.
3. To restore "lost" vertical dimension in a severely worn occlusion.
4. To get rid of facial wrinkles.

None of these reasons is valid.

Increasing the vertical in each of these situations is based on erroneous concepts and may in fact be harmful. It is almost always contraindicated. A better perception of each of these problems should be gained before any treatment is considered.

Bite raising for temporomandibular joint disorders. The vertical dimension of occlusion has in itself nothing to do with temporomandibular disorders. If the pain is from a true pathosis, vertical changes could actually increase the muscular loading of compromised tissues. The pain and dysfunction associated with occluso-muscle imbalances can be resolved at any vertical dimension up to the point of condylar translation or closed down to the point of coronoid impingement. As long as the correctly aligned condyle-disk assemblies are free to go to the most superior position against the eminentiae, the pain of muscle incoordination can be relieved. Condylar access to centric relation is not dependent on any given vertical dimension because the condyles are free to rotate on a fixed axis.

Dentists who have accomplished relief of occluso-muscle pain with the use of bite-raising appliances may erroneously give the credit to the increased vertical dimension. Actually, the same symptoms could have been relieved at a closed vertical as long as the articulation is noninterfering with the centric relation axis of the joints.

Correcting the occlusion at an increased vertical may indeed eliminate the patient's discomfort, but it appears that the increased vertical amost always reverts to its original dimen-

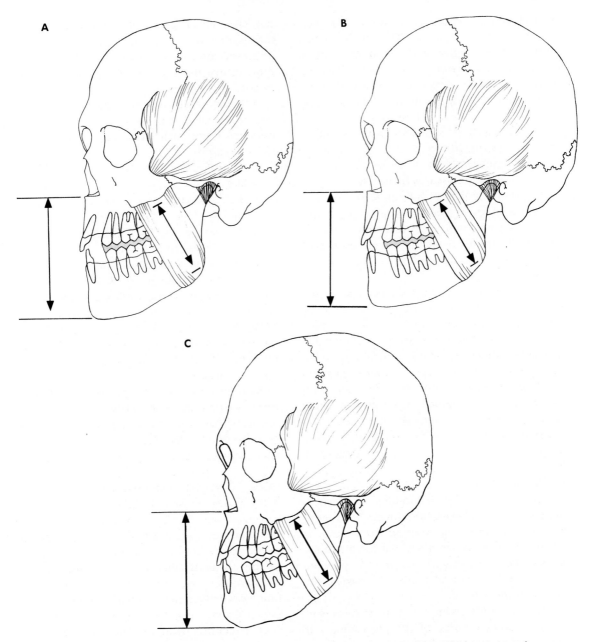

Fig. 5-4. Bite-raising appliances increase the jaw-to-jaw dimension and interfere with the contracted length of the elevator muscle, **A.** The muscles can be expected to regain a vertical jaw relationship that is consistent with their contracted length. This occurs by intrusion of the covered teeth by an amount equal to the thickness of the bite plane, **B.** When the posterior bite-raising appliance is removed, the teeth it covered will be out of contact, **C.**

sion by intrusion of the teeth that have been increased in height (Figs. 5-4 and 5-5). If vertical stability is one of the goals of occlusal treatment, it seems more logical to work to the correct vertical to start with, rather than to increase it and then wait for it to change back to where it was.

"Unloading" the temporomandibular joints. Increasing the vertical dimension does not "unload" the joints. This is a common misconception based on another erroneous concept that the condyles should be *supported* by the occlusion. The condyles are not supported by the teeth, and the condyles are not posi-

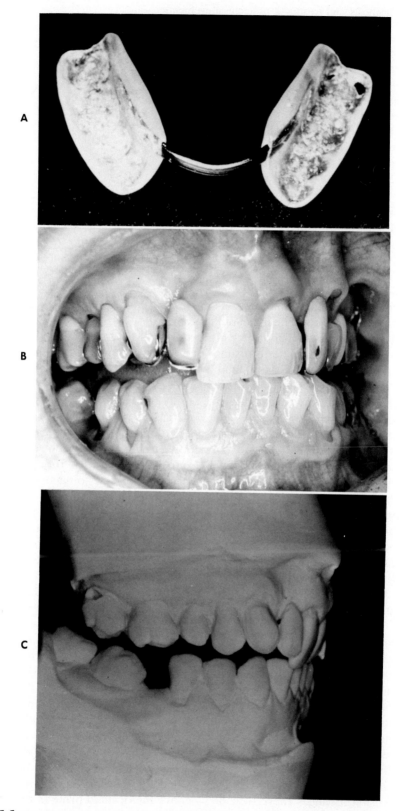

Fig. 5-5. Typical example of the effect of bite raising using a posterior appliance. **A,** As the contracted length of the elevator muscles regains equilibrium with the vertical jaw position, the posterior teeth are intruded by an amount that equals the added-on dimension of the splint thickness, **B.** Casts mounted in centric relation, **C,** show how the upper anterior teeth have been inclined lingually. It results because the anterior teeth are separated when the appliance is placed. The lower anterior teeth thus block forward pressure from the tongue from counterbalancing the lingualizing pressure from the lips. This is a routine observation when posterior bite-raising appliances are used for extended periods.

tioned by the teeth in a centered relationship with "space" around the condyle. That "space" is merely radiolucent tissue that is *loaded* by the elevator muscles, all of which are between the posterior teeth and the condyles.

Bite raising increases the vertical, not by lifting the condyles away from the eminence, but rather by rotation of the condyles, *which remain loaded during the opening rotation.* If the bite-raising appliance attempts to distract the condyles away from their seated position, the elevator muscles will simply elevate the condyles against the eminentiae at whatever position may be dictated by the erroneous occlusal inclines. The most posterior tooth contact becomes the pivotal point in the dentition, and the elevator muscles behind that point elevate the condyles toward the eminentiae until they are loaded. If the bite-raising appliance is made at centric relation, the condyles can simply rotate the jaw more open, without joint displacement. The joints will still be loaded.

Increasing the vertical, even though no discomfort results, can have detrimental effects. Depression of the teeth can create excessive stresses on the periodontium and result in instability of the occlusion. Instability can lead to occlusal interferences that activate muscle incoordination and its detrimental consequences. Whenever possible, occlusal treatment should be performed as close to the original vertical dimension as possible. The vertical dimension the patient presents with has already stabilized in relation to contracted muscle length. Any changes will require adaptation that would be better to avoid whenever possible.

Other temporomandibular disorders, such as disk derangements and other intra-articular problems, do not benefit directly by changes in vertical dimension. The effects of various types of bite planes are the result of either permitting condylar access to centric relation or directing the condyles to a treatment position. The ability of the condyles to rotate from any position along their border paths enables them to assume any of those positions irrespective of vertical dimension. Changes in vertical dimension would rarely be a direct factor in the treatment of joint disorders.

Restoring "lost" vertical dimension.
More study is needed, but much clinical evidence indicates that even severely worn occlusions do not lose vertical dimension. Restoring

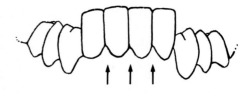

Fig. 5-6. When teeth have no holding contacts, they erupt until they meet resistance that equals the eruptive force. Eruption takes place by elongation of the alveolar process. Notice that the level of the alveolar bone in relation to the cementoenamel junctions of teeth that have not had acceptable stops. Compare bone height with that around teeth that have occlusal stops.

"lost" vertical dimension in a worn occlusion really amounts to opening the bite because wear does not normally produce a loss of vertical dimension. Patients can wear their teeth down to the gum line and still not lose vertical dimension because the eruptive process matches the wear to maintain the original vertical dimension.

This process of eruption and alveolar development may continue throughout life as teeth are worn because of the continual addition of layers of cementum on the root and concurrent elongation of the alveolar process. So even with wear, the jaw-to-jaw relationship remains the same when the teeth are together.

The idea that eruption keeps up with wear comes as a surprise to some dentists, but it can be observed in many different ways. We notice what happens to the lower anterior teeth when they are not met by the upper teeth in some deep overbite situations. If the tongue does not substitute for the missing contact, the teeth erupt up into the palate. Do they erupt out of the alveolar bone? Of course not; the bone develops vertically on up with the teeth. Often the level of the anterior bone expands above the occlusal plane of the posterior teeth (Fig. 5-6). As another example, we notice how the tuberosity enlarges and grows down with an unopposed upper molar.

We have noticed what happens to natural teeth when they are opposed by plastic teeth on a bridge or partial restoration. As the plastic teeth wear, the natural teeth erupt. We have all probably seen teeth that have worn all the way through a plastic partial restoration so that the erupted teeth were contacting the opposing ridge. Such problems are sometimes difficult to solve because the properly opposed teeth maintain their position as the others erupt and the occlusal plane ends up all out of harmony.

It might be asked whether there are not exceptions to the rule. What about the tobacco chewer who wears his teeth down rapidly? Surely the eruptive process cannot keep up with that kind of wear. There is some evidence to suggest that the ability of the alveolar process to compensate for lost vertical dimension diminishes in later years, but it is safer not to count on this loss even when rapid and extensive wear has occurred.

Anyone who has ever observed what happens when a patient loses the temporary restoration on an onlay preparation has seen first-hand how quickly teeth can erupt. In some cases, the prepared tooth may erupt all the way to contact within a couple of weeks' time. It is almost a certainty that the restoration will be quite "high" any time a prepared tooth is not stabilized with a properly occluding temporary restoration.

We must not be fooled by worn teeth into believing the bite has closed. Restoring "lost" vertical dimension is most often really bite raising when it is done on natural teeth. It is true that some occlusions are worn so badly that we have no logical alternative but to increase the vertical dimension slightly. When we do it, we must remember that the patient who wears the teeth badly is the one who can least afford to have any impingement on the freeway space. Luckily, it is rarely necessary.

Opening the bite to eliminate facial wrinkles. On patients with natural opposing teeth, this procedure may have very detrimental effects. *When the masticatory and facial muscles are at rest, the teeth should not be in contact.* Increasing the vertical dimension to the extent of stretching the wrinkles out puts such an unnatural demand on the stretched muscles that it may actually accelerate further wrinkling. The increased length of the teeth positions them in continuous interference to both normal contracting and resting lengths of the muscles. Such continuous stretch stimulation may cause reflex contraction of the mus-

cles with damaging results to the teeth and supporting structures. The stresses exerted on the teeth are amplified by unfavorable crown-root ratios that result from increasing the length of the clinical crowns. Furthermore, the effect on the continuously stretched muscle is to "age" it faster and produce worse wrinkles.

Patients who have previously had bite-raising procedures to eliminate wrinkles are often very insistent about further increases. As the teeth depress or the wrinkles return, they express the need for more and more increase in vertical dimension. Some patients tell us they were more comfortable when the bite was first raised and they would like to regain that comfort. It is difficult not to give in to such a request because it sounds so reasonable. If we understand that their early comfort was the result of an improved occlusion relationship rather than the increased vertical dimension, we can almost always regain the comfort by equilibration without further increase of vertical dimension.

The patient must be made to understand that the muscles should be allowed to position the jaw without interference from the teeth. "Support" from the teeth at an opened vertical dimension constitutes an interference to the contracted muscle in a normal power stroke.

Rather than trying to solve the wrinkle problem with a potentially destructive "solution," it would be far better to refer the patient to a plastic surgeon for cosmetic surgery. Cosmetic surgery techniques are quite successful when they are done by competent surgeons, and since such techniques do not involve the masticatory muscles, they have little if any effect on the occlusal vertical dimension.

Several studies have shown that there is a significant relationship between the "power point" of muscular contraction and repeatable phonetic and comfort measurements. Tueller,[7] using electronic means on dentures, found an average variation of less than 0.5 mm from the vertical established at the muscular power point when compared with either preextraction records or phonetic methods.

Silverman[8] has reported consistent results in measuring the vertical dimension of occlusion by phonetic methods. When a patient has lost natural occlusal stops for recording the vertical, we have found that Silverman's closest speaking technique has provided consistently reliable results. The vertical dimension established in this manner is repeatable with extreme accuracy, even over a period of months.

PHONETIC METHOD OF MEASURING OCCLUSAL VERTICAL DIMENSION

It must be emphasized that patients with opposing natural teeth should be maintained at the vertical of their maximum intercuspation position. The phonetic technique is used when there are no opposing teeth in contact. It is an ideal method for use in full denture construction but has equal value for the restorative dentist when a restored arch is opposed by a denture, when the vertical has been altered by improper restorations, or in any relationship without adequate opposing tooth contacts.

To understand the principle, one may perform the following steps, as outlined by Silverman, on a patient with opposing teeth.

1. The patient is seated in an upright position with the occlusal plane parallel to the floor. He is asked to close firmly (centric occlusion), and a line is drawn on a lower anterior tooth at the exact level of the upper incisal edge (Fig. 5-7, *A*). This line is called the *centric occlusion line.*

2. Now the patient says *yes* and continues the *s* sound like *yessssss*. While he is pronouncing the *s* sound, a line is again drawn on the same lower anterior tooth at the level of the upper incisal edge. This line is called the *closest speaking line* (Fig. 5-7, *B*). The space between the lower centric occlusion line and the upper closest speaking line is called the *closest speaking space.*

3. To analyze how repeatable this record is, the patient should be asked to count from 60 to 66. One should notice how the upper incisal edge comes right back to the closest speaking line with the pronunciation of each *s* sound. If it does not, the line should be altered slightly to match the *s* position when the patient reads or talks fairly rapidly.

4. If such a measurement is to serve as a preextraction record, the difference between the closest speaking line and the centric occlusion line is recorded. The closest speaking space must be maintained in the finished denture.

5. If the determinations are being made on a patient who has already lost the natural occlusal vertical dimension, the missing teeth can be substituted for on temporary restorations or on fabricated bases. After proper lip support, esthetics, and incisal-edge position have been determined, the phonetic method can be used to establish the vertical dimension. Since the vertical dimension of occlusion is unknown, we determine the closest speaking position first and then close the vertical 1 mm from that point. A wax esthetic control rim (Fig. 5-8) can be used in place of upper teeth. It can be attached to the upper denture base and adjusted for lip support, smile-line esthetics, and the like. If it interfers during the phonetic exercises, it can be easily corrected. By placing several marks on the lower anterior teeth, we can observe which mark aligns with the incisal edge of the esthetic control rim or the artificial upper anterior teeth (Figs. 5-9 and 5-10) when the *s* sounds are made.

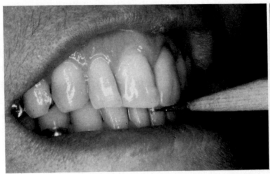 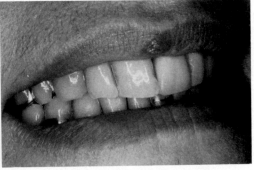

A   B

Fig. 5-7. A, *Centric occlusion line.* With the patient's teeth in maximum occlusal contact a line is drawn on a lower anterior tooth at the exact level of the upper incisal edge. This is referred to as the "centric occlusion line." **B,** The position of the line when the patient says *yessssss.* Notice that the distance from the line to the incisal edge on the *s* sound is about 1 mm. A new line is drawn at the incisal edge position that is repeated during the *s* sound. This is called the *closest speaking line.* Observe how precisely the closest speaking line is repeatedly aligned with the upper incisal edge on *s* sounds.

There should be no bumping of the teeth during speaking. Such contacts would indicate either interference to the correct vertical dimension or insufficient overjet. When normal phonetic function can take place comfortably, the closest speaking level should be noted and the centric bite record should be made by closing 1 mm farther to the vertical dimension of occlusion.

The vertical dimension has long been regarded as one of the variables of occlusion, but with time more and more evidence has been found that points to a need for more preciseness. Perhaps some of the confusion comes from the loss of vertical dimension that occurs in denture patients as the ridges resorb. However, natural teeth do not react the same as edentulous ridges. More scientific study is needed, but on the basis of clinical evidence and studies of muscle physiology, the safest approach for restorative patients with natural teeth is, Work as close to the existing vertical dimension of occlusion as possible.

WHEN THE VERTICAL MUST BE CHANGED

There are some problems of occlusion that would be very difficult to solve without increasing the vertical dimension. It is not always possible to restore an extremely worn occlusion without some increase, and sometimes the choice may be to either increase the vertical dimension or perform multiple pulp extirpations and endodontics to provide enough room for restorations. In some cases, the esthetic needs of the patient cannot be satisfied without the crown length being increased and the choices may be either surgical crown-lengthening procedures versus increasing the vertical dimension. Some orthodontic results may be difficult to achieve without increasing the vertical dimension. The same may be true when one is restoring some severe arch malrelationships or extreme occlusal plane problems.

There are other types of occlusal problems such as anterior open bite that require a *reduction* of the vertical dimension in order to get

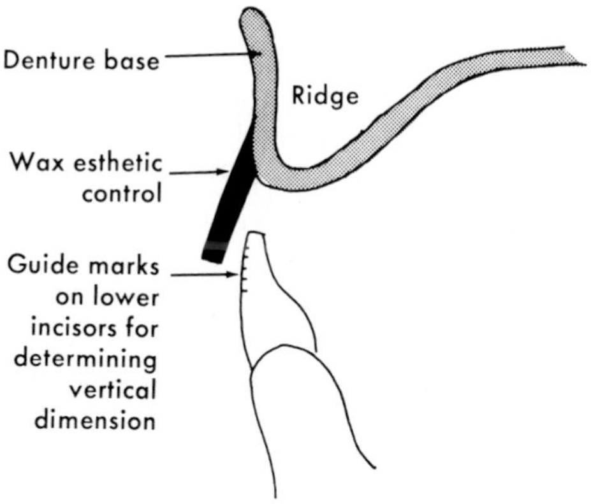

Fig. 5-8. Determining the vertical dimension when the upper arch is edentulous. A wax esthetic control rim is added to the labial of a processed acrylic denture base. The esthetic control rim is used to establish correct lip support and incisal edge position. When this is accomplished, several lines are drawn 1 mm apart on the lower incisors. On s sounds, the line that repeatedly aligns with the incisal edge of the esthetic control rim is selected as the closest speaking line. The centric bite record is then made with the vertical dimension closed 1 mm from the closest speaking line, and that vertical is accepted as the correct vertical dimension of occlusion.

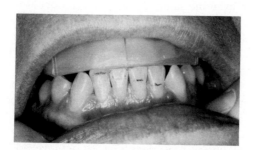

Fig. 5-9. An esthetic control rim in place. Length and lip support have been determined so that the lower edge of the rim represents the precise incisal edge position. Lines are drawn on the lower incisors so that it will be easy to determine which line is repeatedly aligned with the edge of the rim when s sounds are made.

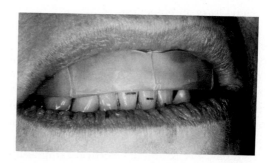

Fig. 5-10. The patient says *yessssss* or counts from sixty to sixty-six. At each s or x sound, the line on the patient's right central aligns with the edge of the control rim. This line is then accepted as the closest speaking line. The vertical dimension of occlusion is set 1 mm closed from this position.

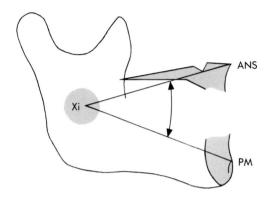

Fig. 5-11. Ricketts' analysis of lower facial height has shown that it stays constant with age. The angle from the Xi point to the anterior nasal spine (ANS point) and the PM point also stays constant as the mandible grows in children.

an acceptable result. When the only alternative would be anterior teeth that are too long or smiles that would be too gummy, closure of the vertical dimension seems to be a far better choice.

Do all changes in vertical dimension lead to eventual problems in the dentition or its supporting structures? We know a bit more today about the adaptive capacity of the alveolar process to changes in vertical dimension, and we now know that in many patients, changes in vertical dimension can be managed. We also feel quite certain that changes in vertical dimension are only temporary. There is growing evidence to indicate that whether the vertical dimension is increased or decreased in adults it will in time return to its pretreatment vertical dimension. This is not surprising if one considers how effectively muscle dominates skeletal form and function.

Ricketts[9] has described lower facial height in adults as staying constant with age. Using the same bony landmarks (Fig. 5-11) to measure the distance between the point on the mandible and the ANS point (at the anterior nasal spine), McAndrews[10] showed that adult orthodontic patients whose vertical dimension had been increased up to 8 mm had reverted to their pretreatment vertical dimension within 1 year. He also observed that *decreases* in vertical of up to 7 mm regained the lost vertical within 1 year.

An even more important finding in the McAndrews study, however, was that the change back to the original vertical did not adversely affect the corrected arch alignments or the intercuspal relationships. This would indicate that changes back to the pretreatment vertical occurred almost entirely within the alveolar bone by either progressive or regressive remodeling.[11] A further indication that changes in vertical were the result of alveolar bone remodeling was the observation that the cementoenamel junction of the teeth retained the same relationship to the crest of bone.

Of great significance in the McAndrews study is the attention paid to achieving holding contacts for all teeth in centric relation. It appears that the response to increased vertical is not the same if contacts are established only on posterior teeth. Where only segments of the occlusion are increased in height, there seems to be a tendency to intrude those teeth into the alveolar bone, whereas if the entire arch contacts simultaneously in centric relation, the changes take place by regressive remodeling of the alveolar process.

What this study and our own clinical observations seem to indicate is that it is permissible to alter the vertical dimension when necessary for achieving an improved occlusal relationship as long as all teeth are properly intercuspated at a correct centric relation. It is also a consistent finding that whenever the vertical dimension is increased, the number of postoperative occlusal adjustments required are noticeably increased and may be required repeatedly for up to a year before the occlusion stabilizes.

Before increasing any vertical dimension, one should evaluate the alveolar bone. Dense sclerotic bone with numerous exostoses does not have the same capacity to remodel as alveolar bone with normal trabeculas. Increasing vertical dimension in such unchangeable bone is contraindicated. (See Chapter 30, Solving Occlusal Wear Problems.)

If the constancy of vertical dimension is perceived in detail, it will be obvious that promiscuous alteration of the vertical is to be avoided. There is no reason to change any vertical unless it is necessary to achieve an acceptable result. If the vertical dimension must be changed, it should be changed as little as necessary because the increased dimension between the jaws will in all probability not be maintained.

Finding a "comfortable" vertical dimension. Many clinicians advocate working with provisional restorations and varying the vertical dimension until a *comfortable* occlusovertical dimension is located. Despite the fact that this is the most popular way to determine vertical dimension for bite-raising procedures and other restorative vertical changes, it is absolutely without merit. There is no recognizable difference in the comfort level through a wide variation of changes in vertical dimension if the condyles are in centric relation when occlusal contact is made bilaterally on nondeviating surfaces.

Regardless of how comfortable a patient may be at an increased vertical, it is not an indication that the vertical is correct.

If opposing, reasonably stable posterior teeth occlude, the jaw relationship at maximum intercuspation is the correct vertical. If that relationship is uncomfortable, it will be because the intercuspation does not occur at centric relation or because of an intra-articular problem or because of a continuous clenching pattern. Correction of any of those problems will permit an optimum level of comfort without increasing the vertical. The same level of comfort can also be achieved at an increased or decreased vertical, and so the use of "comfort" as an indication of correct vertical is not valid.

Intrusions into the interocclusal space. If the vertical dimension is perceived to be a jaw-to-jaw relationship, it will be apparent that there is only so much space between the jaws to accommodate the teeth. If any object is placed between the teeth for an extended period, the teeth will be intruded by the thickness of the object so that the dimension between the jaws can remain the same.[12]

Whether the intruding object is a bite plane, a high crown, or a tongue, the result is the same. The muscles will eventually bring the mandible back to its original vertical relationship to the maxilla, and the teeth will be intruded by whatever amount is necessary to allow that to happen. The length of the contracted muscle will prevail. The teeth, being the most movable part of the masticatory system, will adapt.

This concept is illustrated dramatically by the thumb-sucking child. Placing the thumb between the anterior teeth may temporarily open the bite, but eventually the mandible regains its normal relationship to the maxilla as the teeth around the thumb are intruded to conform to the shape of the thumb. Notice also that the alveolar process conforms to the position of the teeth. The basal bone of the mandible and maxilla retains a fairly constant relationship to the contracted elevator muscles, whereas the teeth and their alveolar bone adapt to conform, sharing the limited space with whatever intrudes into that set dimension.

WHY NOT INCREASE VERTICAL DIMENSION

A major goal of all occlusal treatment is to develop harmony in the masticatory system. Any disharmony in the system provokes adaptive responses designed to return the system to equilibrium. There is always some price to pay for adaptation, and even though the adaptive process may be beneficial, it is not always predictable. Adaptive responses to increased vertical dimension may simply cause the lengthened teeth to intrude into the alveolar bone to regain the original jaw-to-jaw relationship, or there may be an attempt to wear away the increased dimension by bruxing. There is increased loading on the lengthened teeth from muscle that is attempting to regain its normal length of contraction, and if that added compression of the supporting tissues exceeds their capacity to remodel acceptably, we will see hypermobility of the teeth and a lowered resistance in the periodontal structures.

With adequate care and attention to the details of a perfected centric relation occlusion, the adaptive responses can be managed and controlled, but if it is not necessary to disturb the equilibrium in the first place, it makes sense to plan treatments that do not require adaptive changes to correct for an increased vertical that was of no benefit to the patient and could not be maintained at the treatment level.

Most increases in vertical dimension have no benefit to the patient whatsoever. If there is no benefit to be derived from the treatment, it is difficult to rationalize doing it. The goal of occlusal therapy is to *minimize* the requirements for adaptation. Unnecessary increases in vertical dimension do the opposite. They increase the requirements for adaptation, and once the adaptive process is in accelerated activity, it is not always completely predictable.

If the increased vertical dimension is achieved by restorations that have no other purpose, the procedure is clearly contraindicated. In dentitions that have no need for extensive restorative dentistry, using restorations to increase the vertical dimension is an unnecessary expense and inconvenience to the patient and has no ultimate benefit, since the increase in vertical cannot be maintained anyway.

Increasing the vertical dimension on only part of the dentition is clearly contraindicated because it leads to an instability of the entire occlusal harmony. Segmental bite raising causes intrusion of the covered teeth and supraeruption of the uncovered teeth. The damage to occlusal harmony is the same whether the segmental coverage is removable or fixed, but the use of fixed restorations to segmentally increase vertical dimension is also an irreversible insult to the teeth themselves that is more difficult and more costly to repair.

If the constancy of vertical dimension is perceived in detail, it will be obvious that promiscuous alteration of the vertical is to be avoided. There is no reason to change any vertical unless an acceptable result cannot be achieved with a logical treatment plan at the patient's given vertical dimension at full articulation. If the vertical dimension must be changed, it should be changed as little as necessary to reduce the requirements for adaptation to the minimum. In all probability the increased vertical will gradually revert to the original jaw-to-jaw measurement.

WHY SOME PATIENTS REQUEST BITE RAISING

Some patients request an increase in vertical dimension based on a feeling of greatly improved comfort if they can have added height to their occlusions. They routinely justify such requests by explaining how uncomfortable they are when their teeth are together. Often there are esthetic implications of a "collapsed" bite or an "old-woman look" with fear that their nose-to-chin distance will continue to close together until they meet, unless the teeth can be built up to stop the closure.

Such observations may be valid if one or both arches are edentulous because the loss of alveolar bone often occurs when the teeth are extracted. Denture wearers do in fact lose vertical height if ridge resorption occurs.

The problem with the dentulous patient, however, is rarely the result of lost vertical height, and increasing the vertical will usually just be the first of a continuing series of bite raisings that eventually close back down to the original dimension. Notice how many of the patients who request such treatment have had it done previously. I have had patients request bite-raising treatment who have had as many as seven previous attempts at increasing the occlusal vertical dimension.

Patients need to understand the consequences of such treatment before it is rendered. They also need to understand the reason for their discomfort at the occluded position as well as their apparent lost facial height.

The primary thing patients (and dentists) must understand is that the teeth should not be in contact except fleetingly during chewing and during swallowing.

The teeth do not and should not *support* the facial height. At the resting jaw position the teeth should be separated. It is the posture of the lower jaw as dictated by the musculature that determines the lower facial profile. Tooth *contact* is not necessary or desirable at the jaw position of best profile appearance.

The feeling of overclosure, or the strained feeling that occurs when the teeth are held together, is a normal response to prolonged elevator muscle contraction. The masticatory muscles are designed for *intermittent* tooth contact. They are not designed for the extended contraction required to hold the teeth together. Patients who feel uncomfortable when they hold their teeth together should be educated to correct jaw posture without tooth contact. The old adage "lips together—teeth apart" is physiologically correct, and patients must often be taught its importance. Some patients are under the mistaken impression that they are supposed to keep the teeth together. Such a position is extremely tiresome.

Building the occlusion up to provide comfortable "support" may make the clenching patient more comfortable during prolonged tooth contact, but the increased vertical will interfere with the normal contracting length of the elevator muscles, and so it will not be maintainable. Furthermore, it is unnecessary because the muscles will actually be more comfortable if the patient allows the mandible to be suspended by the resting musculature without tooth contact.

There is such a wide variation between resting and contracted muscle length in different patients that there also may be some patient-to-patient variation in the response to increasing the vertical dimension. More research is needed to analyze these differences more critically, but in some patients the chance for successfully increasing vertical dimension may increase proportionately as the freeway space increases. It is doubtful that such increases will be maintained, but they do not seem to cause problems for patients. Adaptation to the increase is usually uneventful.

If this observation is correct, it may be related to the differences in morphology of the masticatory muscles. Patients should always be examined carefully to notice the type of musculature. Any evidence of hypertrophy or the effects of strong muscle pull on the bony parts should alert the examiner to avoid any increases in vertical if there is any way to plan the treatment at the given occlusal vertical dimension.

Patients with minimal freeway space often have shorter thicker muscles with a smaller range of difference between the contracted length and the resting length. On palpation, the muscles appear firmer and more unyielding than normal, and the gonial angle may be more acute. Evidence of strong masseter and internal pterygoid complex may be related to formation of an *antegonial notch* (Fig. 5-12). The concavity at the base of the mandible is evidence of the limiting power of the contracted elevator muscles. When it is present, the vertical dimension should not be increased regardless of how much freeway space is present.

Patients with greater freeway space may or may not accept an increased vertical, depending on the character of their muscle contraction. We have seen patients with the appearance of a long, lean musculature who had masseteric hypertrophy and a severe antegonial notch but an obvious freeway space of over 10 mm. Regardless of the high interocclusal dimension at rest, the contracting force of the muscle would overpower even the slightest extension of teeth into the vertical dimension at full contraction.

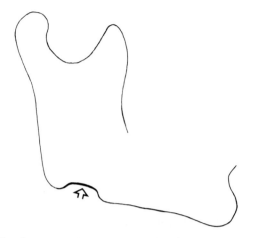

Fig. 5-12. Formation of an antegonial notch indicates a strong limiting influence on vertically directed bone growth. It is generally found in combination with strong, hypertrophic masseter muscles. It is a signal to avoid any attempts at increasing the vertical dimension.

The amount of freeway space at rest is not an automatic indication of whether the vertical dimension can be increased. But if the musculature is fairly weak and not too resistive to palpation, there may be a better chance of maintaining an increase in vertical if there is ample freeway space to permit. But here's the rub—patients with weak muscles and large freeway space rarely need an increae in vertical.

CLOSING THE VERTICAL DIMENSION

Unless it results in labially directed stress on the upper anterior teeth, there do not appear to be any problems associated with closing the vertical dimension on natural teeth. It does not produce stress because a closed vertical dimension does not interfere with muscle lengths.

It appears that even when a natural occlusion is closed down all at once, it eventually regains its original vertical dimension, probably in less than a year. We know that slight reductions in vertical dimension often permit us to harmonize an occlusion with reduced need for restorations. When all the teeth are in harmonious contact, any readjustment of the vertical seems to take place with minimal disturbance to that harmony. At least it does not normally present any clinical problems.

Closing the vertical dimension to an extreme degree could cause coronoid impingement against the zygoma, but it is highly unlikely that there would ever be a need for that much closure. Tenderness to palpation in the zygoma area would alert us to this.

Relationship of the anterior teeth to vertical dimension

One of the most important considerations in any change of vertical dimension is the direction of the arc of closure. As the mandible is elevated, the lower incisors travel *forward* on the closing arc. Any time the vertical dimension of occlusion is reduced, the lower incisal edges are automatically moved forward at the more closed vertical dimension.

If the lingual surfaces of the upper anterior teeth are in the way of this forward movement of the lower teeth, it results in horizontal stress directed labially against the upper anterior teeth and lingually against the lower anterior teeth. As obvious as this stressful relationship may seem, it is easily missed by many dentists because of carelessness in recording the correct vertical dimension and failure to record the correct horizontal axis with a facebow.

The axis of closure on most simple articulators is much closer to the occlusal plane level than the true condylar axis (which is higher). The arc of closure on the erroneous "simple" articulators is nearly vertical, rather than forward. If the bite is closed during restorative procedures, the interference to the front teeth is not noticed on the improperly mounted models.

If such restorations are placed in the mouth, the resultant stress against the anterior teeth is not easily picked up without digital examination. The incline contacts are so steep and the vector of force is so horizontal that the upper anterior teeth are forced out of the way and the lower anterior teeth are forced inward. The result is continuous complaints by the patient that the front teeth "hit too hard." If the upper lingual surfaces have been restored, it is often necessary to grind completely through the metal to adjust the anterior occlusion on such closed vertical cases. If the vertical has been closed enough, it may be impossible to

reduce the horizontal stress on the anterior teeth without restoring the posterior teeth back to a correct vertical dimension or inducing their eruption by using an anterior bite plane.

The vertical dimension can sometimes be closed to *improve* anterior relationships in anterior overjet problems. Closing the vertical dimension may arc the lower incisors forward into contact that they did not have at their original occlusal vertical dimension.

Regardless of whether teeth are being restored or equilibrated, care must be taken to assure that the harmonious relationship of the anterior teeth is never disturbed by imprudent or careless changes in vertical dimension.

SUMMARY

The vertical dimension of occlusion is established by muscular placement of the mandible. The optimum length of contraction for the closing muscles repeatedly positions the jaw when the muscles go through their maximum power cycle. Teeth erupt until they are met by their contraposed teeth at the point of optimum muscle contraction. This is the *occlusal vertical dimension.* More scientific study is needed, but it apparently stays remarkably stable over a period of years, even when the teeth wear. Occlusal contours should be restored to this vertical dimension. Any increase in clinical crown length places the teeth in direct conflict with the optimum power cycle of the muscles and often results in damaging stress to the teeth and supporting structures.

The *rest position* refers to the relationship of the arches when the muscles are at their optimum resting length. It is an unreliable dimension to record and should not be used to determine the occlusal vertical dimension.

The *freeway space* is the space difference between the occlusal vertical dimension and the rest position of the mandible. It varies greatly from one patient to the next. It should not be interfered with regardless of how great or small its dimension may be. It is a totally unreliable determinant of occlusal vertical dimension. It will automatically be correct when the occlusal vertical dimension is correct.

REFERENCES

1. Niswonger, M.E.: Rest position of the mandible and centric relation, J. Prosthet. Dent. Assoc. **21:**1572, 1934.
2. Atwood, D.A.: A critique of research of the rest position of the mandible, J. Prosthet. Dent. **16:**848, 1966.
3. Boos, R.H.: Intermaxillary relation established by biting power, J. Am. Dent. Assoc. **27:**1192, 1940.
4. Gibbs, C.H., Mahan, P.E., et al.: Occlusal forces during chewing: the influences of biting strength and food consistency, J. Prosthet. Dent. **46(**5**):**561, 1981.
5. Williamson, E.H.: Myomonitor rest position in the presence and absence of stress, Facial Orthop. Temporomandibular Arthrol. **3(**2**):**14, 1986.
6. Rugh, J.D.: Vertical dimension, a study of clinical rest position and jaw muscle activity, J. Prosthet. Dent. **45:**670, 1981.
7. Tueller, V.M.: The relationship between the vertical dimension of occlusion and forces generated by closing muscles of mastication, J. Prosthet. Dent. **22:**284, 1969.
8. Silverman, M.M.: Determination of vertical dimension by phonetics, J. Prosthet. Dent. **6:**463, 1956.
9. Ricketts, R.M.: Orthodontic diagnosis and planning, their roles in preventative and rehabilitative dentistry, Denver, 1982, Rocky Mountain Orthodontic Publishers.
10. McAndrews, J.: Presentation to Florida Prosthodontic Seminar, Miami, Florida, Oct. 1984.
11. Suga, S.: Bone remodeling in oral region, J. Dent. Res. **64(**4**):**736, 1985. (Abstract.)
12. Ramfjord, S.P., and Blankenship, J.R.: Increased occlusal vertical dimension in adult monkeys, J. Prosthet. Dent. **45:**74, 1981.

SUGGESTED READINGS

Dawson, P.E.: Determining the determinants of occlusion, Int. J. Periodontics Restorative Dent. **6:**9, 1983.
Nairin, R.I.: The concept of occlusal vertical dimension and its importance in clinical practice. In Anderson, D.J., and Jatthews, B.: Mastication, Bristol, 1976, John Wright & Sons Ltd., p. 58.
Schuyler, C.H.: Problems associated with opening the bite that would contraindicate it as a general practice, J. Am. Dent. Assoc. **72:**1448, 1966.
Sicher, H., and DeBrul, E.L.: Oral anatomy, ed. 6, St. Louis, 1975, The C.V. Mosby Co.
Weijs, W.A., and Hillen, B.: An analysis of the pattern of correlations between the size of the masticatory muscles and shape of the facial skeleton, J. Oral Rehabil. **12:**530, 1985. (Abstract.)
Weinberg, L.A.: Vertical dimension, a research and clinical analysis, J. Prosthet. Dent. **47:**290, 1982.

6

The neutral zone

As each tooth erupts into position within its respective arch, it is guided into a narrow zone located between horizontally directed forces. The outward pressure of the tongue versus the inward pressure of the perioral musculature defines the neutral zone (Fig. 6-1). The zone of neutrality between these opposing forces is positioned where outward pressure from the tongue is equal to the inward pressure from the buccinator–orbicularis oris band of muscle (Fig. 6-2). The neutral zone determines the position of each tooth and establishes the dimensions of the entire arch, *including the shape and position of the alveolar processes.*

In effect, the boundaries of the neutral zone form a matrix for the dental arches. Any attempt to move any part of the dental arch, including the alveolar structures outside the neutral zone, will result in increased pressure against the part that intrudes. There is no occlusal scheme that can stabilize teeth if they are in an unbalanced relationship with muscular forces against them.

The neutral zone has not been given enough importance in the literature, but as a determinant of occlusion it cannot be ignored. Understanding of the neutral zone would make it readily apparent why so many orthodontic results do not remain stable. It also explains why many postrestorative problems occur and even why some periodontal procedures are unsuccessful. Relapses with orthognathic surgery can almost always be explained by neutral zone imbalance. And complete or partial denture failures are often related to noncompliance with neutral zone factors.

Regardless of the method of treatment, any part of the dentition out of harmony with the neutral zone will result in instability, interference with function, or some degree of discomfort or will bother the patient. Thus the neutral zone must be evaluated as an important factor before one makes any changes in arch form or alignment of teeth.

The landmark work regarding the limiting effect on arch size was done by Sidney Frederick.[1] He showed that the perioral musculature was erroneously described in the majority of anatomy texts. He also observed the effects of muscle pressure against the dentoalveolar structures in hundreds of patients. His findings are important to every phase of dental treatment that deals with arch contour or tooth alignment. Understanding of the neutral zone is incomplete without knowledge of Frederick's contributions regarding the perioral musculature.

The outer limits of the neutral zone are determined by the perioral musculature. The main determinant of length, strength, and position of the perioral musculature is the buccinator muscle (Figs. 6-3 and 6-4). The buccinator is a flat, thin muscle composed of three bands.

The *upper band* has a wide bony origin that starts at the base of the alveolar process above the first molar and extends distally on the skel-

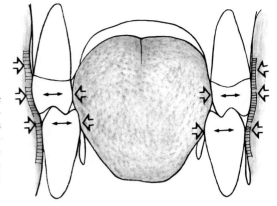

Fig. 6-1. The outward pressure of the tongue versus the inward pressure of the three bands of the buccinator muscle determine where the corridor of neutral pressure is positioned. As the teeth erupt, they are directed into position horizontally by these opposing forces. The size of the tongue and the strength of the perioral muscles influence the position of this neutral zone, as does any habit pattern that affects tongue or lip pressures.

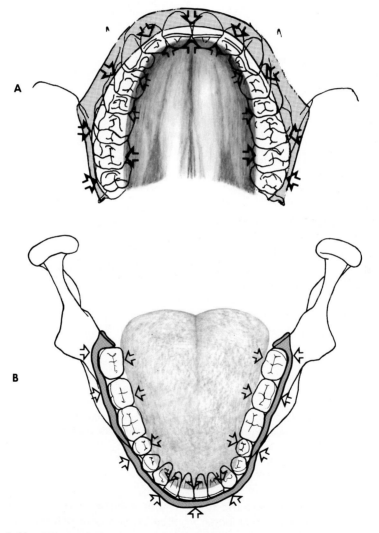

Fig. 6-2. A, The upper band of the buccinator extends around the arch from origin to origin, and even though it becomes part of the orbicularis oris muscle, it is effectively one band of muscle. Thus it influences the dimensions of the arch to the limits of its repetitive contracted length. The tongue is postured in direct opposition. **B,** The lower band of the buccinator is often a strong band that, like the upper band, extends from origin to origin. If tongue size and posture is normal, it has the effect of resisting the inward force to form the neutral zone in between the opposing pressures. Notice how the buccinator origin extends from the external oblique line around the posterior teeth onto the internal oblique line. At this molar position the widest, strongest part of the tongue resists the strongest part of the buccinator.

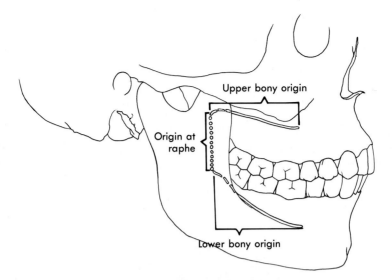

Fig. 6-3. Origin of the three bands of the buccinator muscle. See text for description. (After Frederick, S.: The buccinator, orbicularis oris complex, Manual prepared for Florida Prosthodontic Seminar, 1987.)

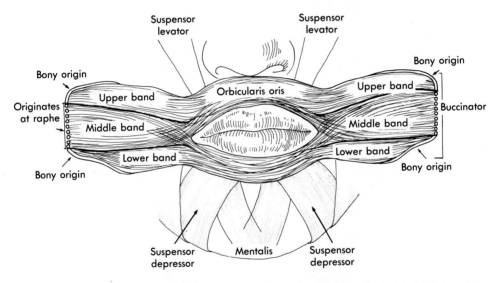

Fig. 6-4. The three bands of the buccinator. See text for description. (After Frederick, S.: The buccinator, orbicularis oris complex, Manual prepared for Florida Prosthodontic Seminar, 1987.)

etal base above the alveolar process to the suture between the maxilla and palatine bone. From that bone, the line extends down to the lower surface of the pyramidal process of the palatine bone and continues on a short ligament to the tip of the pterygoid hamulus.

The *lower band* also has a wide bony origin that starts at the skeletal base below the alveolar process at the first molar. It extends back and up along the external oblique line where it then crosses over behind the last molar at the lower end of the retromolar fossa and proceeds onto the internal oblique line. Its bony origin stops where the middle band starts at the end of the internal oblique line.

The *middle band* fibers originate from the pterygomandibular raphe, a ligament that extends from the tip of the pterygoid hamulus down to the posterior extremity of the internal oblique line on the mandible. This middle band does not have a bony origin like the upper and lower bands, and because of its soft origin, it cannot exert the strength of contraction that the upper and lower bands can apply to their underlying structures.

The combined width of the three bands covers the entire outer surface of the dentoalveolar structures, that is, the teeth, alveolar process, and gingival tissues (Fig. 6-5).

The upper and lower bands are continuous from side to side without decussation. The middle band fibers decussate and join into the fibers of the orbicularis oris. Because the muscle fibers form a continuous band from origin to origin, the size of the arch is limited by the length of the muscles when they are contracted repetitiously. The tonus of the buccinator—orbicularis oris muscle band may very well be controlled by the central nervous system, but regardless of the reason for variations in muscle tonus in different patients, the strength of that contractile force, at the length of the muscle band during contraction, forms an inviolate outer limit for arch size.

Problems of alignment occur when the size of the teeth are too large to fit into the arch-size dimension dictated by a constrictive perioral musculature.

The effects of neutral zone confinement on the dentoalveolar structures can also play a critical role as a determinant of facial profile. A restrictive perioral musculature may prevent the dentoalveolar arches from expanding to a normal alignment with the skeletal base. Thus mandibular skeletal growth may extend the chin point forward while the dental arches are restricted by the band of muscles that prevent them from growing commensurately with their skeletal base (Fig. 6-6).

Variations in length and strength of the three bands of the buccinator can further affect the profile by controlling the axial inclinations of the anterior teeth, especially when combined with the myriad variations of tongue size and pressure.

Other factors, such as the size of the mouth, must also be evaluated when a change in arch size is being contemplated. A very small orifice is far more restrictive than a large broad opening that exposes the dentition all the way around to the molars.

A series of statements may give perspective

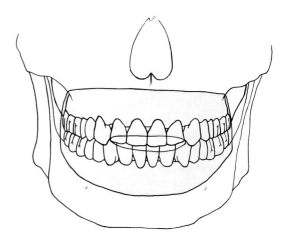

Fig. 6-5. The combined width of the three bands of the buccinator cover both the teeth and the alveolar processes. The size of the orifice is also an important factor in regard to the limiting effect of the perioral musculature. The smaller the orifice, the stronger is the limiting effect on arch size and incisor inclination.

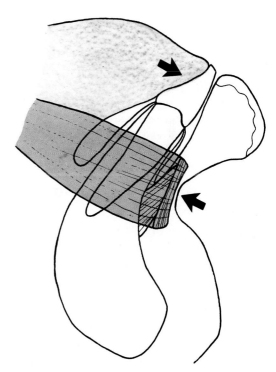

Fig. 6-6. The combination of buccinator position and strength relates to tongue position and strength to determine the inclination of the incisors. A strong lower band may limit arch size of the dentoalveolar process while the skeletal bone below it continues to grow, forming a button chin. If a strong lower band is placed low, it presses the roots back. A strong tongue can simultaneously press the crown forward. Various combinations in position and strength of the three bands versus differences in tongue size and position can produce a variety of incisor inclinations.

to an evaluation of neutral zone consider-ations:

1. The teeth and their alveolar process are the most adaptive part of the masticatory system. They can be moved horizontally or vertically by light forces.
2. There is a neutral zone within which muscular pressure against the dentition is equalized from opposite directions. The entire arch form falls within that zone of neutral pressure.
3. If irregularities of tooth position, alignment, or contour can be corrected within the neutral zone, the prognosis for long-term stability is good.
4. A problem occurs when the neutral zone is not where we want the teeth to be.
5. A treatment decision then must allow determination of if and how we can change the neutral zone to orient it where we want the teeth to be.

Because the neutral zone can assume so many variations of form from different types of confinement by the same musculature, any irregular dental alignment or arch form should be evaluated in relation to the directional pressures exerted by the tongue, the lips, and the cheeks. It should be determined *why* the dental arches are where they are before it can be determined if they can be altered. Several different arch configurations may be possible without any changes in muscle lengths.

RELATING MALOCCLUSION TO THE NEUTRAL ZONE

The high-vaulted, constricted maxillary arch is a good illustration of how aberrant pressures relate to the configuration of the dentoalveolar arches. It also serves as an example of the cause-and-effect influence by muscle pressures, explaining both why the problem occurs and how it can be treated. In the case of a patient with a high, narrow vault the maxillary arch is squeezed inwardly by buccinator muscle pressure that is unopposed by outward tongue pressure.

The reason for the lack of outward tongue pressure against the posterior arch segments is a forward tongue posture that possibly developed as the effect of an inadequate airway space. With enlarged tonsils or adenoids, there is no room for the posterior width of the tongue in its normal position, and so it must be postured forward to provide an airway.

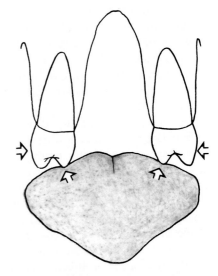

Fig. 6-7. An airway problem often results in a forward tongue posture in the growing child. The forward tongue thrust moves the wide part of the tongue forward out of the vault. This changes the direction and position of tongue pressure against the posterior teeth and reduces resistance to the inward force of the buccinator muscle. The result is a collapsed posterior arch. Simultaneously, the forward tongue position moves the anterior segment forward.

The forward tongue posture causes two effects. It pushes the anterior teeth forward, and it evacuates its normal space up in the vault, thus eliminating the outward tongue pressure as resistance to buccinator pressure against the posterior teeth (Fig. 6-7). The narrowing of the arch form in back also permits a lengthening of the arch forward, without altering the length of the perioral musculature.

The arch configuration is determined by the pressures exerted against the dentoalveolar structures during eruption of the teeth, and even though the airway space may be enlarged during growth, permitting a more posterior tongue posture, the narrowed space between the posterior segments will not permit a normal tongue position up in the vault. Thus the arch malformation will persist along with an aberrant neutral zone.

One can correct both the narrow arch and the anterior disharmony by changing the neutral zone orthodontically. Expansion of the dentoalveolar arch width at the posterior segments creates room for the tongue to fit up into the vault where it can then direct outward pressure against the posterior teeth to resist the inward buccinator pressure (Fig. 6-8).

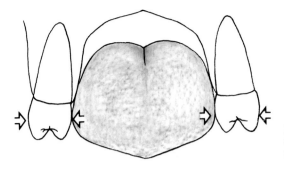

Fig. 6-8. Expansion of the arch permits the tongue to fit up in the vault and into a position whereby it can resist the inward force of the buccinators. When the tongue is permitted to drop back, the forward pressure against the anterior teeth is reduced, allowing them to be repositioned back into a better alignment.

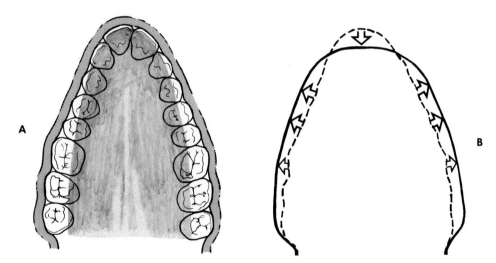

Fig. 6-9. A, The arch form that results from an airway problem because of the forward tongue thrust. The linear dimension of the perioral muscle bands is limited to its contraction length, but it can be altered in shape. This arch form resulted from a malposed neutral zone. **B,** Expansion of arch width can result in a stable arch form by altering the neutral zone position without altering the linear dimension. The wider arch form also accommodates the tongue in the vault to resist the inward forces of the buccinator.

As the posterior arch width is expanded, the perioral band of muscle pulls back on the anterior teeth thus allowing for correction of the pointed protrusion in the anterior segment (Fig. 6-9). The corrected arch form can then be quite stable because the widened vault not only permits normalized outward tongue pressure against the posterior teeth, but it also reduces the forward pressure against the anterior teeth as the tongue is allowed to posture back into the widened vault space. The combination of firmer perioral muscle pressure against the anterior teeth versus lessened forward tongue pressure results in a changed neutral zone position that is consistent with the corrected arch form.

The above correction also alters the *direction* of lip pressures against the upper anterior teeth. When the upper anterior segment is protruded, the lower lip tucks in against their lingual and incisal edges with forwardly directed pressure (Fig. 6-10). Correction of the overjet alters the neutral zone by allowing the lower lip to pass in front of the labial surfaces and thus reverse the lip pressure to hold the teeth in the improved alignment (Fig. 6-11).

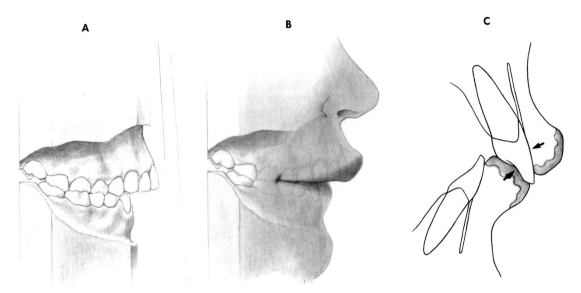

Fig. 6-10. Analysis of any malocclusion should include analysis of the neutral zone that contributed to the malrelationship to see if the neutral zone can be changed. Diagnostic casts, **A,** tell only part of the story. Observation of lip position in relation to the anterior teeth, **B,** is essential. When the lower lip has insufficient linear dimension to posture in front of the upper incisors, it takes a position behind them and contributes further to the malposition, **C.**

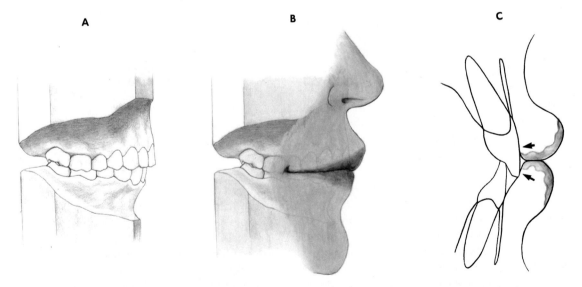

Fig. 6-11. Repositioning the anterior teeth back, **A,** makes it possible for the lower lip to bypass the upper incisors to form a proper lip seal, **B.** This in turn postures the lips to resist the forward tongue pressure, **C,** which is also reduced by the expansion of the arch width at the posterior segments.

Determining the neutral zone clinically

In dentulous patients the position and angulation of the teeth is the best indicator of the current neutral zone position if the teeth appear to be stable.

The strength and position of the three bands of the buccinator can be determined by observation of the location and contour of the line of demarcation where the bound-down gingiva separates from the underlying bone. The upper border of the lower band of the buccinator aligns with the lower border of the bound-down tissue on the labial surfaces of the mandible, and the lower border of the upper band of the buccinator relates to the upper border of bound-down tissue on the maxillary arch. The middle band is a much weaker band and covers the teeth and the attached gingiva (Fig. 6-12).

If the contour of the alveolar process is observed at the border of attached tissue, the strength and length of the buccinator band can be evaluated. A deep ledge indicates that a strong band is exerting firm pressure against the underlying structures (Fig. 6-13). In some instances, the pressure is so great that there are deep indentations around the roots and the roots may be jammed back against the lingual plate. The labial bone around the roots may be thinner than normal. Depending on tongue pressure variances against the crowns of the teeth, the incisors may be flared out at the incisal edges.

If the lower band covers the incisal edges of the upper anterior teeth or there is an enlarged mentalis muscle underlying the buccinator–orbicularis oris complex, there will be a tendency to press back on the crowns of the upper teeth and verticalize their inclination.

A strong lower band combined with a short upper lip results in even greater lingualized inclination of the upper incisors because the lower lip must reach up further to seal during swallowing.

Clinically, the observation of a deep cleft and a button chin is a sign of a tight, strong neutral zone, which will almost always result in a vertical or lingual inclination of the anterior teeth (Fig. 6-14).

Observation of a deeply indented alveolar process can have a significant effect on diagnosis and treatment selection on the posterior segments as well as the anterior teeth. A deep indentation indicates a strong band of muscle that should not be encroached on if it is possible to avoid it. Partial denture bases that extend improperly into conflict with the muscle bands are easily dislodged by normal muscle function (Fig. 6-15).

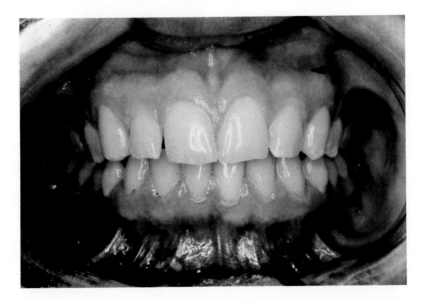

Fig. 6-12. Normal, stable neutral zone showing demarcation of upper and lower bands of the buccinator. Lower border of the upper band aligns with the upper border of attached gingiva. Upper border of the lower band aligns with the lower border of attached gingiva. Middle band covers attached tissue. Height of the bands is altered during lip seal.

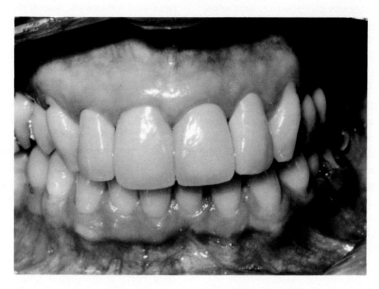

Fig. 6-13. Notice the effect of a strong lower band on the alveolar process. A deep ledge with fairly sharp indentation indicates strong pressure against the dentoalveolar process. Expansion of the arch into such pressure would be unstable.

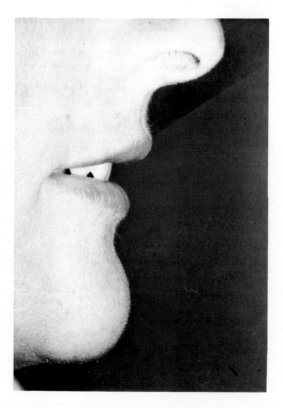

Fig. 6-14. A deep cleft and button chin is a sign of a tight neutral zone that is limited by a strong perioral musculature. This combination almost always results in lingually inclined upper incisors. The lingual inclination is needed to permit the lower lip to close to a seal without interference from the upper incisal edges. This is a stable relationship as long as holding contacts are present.

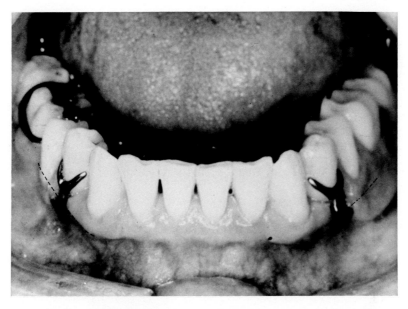

Fig. 6-15. Example of a partial denture base that interferes with a strong lower band of the buccinator, **A.** Notice how the base extends below the ledge line that indicates the upper edge of the buccinator band, **B.** Many prosthetic failures can be traced to interference with the neutral zone. This patient complained of constant dislodgment.

Determining the posterior neutral zone

Unless posterior teeth have been recently moved or restored, they will be in their current neutral-zone relationship. Teeth will never spontaneously move either vertically or horizontally out of neutral-zone harmony. If muscle pressures change in intensity or direction, the teeth will change position to accommodate. Thus any tooth that has remained in a stable position is in neutral-zone harmony. This position should be carefully evaluated in relation to muscle forces before one makes any decision to alter shape or position.

Inclination and alignment of second and third molars are particularly subjected to the strongest pressures from the widest part of the tongue versus the most unyielding part of the buccinator muscle near its origin. Attempts at uprighting or perfecting alignment in this segment are often unsuccessful because the neutral zone does not conform to the textbook norm. Pretreatment observation can be very enlightening regarding the location of the neutral zone, and if realignment can take place within that established zone, the prognosis for stability will be excellent.

In replacement of teeth on posterior edentulous ridges, there are no teeth to indicate the neutral zone location, but one can precisely determine it by allowing the musculature to form a moldable material during swallowing. The procedure is described in Fig. 6-16.

Observation of several neutral-zone recordings is a convincing exercise that is highly recommended. One will notice the consistency in the width of the recorded neutral zones, and it will be apparent that it relates to the normal width of natural teeth. It will also be apparent that even in mouths that have been without posterior teeth for extended time periods, the outward tongue pressure is still resisted by inward buccinator pressure that is sufficiently strong to position the neutral zone in a reasonably normal alignment over the ridge. This repeated finding raises doubt about the popular belief that the tongue expands when teeth are lost.

The effectiveness of some functional appliances is based on blocking the pressure from one side of the neutral zone. By placing a shield on the cheek side to prevent inward pressure, one can see that the unopposed tongue forces then move the teeth toward the cheek. Regardless of the method of creating uneven pressure, teeth will move toward the

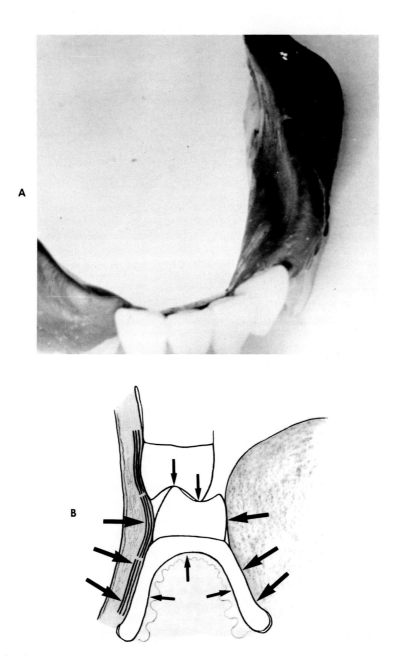

Fig. 6-16. The neutral zone for an edentulous ridge can be formed in moldable compound during swallowing. Notice how the tongue pressure has formed the lingual contour. Pressure from the buccinator forms the buccal contour and defines the neutral zone where the posterior teeth should be placed. **B,** A lower denture in harmony with the neutral zone is stabilized as much by the tongue and cheek musculature as it is by the adaptation on the ridge. When both vertical and horizontal harmony is achieved, there are no dislodging forces.

negative side of imbalanced forces and away from the side with stronger pressure. The long-term effectiveness of functional appliances is ultimately related to the balance of pressures at the completion of treatment. If the parts of the system can be related to the variety of spacial accommodations that must conform to the length of muscles and the bulk of the tongue, the results of treatment can be predicted more accurately.

Determining the neutral zone for anterior teeth

Because the neutral zone is determined by the functional relationship of the tongue versus the perioral musculature, locating an unknown neutral zone starts by observation of the positional relationships of these structures during specific functions. There are several different functions that require rather precise mechanical interrelationships between the teeth, the tongue, and the lips in order to perform the function correctly. The value of understanding how these interrelationships work *mechanically* is that it provides known reference points for determining how the teeth must interrelate in order for correct function to occur. Functional harmony and anatomic harmony are almost always coincidental.

Phonetic methods can be used with a high degree of accuracy because the shaping of sounds results from such approximation of upper and lower teeth with each other, with the lips, and with the tongue. The near contact of structures that constrict the airflow into particular sound forms can also be used as guidelines for incisal edge position and the entire incisal plane. The lip closure path can be used to determine labial contours, and methods for determining the anterior guidance can direct the contouring of the upper lingual surfaces. When all these functional relationships are correct, the teeth will be in harmony with the neutral zone.

The methods for determining all the necessary anterior relationships are described in detail in Chapters 16 to 18.

Methods for altering the neutral zone

The neutral zone may be altered in several ways, as follows.

Orthodontics. By realigning the teeth for improved balance between the tongue and the perioral musculature, one can most often improve it without the need for lengthening muscle.

Elimination of noxious habits. Thumb-sucking, lip-biting, or forward tongue-posturing all tend to increase outward pressure against the perioral musculature, thus moving the neutral zone accordingly. Elimination of such habit patterns allows the perioral muscles to move the teeth back into harmony with normal tongue position. It should be noted however that success in changing habit patterns is often difficult or impossible if they involve long-standing tongue-thrust patterns.

Myofunctional therapy. If lip pressure can be increased by strenthening the perioral musculature, the neutral zone will move accordingly. Any change in muscle pressure will affect the neutral zone, but results are often disappointing for long-term effectiveness in mature adults.

Reduction of tongue size. Surgical reduction of tongue size will reduce outward pressure and allow the perioral muscles to move the teeth lingually into a new neutral zone. For some reason this procedure has not had popular acceptance.

Surgical lengthening of the buccinator band. Surgical lengthening of the buccinator band can be used to reduce restrictive pressure that limits arch size. Frederick has reported increased thickness of labial tissues over the roots of teeth, along with increased stability of the teeth after arch expansion when restrictive muscle pressure is released. It is usually done to lengthen the lower band of the buccinator.

The procedure involves four steps:
1. Surgically cut through the mucosa with a vertical incision.
2. Vertically cut through the lower band of the buccinator muscle on each side.
3. Suture the mucosa only. Leave the muscle segments unattached.
4. Add lip pressure to increase the length of muscle with a Frankel type of appliance.

Scar tissue will fill in between the two cut ends effectively lengthening the perioral band around the arch.

Vestibuloplasty. A vestibuloplasty either alone or in combination with the muscle-lengthening procedures appears to cause a reduction of perioral pressure. It should extend around the anterior arch to the bicuspid area.

More study is needed to evaluate the full effect of the surgical approach. However clinical results appear to be beneficial in reducing the thinning out and clefting of labial tissues when arches are expanded beyond the normal boundaries of a tight neutral zone.

Neutral zone considerations in orthognathic surgery

Surgical advancements tend to relapse if the advanced section causes extension of any connected muscle or interferes with the length of the perioral musculature. Modern surgical techniques all consider muscle relationships and either move the muscle origin or insertion to compensate for the change in position of the skeletal part.

REFERENCE

1. Frederick, S.: The buccinator, orbicularis oris complex, Manual prepared for Florida Prosthodontic Seminar, 1987.

SUGGESTED READINGS

Beresin, V.E., and Scheesser, F.J.: The neutral zone in complete dentures, J. Prosthet. Dent. **36**:356, 1976.

Fish, E.W.: An analysis of the stabilizing factors in full denture construction, Br. Dent. J. **52**:559, 1931.

Frederick, S.: The buccinator muscle and alveolar process. Unpublished article, Lafayette, La.

Goldspink, G.: Sarcomere length during post natal growth of mammalian muscle fibers, J. Cell Sci. **3**:539, 1968.

Singer, C.P.: The depth of the mandibular antegonial notch as an indicator of mandibular growth potential, Am. J. Orthod. **89**:528, 1986. (Abstract.)

Weijs, W., and Hillen, B.: An analysis of the patterns of correlations between the size of the masticatory muscles and shape of the facial skeleton, J. Oral Rehabil. **12**:530, 1985. (Abstract.)

7

The occlusal plane

The configuration of the occlusal plane is one of the most beautiful examples of design that can be found in nature. The conformity to that design by the other parts of the masticatory system is so subtle it is often missed. But the logic of these interrelationships is important to understand because even slight variations from this intended configuration can lead to unexplained occlusal instability. The irritating reductions in comfort or function that bother the patient and frustrate the dentist are often related to unnoticed occlusal plane problems.

Because of the importance of the occlusal plane to the total harmony of the masticatory system, I have elected to divide the discussion into two separated chapters. This chapter describes the design and purpose of the plane so that its relevance can be coordinated with other aspects of masticatory system function. I will then discuss the diagnosis and treatment of occlusal plane variations in a separate chapter so that it can relate better to the particular sequencing of occlusal treatment.

The *plane of occlusion* refers to an imaginary surface that theoretically touches the incisal edges of the incisors and the tips of the occluding surfaces of the posterior teeth. Because the term "plane" refers geometrically to a flat surface, it is not entirely correct to describe the occlusal surface as following a true plane. Instead of a flat surface, the plane of occlusion represents the average curvature of the occlusal surface. Despite the problem of se-

mantics, it is probably the most practical way of relating the occlusal surfaces of the teeth to one another and to other structures of the head. Each curvature of the plane is related to specific effects it should produce. Its acceptability should be analyzed on that functional basis rather than on its conformity to a set ideal.

The curvatures of the anterior teeth are determined by establishment of the esthetically correct smile line on the upper and the relationship of the lower incisal edges to the anterior guidance and the requirements for phonetics. These factors are covered in Chapter 17.

The curvatures of the posterior plane of occlusion are divided into (1) an anteroposterior curve called the *curve of Spee* (Fig. 7-1) and (2) a mediolateral curve, referred to as the *curve of Wilson* (Fig. 7-2).

Together, the composite of the curve of Spee, the curve of Wilson, and the curve of the incisal edges is properly referred to as the *curve of occlusion*. Popular usage combines both the curve of occlusion and its relationship to the cranium into the *plane of occlusion* (Fig. 7-3). I will discuss each aspect of it individually.

CURVE OF SPEE

The *curve of Spee* refers to the anteroposterior curvature of the occlusal surfaces, beginning at the tip of the lower cuspid and following the buccal cusp tips of the bicuspids and

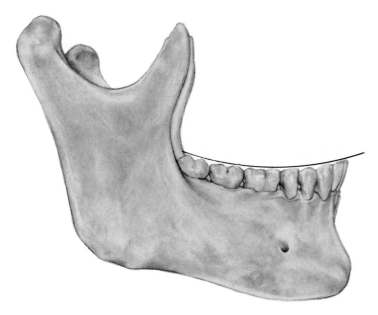

Fig. 7-1. The *curve of Spee* begins at the top of the cuspid and touches the tips of the cusp tips of all the posterior teeth.

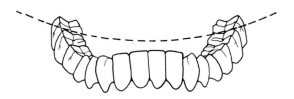

Fig. 7-2. The *curve of Wilson* is the mediolateral curve that contacts the buccal and lingual cusp tips on each side of the arch.

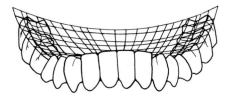

Fig. 7-3. The *curve of occlusion* combines a composite of the curve of Spee, the curve of Wilson, and the curve of the incisal edges. It is more often called the *plane of occlusion* when it is related to the cranium.

molars and continuing to the anterior border of the ramus. If the curved line continued further back, it would ideally follow an arc through the condyle (Fig. 7-4). The curvature of the arc would relate, on average, to part of a circle with a 4-inch radius.

There is a purpose behind the curve of Spee design as well as its location in relation to the condyle. The curve results from variations in axial alignment of the lower teeth. To align each tooth for maximum resistance to functional loading, the long axis of each lower tooth is aligned nearly parallel to its individual arc of closure around the condylar axis (Fig. 7-5). This requires the last molar to be tilted forward at the greatest angle and the forward tooth to be at the least angle. This progression positions the cusp tips on a curve that is di-

rectly related to the condylar axis by a progressive series of tangents.

The relationship of the curve of occlusion to the condylar axis also relates to the condylar path in protrusion. If the occlusal plane is on an arc that passes through the condyle, the posterior part of the occlusal plane will always be flat enough and low enough to be discluded by the normal condylar path on its steeper eminentia (Fig. 7-6). Thus even with a flat zero-degree anterior guidance in protrusion the occlusal plane on the lower will be discluded by the forward movement of the condyle that is directed downward at an angle that is steeper than the posterior part of the occlusal plane.

It is because of this geometric design that the 4-inch radius of the Monson curve works so effectively if the condyle is used for a sur-

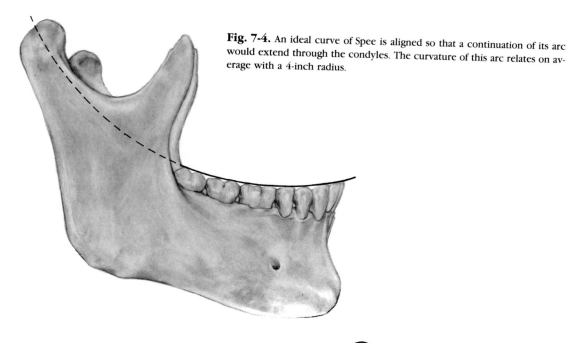

Fig. 7-4. An ideal curve of Spee is aligned so that a continuation of its arc would extend through the condyles. The curvature of this arc relates on average with a 4-inch radius.

Fig. 7-5. The curve of Spee results, in part, from aligning each lower tooth parallel to its arc of closure. This requires the last molar to be inclinded at the greatest angle.

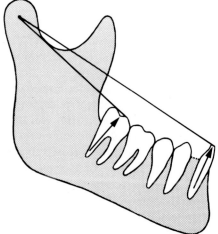

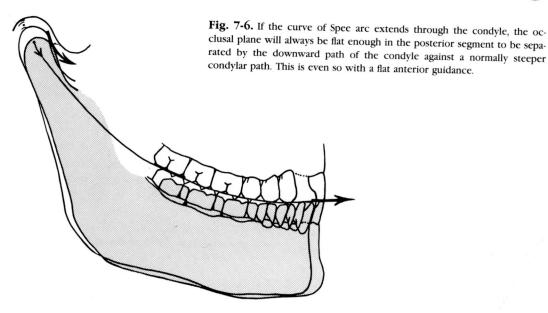

Fig. 7-6. If the curve of Spee arc extends through the condyle, the occlusal plane will always be flat enough in the posterior segment to be separated by the downward path of the condyle against a normally steeper condylar path. This is even so with a flat anterior guidance.

vey point, as it is in the PMS technique described in Chapter 14.

The anteroposterior curvature of the occlusal plane is designed to permit protrusive disclusion of the posterior teeth by the combination of anterior guidance and condylar guidance. The separation of posterior teeth during excursive contact of the anterior teeth results in more efficient incisive function as the anterior teeth slide past each other to the overlapped relationship that makes the shearing action possible.

To separate the posterior teeth for better incisive function during protrusive excursions, all forces of the elevator muscles must be loaded entirely onto the condyle and the anterior teeth. This results in a strong horizontal component against the upper anterior teeth, since all the contacts are against their lingual surfaces. To protect the anterior teeth from being overloaded, an ingeniously designed sensor system shuts off most of the elevator muscle activity at the precise moment of complete posterior disclusion. This reduction of pressure against the anterior teeth depends on a correct occlusal plane because if there is any interfering tooth contact posterior to the canines during excursions the elevator muscles are triggered into *hyper*contraction.

This prevention of increased muscle loading on the teeth and the joints is the dominant reason for making certain the occlusal plane is correctly evaluated as a part of every complete examination. If it does not permit the anterior guidance to separate the posterior teeth in excursive movements, there is a real possibility of eventual damage to the teeth, the joints, and the periodontal structure.

CURVE OF WILSON

The curve of Wilson is the mediolateral curve that contacts the buccal and lingual cusp tips on each side of the arch. It results from inward inclination of the lower posterior teeth, making the lingual cusps lower than the buccal cusps on the mandibular arch; the buccal cusps are higher than the lingual cusps on the maxillary arch because of the outward inclination of the upper posterior teeth.

There are two reasons for this inclination of posterior teeth. One has to do with resistance to loading, and the second has to do with masticatory function.

If the buccolingual inclination of the posterior teeth is analyzed in relation to the dominant direction of muscle force against them, it will be apparent that the axial alignment of all posterior teeth is nearly parallel with the strong inward pull of the internal pterygoid muscles (Fig. 7-7). The strongest component of lateral function occurs from the outside in, nearly parallel with the direction of the internal pterygoid muscles, which bilaterally pull the condyles medially to the midmost position of centric relation. Aligning both upper and lower posterior teeth with the principle direction of muscle contraction produces the greatest resistance to masticatory forces and creates the inclinations that form the curve of Wilson (Fig. 7-8).

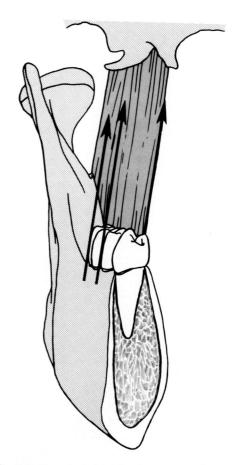

Fig. 7-7. The principal loading force against the posterior teeth occurs during outside-inward chewing stroke. The posterior teeth are thus aligned parallel to the internal pterygoid muscles for optimum resistance to that functional stress.

There is another reason for the curve of Wilson that relates it definitively to masticatory function. Because the tongue and the buccinator complex must repetitively place each bite of food onto the occlusal surfaces for mastication, there must be easy access for the food to get to the occlusal table. The inward inclination of the lower occlusal table is designed for direct access from the lingual, with no blockage by lower lingual cusps (Fig. 7-9).

The outward inclination of the upper occlusal table provides access from the buccal for the food to be tossed directly onto the occlusal table by the action of the bands of the buccinator muscle (Fig. 7-10). The longer lingual cusps of the upper posterior teeth serve as a baffle for food tossed on from the buccal; and the lower buccal cusp serves the same purpose for food tossed on by the tongue.

When the curve of Wilson is made too flat, ease of masticatory function may be impaired because of increased activity required to get the food onto the occlusal table. The greater the relative height of the lower lingual cusps, the greater the problem of chewing efficiency may become. Unless the problem is understood, it is easily missed because patient complaints do not pinpoint the problem.

The inclination of the posterior teeth coordinates their masticatory function with the necessary function of the tongue and cheeks to put the food where it can be chewed. This coordination of functional design creates a need for further design coordination in the articulation of the jaw joints. The upper lingual cusps would be in jeopardy of great horizontal stress from the lower buccal cusps if the lower teeth are permitted to move horizontally toward the midline. The articulation of the medial pole of the condyle is designed to prevent that from happening. The same configuration of the fossae that brace the condyle-disk assemblies in the midmost position also prevent them from traveling medially without first moving downward (Fig. 7-11). In short, the lower posterior teeth *must* travel down before they can shift medially. This important aspect of design makes it possible to have a curve of Wilson without creating balancing incline interferences.

The concept of an immediate side shift, which allows the condyles to translate horizontally before any rotation occurs, was a pop-

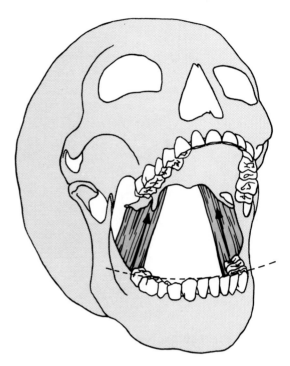

Fig. 7-8. Alignment of the posterior teeth to parallel the direction of loading from the internal pterygoid muscles results in the curve of Wilson.

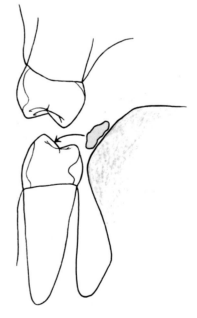

Fig. 7-9. The lingual inclination of the lower posterior teeth positions the lingual cusps lower than the buccal cusps. This design permits easy access to the occlusal table. As the tongue lays the food on the occlusal surfaces, it is stopped from going past the chewing position by the taller buccal cusps.

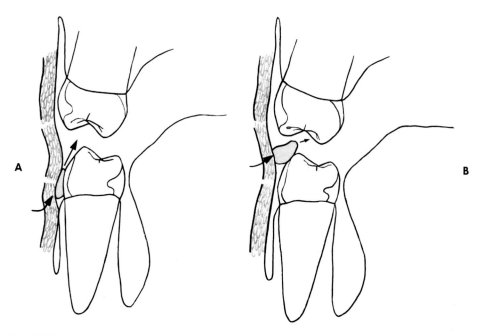

Fig. 7-10. The outer inclination of the upper teeth positions the buccal cusp higher for easier access from the buccal corridor. The action of the lower band of the buccinator squeezes the bolus up, **A,** where it can then be pressed on to the food table by the middle band, **B,** The longer lingual cusp stops it on the occlusal surface.

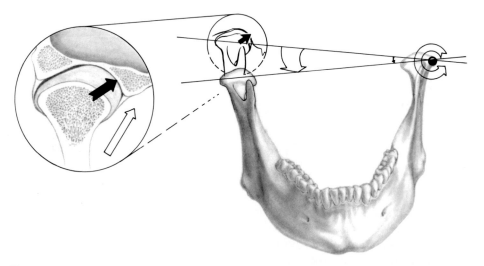

Fig. 7-11. The design of the functional curve of Wilson would not work if the lower posterior teeth could travel horizontally toward the midline because the longer lower buccal cusps would clash with the longer upper lingual cusps. The medial pole bony stop prevents any side shift until after the condyle has moved down the eminentia and permits the curve of Wilson design to function without interference. This necessary functional relationship of the joints is also responsible for the solid "midmost" position in centric relation. It also explains why the concept of an immediate side shift is wrong.

ular notion, but it cannot occur in a healthy
joint if the condyles are in centric relation at
the start of motion. If it could occur, the curve
of Wilson would result in balancing incline interferences. The only way this can occur is if
there is severe alteration of the shape of the articulating surfaces.

It would be very unlikely to have flattening
of the condyle and eminence without similar
adaptation of the curve of Wilson. The *effect* of
such changes in the joints is seen in the flattening of the curve of Wilson by wearing away
of the upper lingual cusps. This type of wear
cannot occur in a correct occlusal plane with
normal, healthy temporomandibular joints.
The presence of severe wear on upper lingual
cusps should alert the diagnostician to adaptive changes in the articular surfaces of the
joint.

The occlusal plane is a marvelous example
of the interplay between form and function.
Analysis of the occlusal plane should be important to any dental examination because of its
importance to coordinated function of the entire masticatory system. Adaptive changes in
the occlusal plane are signals of possible dysfunction somewhere in the system.

SUMMARY

The form of the occlusal plane is directly related to specific functional requirements. In addition to alignment of teeth in relationship to
the arc of closure for best resistance to loading, it should permit ease of access for positioning of the food on the occlusal surfaces. If
these two functional requirements are met, an
occlusal plane is acceptable if it permits the
anterior guidance to do its job.

The relationship of the occlusal plane to
skeletal points and planes is described in Chapter 38.

The relationship of the anterior teeth to the
occlusal plane is described in Chapter 17.

Methods for determining the occlusal plane
are discussed in Chapter 20.

The methods for mounting casts in relation
to a correct occlusal plane are discussed in
Chapter 13.

All the above references are important to a
full understanding of evaluation, diagnosis, and
treatment of occlusal plane problems.

SUGGESTED READINGS

Boucher, D.O.: Current status of prosthodontics, J. Prosthet. Dent. **10**:418, 1960.

Mann, A.W., and Pankey, L.D.: Use of the Pankey-Mann instrument in treatment planning and in restoring the
lower posterior teeth, J. Prosthet. Dent. **10**:135, 1980.

Monson, G.S.: Applied mechanics to the theory of mandibular movements, Dent. Cosmos **74**:1039, 1932.

Spee, F.G.: Prosthetic dentistry, ed. 4, Chicago, 1928, Med-
ico-dental Publishing Co.

Wilson, G.H.: Dental prosthetics, Philadelphia, 1917, Lea &
Febiger.

8

Differential diagnosis of temporomandibular disorders

Functional harmony of the occlusion cannot be achieved if it is aligned with a disturbed temporomandibular articulation. Competence with occlusal therapy requires the ability to differentiate the different disorders that occur with the temporomandibular articulation so that they can be treated *before* the intercuspal relationship of the teeth is determined.

The procedures for diagnosing temporomandibular disorders have gone through a continuing evolution during the past few years. The most important advancements have been made in the recognition of more definitive cause-and-effect relationships and the rejection of the all-inclusive syndrome approach, which fails to relate specific causes to specific signs and symptoms.

Improved information about the anatomy and physiology of the temporomandibular joints has been combined with new insights into the adaptive responses of the involved tissues and a better understanding of the varying capacities of the different tissues for repair. Research directed toward objective analysis has eliminated the need for subjective opinions and has encouraged more specificity regarding what is wrong in the joint or the elements that relate to it. Thus the clinician can design treat-

ment approaches aimed at correcting specific causes rather than treating symptoms.

Symptomatic treatment will not correct what is wrong, and so the following questions should be asked before treatment is initiated:

1. Is this treatment specifically aimed at correcting the cause of the problem, or is it merely repairing effects?
2. Will the treatment leave the system in a state of harmony that will foster healing and *maintainable* health, or will it just provide a transient relief of symptoms?

To be able to answer the above questions, a systematic examination is required to do the following:

1. Determine specific signs and symptoms.
2. Note combinations of signs and symptoms.
3. Evaluate *all* possible causes for each sign and each symptom.
4. Evaluate all possible combinations of direct causes as well as indirect contributing factors.
5. Test your premise. Use reversible methods whenever practical.
6. Evaluate all possible reasons for every response to treatment or diagnostic testing. Know *why* each response occurs.

7. Based on the age and health of the patient, determine whether the effect of the disorder is sufficiently serious to warrant extensive treatment. In other words, would the treatment be worse than the disorder? If so, is there a logical palliative alternative? In some situations symptomatic treatment may be the treatment of choice.

ROUTINE SCREENING PROCEDURES FOR TEMPOROMANDIBULAR DISORDERS

The initial examination for routine dental patients should include procedures and history to determine whether any temporomandibular disorders exist. Many patients have problems that should be corrected, but they are not aware of the relationship of the temporomandibular joints to the health and stability of the dentition and vice versa. A simple screening should be done on every dental patient as part of a complete examination. The results should be noted on the patient's chart and should include the following information:

SCREENING EXAMINATION

1. Can the mandible be positioned in centric relation with no sign of discomfort? Does upward pressure toward the joints elicit any response of tenderness or tension in centric relation?
2. Can the mandible hinge freely in centric relation? Can the joints resist firm upward pressure while hinging with no sign of discomfort?
3. Can the patient open the mouth without difficulty? Any deviations?
4. Are there any grating sounds, clicks, or discoordination in either joint during jaw movement or function?
5. Does palpation of the masticatory muscles cause any tenderness or pain?
6. Is the intercuspation of the teeth in harmony with centric relation?
7. Does firm clenching of the teeth elicit any sign of tenderness in either joint area or in any tooth?
8. Does any part of the dentition show signs of excessive wear, or hypermobility of teeth?

SCREENING HISTORY

It is helpful to complete the screening examination before the history is taken because the examination often turns up signs of suspected disorders that the examiner can relate to when quizzing patients about their history. Whether the examination reveals any suspected disorders, the screening history should still be taken.

The following questions were recommended as a basic screening history by the consensus of conferees at the American Dental Association President's Conference on Examination, Diagnosis, and Management of Temporomandibular Disorders (1982):

- Do you have difficulty opening your mouth?
- Do you hear noises from the jaw joints?
- Does your jaw ever get "stuck" or "locked" or "go out"?
- Do you have pain in or about the ears or cheeks?
- Do you have pain on chewing, yawning, or wide opening?
- Does your bite feel uncomfortable or unusual?
- Have you ever had an injury to your jaw, head, or neck?
- Have you ever had arthritis?
- Have you previously been treated for a temporomandibular disorder? If so, when, what, how, and by whom?

To this list, I would add questions related to headache history: Are you bothered with frequent headaches? If so, where? How often? How severe? When do they occur?

The above examination and screening history should be a routine part of a complete dental examination. If any positive findings are turned up, a more comprehensive examination should be directed at the specific signs and symptoms.

CLASSIFYING TEMPOROMANDIBULAR DISORDERS

Temporomandibular disorders should be classified into specific cause-and-effect categories. Poor terminology such as "myofascial pain dysfunction syndrome" (MPD), or "TMJ syndrome," has mislead many practitioners into simplistic treatments in the belief that pain or dysfunction in the TMJ region is part of a broad, nonspecific group of symptoms. If the practitioner believes that limited opening, clicking, and joint tenderness is one syndrome caused by psychologic stress, he will probably treat the group of symptoms by counseling or by prescribing drugs. If the practitioner believes the symptoms are always part of a syndrome caused by malocclusion, he may routinely use bite planes or equilibration empirically. If proper diagnostic procedures are used, however, each specific sign or symptom must be evaluated and related to a cause before treatment begins. Improved classification of temporomandibular disorders has made differential diagnosis a more logical process. Such disorders should first be separated into three broad categories, and then each category can be studied in detail.

Temporomandibular disorders can be classified broadly, as follows:

1. Masticatory muscle disorders
2. Intra-articular problems
3. Conditions that mimick temporomandibular disorders

It is imperative that all three categories be considered when one is evaluating any temporomandibular disorder because combinations of two or all three problems can and do occur. Furthermore, one type of problem can cause or be caused by a different type of problem. As an example, a disk derangement will virtually always be accompanied by masticatory muscle spasm. It must be determined whether the muscle spasm caused the disk derangement or vice versa.

At the ADA President's Conference on temporomandibular disorders (1982), guidelines were suggested for classifying temporomandibular disorders. They are based on the classification developed by Weldon Bell. Use of such a logical classification system benefits diagnostic capability as well as communication within the profession. The following outline is compiled with minor modifications from those guidelines:

Masticatory muscle disorders
1. Protective muscle splinting
2. Muscle hyperactivity or spasm
3. Myositis (muscle inflammation)

Problems involving derangement of the temporomandibular joint
1. Incoordination
2. Clicking
3. Partial disk derangement
4. Anterior disk displacement with reduction (clicking)
5. Anterior disk displacement without reduction (closed lock)

Problems that result from extrinsic trauma
1. Traumatic arthritis
2. Dislocation
3. Fracture
4. Disk derangement
5. Myositis
6. Myospasm
7. Tendinitis

Degenerative joint disease
1. Arthrosis (noninflammatory phase)
2. Osteoarthritis (inflammatory phase)

Inflammatory joint disorders
1. Rheumatoid arthritis
2. Infectious arthritis
3. Metabolic arthritis

Chronic mandibular hypomobility
1. Ankylosis (fibrous or osseous)
2. Fibrosis of articular capsule
3. Contracture of elevator muscles (myostatic or myofibrotic contracture)
4. Internal disk derangement (closed lock)

Growth disorders of the joint
1. Developmental disorders
2. Acquired disorders
3. Neoplastic disorders

Postsurgical problems

Although the above list includes classifications for all types of temporomandibular disorders, many patients report with a chief complaint of *pain* in the region of the temporomandibular joint who do not have a problem with the joint itself. Many patients have craniofacial pain that is not related to any type of temporomandibular disorder.

Since the dentist has become a primary source of diagnosis for all symptoms in this area, including pain, the recognition and differentiation of a wide range of craniomandibular pain should be considered an important element of thorough diagnosis.

Although most of the patients who complain of pain or dysfunction in the temporomandibular region will have pain that is related to muscle, we should evaluate other potential causes for pain, even when masticatory muscle pain is evident. The following check list is simple but practical. If it alerts us to a potential causative factor, we should then explore further.

POTENTIAL CAUSES OF PAIN IN THE TMJ AREA

1. Trauma
2. Masticatory muscle disturbances
3. Intra-articular problems
4. Pathologic factors
5. Neurologic factors
6. Psychologic factors

Craniofacial pain can be very elusive, and because even severe pain can be so often related to muscle incoordination, it is a practical approach to start the evaluation of craniofacial pain with a step-by-step procedure for determining whether the cause of the problem is masticatory muscle pain resulting from occlusal disharmony (occluso-muscle pain). If it is not, the source of the pain must be found in one or more of the other classifications.

DIAGNOSING OCCLUSO-MUSCLE PAIN (MASTICATORY MUSCLE PAIN RESULTING FROM OCCLUSAL DISHARMONY)

There is no need for masticatory muscle pain to be treated in an empiric manner though it is far too common to do so. Nor should it ever be considered as the exclusive cause of pain or dysfunction without a thorough examination to rule out all other potential causative factors, even in the presence of muscle pain. If the following procedures are followed consistently and in proper sequence, they will serve as a practical method for evaluating each patient. The procedures have been designed to isolate specific problem categories so that they can either be discovered as a possible cause or ruled out as a causative or contributing factor. This same diagnostic sequence has been used in our practice for many years and has passed the test of time as a practical screening procedure for masticatory muscle pain of occlusal cause. One of the primary advantages to the system is that it enables the practitioner to quickly determine whether occluso-muscle pain or dysfunction is or is not a factor of importance. Thus the indiscriminate, empiric use of occlusal therapy is never considered. If occlusal treatment of any kind is used, it will be prescribed for a specific and completely understandable reason.

The steps for diagnosing occluso-muscle pain are as follows:

Step 1. Determine whether muscle is involved in the pain.

Step 2. Rule out intra-articular problems.

Step 3. Relate the specific muscle pain to occlusal contacts.

Step 4. Verify the acceptability of condyle-fossa health and position with TMJ radiographs (if any problem is suspected).

Step 5. Rule out gross bone pathosis with radiographs.

Step 6. Rule out pulpal or periodontal pathosis as sources of pain.

Step 7. Correct the cause of the problem.

Occluso-muscle pain and dysfunction *can* be differentiated from other craniomandibular pain and even in the presence of a combination of other complex problems, it can be diagnosed and treated with a high degree of predictability. It can also be ruled *out* very early as a possible cause of pain, so that attention can then be directed toward isolation of other potential causes.

The first step is to determine whether muscle is involved with the pain. This evaluation must be executed with expertise but, once learned, is a consistently dependable procedure.

Evaluating muscle tenderness

Any factor that disturbs the tonus of one muscle will also disturb the tonus of any muscle that opposes its action. Thus any stimulus to muscle hyperactivity will create a rational pattern of hyperactivity in specifically related muscles.

Because specific skeletal muscles move their skeletal components in well-defined directions, aberrant movements can be analyzed to determine which muscles must be involved to make such movements. Deviations in skeletal *alignment* can likewise be analyzed because regardless of the cause of the misalignment the muscles that are attached to the misaligned parts will be affected adversely. When the muscles are unable to adjust to achieve harmonious action in producing complex movements, *muscle incoordination* is the result.

Muscles are always in some degree of contraction. Even at rest a muscle maintains a certain tonicity by keeping some of its fibers contracted. This postural contraction of opposing muscles is responsible for maintaining skeletal alignment during resting posture and can be considered the base line for *normal tonicity.* Muscles that are not in a normal state of tonicity are either *hypotonic* or *hypertonic.*

In the normal state of resting tonicity, a muscle in its entirety never fatigues. Because of the "all or none" law of muscle contraction, individual fiber bundles of muscle contract completely or not at all. Because the contraction requires a mechanochemical action, the normal time of contraction of each fiber is limited to the time required for the chemical action to occur, at which point the fiber bundle must rest to permit a recycling of the chemicals and the elimination of the waste chemical byproducts, including lactic acid. Because only a small percentage of the fiber bundles contract at one time during resting posture, there are enough muscle fibers on reserve to maintain normal muscle tonus. By allowing alternating fiber bundles to rest and contract, the muscle can maintain the strength of contraction needed for postural alignment without fatigue.

As demands are increased on any muscle, the ratio of contracting fibers to resting fibers increases. If the duration and intensity of the demands are greater than the muscle can handle by alternation of working and resting fibers, the entire muscle becomes fatigued. Prolonged fatigue leads to incoordination and muscle spasm.

The fatigue or spasm that occurs from prolonged hyperactivity often produces pain in the muscle. Sensory nerve endings in the muscles are highly sensitive to lactic acid buildup and also to ischemia. When the nerve endings are stimulated, they report such stimulation as pain. Ischemia can occur in the muscle because of the tight spastic contraction around its own blood supply while the formation of lactic acid takes up much of the remaining available oxygen. So reduced oxygen to the muscle and its sensory pain fibers occurs from both chemical and mechanical reasons, occurring simultaneously. Anyone who has experienced the intense pain of cramping in a leg or foot muscle can relate to the effect of ischemic muscle pain, which is compounded by pain fibers in the stretched tendons. When such painful spasm occurs in the richly innervated masticatory muscles, the pain can be excruciating.

Fortunately, the muscle-related pain can also be diagnostic because if it can be determined that the patient's pain is related to a muscle or group of muscles it is usually a simple procedure to determine the source of stimulation that requires those specific muscles to stay in contraction beyond their physiologically acceptable limits.

Not all hyperactive muscles are painful, but tenderness to palpation is one of the most consistent signs that we find in masticatory muscles that are forced into prolonged activity. We can simplify the differential diagnosis of occluso-muscle pain if we are aware that in any deviation of the condyles from centric relation the lateral pterygoid muscles are always involved. Soreness of the pterygoid musculature is almost always indicative of abnormal function. It will result when prolonged contraction is required to position the mandible forward of centric relation, and it will also occur from prolonged stretching if the mandible is forced distal to centric relation.

Tenderness to palpation may be observed in any pterygoid muscle that is in a long-term forced contraction or stretch-reflex contraction whether the patient has noticeable masticatory muscle pain. The exceptions to this are so rare that tenderness to palpation may be used as a reliable indicator that there is some form of mandibular displacement present. Any exceptions to this rule will be automatically picked up as the subsequent procedural steps of the differential diagnosis are carried out, but regardless of the cause, the first step in differential diagnosis is to determine whether muscle is or is not involved in the pain.

Like so many other aspects of diagnosis, the technique for palpation must be performed correctly. The lateral pterygoid muscles are important because they are *always* involved with any deviation of the mandible. They are uniquely responsive to the reflex pressure receptors around the teeth, and the elimination of pterygoid tenderness eliminates the occlusion as a causative factor.

Despite the direct relationship of the lateral pterygoid muscles, the most reliable palpation area is on the *medial* pterygoid muscle. The reason for this is the ease of palpating the medial pterygoid, which, being an antagonist to the lateral pterygoid, is always involved whenever the lateral pterygoid is hypertonic. Furthermore, electromyographic studies have shown that the internal pterygoid becomes hyperactive in the presence of occlusal interferences. It is also possible that pressure against the medial pterygoid presses it into the underlying lateral pterygoid, and so at least part of the response might come from it.

Technique of pterygoid palpation. Palpation of the medial pterygoid muscle is done to determine whether the muscle is hypertonic. A hypertonic muscle is very firm to the touch, whereas a muscle with normal tonicity is easily indented with little resistance.

To palpate the pterygoid complex, have the patient open as wide as possible. The tip of the index finger is then moved gently up the anterior border of the ascending ramus and into the pterygomandibular raphe to the same spot that would be entered for a mandibular injection. The medial border of this indentation is formed by the anterior border of the medial pterygoid muscle. At the level of the hamular notch, move the fingertip medially across the border of the muscle and approximatley 1 cm toward the uvula. With the mouth open, the anterior margin of the muscle often feels like a tight string. Hook the finger around that border and direct light pressure back and up through an imaginary line that goes through the center of the ear (Fig. 8-1).

Care should be taken not to press too firmly if the muscle is tender. In some acute spasms, merely touching the muscle elicits a painful response; however, *any* tenderness to palpation has significance. Common sense should be the guide in applying pressure. Once it has been determined that a muscle is tender to palpation, the procedure should not be repeated, since continual pressure on a sore muscle can prod it into a more intense spasm with increased pain.

As proficiency is developed, variations in the feel of the muscles will become more apparent. A muscle with normal tonicity can be indented easily 5 to 10 mm or more with little resistance and no sign of tenderness. A spastic muscle will feel hard to the touch. Experience will enable the dentist to make a diagnosis quite often just from the state of tension or flaccidity of the muscle. Some spastic muscles will tense up into a series of knots. These variations will have more significance when experience has related them repeatedly to symptoms.

It is not always necessary to ask a patient to verbally respond regarding palpation effects. A response to muscle tenderness is usually apparent when the eyes are watched or a flinch or some noticeable reaction in the facial muscles is observed. It is sometimes wise *not* to ask for a response when psychologic factors are suspected, since some patients may give the response that they believe is expected.

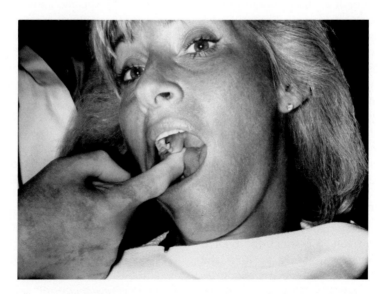

Fig. 8-1. Palpation of the medial pterygoid muscle is best accomplished when you hook the tip of the index finger on the anterior border of the muscle and press back and up toward the center of the ear. Indent the muscle about 5 to 10 mm. Use less pressure if the muscle feels hard because that is an indication of hypercontraction.

Some psychotic or neurotic patients use pain to strengthen their story of how miserable they are, and so in the interest of diagnostic accuracy it is better to avoid suggesting any pain locations.

In cases of severe trismus, it may be difficult to reach the palpation point just described. Trismus is an indication in itself of muscle spasm, but to verify that the pterygoids are involved, it is usually possible to slip the fingertip or at least a mouth mirror into position to press on the anterior border of the internal pterygoid. A response to that confirms that muscle spasm is present.

Palpation of other muscles. The pterygoid complex is directly related to all mandibular deviations from centric relation, and so it is the primary diagnostic site for palpation when occlusal factors are suspected. Other masticatory muscles may also be responsible for facial pain, and it is helpful to know which ones are contributing to the symptoms. It is also common to find muscle pain in the neck, shoulders, and back, and it must be remembered that cervical misalignment can also cause muscle incoordination of this region. When cervical misalignment is suspected, referral to an orthopedic physician or a physical therapist is in order. Cervical area disorders must be differentiated from occlusal disorders. Occlusal interferences to central relation cannot be resolved with physical therapy, and it is doubtful if most cervical misalignment can be resolved with occlusal therapy. Each must be evaluated separately, even though there can be a crossover of symptoms in the musculature of each region. Muscle palpation is the best clinical method for quickly determining when and where misalignments and incoordinations exist. When the symptom of muscle incoordination has been observed, it will then be necessary to determine the cause. Finding the cause of muscle tenderness is always easier when the search can be related to specific muscles.

Ruling out intra-articular problems

If pterygoid muscle tenderness is noted on either side, it will almost certainly be related to protective muscle splinting to hold the condyle-disk assembly in a braced position inferior to centric relation. This is usually required because of occlusal relationships that are not in harmony with centric relation, but it may also be a protective response to prevent excessive loading on a damaged joint or a misaligned condyle-disk relationship. Before occlusal interference can be determined as the cause of muscle incoordination, it is axiomatic that intra-articular problems must be ruled out. In fact, intra-articular problems must be ruled out before it is even possible to evaluate an occlusion because occlusal analysis depends on relating the occlusion to a correct centric relation.

Intra-articular problems are ruled out by testing of the joint with very firm upward pressure after the condyles are gently positioned into what the operator feels is centric relation (follow the method described in Chapter 4). If there is *any sign* of pain, tenderness, or even tension in the joint area when pressure is applied, that position cannot be accepted as centric relation. It is essential that the cause of the discomfort be determined before one proceeds with occlusal diagnosis or treatment.

Testing the joint with pressure is one of the most reliable clinical procedures that can be used. If any discomfort is noticed from the pressure, the cause of the discomfort will be from either muscle bracing, condyle-disk misalignment, or some pathologic or inflammatory problem within the joint. If it is determined that the source of the craniomandibular pain is within the joint structures, the pain will be treated as a joint problem and the differential diagnostic procedures should be carried out to pin down the specific nature of the intra-articular disorder. If there is no sign of discomfort or tension within the joint when upward pressure is applied as outlined, it has been our consistent finding that intra-articular problems can be ruled out as the primary cause of the craniofacial pain.

For the sake of clarity, several points should be emphasized regarding the test for intra-articular problems, as follows:

1. Pressure is not applied until *after* the joints are seated into a freely hinging position.
2. Pressure must be directed upwardly through the condyles. This can be achieved with bilateral manipulation or the pressure can be exerted by the patient's own elevator muscle contraction if a *nondeviating* anterior stop is in place.
3. Pressure must be *firm.* It must be sufficient to test the structures of the joint. A

properly aligned, healthy joint can resist very firm pressure with total comfort.

4. Pressure must be applied in both a static and a hinging relationship. All bearing surfaces should be tested as the condyles rotate in centric relation. This is done best with bilateral manipulation because the upward pressure can be maintained during opening and closing of the mandible.

5. If pressure produces discomfort in either joint, it should be considered as a signal that there is some problem present regardless of how freely the jaw may hinge, regardless of how well centered the condyles are radiographically, or regardless of the apparent absence of any other sign or symptom. A closer look will almost always locate a specific reason for this discomfort.

The potential causes for discomfort to pressure are outlined in Chapter 4, and they are discussed separately in more detail here. It has been our experience, however, that a very small percentage are actually pathologic disorders or derangements that do not respond to conservative treatment in a rather short time span. The uncomfortable disorder is usually no more than transient muscle bracing that can be released with judicious, gentle manipulation to centric relation. Those joints that cannot be successfully manipulated into a comfortable position should be tested again after attempts have been made to deprogram the spastic musculature. If an intra-articular problem is not present, the muscle spasm can often be released by simple placement of cotton rolls between the teeth for a few minutes. By separating the teeth with the soft material, one can prevent the interfering inclines from programming the muscles. When the protective muscle contraction is released, the mandible can then be easily manipulated into a comfortable centric relation.

Perhaps the best method for distinguishing between an intra-articular problem and an occluso-muscle problem is through the use of an anterior bite plane that separates all posterior teeth. The bite plane aids the diagnosis in two ways:

1. By eliminating occlusal interferences, it eliminates the need for lateral pterygoid bracing and allows the condyles free access to centric relation.

2. By taking away all posterior support from the teeth, it effectively tests the joints for responses to pressure.

If there are no intra-articular disorders present, the overnight use of an anterior bite plane should relieve the muscle bracing and make it possible for the joints to resist pressure comfortably. If the anterior bite plane fails to relieve the discomfort in the joint or makes it worse, the probability of an intra-articular problem is increased.

In reducible condyle-disk derangements with clicks, an anterior bite plane can help distinguish which derangements are caused by muscle incoordination or by mechanical distalization. Comfort with an anterior bite plane is a virtual guarantee that the disk alignment will hold if the occlusion is corrected. CAUTION: An anterior bite plane should never be used in a nonreducible disk derangement. It should only be considered when the condyle can be positioned on the disk, and then the condyle-disk assembly can be moved together to centric relation and verified. It should be retested with pressure after a day or two of wearing the bite plane. If it is still comfortable, one may conclude that its cause was occluso-muscle imbalance.

It is critically important that the anterior bite plane be constructed properly (see Chapter 11). We see many such bite planes that have deviating inclines built into the bite plane surface. If the surface is not smooth enough and flat enough to permit free sliding access of the mandible to centric relation, it will perpetuate the muscle bracing, or may actually create new deviations that intensify the muscle spasm.

The important consideraton here is that muscle bracing must be eliminated before the joint itself can be tested. If reasonable attempts to deprogram the muscles through disengagement of occlusal inclines does not relieve the discomfort in the joint, the examination should then focus on the joint itself.

If there is any question about the condition of the articulating surfaces or the alignment of the condyle-disk relationship, Doppler auscultation (described in Chapters 9 and 10) is one of the most reliable methods for noninvasive analysis. A Dopplergram recording can also serve as a permanent record of the condition of the joint before one initiates occlusal changes.

If intra-articular problems can be ruled out in a patient with masticatory muscle tenderness, the next step in diagnosis is to relate the muscle pain to specific occlusal contacts. In other words, find the cause of the muscle incoordination.

Finding the trigger for occluso-muscle pain

The importance of learning to precisely manipulate the mandible into centric relation should be apparent if occlusal interferences are to be detected accurately. After determining specifically which muscles are involved in the pain and after verifying that the condyles can hinge freely with complete comfort in centric relation, you must close the mandible on the centric relation axis to the first tooth contact. Maintain the upward pressure on the joints while closing to the first point of tooth contact. Observe the lower midline position at first contact, and then ask the patient to squeeze the teeth together into maximum contact. By noting the direction which the lower midline moves to go from first point of contact to maximum contact, it is easy to determine which muscles would be required to move the jaw in that direction. If the slide from centric relation to centric occlusion is to the left, the right pterygoid complex would be involved. If those muscles are the ones that were most tender to palpation, a direct relationship between cause and effect will have been established.

It is not necessary to have a slide to produce muscle hyperactivity. Even a vertically loaded premature tooth contact can activate protective muscle splinting. Often such interferences merely depress the prematurely contacting tooth without causing a shift of the mandible. Such interferences can be difficult to discern, but if casts are mounted with a carefully made centric bite record, the interference can be found easily. The stone cast will not allow movement of the teeth, and so premature contacts will show up clearly.

The use of diagnostic casts, related in a *verified* centric relation record and mounted with a facebow transfer should be a standard procedure for suspected occluso-muscle disorders. The correct intra-arch relationship must be known, along with the arc of closure from the first point of tooth contact to the most closed position in centric relation before an adequate treatment plan can be devised. It is most often necessary to equilibrate the mounted casts to learn the correct tooth-to-tooth relationships in centric relation at the correct vertical. Until this information is clearly defined, the choice of treatment is based on guesswork only. If orthodontics or restorative procedures can improve the occlusion or equilibration would result in exposure of dentin, this should be known in advance and explained to the patient. The mounted casts can also be used for fabrication of bite-plane appliances or occlusal splints if they are deemed necessary for treatment. If the above first three steps are followed, it is possible to determine very clearly whether the patient's pain is a result of occluso-muscle imbalance, but the diagnosis should not stop here. Many patients with occluso-muscle pain also have other active problems that can contribute to the pain. These problems can be easily missed if the total focus is on occlusion. The examination should continue in order to rule out other factors, even when occluso-muscle pain has been diagnosed.

Verifying condyle health and position radiographically

The clinical procedures just described are so dependable it would be highly unlikely to find radiographic evidence of a problem if the condyles passed the test of pressure. If the joint assemblies can be positioned into a verified centric relation, can hinge freely and resist pressure with no sign of discomfort, and can move without restriction or deviation, there is no need to take radiographs of the temporomandibular joints.

TMJ radiographs should be used:

1. If there are any signs of discomfort in the joint that cannot be resolved.
2. If there are joint sounds of crepitus or clicking.
3. If there is any limitation or deviation of normal function movements.
4. If the positional relationship of the condyles is in question.
5. If there is any suspicion of injury or pathosis.

There is no radiographic technique that can *determine* centric relation. Because occluso-muscle pain can result from tooth interferences that deviate the condyles a fraction of a millimeter, almost imperceptible variations in condyle positioning can make the difference between success or failure of occlusal treatment.

The location of such a precise position cannot be determined by a radiograph alone. There is so much variation in the shape of condyles and fossae that any radiographic method based on centering the condyle in the fossa is too crude to accept as a final position. It can however have merit because gross misalignments can alert the dentist to the possibility of a problem. The final determination of condyle position, though, must be where the joint can function and resist pressure with complete comfort. In joints with degenerative changes, radiographs can be used to help find a tentative treatment position, but final refinement of that position will still be necessary as joint changes occur.

TMJ radiographs can be used advantageously to detect fairly small comparative position changes of the condyle if the head is stabilized. Comparative condyle positions can be recorded using a variety of head-holder devices such as the Accurad, or Craniostat. Recording the comparative position requires the use of a hard-material centric relation record for holding the mandible in centric relation for one exposure and then removal of the bite record for a second exposure with the patient biting firmly in centric occlusion. If the head is in the same position for both exposures, it will be simple to compare which direction the condyle travels from centric relation to maximum intercuspation (Fig. 8-2). This procedure

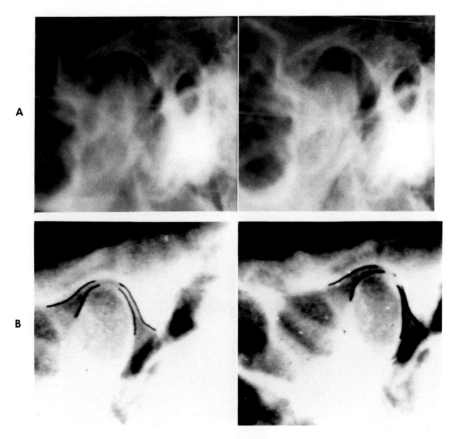

Fig. 8-2. Comparative transcranial radiographs showing, **A,** the difference in condyle position between CR and CO when the condyle is displaced forward. **B** shows comparative positions when the condyle is displaced distally. In both patients a verifiable centric relation was achievable, and the CR radiographs were made with a centric bite record in place. The CO radiographs were made at maximum intercuspation. The head did not move between the CR and CO exposures.

is particularly useful when a possible disk derangement is suspected. A third exposure made at maximum opening shows the range of condylar movement and can be used to rule out ankylosis and to evaluate the integrity of the joint surfaces from a lateral viewpoint.

Radiographic techniques have great value in differential diagnosis of intra-articular problems. The practical approach to using TMJ radiographic techniques is to first determine clinically that there is an intra-articular problem. Then use the radiographic technique that best fits the type of suspected problem. Radiography of the TMJ is discussed in more detail in Chapters 9 and 40. In the absence of a suspected intra-articular problem, the American Dental Association has taken the position that the routine use of TMJ radiographs is contraindicated.

Ruling out gross bone pathosis with radiographs

If the joints cannot be positioned into a *verified*, comfortable centric relation, an intra-articular problem is suspected. If intra-articular problems can be ruled out, it is still a wise idea to scan the entire temporomandibular region radiographically for the presence of bone pathosis or alterations of structure when patients with suspected occluso-muscle pain are analyzed.

A panoramic radiograph gives an overall view of the bony parts involved and in some instances, because of its availability to the general practitioner, is the only way in which specific problems are detected.

Cysts, fractures, tumors, abscesses, and some generalized bone changes can be observed in panoramic films that could easily be missed in a routine dental examination. Far too commonly have we seen patients treated with long-term bite planes or occlusal grinding who had a pathosis that was unrelated to occlusion. When patients with chronic pain present with an obvious occluso-muscle problem, it is dangerous to assume that there are no other causative factors present without thorough analysis of any symptoms or signs that cannot be specifically isolated as occluso-muscle in origin.

If pain persists in the absence of palpable muscle tenderness and no occlusal deviations can be noticed, a panoramic radiograph is indicated to help rule out bone pathosis as part of a differential diagnosis.

Although not common, cysts of varying sizes (Fig. 8-3) are sometimes found to be the source of jaw pain. Some panoramic radiographs also give a clear view of the nasal septum, which, if deviated, can cause sinus pressures to develop because of blockage (Fig. 8-4). A blocked sinus can cause pressure against

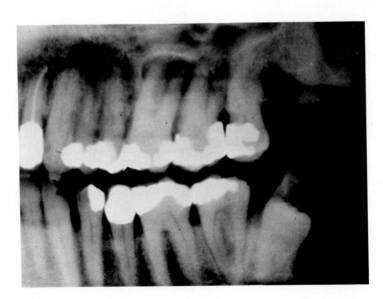

Fig. 8-3. Panoramic film showing presence of a large cyst in the ramus in a patient who had been treated for nearly 2 years with occlusal bite plane therapy and equilibration. Notice the periapical abscess on the upper first molar that was also previously missed. Panoramic films are indicated as a scan for any patient with long-term jaw pain.

the bone around the roots that can move the upper teeth and create occlusal interferences. When muscle pain develops because of such an altered occlusion, the muscle spasm can combine with the pain of the sinus pressure and become severe. Correction of the sinusitis is necessary before the occlusion can be refined.

Panoramic radiography can also be used to get a different viewpoint of the temporomandibular joints. Pathologic or structural changes in the condyle or the fossa may be detected or confirmed from some panoramic radiographs, though it is not the most reliable method for making a primary diagnosis when intraarticular problems are suspected.

Ruling out pulpal or periodontal pathosis as sources of pain

Oddly enough, one of the most commonly missed diagnoses related to craniofacial pain is odontitis. Pulpitis, dying pulps, split teeth, and obvious periapical abscesses too often go undiagnoses while the patient is treated with various forms of occlusal treatment, drugs, or other therapies. The diagnosis is apparently missed because of the intensified muscle response to an occlusal interference from a tooth that also has pulpal involvement. A hypersensitive tooth provokes, by way of its periodontal receptors, a more active avoidance pattern in the musculature. Because of this intensified muscle activity to protect the sensitive tooth, the muscle itself becomes painful. As uncomfortable as an abscessed tooth may be, it is not uncommon for the muscle pain to be more intense, actually blending together with the pain from the tooth, to form a generalized area that creates more of a facial pain than the usual isolated toothache.

The dentist who does not completely evaluate this type of problem may be misled by the obvious diagnosis of occluso-muscle pain. The mistake is often perpetuated because if the occlusion is corrected the pain is relieved dramatically and in most cases immediately. The occlusal correction relieves not only the muscle hyperactivity, but also the excessive occlusal pressure on the sore tooth. The problem is that such relief is transitory unless the pulpal problem is also corrected.

Often the pain will clearly focus in on the involved tooth after the muscle pain is eliminated. When this occurs, the diagnosis becomes obvious and the pulpal problem can be resolved. If, however, the tooth is moved back into hyperocclusion by the inflammation around its root, it may reactivate the painful cycle of occluso-muscle incoordination, without a focus of pain in the tooth itself. The apparently logical but incorrect assumption then is to use the same treatment approach that

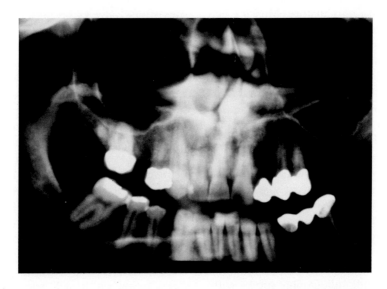

Fig. 8-4. Panoramic film of patient with a severely deviated septum. Although not a dental problem, blockage of sinus cavities can result in a pressure buildup that moves teeth and causes occluso-muscle problems. The dentist is often in a position to discover the problem and refer the patient for needed treatment.

worked before. Since the patient gets a measure of relief each time the occlusion is corrected, the process goes on and on until the pain becomes too intense to bear.

It is difficult to understand how the one thing dentists are trained to do best, that is, diagnosis of a toothache, is the very thing that gets missed so commonly, but the above scenario is commonplace in the patients I have seen who were referred for "TMJ pain" that could not be resolved. Many of these patients were referred by better than average dentists who were frustrated at their inability to solve this particular problem when they had been having such good success in treating the other TMJ patients. This apparently gets to the crux of the diagnostic puzzle. So much patient discomfort *is* caused by occluso-muscle disharmony that it is easy for a dentist who is successful with occlusal therapy to develop "tunnel vision" and overlook the fact that there can be more than one cause for craniomandibular pain. Odontitis is always a possible cause. It should be ruled out as a routine part of the differential diagnosis.

Pulpitis, split teeth, and dying pulps can, in combination with occluso-muscle pain, cause some bizarre symptoms. A high percentage of the patients referred to my office for confirmation or diagnosis of an apparent tic douloureux do not have tic douloureux. It is common to find the classic trigger zone resulting from muscle spasticity that provokes a chain reaction into the facial musculature. Muscles become so hyperactive that even touching them stimulates them into spastic contraction. At the same time, the dying pulp or split tooth can elicit a typical paroxysmal spasm of pain when combined with the muscle hypercontraction. Relief is dramatic and rapid when occluso-muscle harmony is regained and the pulpal problem resolved.

Both an occlusal examination and vitality tests should always be a routine part of the differential diagnosis for any patient suspected of having tic douloureux. Vitality tests should also be a routine test of the examination of any patient with chronic craniofacial pain if the pain cannot specifically be *isolated* within muscle.

A complete mouth radiographic survey with periapical films should be a standard requirement when one is examining the patient with facial pain, just as it should be part of a complete dental examination for any new patient.

Since pulpal abscesses can occur within the confines of the root, they are not always visible in a periapical film. Consequently, vitality tests should be used in addition to the radiographs whenever there is a doubt.

Periodontal pathosis usually does not elicit a painful response in itself, but combined with an occlusal interference, they can activate an intensified protective muscle response, especially in teeth that are not particularly hypermobile. Very loose teeth generally just move out of the way, and so they usually do not cause the severe degree of muscle splinting that occurs when the interfering tooth is firm. If the periodontal abscess is confined in a furcation, occlusal pressure is intensified as the tooth is lifted into interference by the infection. Just as with the pulpally involved tooth, the periodontitis discomfort, amplified by excessive pressure from painful muscles, combines to cause a generalized facial pain that can sometimes focus more in the muscles than in the tooth.

We have seen patients develop unusually severe occluso-muscle discomfort combined with soreness or pain in the supporting tissues. Complete relief could not be achieved without removal of subgingival calculus and in some instances root planing. It appears that subgingival calculus in some patients can activate bruxing, clenching habit patterns, especially when combined with occlusal interferences.

A careful evaluation of the supporting tissues should always be done to rule out periodontal pathosis as a source of pain or as a trigger for muscle hyperactivity.

Split teeth can be potent triggers for protective muscle splinting and can be difficult to diagnose because they often do not show the split on a radiograph. If the split tooth has an incline interference, occlusal contact can wedge the split open and cause very noticeable pain in the tooth itself while simultaneously intensifying muscle hyperactivity to protect it. If the split occurs in a dentition with a perfected occlusion, the muscles will not be involved, and it will be impossible to make the tooth hurt by biting unless something is placed between the teeth. The rubber stopper from an anesthetic carpule is ideal, since biting on it will spread the split and make it easy to locate the specific problem. The use of fiberoptic light is also an excellent diagnostic tool for locating splits.

A full crown or onlay is usually the treatment of choice for split teeth if the split has not penetrated too far. I am convinced that the majority of split teeth could be prevented if excessive occlusal loads against tooth inclines are corrected early enough.

A fiberoptic examination to detect split teeth is a wise procedure to include in the examination of patients with unexplained orofacial pain or suspected occluso-muscle pain.

Correcting the cause of occluso-muscle pain

If the diagnosis of occluso-muscle disharmony confirms that occlusal interferences are the cause of muscle incoordination, treatment then consists in correcting the occlusal relationships to provide unimpeded access to stable occlusal stops in harmony with centric relation. When centric occlusion is made to coincide with centric relation, the demands on the musculature to hold the mandible at the intercuspal position are eliminated. The goal of a peaceful neuromusculature can be achieved in several ways. Selection of the best treatment method must be based on several considerations including the type of occlusal problem and the patient's health, finances, and psychologic state.

Occlusal interferences to centric relation can be eliminated in a reversible or an irreversible manner. Whether a treatment is reversible is only critical when the outcome of treatment is in doubt. Thus reversible methods of treatment realistically fall more into the category of diagnostic procedures. It's really a way of testing a treatment hypothesis to see if it works before we proceed to do something of an invasive nature. Even used in this context, so-called reversible procedures can lead to erroneous treatment because the elimination of symptoms is not *in itself* a reliable indicator of long-term prognosis and the reason for the result can be easily misinterpreted. The result of any diagnostic procedure has informational reliability only if the diagnostician understands how the physiologic response to the procedure is produced. The closer we can get to the cellular level when analyzing responses, the less need there will be for trial-and-error, empiric treatment.

Empiric treatment is never necessary if a verified diagnosis can be made. There are, however, valid reasons for considering reversible procedures, even when the cause-and-effect relationship has been determined.

The skill and experience of the dentist in treating occlusal problems should always be an important factor. Any dentist who does not have complete confidence in his own ability with occlusal therapy should work first with reversible procedures until those skills are perfected. If there is any question about the health, position, or alignment of the condyle-disk assemblies, alteration of the occlusion should be made on removable occlusal splints until the centric relation position can be confirmed. The use and abuse of occlusal splints is described in detail in Chapter 11. If a positive diagnosis of occluso-muscle disharmony has been verified and there are no intra-articular problems of the temporomandibular joints, careful analysis should be made with mounted diagnostic casts to determine the best method for achieving the desired harmony between the occlusion and the centric relation of the joints.

All treatment planning for occlusal disharmony starts with correct positioning and alignment of the temporomandibular joints. When the casts are mounted in relation to that correct position, the occlusal relationship becomes the variable. The treatment planning efforts are then directed to alter the occlusion so that it conforms with the physiologic position of the joints in centric relation. There are several ways of achieving this, as follows:

1. Selective reshaping of the occlusal surfaces by grinding (equilibration, discussed in Chapter 24)
2. Repositioning teeth so that the intercuspal relationships conform to centric relation (orthodontics)
3. Restorative procedures for changing the contour or position of cusps and fossae to harmonize with centric relation
4. Prosthetic procedures for correcting disharmonies that require replacement of missing teeth, or for some major alterations of form
5. Orthopedic procedures for controlling or directing growth (in children)
6. Surgical procedures for repositioning entire segments of either arch into more ideal arch-to-arch relationships that permit harmony of the intercuspal position with centric relation

Each of the above treatment modalities should be considered when one is analyzing a problem of occlusion. The method or combination of methods that achieves the best result in the most practical manner should be selected as a starting point. The pros and cons of alternative treatment approaches should also be evaluated in light of special needs or desires of the patient before one decides on a choice of treatment.

The analysis of each problem occlusion is based on recognition of the requirements for occlusal stability. These requirements form the basis for both diagnosis and treatment. They are explained in Chapter 27 along with a sequence of procedures that is the key to evaluation of even the most complex problems of occlusion. Further chapters describe each different type of occlusal malrelationship and discuss the treatment considerations that are most applicable for each type of problem. These chapters should be studied carefully and then used as a reference for the specific type of problem when it is encountered.

It should be emphasized one more time that the correction of any occlusal problem is dependent on the proper position and alignment of healthy temporomandibular joints. If there are intra-articular problems that prevent physiologic positioning of the joints in centric relation, the treatment should give priority to correction of the joint problem before treatment of the occlusion is finalized.

REFERENCES

1. Bell, W.: Temporomandibular disorders: classification, diagnosis, management, ed. 2, Chicago, 1986, Year Book Medical Publishers, Inc.
2. Laskin, D.M., et al., editors: The President's Conference on the Examination, Diagnosis and Management of Temporomandibular Disorders, Chicago, 1983, American Dental Association.

SUGGESTED READINGS

Blaustein, D.I., and Scapino, R.P.: Remodeling of the temporomandibular joint disk and posterior attachment in disk displacement specimens in relation to glycosaminoglycan content, Plast. Reconstr. Surg. 78:756, 1986.

Campbell, J.H.: Histopathology of the temporomandibular disk, J. Oral Maxillofac. Surg. 45:M4, 1987. (Abstract.)

Eriksson, L., and Westesson, P.L.: Long term evaluation of meniscectomy of the temporomandibular joint, J. Oral Maxillofac. Surg. 43:263, 1985.

Eriksson, L., and Westesson, P.L.: Clinical and radiological study of patients with anterior disc displacement, Swed. Dent. J. 7:55, 1983.

Isberg, A., and Isacsson, G.: TMJ tissue reactions following retrusive guidance of the mandible, J. Dent. Res. 64(4):764, 1985. (Abstract.)

Kobayashi, Y., Takeda, Y., and Ishihara, H.: The influence of experimental occlusal interference on psychoendocrine responses, J. Dent. Res. 64(4):746, 1985. (Abstract.)

Laskin, D., et al., editors: The President's Conference on the Examination, Diagnosis and Management of Temporomandibular Disorders, Chicago, 1983, American Dental Association.

Lundeen, H.C., and Gibbs, C.H.: Advances in occlusion, Boston, 1982, John Wright–PSG Inc.

Piper, M.A.: Meniscal repositioning in the TMJ after mandibular division nerve block, Washington, D.C., Oct. 1985, Case Reports and Outlines of Scientific Sessions, A.A.O.M.S., p. 94.

Ramfjord, S.P., and Ash, M.M., Jr.: Occlusion, ed. 3, Philadelphia, 1983, W.B. Saunders Co.

Solberg, W.K., Clark, G.T., and Mahan, P.E., editors: Temporomandibular joint problems, Chicago, 1980, Quintessence Publishing Co., Inc.

Ward, D.M.: Changes in synovial fluid pressure due to altered mandibular positions, Am. J. Orthod. 88:86, 1985.

Westesson, P.L.: Structural hard tissue changes in temporomandibular joints with internal derangements, Oral Surg. Oral Med. Oral Pathol. 59:220, 1985.

9

Understanding
and diagnosing
intra-articular problems

It has been my clinical experience that less than 3% of all temporomandibular disorders are primary problems of pathosis of the joint itself. Nearly all but this small percentage of joint disorders result from a primary cause of masticatory muscle incoordination, which may or may not be related to varying degrees of trauma. The presence of abnormally contoured joints is almost always an indication that excessive, *prolonged* forces have been overloading the articular components. The altered contour is usually an adaptive response that can occur in the absence of pathosis or noticeably altered function and is not necessarily a sign of irreversible damage to the joint structures. Although some alteration of connective tissue is an essential precursor to disk derangements, the connective tissue changes are in most instances the result of incoordinated muscle overload and are reversible if the cause of the muscle incoordination can be corrected in time.

Prolonged bruxing or clenching causes a direct adaptive effect on all the bearing areas of the joint, including the disk. Mongini[1] has shown a direct relationship between the wear patterns on the teeth and the remodeling patterns of the reshaped joints. I have observed repeatedly a direct correlation between severe abrasive wear and flattening or lipping of the condyles, with corresponding flattening of the normally convex eminence. These changes in the joints, however, should be considered as the *effects* of incoordinated function rather than cause.

Even though I see many joints with radiographic evidence of altered shape, I have learned that most of these remodeled joints can still function, even while loaded, with complete comfort if they are allowed unimpeded access to centric relation, and excessive muscle forces are reduced to normal tonicity.

If a peaceful neuromusculature is established before adaptive changes in the joint become destructive, even a misshapened joint can function without adverse signs or symptoms. When treating patients with complaints of pain in the region of the joints, we should always suspect the possibility of an intra-articular problem and test to determine if one is present. If we cannot rule out a problem within the joint, we must use whatever diagnostic procedures are indicated to determine the specific type of problem we are dealing with.

UNDERSTANDING DISK DERANGEMENTS

The correct alignment of the condyle-disk assembly is so important to the health and function of the temporomandibular joint that we have included it as a requirement for centric relation. In the differential diagnosis of temporomandibular disorders, five determinations must be made regarding condyle-disk alignment before any treatment modality can be logically selected:

1. Are the condyle and disk correctly aligned in centric relation?
2. If the condyle and disk are not correctly aligned, can the disk be reduced or realigned at any position against the eminentia?
3. If a deranged disk can be correctly realigned in an eccentric position, can the realigned condyle-disk assembly move to the uppermost centric relation position against the eminentia without losing the alignment?
4. If the disk is deranged, what is the cause of the derangement?
5. If correct realignment is achieved, will it hold in function?

Although bilateral load testing of the joints can alert us to an intra-articular problem, it cannot provide all the needed answers to the above questions. Because so many condyle-disk derangements are directly caused by masticatory muscle incoordination, a realistic assessment must be made regarding the role of muscle in each derangement problem. Procedures should be followed to determine whether the problem is truly an intra-articular problem or whether it is primarily an occluso-muscle disorder.

The simplest, most direct method for verifying whether there is an intra-articular problem is by testing with an anterior bite plane. It can also be used to test the stability of condyle-disk alignment in function.

Anterior bite planes test the joints by preventing occlusal surfaces from contacting. If the bite plane is flat and smooth, the anterior teeth can slide horizontally in any direction. This allows the mandible to move unimpeded to the centric relation position if the condyles are capable of moving there. Both vertically loaded occlusal interferences and lateral deviations are discluded by an anterior bite plane, so if tooth interferences of any kind are responsible for the muscle incoordination, harmonious muscle function will be restored when the occlusal interferences are separated. If muscle incoordination was responsible for the disk derangement, the disk will return to correct alignment in function *unless there is structural alteration in the joint that prevents it.*

If the temporomandibular joints can function with complete comfort and harmony while the patient is wearing an anterior bite plane, the prognosis for correcting the intra-articular disorder is excellent when the occlusal interferences are eliminated. If damage has been done to the condyle-disk apparatus that prevents normal joint function from occurring, the anterior bite plane will make the joint *more uncomfortable.* Increased discomfort in the joint while an anterior bite plane is worn requires further analysis to determine whether the discomfort is the result of the condyle-disk derangement or it is caused by pathosis in the joint structure. Each of these two types of potential intra-articular problems is a many-faceted challenge of diagnosis and treatment, but for every type of specific problem that occurs within the joint, there is a specific cause, or combination of causes, and so treatment of such problems can also be specific.

Condyle-disk derangements are understood best if the sequence of events that leads to derangement is understood, along with the potential causative factors that can be responsible for each sequel.

The most commonly discussed type of disk derangement is anterior displacement, meaning the condyle has slipped distally past the posterior band of the disk, or the disk has become displaced forward of the condyle. When this occurs, the condyle loads against the innervated, vascular tissues behind the disk.

Anterior displacement of the disk is usually accompanied by a double click, with one click occurring as the mouth is opened and then a reciprocal click during closing. The clicking sounds are the result of the condyle slipping on and off the disk as the condyle moves forward and back on the slope of the eminence (Fig. 9-1). When a reciprocal click occurs, it may or may not be caused by complete anterior displacement of the disk, and so it is important to determine whether the disk is completely displaced or partially displaced, or whether the clicks are the result of alterations of form at the bearing surfaces. Determination of the specific problem is essential before

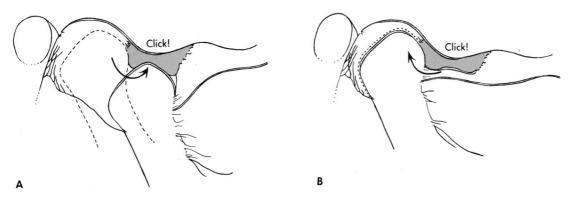

Fig. 9-1. A *reciprocal click* occurs when the condyle clicks onto the disk from a position behind the posterior band of the disk, **A**, and then clicks off the disk, **B**, when the condyle moves back. This occurs as the condyle translates forward and back in opening and closing movements.

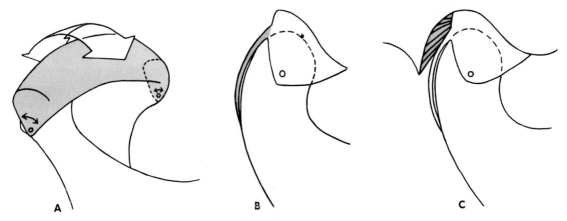

Fig. 9-2. A, The disk is firmly attached to the medial and lateral poles of the condyle by the diskal ligaments. The placement of these attachments permits the disk to rotate from the top of the condyle to the front and back to the top. This allows the disk to stay aligned with the direction of force as the condyle moves up and down the curved eminentia. **B,** The disk is tethered to the back of the condyle by an inelastic band of collagen fibers. The purpose of this ligamentous tether is to prevent the disk from rotating too far forward. Yet it permits the disk to rotate to the top of the condyle. **C,** The superior stratum of the posterior attachment of the disk binds the disk to the temporal bone behind it. The diskal attachment is primarily elastic fibers that keep tension on the disk toward the distal side.

treatment can be selected, but it is only one of the important steps in diagnosis. It is just as essential to determine the specific *cause* of the derangement because different causative factors require different treatment approaches.

The first thing that must be understood about condyle-disk derangements is that muscle must always be involved at some stage, whenever there is incoordination of diskal movement with the condyle. In a healthy joint it is virtually impossible to achieve an anterior displacement of the disk without hypercontraction of the superior lateral pterygoid muscle, and this is even so when the displacement results from a distalizing, traumatic blow to the jaw. The reason for this is that the disk will always move back with the condyle unless it is specifically held forward with a force that is counter to the retrusive movement.

The disk is snugly attached by diskal ligaments that bind it to the condyle at its medial and lateral poles and from its posterior border, and so any movement of the condyle, either up or down the eminence, necessarily pulls the disk along with it (Fig. 9-2). The disk is capable, though, of rotation around the medial and lateral pole attachments, so it can slide from the front of the condyle in centric rela-

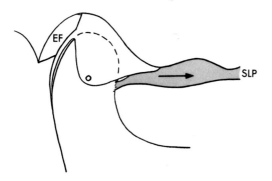

Fig. 9-3. The only forward pulling force that can either pull the disk forward or hold it forward when the condyle moves distally is the superior lateral pterygoid muscle, *SLP*. It is a long muscle and has the capacity to contract to a much shortened length. Its attachment to both the disk and the condyle provides a front tether for the disk, which prevents it from being displaced distally. Contraction of the superior pterygoid is resisted by the constant pull of the elastic fibers, *EF*, that attach to the back of the disk.

tion to the top of the condyle in protrusive. Since the backward pull on the disk from the elastic fibers is constant, the only way the disk can be displaced anteriorly is through superior lateral pterygoid muscle contraction, which must either pull the disk forward of the condyle, or hold it too far forward while the condyle goes backward. There is no other source of anterior pull on the disk other than the muscle that attaches to it (Fig. 9-3).

For a complete anterior displacement of the disk, the superior lateral pterygoid muscle contraction must overpower:

1. The rearward pull of the elastic fibers that attach the disk to the temporal bone and from the superior stratum of the posterior attachment.
2. The inelastic sheet of collagen fibers that attaches the disk to the posterior surface of the condyle and forms the inferior stratum of the posterior attachment.
3. The diskal ligaments that attach the disk to the medial and lateral poles of the condyle.

The superior lateral pterygoid muscle contraction would have to pull forward on the disk as the condyle is moved distally (Fig. 9-3). Otherwise, the disk will simply move distally with the condyle. When masticatory muscle incoordination causes spastic contraction of the superior lateral pterygoid muscle, it unfortunately can provide the forward holding power

on the disk. If the spastic muscle refuses to correctly release the disk as the condyle moves distally, we will have the necessary antagonistic forces in play to *start* the beginning derangement that in time can result in complete displacement of the disk. *Displacement cannot occur however until the connective tissues that bind the disk are torn, stretched, or displaced enough to permit the disk to be pulled off the condyle.*

Since forced distalization of the condyle from improper occlusal inclines can, in itself, be a potent trigger for muscle incoordination, the combined effect of the resultant muscle spasm holding the disk forward, while occlusal interferences force the condyle back, will almost certainly result in a disk derangement if the condition prevails for a period of time. Damage to the disk and its attachments will then contribute to complete anterior displacement.

Mechanical distalization of the condyle is not however a necessary condition for causing a deranged disk. Careful observation will show that the majority of clicking, deranged joints occur with occlusal interferences that displace the condyle *forward* from centric relation. It is difficult to explain how a forwardly displaced condyle can cause its disk to be displaced even further forward so that it ends up completely in front of the condyle. There does not appear to be any mechanical explanation that is related to this common clinical finding, but there is a functional explanation. The incoordinated muscle contraction that occurs with any type of occlusal interference can in itself activate a derangement of the disk. If the superior lateral pterygoid muscle fails to release its contraction, the disk may be subjected to a continuous forward pull that upsets its alignment with the condyle. With hyperactivated muscles pulling the disk forward while similarly hyperactivated muscles pull the condyle back, there is sufficient tension applied to the diskal ligaments to make the disk derangement progress in relation to time and intensity of the pull of the antagonistic muscles.

DIAGNOSING ANTERIOR DISK DISPLACEMENT

A positive diagnosis of anterior disk displacement can be made if:

1. From an open position, the joint clicks during closure or retrusion, and

2. After the click, upward pressure toward the joint causes discomfort, and

3. The joint clicks again on opening or protrusion, and

4. After that click, the joint is more comfortable when upward pressure is applied, and

5. A transcranial radiograph of the joint in the uncomfortable position shows it to be distalized in the fossa.

If all five of the above signs or symptoms can be verified, a positive diagnosis of anteriorly displaced disk is confirmed. The lack of any of these signs, however, does not constitute a negative diagnosis. If testing with upward pressure causes discomfort, the disk may be displaced, even if there is no click and even if the radiograph shows a perfectly centered condyle. Tenderness to pressure indicates a problem in the joint that requires differentiation. Until it is specifically ruled out with other tests, disk displacement must be considered a possibility.

HOW THE DISK BECOMES DISPLACED

Diagnostic accuracy depends on an understanding of the causes and the sequence of events that lead to internal derangements. Let's follow the evolution of disk derangements and relate each type of problem to possible causes. Since distal displacement of the condyle is a commonly found causative factor, it is a good starting point for understanding the mechanics of internal derangements.

DISTAL DISPLACEMENT

One of the most inevitable causes of anterior disk displacement is forced distalization of the condyles. Unfortunately, the concept of a "most retruded" centric relation has contributed to the problem, but several other less obvious causative factors can also be indicted, and most of them are the result of disregarding basic principles of occlusal harmony.

Some leading causes of distalized condyles are the following:

Improper recording of centric relation. If too much pressure is applied to retrude the mandible when centric relation is being recorded, restorative procedures or equilibration will be harmonized to that retruded position and will tend to perpetuate it.

Improper contouring of upper anterior restorations. Thick, convex lingual contours on upper anterior teeth create steep distalizing inclines for the lower anterior teeth to wedge against (Fig. 9-4).

Improper positioning of lower incisal edges. If incisal edges are too thick or are positioned too far forward, they will wedge against upper lingual inclines, forcing the mandible distally.

Failure to mount working casts with a facebow. The more the condylar axis is missed downwardly, the more the arc of closure of the lower cast moves distally. This results in distalizing incline interferences on posterior restorations, thicker upper lingual resto-

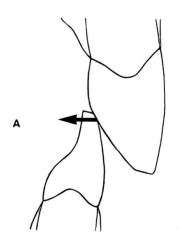
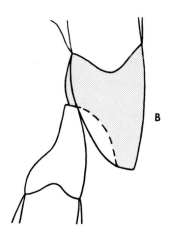

Fig. 9-4. A common cause of distal displacement is improper lingual contour on upper anterior restorations, **A**. Convex lingual surfaces force the mandible distally if contact occurs before full closure. This is a common result of using articulators that have an axis lower than the true condylar axis. Correction of the problem requires reshaping to provide a correct vertical stop, **B**.

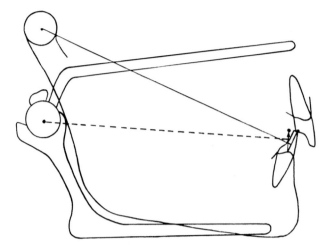

Fig. 9-5. Notice the error in the closing arc when the axis on the articulator is lower than the axis through the condyle. If an open bite record is used for recording centric relation, the error in closure back to the original vertical can be substantial. This illustration compares axis position with one of the most commonly used articulators. Anterior restorations made on such mountings are routinely made too thick in order to engage contact with the improperly positioned lower incisors, which are distal to their correct closing arc.

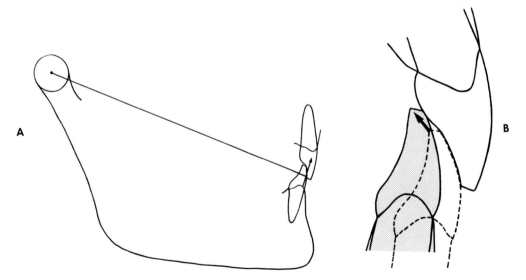

Fig. 9-6. Closing vertical on a deep overbite directs the forward arcing anteriors into a steep incline, **A.** Because closure cannot be completed on the correct arc, the condyles must be displaced distally in order to complete closure, **B.** Anterior tooth mobility is also a possibility.

rations, or forwardly positioned lower incisal edges because when casts are related with an open bite record the lower cast is distal to centric relation when the articulator is closed (Fig. 9-5).

Overclosure of deep overbite. When an anterior deep overbite relationship loses vertical dimension by overgrinding in equilibration or by posterior restorations that do not maintain the correct vertical, the closing arc of the mandible directs the lower anterior teeth into steep upper lingual inclines that produce a distalizing effect on the mandible (Fig. 9-6).

Failure to provide stable holding contacts on anterior teeth. If the lower incisors meet an incline instead of a holding stop, the lower incisal edge has a tendency to wear at a sharp angle, which becomes a distalizing force (Fig. 9-7).

Extraoral orthopedic procedures that result in distalizing force on the mandible. Orthodontic procedures should be related to a centrically related condyle, not a distalized one. Upper teeth that are positioned so that their distal inclines interfere with centric relation closure have the effect of forcing the mandible distally.

Extended use of segmental bite planes. If only part of the dentition is covered with a bite plane at an increased vertical, the covered part is intruded and the uncovered part erupts. If the bite-raising appliance covers the posterior teeth only, the anterior teeth are separated allowing the inward force of the lips to move the upper incisors lingually. As the covered posterior teeth are intruded back to the original vertical, the lower anterior teeth contact against steep inclines, which force the mandible distally (Fig. 9-8).

Loss of posterior support. If posterior support is lost, leaving only incline contacts on anterior teeth, the upper lingual inclines will tend to wedge the mandible distally (Fig. 9-9). This will not be so likely to happen if the anterior teeth are loose, or if anterior contacts are correctly formed to direct forces vertically.

Loss of holding contacts on one side. Lingual incline contacts on one side that deviate the mandible toward the unsupported side can cause distalization of the condyle on the side with no holding contacts (Fig. 9-10).

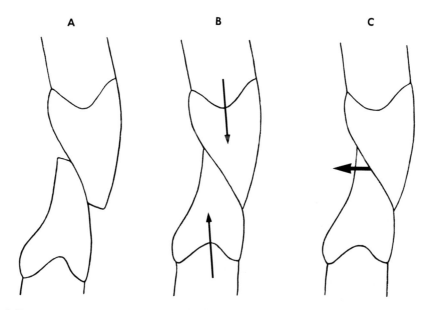

Fig. 9-7. Progressive pattern of wear that commonly occurs when a tight neutral zone is combined with lack of a holding contact on the incisors, **A.** Loss of the labio-incisal line angle resuls in a steep surface-to-surface contact, **B,** with a near-horizontal vector of force when combined with loss of posterior stops, **C.**

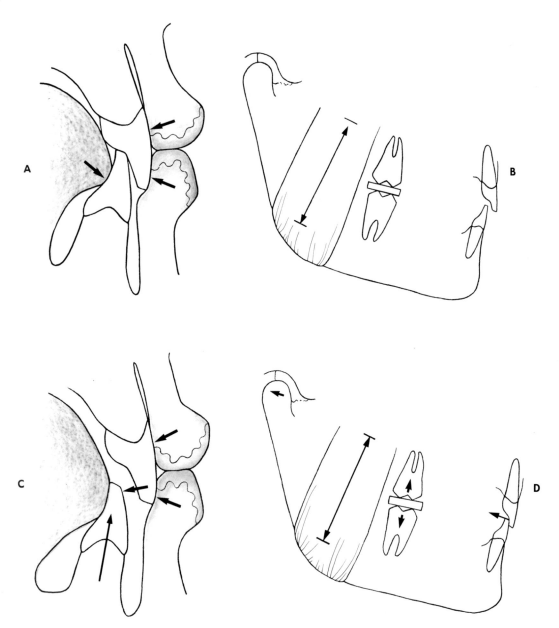

Fig. 9-8. Sequence of changes that occur with extended use of posterior bite planes: **A,** Normal neutral zone position of anterior teeth in a stable relationship with lips and tongue. **B,** Posterior bite-raising appliance separates the anterior teeth and blocks the tongue from resisting lip pressure against the upper anterior teeth. Simultaneously, the elevator muscles are prevented from contracting to their normal power cycle length of contraction, a condition that the muscles will attempt to change by intruding the teeth that are covered by the splint. **C,** With resistance to the inward lip pressure blocked, the lower lip particularly starts to move the upper incisors lingually. The lower incisors may also be moved labially and might erupt slightly because of the loss of their stable holding contacts. **D,** The elevator muscles eventually intrude the posterior teeth so that the mandible-to-maxilla dimension is reestablished, but now the contact is against lingualized upper incisors, which interfere with the arc of closure, forcing the condyles to distalize in order to complete the closure.

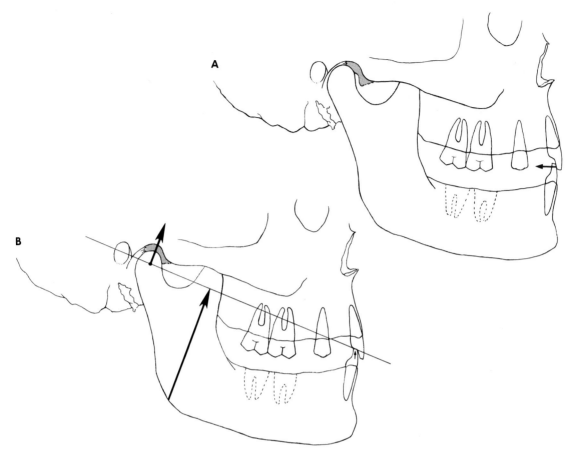

Fig. 9-9. Loss of posterior support has a tendency to distalize the condyles if the lower anterior teeth strike a distalizing incline, **A**. Loss of posterior support is not in itself a cause of distal displacement. If there are stable holding stops on the anterior teeth, **B**, there will be no tendency to distalization of the condyles. The vectors of force will tend to seat the condyles up and forward even in the absence of posterior support.

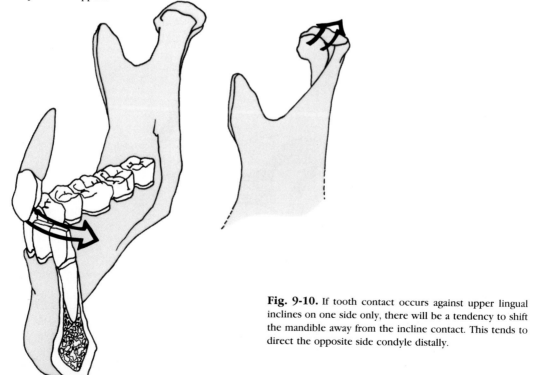

Fig. 9-10. If tooth contact occurs against upper lingual inclines on one side only, there will be a tendency to shift the mandible away from the incline contact. This tends to direct the opposite side condyle distally.

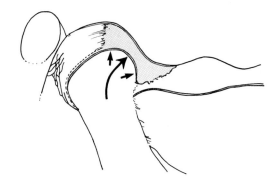

Fig. 9-11. Normal self-centering of the disk takes place if disk and connective tissues are intact and the related musculature is coordinated in function. The biconcave shape of the disk tends to center it on the condyle when the condyle is loaded toward the eminence.

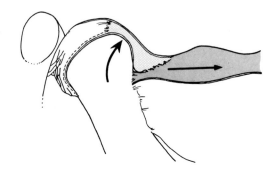

Fig. 9-12. As the disk is pulled forward by a contracted superior pterygoid muscle, its displacement is limited to the extent that its connective tissue attachments allow. But even minimal forward displacement can result in initiating a flattening of the posterior band. As the posterior band thins, it elongates, allowing more forward displacement of the disk.

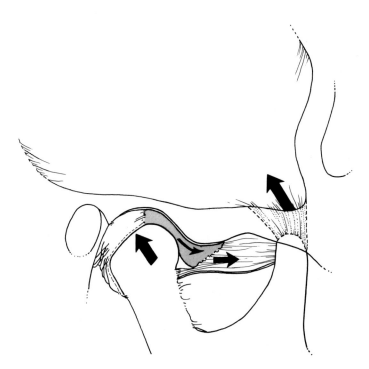

Fig. 9-13. As the posterior band thins, the disk is pulled farther and farther forward by the hyperactivity of the superior lateral pterygoid muscle, while the hyperactivity of the elevator muscles, especially the temporalis, are pulling the condyle back up the posterior slope of the eminentia.

What happens to the disk when the condyle is forced distally?

If you remember that the normal disk has a bi-concave shape with a thick posterior band, it will be obvious that normal elevator muscle contraction would tend to center the condyle into the concave bearing area at the center of the disk (Fig. 9-11). Since elevator muscle contraction pulls the condyles in a *forward,* upward direction against the eminence, normal, coordinated muscle function would always tend toward self-centering of the disk. The concept of squeezing the disk forward like a watermelon seed can occur only if one or both of two things happen: First, the thick posterior band must be flattened to change the biconcave disk so that its posterior border is more convex (Fig. 9-12), or, second, the superior lateral pterygoid muscle must pull or hold the disk forward of its properly aligned relationship with the condyle (Fig. 9-13). Forced distalization of the condyle contributes to both the flattening of the posterior band of the disk (Fig. 9-14) and the muscle incoordination that

displaces the disk anteriorly. When this combination of misdirected forces occurs in the condyle-disk assembly, a sequence of deleterious effects is begun. The amount of damage done is directly related to time and intensity of muscle hyperfunction. It does not occur suddenly. It occurs progressively as connective tissue changes permit more and more displacement of the disk.

If the mandible is forced distally when the interocclusal bite record is made, either of two malrelationships result. If the diskal ligaments are unyielding, the tightly bound disk will move with the condyle as both are forced back and down from centric relation. If restorations are coordinated to this position the distalization of the condyle, combined with the now incoordinated forward pull on the disk from the resultant muscle spasm, puts constant tension on the diskal ligaments. If either diskal ligament becomes stretched or weakened, the condyle can be forced onto the posterior band of the disk.

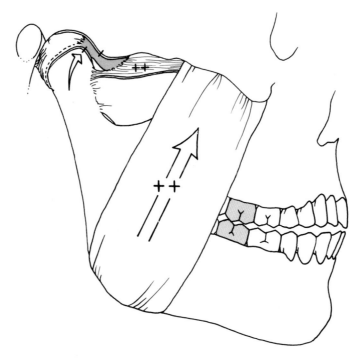

Fig. 9-14. A premature occlusal contact that displaces the mandible distally can intensify the problem of disk derangement because it not only forces the jaw back, but also hyperactivates masticatory muscles to incoordinated contraction. Thus it loads the condyle with extra force against the deranged disk and contributes to progressive further damage to both the disk and its connective tissue attachments.

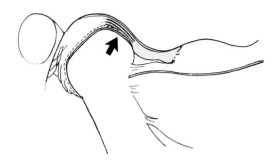

Fig. 9-15. If anterior displacement of the disk progresses slowly enough, it is possible for the vascular retrodiskal tissue to be converted to a fibrous extension of the original disk. This fibrous extension may function acceptably as a new bearing surface for the condyle.

If the mandible is forced into a distalized position by improperly made restorations (or improper equilibration, orthodontics, bite plane therapy, or surgery), the posterior band of the disk in some instances begins to flatten. Because of the triggered elevator muscle hypercontraction, both the intensity and duration of loading on the disk is increased. Clenching or bruxing accelerates the damage done to the disk, and the posterior band is compressed thinner and thinner. The flattening of the posterior band has a lengthening effect on the inferior bilaminar ligament, which allows the disk to move forward. As the posterior band of the disk is flattened by the excessive load on a part of the disk that was not designed for load bearing, two possible reactions can occur in response to the load. Either the tissues can continue to break down or the increased pressure can activate an adaptive response in the cellular components to augment and actually alter the retrodiskal tissues to make them more resistant to the forces now bearing on them. By stimulating the formation of new collagen fibers plus the activation of chondrocytes, a new bearing area can become tough and scar-like and can form as an extension of the disk and provide a comfortable, avascular noninnervated new pad for the condyle (Fig. 9-15). If the condyle can function comfortably against this new extension of the disk, it can be treated in most cases just as if it were a normal joint. Transcranial radiographs often show reduced joint space, but testing the joint with pressure provides the answer to whether the joint relationship is acceptable as a starting point for occlusal treatment. If the joint can re-

sist firm upward pressure and can hinge freely with no sign of tenderness or tension, we have not seen any clinical problems result from harmonizing occlusions to that relationship.

Most joints, however, are not able to adapt to the combination of distalization and muscle incoordination without progressive damage to the articular components. The extent of the damage depends on at which stage the problem is diagnosed and corrected. Conservative treatment is usually successful if causative factors are intercepted and treated early enough. Therapy should always be specifically related to the particular sequential phase that the derangement is in at the time of treatment.

Beginning stage—partial derangement

Until the past few years, the importance of proper condyle-disk alignment was not given enough significance when centric relation was being determined. Many early-stage derangements either went unnoticed because of failure to test the joints with pressure or were actually caused when the mandible was forced back with chin-point manipulation. When the use of arthrograms made it possible to see the disk on a radiograph, it became obvious that disk displacements do occur, and when they do, they must be reckoned with before centric relation can be achieved. From this early awareness of disk displacement grew a disproportionate tendency to treat *most* TMJ disorders as disk displacement problems. Some clinicians were claiming that disk displacement was the cause of more than 80% of all TMJ disorders, but these high percentages were not in line with the clinical experience of many other clinicians who were finding intra-articular problems (other than early muscle incoordination derangements) in approximately 3% of patients with TMJ disorders. I have no doubt that before better diagnostic procedures were developed even highly successful clinicians sometimes failed to recognize internal derangements, but their problems from occlusal treatment would not even remotely approach the 80 percentile failure rate that would be expected if undiagnosed disk displacements were actually as prevalent as claimed.

Although there now seems to be little or no disagreement about the types of internal derangements that occur, there is still some controversy on both the cause and the ratio of occurrence of disk displacements. A better understanding of the beginning stages of disk derangement might shed some light on the confusion because what the dentist does during the early stage of derangement can either correct the derangement or it can cause a slightly deranged disk to become completely displaced.

Since all or most disk displacements (except from trauma) start with a partial derangement of the condyle-disk assembly, a cause-and-effect–based rationale for diagnosis and realignment of partial derangements can affect overall clinical observations by a sizable degree. If the causative factors are understood, disk derangements can not only be corrected, they can also be in most cases prevented.

The method of manipulating the mandible to record centric relation is a key factor in the detection and correction of beginning derangements. Using arthrography combined with fluoroscopy, Gilboe[2] has shown how different forces on the mandible affect the alignment of a partially deranged disk during attempts to record centric relation. Although chin-point guidance can force the condyle completely off the disk (Fig. 9-16), bilateral manipulation can effectively recapture the alignment (Fig. 9-17). Because of the forward component of pressure on the condyle as the mandible is properly retruded up the emi-

nence, the condyle can be pressed against the forward incline of the posterior band of the disk. Pressure against the posterior band forces the deranged disk back and has a tendency to recenter the disk back on the condyle (Fig. 9-17). A slight muffled click is sometimes heard when the disk snaps back onto its concave central bearing area.

My clinical experience has consistently shown that when I find a beginning disk derangement I will almost always find muscular incoordination associated with it, and the muscular incoordination may be the result of occlusal interferences that displace the mandible *either* anteriorly or posteriorly.

If the condyle-disk realignment can be achieved with judicious manipulation and then maintained in comfort overnight with an anterior bite plane, the derangement can definitely be related to muscle incoordination. Analysis of the occlusion should then be done on face-bow-mounted casts related in a verified centric relation to see what must be done to correct the disharmony between the occlusion and the centric relation of the joint. In the absence of pathosis, correction of the occlusion provides an almost immediate response of muscle coordination with stability of condyle-disk alignment if the problem is intercepted at the beginning stage of derangement.

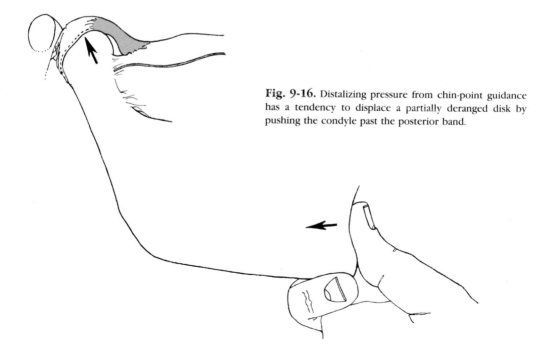

Fig. 9-16. Distalizing pressure from chin-point guidance has a tendency to displace a partially deranged disk by pushing the condyle past the posterior band.

A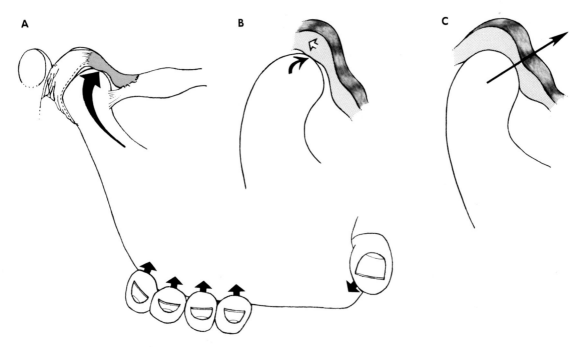

B

C

Fig. 9-17. Proper bilateral manipulation directs the condyle up and *forward*, **A**. This has the effect of engaging the anterior slope of the posterior band, **B**, and wedging the disk back into a centered position on the condyle, which is where it is supposed to function, **C**.

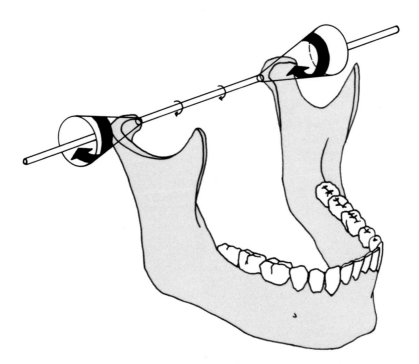

Fig. 9-18. Because the condylar axis is not parallel with the rotational axis through the medial poles, the lateral pole translates forward and downward, even during pure hinge rotation in centric relation. The movement of the lateral pole is reversed on closure. To stay aligned, the lateral border of the disk must rotate forward and back with the lateral pole, while the medial part of the disk stays centered in the medial fossa.

Lateral pole derangement. A large number of beginning disk derangements are the result of slight anterior displacement of the *lateral* part of the disk. I suspect that a major cause of this type of derangement is incoordination of the muscles that are responsible for keeping the disk aligned with the lateral pole of the condyle as it translates during condylar rotation. The lateral poles of the condyles translate on an arcing movement around the rotational axis of the medial poles because the condyles are at an angle to the rotational axis. Even pure opening rotation on the fixed centric relation axis requires a forward, downward translation of the lateral pole as the medial pole remains on a stationary axis (Fig. 9-19).

To maintain its relationship with the condyle in function, the lateral edge of the disk must rotate forward in unison with the lateral pole of the condyle as the mouth opens. It must then rotate back as the lateral pole arcs back and up on closure. Until recently, the mechanism for rotation of the disk on the horizontal plane was not known, but Koritzer's discovery[3] of the mandibular capsular muscle explained how the disk is rotated (Fig. 9-20). The muscle originates at the distal half of the hamular notch and inserts into the anterolateral aspect of the capsule. Its contraction pulls the lateral aspect of the disk and capsule medioanteriorly—the same path that the lateral pole travels on opening.

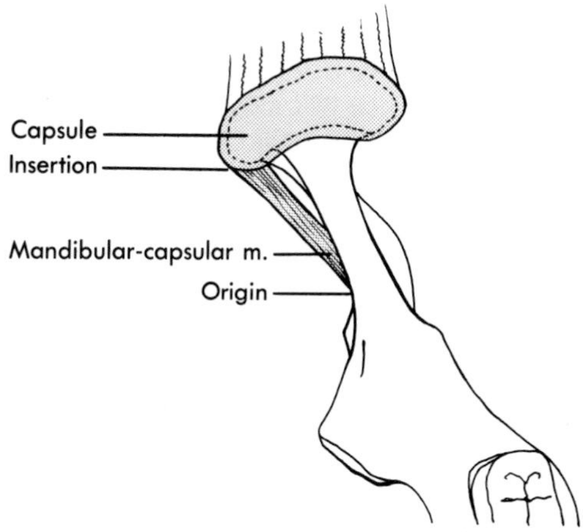

Fig. 9-19. To aid the vertical rotation of the disk, the *mandibular capsular muscle* originates at the distal half of the hamular notch and inserts into the anterolateral aspect of the capsule. Contraction of the muscle pulls the lateral part of the disk down and forward toward its origin. This matches the movement of the lateral pole of the condyle during rotation even on a fixed centric relation axis.

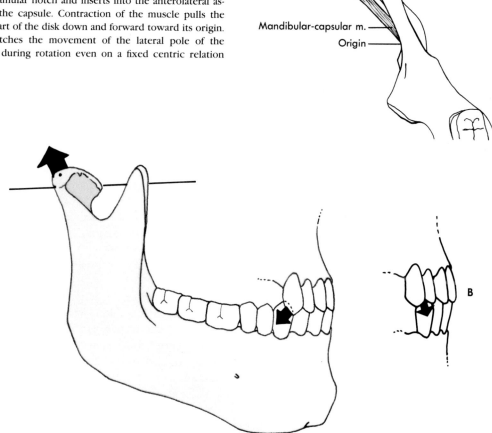

Fig. 9-20. A common cause of lateral pole disk displacement is inclines that direct working-side excursions distally, **A.** Such distalizing functional inclines force the lateral pole back and injure the lateral pole diskal attachments, which allows the disk to then be rotated too far in a medioanterior direction. Correction of the occlusal interference permits lateral excursions in a more anterior direction. **B,** Lateral pole clicks often disappear as soon as this correction is made.

Spastic contraction of the mandibular-capsular muscle has the effect of holding the lateral edge of the disk into a locked forward position. When the mouth is opened, the lateral pole of the condyle clicks into alignment with the disk, but on closure the lateral pole rotates back and off the lateral posterior edge of the disk. Thus opening and closing clicks can be audible even though the medial pole is still centered in its part of the disk because the lateral pole can click each time it crosses the lateral posterior band of the disk. It is not at all uncommon for such beginning disk derangements to occur, accompanied by loud reciprocal clicks, as the result of occlusal interferences that deviate the condyle *forward* of centric relation. It appears that the most common location for interferences that cause such muscle incoordination, is on steep inclines of second or third molars. It is possible that up to 75% to 85% of reciprocal clicks are the result of this type of partial disk displacement, and it would explain why so many clicks disappear when all occlusal interferences to centric relation are eliminated.

Another type of occlusal interference may also initiate a lateral pole displacement often accompanied by a loud pop when the mandible moves laterally. Incline interferences that displace the working-side condyle distally during lateral excursions will directly load the lateral pole with a distalizing force. Such an overload can cause adaptive changes in the shape of the posterior band of the disk on the lateral half. The lateral diskal ligament would also be subjected to stretching or tearing tension by the distalizing force against the lateral pole.

The location for distalizing inclines in lateral excursions can be easily detected with marking ribbon when one guides the mandible into left and right excursions while holding the condyles against the eminentiae. Bilateral manipulation can be used to verify centric relation, and then firm loading pressure should be used to hold the condyles against the slope of the eminentiae during lateral rotation. Any marks on upper distal inclines or lower mesial inclines should be cleared.

Although lateral excursion interferences may be found on any tooth, one of the most common sites for lateral excursion distalizing inclines is at the canines (Fig. 9-20). Especially in a dentition with a steep canine guidance that travels on the distal half of the upper canine, the distalizing effect is easily missed, since it can appear as a normal lateral excursion unless evaluated carefully. It is not uncommon for the loud click or pop to disappear completely as soon as the interferences are corrected.

The effect of muscle incoordination on lateral pole alignment with the disk may also explain in part why damage to the lateral part of the disk is so common and why medial pole damage is so unusual.

In fact, it may also explain a rather typical pattern of disk deformity that maintains the anterior and posterior bands of the disk as separate thickened borders at the medial segment of the disk but gradually coalescing into a single mass at the lateral half of the disk. This would indicate that the medial pole of the condyle is functioning in its proper central bearing area between the two bands of the disk while the lateral half of the disk is locked in front of the lateral pole of the condyle. As the lateral diskal ligament is stretched or torn, the disk rotates more anteromedially into a bunched-up mass that is incoordinated with the lateral pole of the condyle while the disk is still reasonably in place over the medial pole.

There are two reasons why the medial-pole relationship with the disk is so much less susceptible to derangement than that of the lateral pole: The first reason relates to the centering of the rotational axis through the medial pole and so there is no need to translate during a hinge opening, and when the condyle does translate out of the centric relation position the medial pole becomes unloaded because the anterior surface of the condyle bears all the load throughout the protrusive range and shares the load with the lateral surface of the working-side condyle during lateral excursions.

The other reason why the medial aspect of the disk is less likely to become misaligned than the lateral part is that the medial part of the glenoid fossa is narrower and more constrictive and so the disk is cradled in between inclines that are more confining. This cradling makes it more difficult for the disk to be displaced from the medial pole of the condyle. Because the triangular fossa fans out to allow lateral pole translation it provides less confinement for the disk around the lateral pole of the condyle. When these anatomic factors are combined with the greater need for muscle coordination to keep the disk aligned with lateral-pole movement, it is not surprising that the effects of muscle incoordination are usually seen first at the lateral pole. It now appears rather conclusively that complete anterior displacement of the disk does not occur suddenly but is part of a rather consistent sequence of events that generally starts with a slight derangement of the lateral pole and progresses with remodeling changes in the soft and hard tissues until the damage can no longer be repaired by the normal adaptive process.

The sequential remodeling changes that lead to a complete, irreducible disk displacement usually occur in stages because the cellular response to excessive loading of a deranged disk appears to follow rather similar patterns whether the disk is partially or completely displaced. So let's look at what happens in a nonreducing disk displacement.

NONREDUCING DISK DISPLACEMENTS

It is generally accepted that when the posterior band of the disk lies anteriorly to the condyle, a remodeling response occurs in the disk itself. Stimulated by the abnormal loading against the distal slope of the posterior band, the transverse fibers that make up much of the bulk of the band are compressed forward, disrupting the normal fiber pattern of the central bearing area of the disk. It appears that new collagen fibers also proliferate into the mass, making the alteration a true remodeling process and not just a mechanical response to loading. Evidence of chondroblastic activity emanating from the junction of the posterior attachment to the disk could also contribute to an increased thickness of the posterior band.

As the posterior band thickens in front of the condyle (Fig. 9-21), it becomes increasingly more difficult for the condyle to move forward without pushing the disk ahead of it, rather than clicking past the posterior band and into the concave central part of the disk. Condylar loading behind the posterior band also starts to break down the elastic fibers, and so their tension on the disk is gradually reduced, permitting the disk to be pushed further down the eminentia before enough tension is developed to pull the disk back onto the condyle. This results in a delayed click. The amount of protrusive movement the condyle travels before clicking back on the disk has diagnostic significance. The further the condyle must travel forward before recapturing the disk, the more difficult it will be to correct the problem because it is a directly related sign of the degree of damage to the posterior ligament, the diskal attachments, and the deformity of the disk itself. A disk that is pushed forward more than 3 mm. Before recapture is, at best, extremely difficult to treat successfully.

When the condyle can no longer get by the enlarged posterior band, the disk locks the condyle behind it, and so the disk must be shoved along in front of the protruding condyle without ever being recaptured. At this point, the click disappears and the disk displacement is said to be nonreducing. The situation is referred to as a "closed lock" (Fig. 9-22).

One can see that from the beginning slight derangement of the disk, when the condyle rests against the anterior slope of the posterior

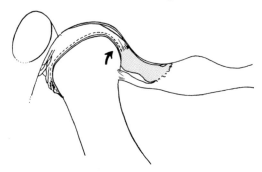

Fig. 9-21. When the condyle slips distally to the posterior band of the disk, elevator muscle pressure loads the condyle against the eminentia, trapping the disk forward. The loading effect is increased by hypercontraction of the incoordinated musculature.

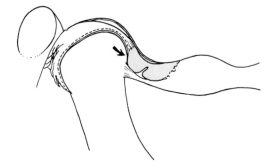

Fig. 9-22. *Closed lock.* The posterior band thickens because of pressure against its distal slope by the forward movement of the condyle, which remains loaded against the retrodiskal tissues. As the retrodiskal tissues are thinned and stretched, the disk is moved ahead of the loaded condyle as it protrudes. Notice how the posterior band is pressured toward the anterior band, eliminating the concave seating area for the condyle.

band, to the partial or complete displacement that gradually becomes irreducibly locked in front of the condyle there is always one necessary component involved in the dysfunction. The essential requirement for progression of internal derangements is incoordination of the musculature. Since incoordination of masticatory muscle function is almost always the result of occlusal interferences, the same occlusal disharmony that displaces the mandible and causes the masticatory muscle incoordination also affects the alignment of the disk. The disk is so dependent on coordinated muscle function to control its alignment on the moving condyle that any incoordination of the musculature can destroy that alignment. Spastic contraction of the muscles attached to the disk pulls the disk forward, rotates the lateral border medially, and then holds it there in direct opposition to the retrusive action of the temporalis muscle. Once the beginning misalignment of the disk occurs, its deformation is perpetuated by hypercontraction of the incoordinated masticatory muscles. In effect, the condyle is being pulled back while the disk is being pulled forward. The articulating surfaces are simultaneously loaded in that malrelated alignment by hyperactive elevator muscles.

Coordination of muscle function depends on precise timing between antagonistic muscles. The timing is necessary to coordinate a smoothly controlled release of contraction to allow a muscle to lengthen as its opposing muscle shortens. Incoordination occurs when the timing of contraction and release is disturbed. The worst incoordination occurs when antagonistic muscles refuse to release at all and thus activate a prolonged contraction against each other. It is precisely this type of muscle incoordination that occurs from occlusally caused displacement of the mandible. It is likewise this type of muscle incoordination that results in the initiation and perpetuation of internal derangements. Consequently, success in treating disk derangements requires the release of muscle hypercontraction and the development of a peaceful, coordinated musculature.

A peaceful neuromuscular system depends on equilibrium of the entire masticatory system. So it cannot be predictably achieved without harmony between the occlusion and the joints. If structural changes have taken place in the joint that prevent it from functioning in centric relation, the problems in the joint must be resolved before occlusal harmony can be achieved. One might wonder how a peaceful neuromuscular system can be attained in the presence of a damaged joint if the occlusal corrections can't be made until the joint problem is resolved. Unless there is a predetermined need for extensive restorative treatment, occlusal changes should be made on occlusal splints until the function of the joint is optimized. Then the necessary refinement can be done directly on the teeth.

Unfortunately, the use of occlusal splints for treating internal derangements is often empiric and unsuccessful. Most of the patients seen in our office for chronic temporomandibular disorders present with several different kinds of occlusal splints, none of which has resolved the problem. When an occlusal appliance is used, it should be prescribed for a definitive cause-and-effect reason, after the specific type of intra-articular problem has been diagnosed and the condition in the joint has been assessed, including the extent of damage.

There are some intra-articular problems that will not respond to any type of occlusal treatment, and so appliance therapy has no value, except as a short-term diagnostic aid or as an adjunct to specific definitive treatment. Nonreducing disk derangements should be evaluated before extended occlusal treatment is initiated to determine:

1. The extent of damage to the disk and its attachments to see if it is too mutilated to respond to noninvasive treatment.
2. The degree of mobility of the disk to see if it is immobilized by adhesions or ankylosis.
3. The role of muscle to see if it is the primary cause of disk immobility.
4. The presence of pathosis to see if it requires direct intervention.
5. The degree of pain or discomfort to determine whether it is tolerable or intolerable.

A combination of diagnostic procedures may be used to learn the true condition in the joint, but even if an obvious internal derangement can be confirmed, there are other factors that must be analyzed before the treatment approach is selected. The level of pain in the joint and the patient's comfort during function are factors that can override other diagnostic findings. The biggest challenge in determining what is best for each patient is in projecting a long-term prognosis if conservative noninvasive treatment is selected for a nonreducible disk derangement.

How does one decide to let a patient function off the disk? The basis for that decision is generally whether function can be restored at a comfortable enough level to be tolerated by the patient. If occluso-muscle harmony can be achieved, adaptive changes in the joint may result in some advantageous remodeling of the articular surfaces. As long as the joint can resist pressure with reasonable comfort and the range of functional movement is acceptable to the patient, we would attempt to treat the problem with occlusal therapy designed to achieve the most peaceful neuromuscular system possible.

When the decision is made to conservatively treat a joint with a nonreducing disk displacement, the patient should be aware that occlusal corrections will have to be made more frequently and over a longer period of time because of the changes that usually occur in the joint as it remodels. As the joint changes, the occlusion must be corrected to the altered position.

The patient should also be aware that degenerative changes in the joint may occur if a disk displacement is not corrected. There can be no guarantee that surgical intervention will not be necessary at a later time.

When should surgery be considered for an internal derangement?

There are two basic reasons for recommending surgery for an internal derangement:

1. *Intolerable pain or discomfort.* Although some patients can function at acceptable comfort levels with a nonreducible disk, many cannot. When acute or chronic pain persists without any expectation of a noninvasive solution and the specific problem can only be resolved surgically, surgery should not be considered a radical treatment.

2. *Conditions that have a high probability of causing progressive degeneration.* Some types of disk derangements tend to cause more degenerative changes than others.

If a safe, simple surgical procedure is all that is needed to correct a problem that would probably cause progressive degeneration, the decision is easier to make. But as the complexity of the surgery increases, the choice of invasive versus noninvasive therapy becomes more difficult.

The inherent reluctance to recommend surgery on the temporomandibular joint is usually based on a very poor record of long-term past surgical success. Several studies have documented that most of the surgerized patients ended up with more problems than the patients who were treated conservatively. The results from surgery were often so disastrous that dentists with experience in treating temporomandibular disorders conservatively were unwilling to risk a surgical invasion of the joint for any reason other than removal of tumors, cysts, or obvious progressive pathosis.

I must admit I was among those who had a very low opinion of surgery as a treatment for TMJ disorders. I still am opposed to the kind of mutilative surgery that was so prevalent. Condylectomies and eminectomies were and still are mutilative treatment, but they were done as routine procedures by some surgeons without any supportable rationale. Condylar shaves and unnecessary meniscectomies have been performed commonly on patients whose only symptom was pain in the region of the joint and the results have not been acceptable. Even when surgery was indicated, it was often done without any regard for postsurgical occlusal harmony, and so patients routinely developed a more intensified muscle incoordination, which accounted for the majority of patients being more uncomfortable 1 year after surgery than they were before.

It would be unfair (and very wrong) to equate today's sophisticated reparative surgical techniques with yesterday's mutilative "cut it off" type of surgery. Just as diagnostic procedures have improved to a highly accurate system of determining precisely what is wrong in the joint, surgical techniques have also been developed to repair defects that cannot heal themselves. The importance of postsurgical care is also better understood now, including the need for occlusal harmony and coordinated muscle function. When an intra-articular problem can be resolved only by surgery, sophisticated diagnostic techniques can verify that decision and so there is no valid reason today for empiric surgery. But there are valid and practical reasons for recommending surgery when it alone can repair a specific defect.

METHODS FOR DIAGNOSING INTERNAL DERANGEMENTS

For treatment to be specifically related to the problem in the joint, the problem must be clearly defined. Sometimes the specific problem is obvious but the *cause* of the problem is obscure, and proper treatment requires knowledge of both cause and effect. There are several methods for diagnosing internal derangements, but a combination of methods is usually necessary to discover all the particulars of the problem in meaningful detail.

Some of the most useful methods, in addition to a detailed history, are as follows:

1. Clinical observation of mandibular movement
2. Manipulative testing
3. Auscultation
4. Palpation
5. Various radiographic techniques
6. Axiography
7. Mounted diagnostic casts
8. Diagnostic occlusal therapy

Clinical observation of mandibular movement

Much information can be learned from careful observation of the path the mandible travels in protrusive and lateral movements in addition to pure opening-closing function.

If the mandible deviates sharply to the side on opening, an anteriorly displaced disk would be suspected on the side to which the mandible deviates. If the patient has difficulty moving toward the opposite side, this would further raise suspicion of closed lock. If the suspected locked side clicks simultaneously with a sudden jerk forward as the condyle protrudes or moves toward the opposite side, it is an almost certain confirmation of an anteriorly displaced disk.

If the mandible follows an erratic figure-S path when attempting a straight protrusion, this could be the result of partial displacement of the disk. If the lateral part of the disk is displaced medially, the condyle must move around the bunched-up segment of the disk. A sudden deviation during any functional jaw movement is an indication of possible disk derangement.

A limited range of movement is an indication that muscle incoordination is involved in the problem, and a progressive deviation on opening would generally be more related to muscle spasm than to a disk derangement.

Manipulation testing

By using bilateral manipulation, one can apply a controlled variation in pressure to load the joints during different jaw movements. By loading the joint through all functional movements, one can find by analysis of pain levels at different positions where the defect is or how the disk is deranged.

Manipulation testing can often be used to distinguish between partial or complete disk displacements with clicking. A reciprocal click on opening and closing can be related either to a complete anterior disk displacement or to partial displacement at the lateral-pole. If bilateral manipulation is used to load the joint while hinging, both the click and the discomfort will disappear if it is a lateral-pole displacement because pressure will tend to hold the disk in place on both poles of the condyles. If it is a complete anterior displacement, loading the joint may eliminate the click, but it will increase the pain because the pressure is directed behind the disk and onto the vascular retrodiskal tissues.

If the lateral part of the disk is displaced and won't reduce but the medial pole is still in place in the disk, loading the joint during a pure hinge movement may not cause discomfort, but lateral movement away from the affected side will cause a buildup of tension and probable pain as the lateral pole compresses the posterior band of the disk in front of the forwardly moving condyle and stretches the lateral posterior ligament while loading them.

Combining manipulative testing with auscultation techniques and with axiographic recordings adds new dimensions to these noninvasive diagnostic methods. If one understands the anatomic changes that occur in pathofunction, structural alterations and misalignments can be detected with a high degree of accuracy.

Auscultation

Much can be learned by listening to the joint. The stethoscope provides a simple method of sound localization that makes quite a few significant joint sounds recognizable. Just as a good cardiologist can detect many different symptoms from listening to the heart, a good diagnostician can learn to relate the joint sounds to specific dysfunction or pathofunction.

TMJ Doppler auscultation is very possibly the most significant contribution to noninvasive differential diagnosis. It is easy to use, is not discomforting to the patient, and is highly accurate when used by a knowledgeable diagnostician. Ultrasound waves are projected into the tissues at a known angle of return so that the depth and location areas of the joint and surrounding tissues can be pinpointed. As the waves return to the transducer, the sound is magnified to become audible. The sound that is generated results from frictional variations of moving tissue parts. The TMJ Doppler method is so sensitive it can detect differences in blood flow. Such sounds are made from the blood cells rubbing against the vessel walls.

Specific areas of the joint can be localized, and with practice, the variations in sound made by different tissues rubbing against each other can be distinguished. The fine crepitus sounds of a slightly deranged disk can be distinguished from a quietly functioning joint that is properly aligned. The coarse, gravelly crepitus of the condyle rubbing against the posterior ligament clearly indicates a displaced disk, and as the tissues break down, the sounds become coarser until they elicit a chirping, squeaky sound indicative of bone-to-bone contact. The sounds heard relate to what is happening in the joint; so once they are learned they are easy to evaluate.

A TMJ Dopplergram (Fig. 9-23) can also

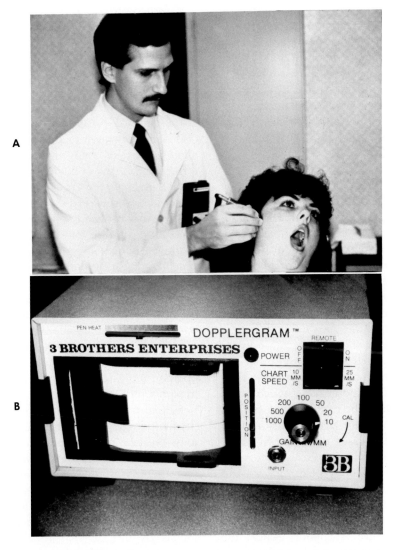

Fig. 9-23. Doppler auscultation is used to listen to joint sounds that result from bouncing ultrasonic waves off moving joint parts and then converting those waves to audible sound, **A**. The Dopplergram produces a hard copy of the wave forms produced, **B**. The feedback is filtered electronically to eliminate nondiagnostic sounds.

serve as a printed record of the sounds in the joint that have definitive diagnostic relationship.

Thanks for this technologic breakthrough in diagnosis must go to Dr. Mark Piper who pioneered the use of Doppler instrumentation and identified the meaning of each sound and each Dopplergram wave series. By comparing the diagnoses made from Doppler auscultation with arthrographic findings and open surgical inspection, he has developed a very reliable correlation between the Doppler sounds and the actual conditions in the joint.

Being noninvasive, the TMJ Dopplergram can be used to monitor the results of treatment as often as desired. It is also a very effective communication device to help patients understand what is happening in their own joint before and after treatment. The TMJ Dopplergram recording can also serve as irrefutable evidence of the condition of any joint at any given time, and it can be used whenever indicated as a part of the patient's permanent record. Later comparative Dopplergrams can be used to evaluate the stability or change that is occurring in the TMJ.

Palpation

As a diagnostic procedure, palpation can be developed to a far greater usefulness than just locating which muscles are tender. The degree of spasm or hyperactivity can be determined, and trigger spots in muscle can be located. Palpation of the lateral and posterior aspects of the joint can alert us to internal derangements or torn diskal ligaments. Palpation can be effective from the skin over the joint or from intraoral vantage points.

Palpation through the earhole is a popular technique but is unreliable because it can easily cause false symptoms of clicking. The tympanic plate of the temporal bone which forms the posterior wall of the mandibular fossa, is a thin curved plate of bone that extends laterally to a position that is easily deformed by finger pressure from the earhole. Pressure forward easily bends the thin bony plate forward and compresses the retrodiskal tissues, forcing the disk forward of its physiologic position. Many normal, healthy joints can be made to click when finger pressure is applied against the tympanic plate, but this does not mean there is a disk derangement.

Radiographic techniques for detecting and analyzing internal derangements

It is not enough to merely know that the disk is deranged. An ideal treatment approach depends on knowing why the disk is deranged and what is necessary to correct the problem. We depend on radiographic techniques as one definitive method for making these determinations but only after we have clinically determined that a problem exists. The radiographic technique should be selected on the basis of a clinical examination that raises specific questions, so that the radiographic technique that will provide specific answers can be selected. The following procedures are used as according to need when an internal derangement is suspected.

Comparative lateral transcranial films. By comparison of the position of the condyle in a verified centric relation with its position in maximum occlusal contact, the direction the condyle moves from centric relation (CR) to centric occlusion (CO) can be a clue to its relation to the disk. *Any* distalization of the condyle in CO indicates the probability of disk derangement or potential disk derangement because of condylar pressure on the posterior band. If the condyle moves *up* from CR to CO, it is an obvious disk displacement. If there is severely reduced space above the condyle in a verified comfortable CR, there is a probability of anterior disk displacement, but adaptive changes may have produced a new, acceptable bearing surface or scar-tissue extension of the disk.

The lateral transcranial films can also be used to show changes in the shape of the condyle or the eminence that are common to complete disk displacement or disintegration.

Observing the films made at maximum jaw opening indicate whether or not ankylosis or hypomobility is a problem.

Simple transcranial films also show most of the pathologic problems that occur on the joint because most pathologic changes occur where the lateral viewpoint can be used to detect them. If simple transcranial radiographs fail to explain the cause of discomfort in the joint and there are reasons for suspecting a probable derangement, arthrograms would be indicated.

Conventional arthrography. The injection of a radiopaque dye into the inferior joint

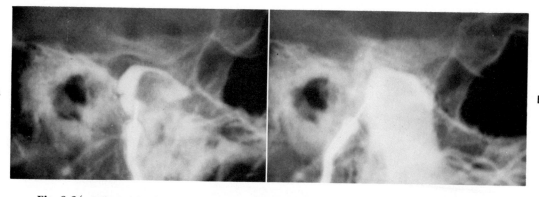

Fig. 9-24. Differential arthrography assesses the role of muscle in disk derangements. **A,** Before nerve block the arthrogram shows disk displacement during attempt to reduce by manipulation. Condyle is forward, but the disk will not reduce. **B,** After blocking the mandibular division of the trigeminal nerve (motor innervation to the lateral pterygoid muscle). Disk has spontaneously reduced even when the condyle is in the fully seated position. This indicates the dominant role of muscle in this derangement.

space between the condyle and the disk makes it possible to see the location of the disk in relation to the condyle. By observing the disk on a fluoroscope as the mandible moves through functional ranges one can learn much about its condition and position in relation to the condyle.

Arthrotomography. By combining arthrography with the laminar assessment capabilities of tomography, it is possible to evaluate the medial-pole relationship to the disk as well as the lateral pole.

Differential arthrography. For assessment of the role of muscle in a disk derangement, the surest, most direct method is the procedure developed by Piper. As soon as a conventional arthrogram is taken, showing the disk to be displaced, the mandibular nerve is anesthetized close to the foramen ovale so that motor innervation to all masticatory muscles is blocked, immediately releasing all masticatory muscle contraction on the side of the injection. If the cause of the disk displacement is muscle spasm that will not release the disk, the disk will immediately move back onto the condyle when the motor nerve is blocked (Fig. 9-24). If the disk spontaneously reduces or if it can be recaptured and kept in place while the condyle returns to centric relation, the disk displacement is then treated as a muscle incoordination problem. If the disk does not move when the injection is made, some type of adhesion or ankylosis of the disk is suspected.

CT scan. Because of its capability to show thin serial slices of the joint area, as well as its capability to depict soft tissue, the computer-

ized tomographic (CT) scan can show views that cannot be seen with conventional radiography. It is also a noninvasive procedure, and so for patients who are allergic to the dye used in arthrography it is possible to evaluate the disk without it. However, at this time it is limited only to static images; so it is questionable if the cost of CT scanning is warranted for joint problems unless there is some special reason for using it (Fig. 9-25).

Axiography

By locating the condylar axis and then precisely tracing the movements of that axis three dimensionally, the movement patterns of each condyle can be analyzed. A healthy, properly aligned condyle-disk assembly follows a classic convex pattern that starts at centric relation and travels a nondeviating protrusive path down the eminentia (Fig. 9-26). Any variation from the norm can be interpreted on the basis of possible causes for the deviated condylar path. Even minute variations can be readily related to structural alterations or misalignments.

With axiography, mandibular function can be analyzed in relation to both the condylar hinge axis and the occlusal relationships. Guided jaw movements can be compared with unguided function, and even the compressibility of the disk can be measured. When axiography is combined with specialized instrumentation, it is possible to relate mounted casts to a condylar treatment position that is predetermined for optimum neuromuscular balance so that adaptive remodeling, realignment, or healing of the articular components will be en-

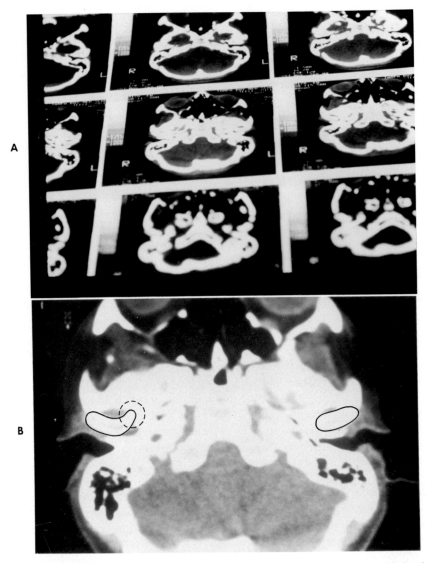

Fig. 9-25. Computerized tomographic scan image of an osteochondroma on the medial pole of the condyle. Routine radiography failed to show a cause for the joint pain, but the patient could not tolerate loading on the joint. Evaluation of horizontal "slices" through the joint showed the problem, which was then successfully treated by surgical removal (by Piper) of the small mass. **A,** Series of slices. **B,** Comparison of condyle shapes. *Condyle's left,* Normal shape; *right,* with extension off medial pole *(circled).*

couraged in degenerating or misaligned condyle-disk assemblies.

Axiographic analysis is one of the most dependable procedures available for determining the precise details of internal derangements. It is also an excellent method for tracking the results of treatment.

Mounted diagnostic casts

Occlusal factors so often play such an unexpected but dominant role in internal derangements it is a mistake to neglect the kind of careful occlusal analysis that is possible only when casts are mounted in centric relation with a facebow transfer.

There is a growing base of scientific data that verify the importance of minute occlusal interferences as triggers for masticatory muscle incoordination. Because of the role that muscle incoordination can play as a causative factor in disk derangements, occlusal interferences that are almost imperceptible can be the primary cause of incoordinated condyle-disk alignment in function. Many of the clicks, pops, and other signs of disk derangements disappear when occlusal interferences ar eliminated, and

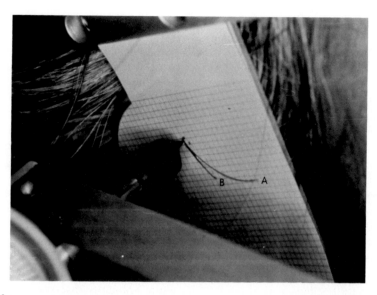

Fig. 9-26. Normal axiograph using SAM system. In protrusion, a healthy joint produces a smooth continuous line from the hinge-axis location down a curved, convex eminentia that normally starts on a steep downward path and then progresses to a near-horizontal pathway *(line A)*. *Line B* represents the path of the condyle as the mandible moves toward the opposite side. A healthy joint tracks the protrusive path for the first 2 to 3 mm before separating into a steeper downward pathway, *line B*. The angle between the two lines is called the Fisher angle.

so a careful occlusal examination should be a routine part of the diagnosis for internal derangements.

When occlusal interferences are on teeth that are loose, the teeth may become depressed or move laterally on contact, making it difficult to find the interference. In fact, it is easy to be fooled because movement of loose teeth is not always observable, especially in the molar area, and when those teeth move out of the way during marking of the interferences, the firmer teeth are often marked erroneously as the premature contacts. Teeth on the stone casts are not depressed or move laterally; so even minute occlusal interferences can be determined precisely if the casts are mounted properly in centric relation.

Dentists who have not been precise in recording and correcting occlusal interferences are generally not aware of the role that minor occlusal deviations can play as potent triggers for muscle incoordination and their effect on condyle-disk alignment.

If a disk displacement is reducible to a verifiable centric relation and when occlusal relationships permit the anterior guidance to disclude the posterior teeth with reasonable correction of posterior inclines, or if there is no evidence of progressive degenerative joint dis-

ease or severe wear problems, occlusal analysis can be done adequately on semiadjustable instrumentation.

If a verifiable centric relation position cannot be found and there is severe abrasive wear on posterior teeth, a more detailed analysis is needed of the joint-occlusion relationship. If there are occlusal plane problems or radiographic evidence of flattened or severely altered joints and the clinical examination shows deviated functional patterns, it may be necessary to start occlusal therapy at a tentative treatment position. The location of that treatment position can be based on axiographic analysis, radiographic interpretation, or clinical judgment. Casts should be mounted in relation to that tentative treatment position for occlusal analysis and fabrication of occlusal splints. For this type of analysis, a more adjustable instrument system has merit.

Diagnostic occlusal therapy

When the problem can be diagnosed as an obvious occluso-muscle imbalance, occlusal correction is a definitive treatment with an expected favorable prognosis. But what about the obvious occluso-muscle imbalance when it is accompanied by an internal derangement, or when there is an expectation of a successful result but with no certainty because of an internal derangement that is caused by suspected muscle imbalance?

If occluso-muscle imbalance is suspected as a definitive part of the total problem, at some point in treatment occlusal harmony must be established. Final occlusal harmony cannot be achieved until the condyle-disk assemblies are in comfortable, physiologic alignment and position. But the reverse is also true: comfortable condyles depend on occlusal harmony to be able to function in that physiologic position. A decision must be made as to how and when the occlusion should be altered. There are three ways to safely alter an occlusion when an intra-articular problem is coincidental to an occlusal problem:

1. Muscle-relaxation splint
2. Diagnostic occlusal equilibration
3. Provisional restorative splint

The selection of which method to use must be based on the conditions present.

Muscle-relaxation splints. Because of the intense nature of some types of muscle spasm, it is extremely difficult to determine accurately the effect of muscle incoordination on derangements of the condyle-disk assembly. This is especially so when structural changes have taken place in the joint. Thus the use of occlusal splints for deprogramming muscle hyperactivity often have great advantage for diagnostic purposes.

The best and most easily fabricated muscle deprogrammer is the anterior bite plane because it discludes all posterior teeth and makes it easier for the condyles to travel up the eminence to centric relation. Its primary value is its effectiveness in distinguishing the difference between an occluso-muscle problem and an intra-articular problem. If muscle incoordination can be ruled out as the source of pain or dysfunction, the joint itself becomes the prime suspect, and diagnostic efforts must then focus on determing what cause-and-effect relationship is responsible for the intra-articular problem. Muscle hyperactivity may still be a factor, but it must now be considered as one part of a combination of factors.

In using any occlusal appliance, the relationship of the disk to the condyle should be determined in advance if at all possible. If a displaced disk can be recaptured and returned to centric relation with the condyle, an anterior bite plane can be used to (1) deprogram the muscles, (2) verify that the condyle-disk alignment is correct, and (3) determine if it will stay that way with coordinated musculature. If the joints get comfortable with an anterior bite plane, a full occlusal splint should then be made immediately, or the occlusion should be corrected directly. The anterior bite plane should not be worn for more than a few days. If comfort can be maintained for a day or so with an anterior bite plane, the diagnosis is made. It is not an intra-articular problem.

If there is radiographic evidence of structural changes in the joint but a tolerable comfort level can be achieved at a determined condyle position, one can fabricate a full occlusal splint to that position to see if adaptive changes will improve the joint structures in a more peaceful neuromuscular environment.

Full occlusal splints used in this manner are partly diagnostic and partly treatment devices because they are made to conform the occlusion to a tentative joint position. The tentative joint position becomes the *treatment position,* and it must be determined very carefully. Information might be gleaned from several different diagnostic methods including axiography and radiography. Careful observation of the most comfortable position and the muscle response to that position are essential to successful treatment.

Since adaptive remodeling of both hard and soft joint structures may progressively alter the tentative joint position, centric relation will continue to change until a point of joint stability is achieved. Thus it is usually more practical to make the necessary occlusal changes in a removable occlusal splint until a stable centric relation is accomplished. Williamson refers to this type of appliance as a superior repositioning splint.

One measurement of the effectiveness of a muscle-relaxation splint should be the degree of comfort it produces. It should not be uncomfortable to wear and should not cause any increase in muscle or joint tenderness. If it does not improve the comfort level, it is not right, and there is no rationale for its use as fabricated. The patient should fully understand the necessity of making occlusal corrections in the splint whenever a comfortable appliance becomes uncomfortable until a final diagnosis of a reasonably stable, comfortable joint position can be verified.

The steps for fabricating muscle-relaxation splints are explained in Chapter 11.

Diagnostic occlusal equilibration. If occlusal corrections are necessary for a dentition that will require extensive restorative treatment, it is often advantageous to the patient to have the corrections done directly on the teeth. This can eliminate the need for wearing an occlusal splint and in many instances can reduce the treatment time. Diagnostic equilibration should be considered only if the following conditions are met:

1. A position of the joint that produces a tolerable level of comfort can be found.
2. Diagnostic casts, mounted to that position, show that direct equilibration can be accomplished with reasonableness.
3. The patient is aware that the equilibration must be followed by restorations that are needed regardless of occlusal factors.
4. The patient is aware that the occlusal treatment may not completely resolve the intra-articular problem. It is a conservative approach with a reasonable expectation of success but no guarantee that further treatment of the joint itself will not be necessary.
5. The patient is aware that corrections will continue to be needed on the occlusion as remodeling changes occur in the joint structures.
6. Final restoration of the teeth will not be attempted until the joint has reached an acceptable level of comfort.

Diagnostic equilibration should not be confused with routine equilibration, related to temporomandibular joints that can be positioned with complete comfort into centric relation. If centric relation can be verified, occlusal corrections can be made on natural teeth, regardless of whether they will need restorations later.

Diagnostic equilibration is usually reserved only for teeth that will later need restoration because an end point of adjustment cannot be accurately predicted with a joint position that is tentative.

Justification for diagnostic equilibration or for delayed restoration of occlusal surfaces includes the following:

1. Teeth that are decayed or damaged or have obsolete operative or restorative dentistry.
2. Teeth that require fixed protheses.
3. Severely worn teeth.
4. Teeth with obvious gross occlusal interferences to the expected final joint position as determined by diagnostic procedures. Such teeth may or may not require restorations at a later time.
5. Teeth that require restorative correction of the occlusal plane.
6. Teeth that require restorative procedures to correct esthetic defects.

Provisional restorative splints. It is not uncommon to find intra-articular problems, including derangements, in patients with grossly unacceptable restorative dentistry. If there is an obvious need for replacement of bridges or multiple restorations, it is sometimes advantageous to remove them and replace them with properly occluded provisional splints on correctly prepared teeth. The provisional splints can be cemented with temporary cement, and all occlusal adjustments can be worked out on them instead of on removable occlusal splints. This method is usually more comfortable for the patient and can be very advantageous to other preliminary mouth preparation needs.

Provisional restorative splints can also be used when periodontal or prosthodontic problems require them as part of preliminary mouth preparations coincidental with therapy for intra-articular problems. The provisional restorative splints can be harmonized to a tentative treatment position just as conveniently as removable splints, and they can be adjusted as needed and can be worn comfortably until the joint-occlusion relationship becomes stabilized.

REFERENCES

1. Mongini, F.: Temporomandibular joint remodeling and degenerative disease, Dent. Clin. North Am. **27**:479-494, 1983.
2. Gilboe, D.: Centric relation as the treatment position, J. Prosthet. Dent. **50**(5):685-689, 1983.
3. Koritzer, R.: Personal communication, Washington, D.C., 1985, Georgetown University.

SUGGESTED READINGS

Dolwick, M.G., and Riggs, R.R.: Diagnosis and treatment of internal derangements of the temporomandibular joint, Dent. Clin. North Am. **27**:561, 1983.

Farrar, W.B., and McCarty, W.L., Jr.: Inferior joint space arthrography and characteristics of condylar paths in internal derangements of the TMJ, J. Prosthet. Dent. **41**:458, 1979.

McCarty, W.: Diagnosis and treatment of internal derangements of the articular disk and mandible condyle. In Solberg, W.K., and Clark, G.T.: Temporomandibular joint problems: biologic diagnosis and treatment, Chicago, 1980, Quintessence Publishing Co., Inc.

Piper, M.A.: Doppler diagnosis for temporomandibular joint disorders, N.E. Dental Seminars Newsletter, Sept. 1985.

Piper, M.A.: Intraoperative assessment of discal position using C-arm arthrography during arthroscopic surgery, J. Oral Maxillofac. Surg. **45**:M3, 1987. (Abstract.)

Piper, M.A.: Meniscal repositioning in the TMJ after mandibular division nerve block, Washington, D.C., Oct. 1985, Case Reports and Outlines of Scientific Sessions, A.A.O.M.S., p. 94.

Wade, M.L.: Assessment of discoplasties and discectomies with alloplastic implants as TMJ surgical procedures, J. Oral Maxillofac. Surg. **45**:M2, 1987. (Abstract.)

Williamson, E.H.: The etiology of temporomandibular pain dysfunction. Part 1. Is it internal derangement? Facial Orthop. Temporomandibular Arthrol. **3**(6):13, 1986.

10

Relating treatment to diagnosis of internal derangements of TMJ

Before treating an internal derangement of the temporomandibular joint, one should diagnose the following:

1. Stage of derangement
2. Cause of derangement
3. Condition of disk and its attachments
4. Condition of bony structures
5. Level of discomfort and dysfunction
6. Potential for further pathosis and its consequences
7. Potential for correction of the problem through adaptive changes

There are many patients who function comfortably with completely displaced disks. There are other patients with almost insignificant beginning derangements who are acutely distressed. Thus the selection of treatment depends not only on the condition of the joint structures, but also on the reaction of the patient to it.

The anticipated prognosis with or without treatment must be related to the choice of therapy. We must determine whether the treatment would be worse than the disease. The age of the patient, the state of health, and the emotional attitude toward the problem are all important considerations in deciding on a course of treatment.

Whenever possible, the safest and most conservative treatment is the adaptive response of the patient in an environment of neuromuscular peacefulness. If damage to the articular parts has not gone beyond the self-repairable stage, treatment will usually consist in correcting structural disharmonies that cause mandibular displacement and its sequel of muscle incoordination. When disk derangements occur, structural disharmonies will be found at both ends of the articulation. Neither the joint nor the occlusion are correctly related, and so both must be reoriented to achieve the necessary harmony in the system. There are many conservative ways this can be accomplished for most patients, but in some patients the disharmony is so great that there are no simple solutions. The goal of treatment, however, remains the same, which is to achieve the best possible harmony between the joints and the occlusion, so that there is no mechanical displacement of the mandible and consequently no stimulus for muscle incoordination that overloads both the joint and the dentition.

If damage to the articulation has progressed beyond the capacity for corrective remodeling, treatment may be required to repair the deformities in the joint in order to achieve an acceptable level of stability or relief of pain.

The most significant improvement in the treatment of internal derangements has come from being able to diagnose more accurately the specific stage of the derangement. Thus treatment can be related to specific causes and effects of a clearly defined problem. The following outline relates each stage of disk derangement to the methods for diagnosing it and the corresponding choices of treatment.

The stages of disk derangement usually occur in a fairly consistent sequence that starts with a beginning partial derangement at the lateral pole. From this stage it is progressive, and the degree of damage in the joint is related to time and the intensity of load that the deranged joint must bear because of incoordinated muscle hypercontraction.

The same type of derangement may occur as the result of different causes. If the selected treatment does not correct the cause of the problem, the effects of treatment will not last. The goal of treatment is to return the system to the best level of equilibrium possible so that the requirements for adaptation are reduced to the minimum.

THE STAGES OF DISK DERANGEMENT

Starting with a healthy, properly aligned condyle-disk assembly, the disk becomes misaligned in stages. The stages result from forces that progressively stretch or tear the ligaments that bind the disk to the condyle. As these ligaments are weakened, the forces against the disk cause it to change shape through adaptive remodeling. The changes in the disk are thus the direct result of misdirected loading by the condyle. Other than extrinsic trauma, the only source of power for loading the joint in any direction is muscle. Coordinated muscle normally loads the joint intermittently, but incoordinated muscle maintains the contracted force against the joint for prolonged periods of time through clenching or bruxing. It is the prolonged loading that causes the adaptive changes to occur in both the hard and soft tissues. The shape these tissues assume is a direct result of the amount and direction of the forces applied through the condyle.

As the disk changes from its normal biconcave shape, its alignment with the condyle becomes less stable until the self-centering concavity is lost entirely and the shape of the disk then becomes itself a major problem. For clarity of understanding and simplicity of communication the progressive joint changes have been divided into *stages*. These stages can apply to either lateral pole derangements or to total condyle-disk derangements. Since most derangements start at the lateral pole, I will discuss that progression first.

LATERAL-POLE DISK DERANGEMENTS

Stage 1. Beginning forward derangement of the lateral part of the disk, the disk is still biconcave in shape.

Stage 2. The posterior band of the disk starts to flatten under the misaligned load of the condyle's lateral pole.

Stage 3. The lateral half of the disk becomes anteriorly displaced in front of the lateral pole of the condyle (reducible).

Stage 4. The posterior band thickens and is pushed forward by the lateral pole of the condyle (lateral pole closed lock).

Stage 5. The posterior band of the disk is folded into the anterior band at the lateral pole. The two bands may then start to coalesce into a single mass. The medial pole is still seated between the two bands on the medial half, but the disk is rotated medioanteriorly.

Stage 6. The disk becomes anteriorly displaced from the medial pole (complete anteriorly displaced disk).

Depending on the amount of distortion of the disk, stages 4 to 6 may be reducible or nonreducible.

The total disk may become displaced by a similar progression, but it appears to be unusual for simultaneous displacement to occur at both poles. The medial collateral ligament is stronger than the lateral attachment of the disk, but regardless of which ligament gives way first, the causative factors may follow a fairly similar pattern.

COMPLETE DISK DISPLACEMENTS

Complete disk displacements can occur in the same pattern as stages 1 and 2.

Stage 1. The condyle loads against the anterior slope of the posterior band of the disk. At this beginning forward derangement of the disk, the disk is still biconcave in shape.

Stage 2. The posterior band of the disk starts to flatten across the full width of the disk.

All the remaining stages of complete anterior disk displacement fall into the variations of stage 6. The progressive changes that occur after the disk is completely displaced forward of the condyle are similar to the changes that occur in lateral-pole displacements, and so the descriptions will not be repeated. An understanding of how adaptive changes relate to the direction and intensity of loading of the joint can be applied to complete disk displacements just as they are to the cause-and-effect sequence of partial disk displacements.

To put diagnosis and treatment into the best perspective, let us start the analysis with the healthy joint. The stages of derangement can then start from that base line.

THE HEALTHY JOINT

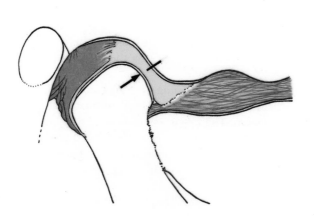
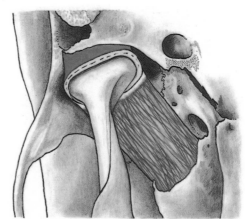

Description. The healthy temporomandibular joint is aligned in the center of its disk. Both condyle and eminence are convex and are covered with intact fibrocartilage over a dense cortical bone layer. The disk is firmly attached to the lateral and medial poles of the condyle. The retrodiskal tissues that compose the bilaminar posterior attachment of the disk are intact, and the superior strata exerts an elastic pull on the disk.

History. Negative. If past symptoms have been observed, they have been corrected satisfactorily. Symptoms of muscle incoordination may be present, even with a healthy joint, and so any muscle problems must be distinguished from signs or symptoms of a true intracapsular disorder.

Clinical observations. Range of motion should be within normal limits. Maximum opening should be in the range of 40 mm or more. Less than a 40 mm opening indicates probable muscle incoordination. Less than a 20 mm opening indicates a possible intracapsular problem. There should be no deviation in protrusive and no restrictions on lateral excursions. There should be no clicks, pops, or grating sounds through the normal range of motion.

Manipulative testing. The joints should be free of any sign of tension or tenderness while firmly loaded by bilateral manipulation. The mandible should be able to hinge freely, protrude, and move laterally while loaded without any sign of discomfort.

Palpation. Negative at joint. Muscles may or may not be tender to palpation.

Auscultation. A healthy joint is well lubricated with synovial fluids. If its fibrocartilaginous surfaces are intact, it should be noiseless in function. TMJ Doppler auscultation produces no crepitus sounds and a TMJ Dopplergram is normal (Fig. 10-1).

Radiographic findings. Condyles are reasonably well centered in fossae on transcranial films. There is a fairly even radiolucent space around the condyles. Both the condyles and the eminence are convex with good cortical bone layer showing (Fig. 10-2).

The use of arthography is reserved for joints that are in probable need of surgery, or when the cause of intracapsular pain cannot be confirmed. Arthrograms of a healthy joint show the disk maintaining proper alignment throughout the range of motion (Fig. 10-3).

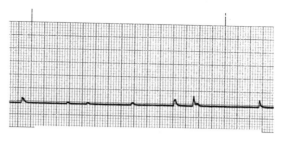

Fig. 10-1. Normal Dopplergram shows a fairly straight base line. This indicates proper alignment of a well-lubricated disk that is intact.

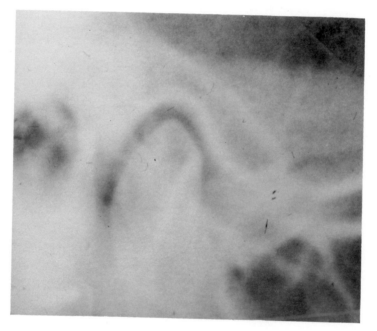

Fig. 10-2. Normal transcranial radiograph.

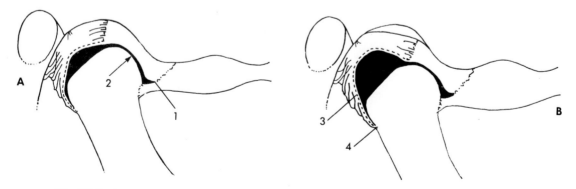

Fig. 10-3. Illustration of an arthrogram of a normal joint shows the extension of the dye in front of the condyle limited to 2 to 3 mm, **A**. The most anterior boundary of the dye represents the attachment of the superior lateral pterygoid muscle to the disk, *1*. The filling of the inferior joint space outlines the contour of the underside of the disk. The normal disk has a concave underside, *2*. As the condyle moves forward, **B**, the disk rotates to the top of the condyle, allowing the dye to bulge out the slackened ligament, *3*, that attaches to the back of the condyle, *4*.

Axiographic recording (Fig. 10-4). The normal, healthy joint starts at centric relation and follows a continuous convex path in protrusive movement. The centric relation point should never be behind the unguided protrusive-path starting point. The orbiting excursive path (balancing side) should track on the protrusive path for 2 to 3 mm before starting the Fisher angle.

Mounted diagnostic casts. If the temporomandibular joints can be positioned into a verifiable centric relation and casts mounted to that position, the occlusion can be related to the physiologic joint position and studied. Problems of malocclusion, muscle incoordination, or excessive tooth wear or mobility often occur before damage to the joint itself, and an occlusal analysis should be done to determine whether correction of the occlusion is needed to reduce the potential for degenerative changes in the joint.

Treatment. From the standpoint of the joint there are no contraindications for starting any necessary treatment of the occlusion.

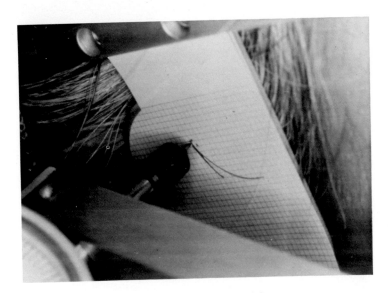

Fig. 10-4. Normal axiograph.

BEGINNING LATERAL-POLE DERANGEMENT

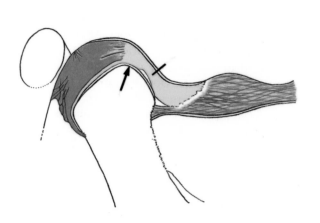

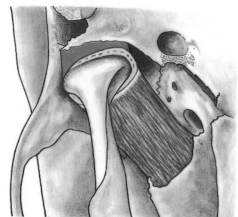

Stage 1. Slight anterior derangement of the lateral part of the disk.

Description. At this earliest stage of derangement, the lateral pole of the condyle loads against the lateral half of the posterior band of the disk. The medial pole is still seated properly in the central bearing area between the anterior and posterior bands of the disk. The lateral border of the disk is held slightly forward of its centered position by muscle contraction that creates tension on the lateral diskal ligament as well as the inferior stratum of the bilaminar zone.

Possible causes. There are at least four ways by which a lateral-pole disk derangement can be initiated:

1. Muscle incoordination
2. Distalization of the working-side condyle in lateral excursions
3. Distalization of the condyle during maximum intercuspation
4. Trauma

The most common cause appears to be muscle incoordination resulting from occlusal interferences, particularly steep incline interferences on second or third molars. But muscle incoordination can result from any occlusal interference including those that displace the condyle forward.

Distalization of the lateral pole of the condyle can occur from occlusal incline interferences that force the rotating condyle back as it moves to a working-side excursion. When this occurs, the major part of the force is loaded onto the lateral pole. However, any occlusal relationship that results in distalizing pressure on a condyle can be a factor. When incoordinated muscle hypercontraction combines with a distalizing displacement of the condyle, the condyle-disk alignment is always in jeopardy, and the lateral diskal ligament appears to be the weakest link.

A lateral blow to the mandible can traumatize the lateral pole on the opposite side, injuring the diskal attachment by compression or sudden stretching. A torn ligament does not hold the disk firmly to the condyle, and so the disk is more susceptible to misalignment from incoordinated muscle contraction.

A blow to the jaw can also compress the retrodiskal tissues, causing edema. The swelling behind the disk can exert a forward pressure against the disk. The lateral half of the disk, being less confined by fossa walls, is more easily displaced slightly forward.

Methods for diagnosing

History. Other than a possible report of trauma, the history is usually uneventful at this stage except for symptoms from muscle incoordination, which can vary from mild to severe. Slight lateral-pole derangements are common in patients with long-standing, undiagnosed TMJ discomfort, but other than an almost unnoticeable, dull click, the joint itself is not generally the specific location of the chief complaint. It is not uncommon for such patients to report multiple attempts at equilibration without ever achieving complete comfort. Complaints of tiredness in the jaw muscles, headaches, and limitation of opening are not uncommon.

Clinical observations. In early stages of lateral-pole derangement the range of motion may appear normal, or it may exhibit any of the typical signs of muscle incoordination such as deviation on opening toward the affected side because of muscle hypercontraction or spasm.

Manipulative testing. With delicate bilateral manipulation a dull, almost imperceptible click may be felt as the jaw is hinged with very light pressure directed through the condyles toward the eminence. After the click occurs, continue to slowly hinge the mandible and test lightly at first for centric relation. If the joint is comfortable and hinging freely, load it with firm pressure to test it. Maintain the loading pressure as the jaw is hinged and tested through the complete range of motion. At this stage of disk derangement, it is rarely a problem to align the disk on the condyle with correctly done manipulation. If severe muscle spasm accompanies the derangement, it may be necessary to deprogram the muscles by separating the teeth with a cotton roll for a few minutes before centric relation can be found and verified. If the disk is correctly aligned, there will be no sign of tenderness or tension when it is loaded.

Palpation. Muscle tenderness to palpation will almost invariably be observed whenever a disk derangement occurs. It will routinely be related directly to the direction of forced displacement of the mandible from occlusal interferences. At this early stage of derangement, palpation of the condyle is generally unremarkable.

Auscultation. Stethoscopic examination is usually negative because the stethoscope is not sensitive enough to transmit the sound of very early derangements. At this stage the posterior band of the disk is still pliable, and there is no staccato to the sound of the shift in the disk. TMJ Doppler auscultation, however, will pick up a fine crepitus sound as the patient opens and closes. The sound produced is similar to rubbing against fine sandpaper. After manipulation into a verified centric relation the joint immediately becomes quiet and reports no sound through the Doppler probe.

A TMJ Dopplergram shows the comparison of wave form before and after manipulation to centric relation (Fig. 10-5).

Radiographic findings. Generally unremarkable. At the early stage the joint is still centered, and no adaptive changes can be noticed on lateral transcranial films.

Axiographic findings (Fig. 10-6). If the mandible is first manipulated into a verified centric relation and that position is used as the starting point for the axiograph, the recording will be normal. If the axiograph is made with no guidance first and then with manipulated movements of the mandible, the axiograph may start out slightly behind the manipulated position. A slight concave path that goes forward even a minute amount before starting down on the convex protrusive path is a nearly certain indication that at least part of the condyle is on the posterior band of the disk rather than in its center. If the clutch is allowed to stay in the mouth long enough to deprogram the muscles, the axiograph will appear normal.

Mounted casts. Casts that are meticulously mounted with facebow and verified centric relation bite record can be expected to show up premature occlusal contacts that displace the condyles from centric relation during maximum intercuspation. The forced deviation may be either forward or backward from centric relation. Any occlusal interference that is capable of causing muscle incoordination is capable of causing a disk misalignment.

Diagnostic occlusal therapy. A flat anterior bite plane adjusted precisely to centric relation can be worn by the patient overnight. If all symptoms of discomfort disappear, the disk derangement was caused by muscle incoordination resulting from occlusal interferences.

Treatment. Occlusal correction is indicated to eliminate all interferences to centric relation and to correct excursive pathways.

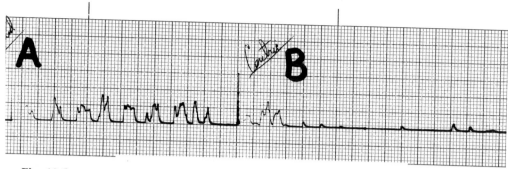

Fig. 10-5. A, Dopplergram shows mild crepitus, which indicates that the condyle is not centered in the disk. Mild crepitus is also indicative of intact bearing surfaces that have not yet begun to break down. This is a common finding with early stages of lateral-pole displacement. **B**, After manipulation into centric relation and separation of the occlusal interferences for a few minutes with a cotton roll between the teeth, the Dopplergram shows a normal base line, indicating a return to proper disk alignment.

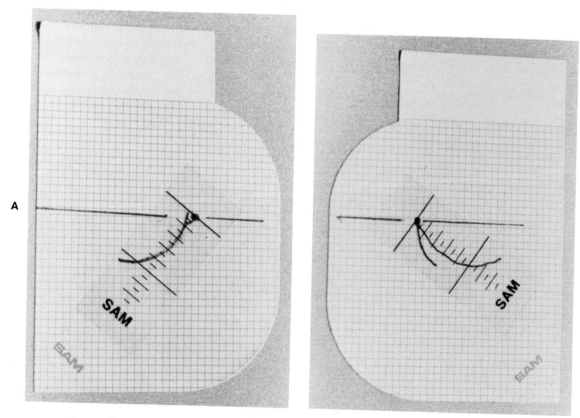

Fig. 10-6. A, Axiograph made without guidance indicates partial derangement with condyle starting out on posterior band of disk. Notice slight concave path at top, which indicates a distalized condyle is moving forward before centering occurs in the disk. After muscle deprogramming by separation of the interference, the axiograph appears normal as shown by the continuous convex path that starts anterior to the original displaced condyle position. **B**, Fisher angle indicates a medial-pole displacement. Lower line, representing the orbiting path, should track on the protrusive path for 3 to 4 mm before separation.

The manipulation into centric relation must be verified to ensure correct disk alignment. The treatment method of choice is selected after analysis of the mounted casts. If interim treatment is needed for some purpose, a full occlusal bite plane can be constructed as a temporary procedure. If a bite plane is used, it should be meticulously adjusted to centric relation, and the anterior guidance on the bite plane should disclude the posterior teeth in all excursions.

Adjunctive treatment for relief of muscle hypercontraction may also be considered, but except in extreme conditions of muscle spasm it is rarely necessary. If a metabolic disorder, nutritional deficiency, or severe emotional stress is related to a lowered resistance to muscle spasm, therapy should be directed accordingly.

Counseling of patients regarding the causes and effects of their disorder is important. The more patients understand about the nature of the problem, the less apprehensive they become. One should start this counseling, however, during the original examination by explaining the symptoms and relating them to the examination procedures.

We have found almost no need for drugs, injections, or any electronic modalities for successful treatment of this stage of disk derangement.

Appliances for positioning the mandible forward are unnecessary at this stage and in fact are contraindicated.

Prognosis. The relief of symptoms and the return to coordinated function usually occurs rapidly and most often within minutes if all interferences to a verified centric relation are eliminated meticulously enough. The patient should be unable to squeeze the teeth together and provoke any tenderness in the joint if correct alignment of the disk has been achieved in harmony with maximum intercuspation at centric relation.

Recurrence of symptoms is common, and the patient should be told to expect some return of the discomfort until both the joint and the teeth stabilize. Follow-up appointments for further refinement of the occlusion should be arranged. This frequency varies greatly depending on the condition of the dentition, but my experience is that a stable comfort level is usually achieved by the third appointment.

At this stage, any stretching of the posterior attachments to the disk or the collateral ligaments appears to be completely reversible.

PROGRESSIVE LATERAL-POLE DERANGEMENT

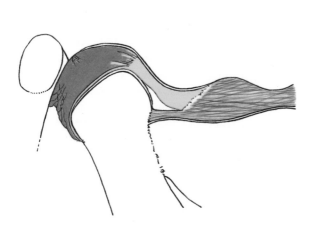 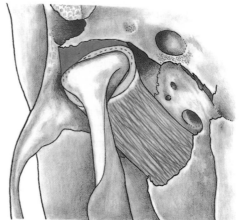

Stage 2. Flattening of the posterior band of the disk.

Description. Because of continuous loading of the posterior band of the disk, it is flattened where it has been compressed by the lateral pole of the condyle. The lateral diskal ligament has been stretched permitting a more medioanterior derangement of the disk, and the flattening of the posterior band also has the effect of lengthening the posterior attachment to let the disk move forward.

Possible causes. The same factors that can cause a beginning derangement at the lateral pole are progressive if not corrected. The flattening of the posterior band is related to the duration and intensity of these same factors (that is, muscle incoordination, distalization of the working condyle in lateral excursions, distalization of the condyle during maximum intercuspation, or trauma).

If distalizing occlusal inclines are present, they should be considered the primary causative factor even though severe muscle incoordination may also be diagnosed. If occlusal interferences displace the condyle forward, muscle incoordination should be suspected as the primary cause of the derangement.

If there is a history of trauma, the derangement may have been initially caused by a torn ligament or by swelling in the retrodiskal tis-

sues. However, normal repair may be hampered by occlusally caused muscle incoordination, and so muscle spasm may be a perpetuating provoker of more serious problems, even though it was not the original cause. Occlusal interference should thus be considered as one of a combination of causes, since it is the principal stimulus for muscle incoordination.

Symptoms. As long as the condyle is still loading the avascular, noninnervated part of the disk, the symptoms will be mostly isolated in muscle. It is doubtful that early flattening of the posterior band will produce pain in the joint itself. Swelling as a result of trauma may produce some intracapsular pain.

Methods for diagnosing

History. For flattening of the posterior band of the disk to occur, the derangement of the disk must have been present for some time. Careful questioning of the patient may reveal a long history of general discomfort, but at this stage most of the signs will be related to muscle. Tiredness from chewing, inability to open wide, occipital or temporal headaches, or any of the myriad symptoms that muscle incoordination can produce may be reported by the patient. Noticeable clicking may be reported but is generally not yet a principal problem.

Patients frequently report multiple equilibrations done by forcing the jaw back. Try to ascertain why the equilibration was done in the first place. Note the patient's comments about the results. Question the patient about when the symptoms first started. If the onset of problems occurred immediately after restorative treatment, we would suspect the introduction of occlusal interferences.

Ask the patient what time of day the symptoms are most noticeable. If discomfort is greatest in the morning, expect a nocturnal bruxing problem. If the patient has worn a segmental bite plane appliance, you will need to determine if it has caused harm.

Clinical observations. The range of motion may be affected as in muscle incoordination.

Look for occlusal wear facets. Particularly look for thick restorations on the lingual of upper anterior teeth as potential distalizing forces.

In patients with deep overbite, look for possible overgrinding that may have closed the vertical into a wedging, distalizing contact on the anterior teeth.

Manipulative testing. Because the medial pole of the condyle is still centered in the disk, it should be possible to manipulate the mandible into centric relation with minimal difficulty. As the jaw is being delicately eased into centric relation, a soft, muffled click can usually be felt as the lateral half of the disk slips back into its centered alignment. If bilateral pressure is then used to load the joints forward against the eminentiae and the pressure is maintained through excursive ranges, there should be no discomfort.

Palpation. Negative except for muscle, unless pathosis or accidental injury induced the derangement. Then joint tenderness may be found.

Auscultation. Loud clicking generally does not occur until the next stage, but there are exceptions. The click at this stage is usually a soft, muffled sound that is easier to feel than it is to hear. Unguided hinging with TMJ Doppler auscultation produces a fine crepitus sound, but such auscultation is quiet with guided, bilateral pressure while hinging is done in a verified centric relation.

Radiographic findings. Still unremarkable.

Axiographic findings. Similar to stage 1, except that the condyle may be further behind the protrusive path line in unguided hinging. Guided pathways will appear normal if centric relation is verified first. By leaving the clutch in for a few minutes, occlusal interferences are disengaged. This deprograms muscle incoordination and may allow the disk to move into correct alignment, even without manipulation. If this occurs, it is a positive indication that the cause of the disk derangement is occlusally caused muscle incoordination.

Mounted casts. Casts mounted in centric relation have, in my experience, invariably shown some occlusal interferences when the disk has been deranged. They should be studied before a treatment approach is selected for correcting the occlusion.

Diagnostic occlusal therapy. If centric relation can be verified, this stage of disk derangement can usually be treated successfully with routine correction of the occlusion. However, whenever changes have taken place in the disk, there may be a corrective remodeling after relief of the incoordinated muscle hypercontraction. These adaptive changes in the disk may slightly alter the position of the condyle in centric relation, thus requiring a corresponding further correction in the occlusion. The potential for joint changes should be considered when occlusal treatment is being planned. Finalization of the occlusion cannot be completed until the joints are stable, and so occlusal splints may be utilized until the stability of the joints can be confirmed (superior repositioning splint).

Treatment. As with stage 1, treatment is directed toward counseling, muscle relaxation, and realignment of the disk. The disk normally aligns automatically when muscle coordination is reestablished. Muscle coordination is almost always reestablished when the occlusion is corrected to permit undeviated access of the properly aligned condyle-disk assembly to centric relation.

Because the condyle has not yet slipped past the posterior band onto the retrodiskal tissues, inflammation of the posterior attachment is rarely a problem that requires treatment unless it was caused by extrinsic trauma.

Prognosis. If muscle coordination is achieved, the prognosis is excellent. All changes in the disk or its attachments seem to be routinely reversible at this stage. The same postoperative considerations apply for both stage 1 or stage 2 derangements.

LATERAL-POLE DISK DISPLACEMENT

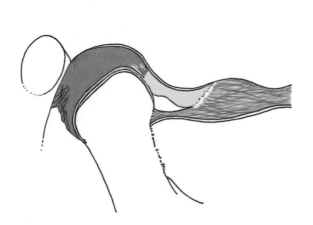

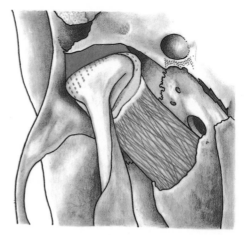

Stage 3. Reducible; displacement of the disk in front of the lateral pole of the condyle.

Description. At this stage of progression, the lateral diskal ligament and the posterior condylar attachment of the disk have been stretched or torn sufficiently to allow the lateral half of the posterior band of the disk to displace completely in front of the lateral pole of the condyle. The lateral pole of the condyle now rests against the vascular, innervated tissue behind the disk. The medial pole is still positioned in its concavity between the anterior and posterior bands of the disk, but from that point laterally the disk has been deranged anteromedially.

As the jaw opens and the lateral pole translates forward and downward, it clicks past the posterior band and recaptures its position in the central bearing area of the disk. Once recaptured, the condyle-disk alignment is maintained until the final closure, at which point the lateral pole snaps past the posterior band and back onto the retrodiskal tissues.

It should be remembered that this lateral pole displacement would not occur without help from incoordinated muscle contraction that tightly holds the disk forward, rather than controlling its timed release as the lateral pole moves back.

Possible causes. Stage 3 results from the same causes that initiated stages 1 and 2. It is the result of progressive damage that occurs when those causative factors are not eliminated in the earlier stages. The degree of damage may be intensified and accelerated by heavy bruxing or clenching, factors that even a conscientious dentist may not completely control.

Signs and symptoms. At this stage, there may be some discomfort in the joint itself, and there will almost always be typical signs and symptoms of muscle incoordination, but the chief complaint is often related to a loud, staccato click or pop when chewing. My current opinion is that the louder the click or pop, the more likely it is that it is a lateral pole disk displacement and not a complete disk displacement. When the disk is held so firmly in place by the medial pole and the confining walls of the fossa at the medial pole, the rigidity of the disk is increased. As the translating lateral pole builds up pressure against the posterior band of the rigidly held disk, it produces a loud pop from the increased friction when it does snap past the thickened posterior band.

Remember that the lateral pole of the condyle must travel forward and downward on opening even if the medial pole stays on a fixed axis of rotation. The angle of the condylar axis in relation to the horizontal axis of rotation will determine how much the lateral pole must move. The shape of the condyle may also influence the signs or symptoms, and certainly the different possibilities of how the posterior band is shaped or flattened by various degrees of loading from the condyle will affect the way it responds to condylar movement. The posterior band may be flattened to a shape that does not produce a noticeable click. There are endless possibilities of remodeling changes that can occur to both the hard and soft tissues of the joint. I diagnose best when I develop a visualization of what is happening in the joint, based on the signs and symptoms that I can correlate. By observing signs of occlusal wear and relating it to a visualization of how the joint would necessarily respond to the mandibular deviations that such faceted inclines would direct, I can generally get a mental picture of the direct relationship between the signs and the symptoms.

Observing signs and symptoms is also critical from a prognosis standpoint. If there are signs of elevator muscle hypertrophy, I know I am dealing with a habitual bruxer or clencher and I also know the joint is subjected to prolonged heavy loading. Thus different patients at the same stage of disk derangements may have different requirements for treatment and may have different expectations for a successful prognosis.

Based on the signs and symptoms, try to form a mental picture of what you think is happening to the joint. Then test your tentative hypothesis with different diagnostic methods until a clear pattern emerges.

History. Similar to stages 1 and 2, except that the patient may have been aware of symptoms longer. The jaw may periodically lock or "go out." Patients sometimes report embarrassment from the pops that occur in the joint during eating.

Clinical observations. Look for the same factors that are evident in the first two stages. Observe the direction of displacement of the mandible as the patient squeezes from the first point of contact. Particularly look for any occlusal configuration that forces the condyle distally when the teeth are intercuspated, or when the mandible moves laterally.

Manipulative testing. At stage 3, the diskal ligaments have now become stretched or torn enough to allow the lateral part of the disk to move in front of the condyle. For this reason the method of manipulation is critical. If the mandible is pushed back, the condyle can easily be forced past a partially deranged disk, completely displacing the disk forward of the condyle. Correct manipulation can, on the other hand, reposition the condyle in the center of the disk. Bilateral manipulation should be done delicately, with the teeth apart. As the jaw opens or moves slightly forward, a click can generally be felt as the lateral pole crosses the posterior band of the disk. As the condyle engages the anterior slope of the posterior band of the disk, upward, forward pressure through the condyle causes the disk to snap back into its centered position.

A characteristic of this stage is that the disk is recapturable. Evidence of recapture is the total absence of any discomfort or tension when loaded, as the jaw goes through a full range of motion. There should be no sign of discomfort at any jaw position after the disk is aligned. If upward pressure is applied *before* the condyle has clicked onto the disk, there should be some evidence of tenderness or tension especially in lateral excursion away from the affected side. This is diagnostic.

Palpation. With the jaw open, external palpation of the posterior surface of the condyle may elicit some tenderness, but, generally, palpable tenderness is confined to the muscles that always seem to be involved in incoordinated function whenever we find a disk derangement.

Auscultation. Clicks on opening and closing can usually be heard through a stethoscope. On TMJ Doppler auscultation there is a fine crepitus as the jaw opens until the lateral pole crosses the posterior band of the disk, and the joint becomes silent until the lateral pole clicks on closure as it crosses back over the band. The crepitus sound is then heard again as the condyle rubs against the posterior ligament.

The combination of Doppler auscultation and manipulation is an excellent diagnostic process for lateral-pole displacement. The joint must be both comfortable and quiet while loaded during hinge movements before we can accept a diagnosis of correct disk alignment. Any crepitus indicates lack of correct alignment. By observing where the crepitus occurs in relation to clicks or to discomfort, we can rather clearly visualize what is happening within the joint regarding condyle-disk alignment.

Radiographic findings. Because the medial pole is still centered in its part of the disk, the condyle will appear properly positioned in the fossa on lateral transcranial films. At this stage, we would not yet commonly see remodeling changes in the condyle or the eminence and so the joint may look normal with routine radiographic techniques.

Axiographic findings. There is a range of possible configurations that may be recorded on an axiograph. If the condyle is distally displaced, there will be a concave path recorded that starts behind the convex protrusive path. But in many condyle-disk misalignments, the disk is held forward by muscle rather than the condyle being distally displaced. In fact, if the medial pole is correctly centered while the lateral half of the disk is anteriorly displaced, the effect on the axiographic tracing may be negligible during this early stage of displacement.

Mounted casts. Other than from accidental injury, I have never seen a condyle-disk derangement initiated in a perfectly occluded dentition. Occlusal interferences can work in two different ways: They can either force one or both condyles distally when the teeth are occluded in maximum intercuspation, or they can displace the condyles forward or lateral to centric relation. Either type of mandibular displacement can be easily missed in the mouth because of tooth mobility, but either type of displacement can cause the muscle incoordination that is necessary for holding the disk forward. Mounted casts permit a three-dimensional analysis of the relationship between the joints and the occlusion. But remember that the accuracy of this analysis is dependent on the accuracy of the verified centric relation bite record used with a facebow.

It is from the analysis of mounted casts that you decide on the choice of occlusal treatment. If you decide on the use of a bite plane, it can be made on the articulated casts.

Diagnostic occlusal therapy. The disk displacement in stage 3 is reducible. You must learn whether it will stay aligned in function after you recapture it. The best way to determine that it is is by use of an anterior bite plane, worn overnight. If the disk does not become displaced while the anterior bite plane is worn for 1 or 2 days, you can safely assume it will stay aligned if the occlusion is corrected.

Treatment. If prolonged use of a bite plane is desired, it should include the full occlusion harmonized to a verified centric relation. Do not use any segmental bite plane for more than a few days. Once the diagnosis is confirmed by the anterior bite plane, it is logical to proceed with your selected occlusal treatment. Finalization of the occlusion may not be possible, however, until some remodeling occurs in the deformed disk. If the occlusion is to be restored, equilibration should be done first until a point of stability is reached. This can be done directly or on a superior repositioning splint.

I evaluate the stability by observing the amount of correction needed at intervals of 2 to 4 weeks. When minimal or no adjustment is required and the joints are comfortable, the final stage of occlusal treatment can be completed.

Prognosis. If a peaceful neuromusculature can be established, the prognosis for stage 1, 2, or 3 is generally excellent. The patient should be checked periodically for any signs of occlusal changes that could trigger a recurrence of the derangement.

LATERAL-POLE CLOSED LOCK

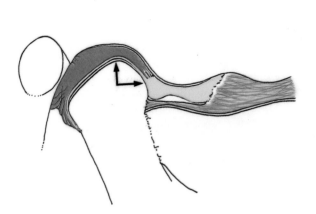

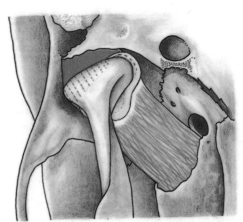

Stage 4. The lateral part of the posterior band thickens and locks in front of the lateral pole of the condyle.

Description. The disk is rotated medioanteriorly so that the medial pole of the condyle is still between the anterior and posterior bands of the disk, but the posterior band crosses over the condyle diagonally, putting the lateral part of the posterior band in front of the condyle. In a continuous progression from stage 3, the condyle starts to push the outer part of the disk forward during function. This causes the posterior band to thicken as it is bunched up in front of the forward-moving lateral condyle pole. Proliferation of fibroblasts and chondrocytes forms a progressively thicker mass, which makes it more difficult for the condyle to get across the posterior band and into the central bearing area of the disk. Elevator muscle hypercontraction holds the condyle so tightly against the retrodiskal tissues that they start to thin. The muscle contraction also makes it more difficult for the condyle to release pressure against the back of the raised posterior band to get past it, and so it pushes the posterior band and the lateral border of the disk forward.

Possible causes. Since this stage is the progressive result of the same untreated factors that started the derangement in the first place, the increased severity of the damage to the joint is in direct proportion to the time

and intensity of muscular loading of the deranged parts. The changes in the joint are merely adaptive. The tissues conform to the direction and amount of overload. Thus at least two causative factors will almost always be present as the articulating mechanism breaks down. They are (1) occlusal surfaces that displace the position or alignment of the condyle-disk assembly and (2) muscle hypercontraction to overload the deranged articulation.

When one looks at the joint and finds the disk locked in front of the condyle, the erroneous assumption is often made that the anteriorly displaced disk is the cause of the patient's problem. The anteriorly displaced disk is not the cause of the problem. It is the result of the problem. Unfortunately, the misplacement of the condyle onto the vascular, innervated retrodiscal tissues does now become a cause of discomfort as well as a cause of breakdown of the posterior ligament and damage to the disk, but it is a secondary causative factor that would not have occurred without the primary cause of muscular overload on a joint that is displaced at maximum intercuspation. This perspective is easier to appreciate if one realizes that there is no loading of the joint when the teeth are apart. When the teeth are together, the condyle must go where maximum intercuspation directs it—or misdirects it. Loading of the joint occurs in that relationship.

Signs and symptoms. At this stage, discomfort in the joint area becomes a rather commonly reported symptom. Deviation toward the affected side on opening, plus an aberrant protrusive path, is common. The clicking or popping that occurred in stage 3 has now stopped, or it may be delayed, and so the click occurs at a wider opening, in protrusive position, or in lateral excursions to the opposite side.

Any of the signs or symptoms related to muscle spasm such as headache, trismus, or retro-ocular pain may be evident. Generally the combination of pressure on the retrodiskal tissue and the pain of muscle spasm commingle to produce a vague discomfort in the generalized area of the joint and all its related musculature. In many instances, this combination of pain is further intensified by odontalgia that results from the same muscle-contraction overload the joint is subjected to, applied to the teeth and supporting structures. Thus, although the basic problem may be the same, the symptoms can vary greatly from patient to patient, depending on which tissue or which part of the system cries the loudest, so to speak. The part that hurts the most is not necessarily the part that has the most damage.

History. Similar to previous stages, except the patient may report having had a click that disappeared.

Clinical observations. The protrusive path will generally be irregular because the condyle must move around the enlarged lateral part of the disk. The range of motion is usually limited but that may be difficult to gage. Clenching often causes some discomfort in the joint. Look for the same occlusal factors that cause earlier stages of derangement.

Manipulative testing. The jaw may hinge freely, an indication of a normal joint, but testing with bilateral manipulation will almost always cause tension or tenderness when the deranged joint is loaded. Even if there is no discomfort when testing at the uppermost hinge position is performed, maintaining the pressure during protrusive or lateral excursion will cause a stretching of the posterior ligament that will have some degree of tenderness as the lateral border of the disk is forced forward ahead of the condyle.

At the early stages of thickening or development of a closed lock, the lateral pole can usually click onto the disk at some point of condyle translation. By using very delicate manipulation, the condyle will not be loaded too firmly to keep pressure on the back of the disk, preventing its recapture. If the disk can be recaptured, pressure should then be applied after the click is felt, to test for alignment (Fig. 10-7). Keep the teeth separated, and hinge the jaw a few times while pressure is applied. Place a 3-inch cotton roll between the teeth covering the biscuspids on both sides so that no tooth contact can be made. Then close the jaw into the cotton roll. Verify that the joint is comfortable, and then have the patient squeeze on the cotton roll. If the joint stays comfortable while squeezing on the cotton roll and the disk does not displace with firm clenching, the chances are good that the disk has not yet been severely damaged and that occlusal correction will be the treatment of choice.

Palpation. Muscle tenderness will normally be found in the pterygoid complex as well as any of the masticatory muscles that are involved with prolonged contraction. Palpation of the lateral pole via the posterior joint space when the jaw is open often reveals some tenderness.

Auscultation. TMJ Doppler auscultation when the disk is displaced will detect different degrees of crepitus that results from the condyle rubbing on the posterior ligament. The greater the breakdown of the ligament or the surfaces of the condyle, the more coarse is the crepitus.

By listening to the joint through Doppler sound magnification while it is being manipulated, you can easily tell when the condyle clicks onto the disk. If it then becomes quiet during rotation of the condyle in the disk, this confirms that the alignment is acceptable. If at any point the condyle loses its alignment with the disk, the crepitus sounds will recur.

Radiographic findings. Even at this stage of displacement of the disk, lateral transcranial radiography may show what appears to be a normal joint. Because the medial pole of the condyle is still reasonably centered in its part of the disk, the relationship of the lateral aspect of the condyle may also appear normal.

Arthrography can be used to show the anteriorly displaced disk but if a transcranial alignment is limited to one angulation, it may appear as if the entire disk is completely displaced, rather than just the lateral half. Tomographic arthrography can be used to evaluate the medial pole alignment for a more accurate

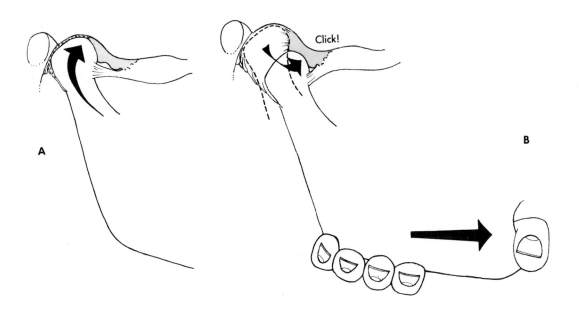

Fig. 10-7. A, Early stage of development of a closed lock. The lateral pole is loaded behind the posterior band of the disk. Elevator muscle hypercontraction locks the condyle against the retrodiskal tissue and the posterior slope of the disk. **B,** *Gentle* manipulation with the teeth separated encourages the jaw to move forward or laterally, or both, until the condyle clicks onto the disk. Recapture is often helped when the jaw is opened wider during excursions. Bilateral hand position should be maintained, but no pressure is applied until after the condyle clicks back onto the disk. **C,** After reduction occurs, the condyle is gently loaded toward the posterior slope of the eminentia. The pressure is gradually increased in an attempt to lock the disk in a centered position on the condyle. *While maintaining forward pressure* against the slope, slide the condyle-disk assembly up the slope with gentle upward pressure applied in small increments. Do not load in any direction quickly because it activates muscle contraction. The condyle should push against the posterior band as it goes up to centric relation. **D,** When it feels as though the condyle-disk assembly is against the bony stop (at the medial pole), test the joint for centric relation by loading. Any sign of tension or tenderness indicates that centric relation has not yet been achieved. When the condyle can rotate while loaded with complete comfort, it is an indication that the disk has stayed in line to the centric relation position. It still must be tested to see if it can stay aligned during function. Biting on a cotton roll, **E,** or use of an anterior bite plane can be used to test.

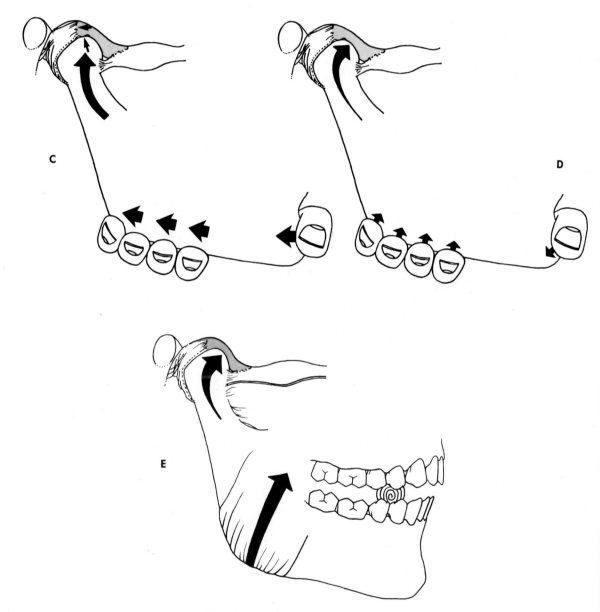

Fig. 10-7. For legend see opposite page.

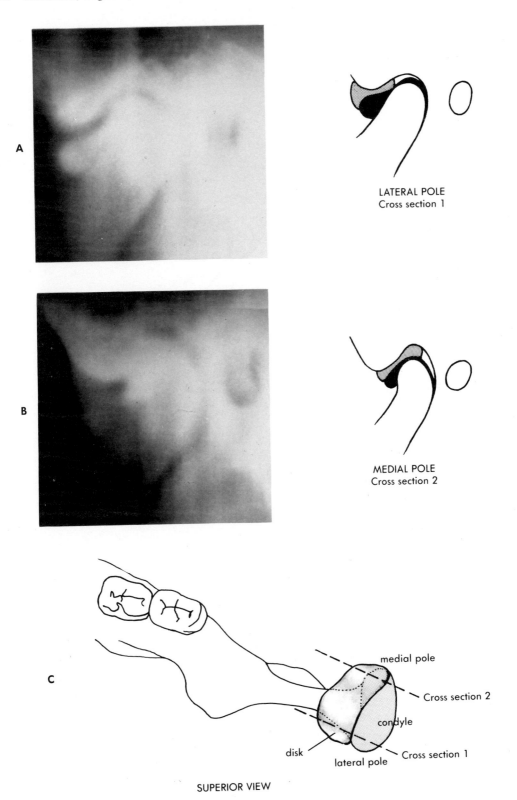

A

LATERAL POLE
Cross section 1

B

MEDIAL POLE
Cross section 2

C

medial pole

Cross section 2

condyle

disk

lateral pole

Cross section 1

SUPERIOR VIEW

Fig. 10-8. A, Arthrotomography of the lateral pole shows a displaced disk. **B,** Medial-pole assessment shows the same condyle with disk reasonably well aligned. **C,** Superior view shows how cross sections are imaged on tomogram.

radiographic survey (Fig. 10-8). A suspicion that only the lateral half of the disk is displaced should be considered whenever there is a disk displacement in a well-centered condyle.

Axiographic findings. Recordings made at this stage may give one or more indications of lateral-pole closed lock if the recordings are made without manipulative guidance.

1. Lateral view of protrusive path will show the point at which the lateral pole crosses over the posterior band.
2. Dorsal view will almost always record a deviation laterally as the condyle negotiates around the thickened lateral border of the disk.
3. The Fisher angle may be steeper than normal for the lateral excursion away from the affected side.

It would be very unusual to find a normal axiograph in all three recordings. A normal recording may be achieved if the condyles are manipulated onto the disk and centric relation is verified. If the recordings are then made while the joints are kept loaded, the axiograph may show normal pathways.

If a normal axiograph can be recorded with bilateral loading of the joints, the patient should then be allowed to make the same movements unassisted. If the unassisted movements then exactly duplicate the guided movements, occlusal treatment can be started with an expected good prognosis. If the patient's unguided movements do not go all the way to the verified centric relation, there are changes in the disk that will require time to correct with adaptive remodeling. In this patient, occlusal therapy would be started at a tentative treatment position. A superior repositioning splint would usually be the choice until the joint stabilizes. If posterior reconstruction is indicated, the occlusal corrections may be made directly in most cases because the teeth will need restorations later regardless of what adjustments are done.

Mounted casts. As changes in the disk occur, the central bearing area of the disk may be altered in shape so that the condyle does not completely seat even though we may achieve a realignment of the condyle in the disk. For this reason, the centric relation bite record must be made with extremely careful verification. If *any* sign of tenderness or tension is present, we cannot consider the bite record as final. Consequently the mounted casts must be re-

lated to a tentative treatment position. That position will change slightly as the condyle-disk assemblies adapt to the realignment. As the joint changes occur and the centric relation position stabilizes, new bite records will be needed. Nevertheless, the mounted casts are necessary for determining what must be done to the occlusion to bring it into harmony with the joints, starting with a tentative treatment position when necessary.

Diagnostic occlusal therapy. The anterior bite plane is still the method of choice for determining whether the joint can function comfortably on the disk if there are no occlusal interferences and the disk can be recaptured. If the disk stays aligned and the joint stays comfortable for a day or two, the bite plane should be changed to a full occlusion. It should be equilibrated meticulously to the comfortable joint position and should be readjusted at intervals of 2 to 4 weeks until the joint appears stable. At that point, final occlusal treatment can be completed.

Treatment. Even though considerable changes have taken place in the joint, the deformation through this stage is transient. Some derangement of fibers may occur in the disk, but it is still elastic enough to revert to its initial fiber pattern if the load is redirected through the central bearing area. In treating this stage of derangement, special care must be taken to ensure that the entire disk has been recaptured and that it stays recaptured during function. Unless the joint is tested carefully with very firm bilateral pressure, it is easy to be misled about the alignment of the disk because the medial pole can still accept most of the load without discomfort. TMJ Doppler auscultation is excellent for verifying that the disk has been completely recaptured because crepitus will be eliminated or barely audible crepitation will be noticed that probably results from some residual changes in the surface of the disk.

Prognosis. Any disk that is recapturable and will stay aligned in function when tested with an anterior bite plane has a good prognosis if the cause of the derangement is eliminated. If realignment is combined with perfected, nondeviating occlusion, both mechanical displacement and muscle incoordination are eliminated as causes. A continued good prognosis depends on maintaining that relationship.

LATERAL-POLE DISK DISPLACEMENT, NONREDUCIBLE

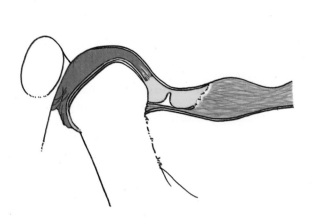
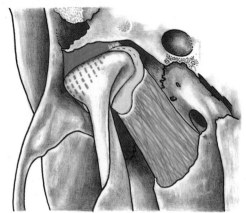

Stage 5. The lateral part of the posterior band is compressed into the anterior band, obliterating the central bearing area for the lateral pole of the condyle.

Description. The combination of pushing the thickened posterior band ahead of the lateral pole, and the damage to the posterior and lateral diskal ligaments from direct loading of the retrodiskal tissues, has caused an irreducible displacement of the lateral segment of the disk. As the two raised bands of the disk are pushed together, they coalesce into a single mass. The lateral pole of the condyle can no longer get past the thickened mass, and if it could, there is no concavity for it to rest in. The lateral border of the disk is now severely rotated medioanteriorly, but the medial pole of the condyle is still seated between the anterior and posterior bands of the disk.

Possible causes. This stage is simply a progressive consequence of leaving the earlier stages untreated. The causes are the same as for the original beginning derangement, compounded by the progressive damage to the ligaments and to the disk. Just as in stage 4, the adaptation of the disk is a response to excessive loading on the misaligned condyle-disk assembly. Understanding of the cause of this problem requires an understanding of each of the previous stages of derangement. When the

progressive nature of the disorder is understood, it will be obvious why early diagnosis and treatment is in the patient's best interest.

Signs and symptoms. Muscle incoordination is virtually always present at this stage, and so any one or more of the muscle-related signs or symptoms are usually present. There is generally some discomfort in the joint, and it may range from mild to severe, depending to a large extent on how much the patient keeps the teeth clenched together.

Patterns of occlusal wear or mobility can generally be related to the joint displacement and the muscle incoordination just as they were in the earlier stages.

Limitation of jaw movements becomes a more common sign as the damage progresses.

History. The patient may or may not be aware of when the problem started, but in many cases he or she will remember the specific episode that started the *acute* phase of discomfort. Unfortunately, many acute phases are stimulated by simple dental procedures. Just keeping the mouth open for a prolonged period of treatment causes a loss of muscle memory patterns to maximum intercuspation. Until those engrams are reestablished the jaw will tend to close into a superior axis closure, and the patient will feel interferences that have been there all the time but were not noticed at the engram pattern of closure into centric occlusion. When the newly found interferences combine with the muscle fatigue from prolonged jaw opening, the result is often acute muscle spasm that in turn intensifies the already advanced stage of the joint disorder. The dentist who may have had nothing to do with causing the major breakdown in the joint gets the full blame for a problem that may have been progressing almost unnoticed for months or years.

The above scenario is avoidable if dentists will follow the advice given repeatedly in this text: Include a screening history and a screening examination of the temporomandibular joints as part of the initial complete examination that should be done on every patient. The routine use of TMJ Doppler auscultation would easily point out and document that a patient had a temporomandibular disorder before any treatment is initiated. The problem can then be discussed with the patient right away; thus this very common accusation is avoided. Furthermore, the dentist is immediately alerted to a problem that should be diagnosed so that the condition of the joint can be considered in the total treatment planning.

Just as causative factors start at stage 1 and progress, the complete history does also. Stage 5 is a continuation of that same history.

Clinical observation. One of the most significant observations to make is the path the mandible follows in straight protrusive. To move forward, the condyle must deviate around the thickened mass at the lateral half of the disk. A sudden lateral movement during protrusive movement is usually followed by a return movement back to the protrusive path. On opening, the jaw may follow a somewhat figure-S path with deviation toward the affected side.

Manipulative testing. Loading the joint at this stage will almost invariably produce some degree of discomfort or at least a feeling of tightness. Oddly enough, the joint may rotate easily during hinging, giving the appearance of normalcy until pressure is applied. If loading does not cause tenderness in a pure hinge movement, it will almost certainly produce discomfort in excursions.

Palpation. When the jaw is opened, the fingertip can be placed into the indentation behind the condyle. From that position the posterior aspect of the condyle can be palpated. The finger can also be rolled around onto the lateral pole as the jaw opens and closes so that light pressure is applied to the ligaments behind the disk. This will generally produce some degree of tenderness if the disk is displaced forward. It may also be possible to feel the aberrant movement of the disk.

Palpation of the masticatory muscles virtually always produces varying degrees of tenderness that relates to the direction of mandibular displacement.

Auscultation. No definite click can be heard at this stage because there is no recapture of the disk. TMJ Doppler auscultation produces definite crepitation through hinging and all excursions. The coarseness of the crepitus sounds vary, increasing as the articulating surfaces progressively break down.

A Dopplergram records a constant pattern of disk misalignment (Fig. 10-9).

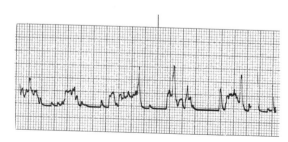

Fig. 10-9. Dopplergram showing moderate crepitus. Notice higher level of wave form with wider base as compared to normal flatter base line or slightly elevated peaks of mild crepitus. Moderate crepitus indicates beginning breakdown of one or more articulating surfaces; most likely site is on the posterior ligament where the displaced condyle is loaded.

Radiographic findings. At stage 5, there is usually some displacement of the condyle, and so lateral transcranial films may show a noncentered relationship with the fossa, but if the medial pole is still reasonably well positioned, the lateral transcranial view may appear normal. The disk derangement can be seen on an arthrogram. Arthrotomography may show the more accurate diagnosis because the medial-pole relationship can be compared with the lateral pole displacement.

Blink mode CT scan can show serial slices of the disk but does not (at this writing) show the dynamic positioning in function that can be seen in arthrography.

Axiographic findings. Because the condyle is nonreducible, it must push the disk ahead of it in protrusive or wide opening movement. This will most often result in a shortened protrusive path on the axiograph unless the lateral diskal ligament has become severely stretched or torn. The horizontal recording is almost always some degree of a figure S.

The condyle may in some instances partially ride down the thickened border, producing a very steep, short protrusive path. The Fisher angle is usually greater whenever the condyle is not traveling normally in its disk.

Mounted casts. It is not possible to record a correct centric relation because proper condyle-disk alignment is not achievable. If casts are taken at this stage, it must be remembered that the jaw relationship is a tentative treatment position and will change if the joint disorder is corrected. Nevertheless, it is often helpful to mount casts at this tentative position in order to study the occlusal relationship. Even with a deranged disk, it may be possible to reduce muscle hyperactivity by improving the occlusion. The casts can be used as a starting point for making a muscle-relaxation occlusal appliance.

Use of special instrumentation (MPI or CMP instruments) for this type of problem enables us to track the positional changes in the joint from the starting-treatment position. It also permits the recording of a treatment position that can be reasonably well determined from interpolation of axiographic and radiographic recordings.

Diagnostic occlusal therapy. Even though we may determine that we are dealing with a stage 5 lateral-pole displacement, we cannot jump to a conclusion that it must be corrected. Many such derangements result in remodeling of the disk with formation of a new and acceptable bearing area on what was formerly vascular retrodiskal tissue. If the condition has been present for a long time and the adaptive response is acceptable, we may do the best service for the patient by working with that altered position to quiet the hyperactive musculature. To test such a hypothesis, a full occlusal bite plane can be made at the joint's most comfortable relationship. Careful monitoring of the bite appliance is necessary to keep it adjusted as changes take place in the joint. If the patient can be made comfortable and functional with such an appliance, occlusal therapy can then be finalized on the dentition as needed. The occlusion should still be harmonized to the most superior position of the condyle-disk assembly against the eminentia.

If the joint discomfort is intolerable or there is a probability of progressive damage in the joint without correction of the disk derangement, occlusal treatment alone would have to be considered as a compromise.

Treatment. If the medial pole of the condyle is still positioned reasonably well between the anterior and posterior bands of the disk, the chances for correcting the problem are still favorable because it is rather certain that enough of the posterior ligament is still intact to maintain disk function if the lateral half of the disk could be recaptured.

At this stage there are four common reasons why recapture of the complete disk may not be achieved:

1. Muscle spasm or fibrotic contracture of the superior pterygoid may be holding the disk forward and will not release it.
2. The lateral diskal ligament and parts of the posterior ligaments may be torn or too stretched or too weak to pull the disk back.
3. The coalesced anterior and posterior bands may have formed a solid mass that leaves no place for the lateral pole to seat.
4. Any combination of the above.

The role of muscle can be assessed by use of the differential arthrography technique described in Chapter 9. Quite often muscle release can be achieved through use of a muscle-relaxation splint.

If the shape of the bunched-up and remodeled disk will not allow recapture, you can surgically reshape it by shaving off layers of the dense fibrocartilagenous buildup (meniscoplasty). Piper has advocated doing this through a surgical microscope so that the contour of the disk can be assessed and corrected all the way to the medial pole. Plication of the posterior ligament must also be done to reposition the disk back on the condyle correctly. All the reshaping is done on the superior surface of the disk and a sheet of Teflon is placed for approximately 5 months in the superior cavity to prevent adhesions from forming between the disk and the eminence. After a new dense fibrous surface layer has organized, the Teflon sheet is removed.

The advantage to such surgery is that it preserves the disk and along with it the synovial lubrication that nourishes the bearing surfaces of the articulation. Without the disk, the bony surfaces must adapt in shape to each other, and so some degree of degenerative joint disease is almost a certainty as the rounded condyle flattens and loses height.

Loss of condylar height appears to be progressive and, as it occurs, continues to load the most posterior teeth in increasing amounts. The classic picture of severely worn upper lingual cusps is a definite indication of a flattened condyle and eminence that typically occurs when the disk is lost and degenerative joint disease has occurred. For that reason, surgical correction, when needed, is a conservative choice of treatment *if it is done meticulously.*

If the comfort level of the patient is not a problem and the age of the patient and suspected duration of the derangement indicate an acceptable remodeling within the articulation, occlusal therapy appears to be the usual treatment of choice. If a peaceful neuromuscular system can be established, damage in the joint is normally reduced to a level that is maintainable by periodic occlusal corrections.

Prognosis. If the disk can be saved and repaired either surgically or through adaptive remodeling, the source of nutrition to the articulating surfaces is preserved in the synovial tissues. Lubrication to the joint is also sustained. Thus, if the disk can be maintained in a peaceful environment of coordinated musculature, the prognosis is good for long-term health and function of the joint.

If the disk is lost or remains displaced, the probability of degenerative joint disease is high though it is often possible to control the degenerative changes at a reduced level if muscle incoordination can be diminished. Reducing the excessive load that results from prolonged hypercontraction often produces dramatic results.

COMPLETE ANTERIOR DISK DISPLACEMENT

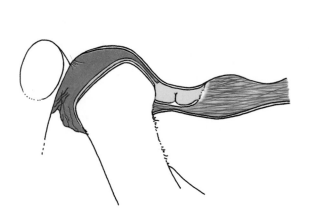

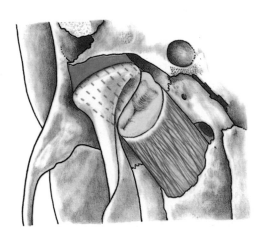

Stage 6. The disk is completely displaced forward of the condyle.

Description. The diskal ligaments to the lateral half of the disk have now been torn or stretched far enough to allow severe medio-anterior displacement of the disk. As this has occurred, more and more of the posterior band of the disk has been progressively forced in front of the condyle until the entire posterior band has become anteriorly displaced. The condyle is now loaded entirely on the vascular, innervated retrodiskal tissues. In protrusive movements of the condyle, there is now a progressive tendency to force the disk ahead of the condyle while compressively loading the entire width of the posterior attachments to the disk.

Scapino has shown that the posterior attachments to the disk may respond to this forward thrust by moving the condylar attachment of the posterior ligament up the posterior surface of the condyle through bony remodeling at the attachment site. A response to excessive traction can occur at both the condylar attachment of the posterior ligament or at the temporal bone attachment of the superior strata of elastic fibers. The apparent reason for moving the anchorage of the elastic fibers forward rather than just allowing them to stretch is probably related to the common finding of fi-

brosis in the elastic fibers of deranged disks. The fibrosis would remarkably reduce the elasticity of the posterior attachment and thus increase the tension on the site of the attachment at the temporal bone. The forward migration of the temporal attachment does not seem to require bony remodeling as is seen in the forward repositioning of the inelastic collagen fibers that attach the disk to the condyle.

This forward attachment of the elastic fibers might also occur as a result of fibrous ankylosis initiated by intracapsular bleeding. Piper reports a fairly common occurrence of such ankylosis or adhesions in the retrodiskal tissues that have been damaged by direct loading from the condyle when the disk is anteriorly displaced.

Variations of disk displacements

There are many variations of complete disk displacement. In the early stages, the medial pole is usually reducible even if the lateral pole is not, because at the medial pole the anterior and posterior raised bands are often still intact and separated long after the lateral part of the disk has become irreducibly altered. The separation of the two bands provides a concave bearing area for the medial pole of the condyle just as long and only as long as the condyle can get past the posterior band and

overcome the forward push of the motive condyle against the disk, the clicks disappear, indicating a closed lock. From that point on, the potential for degenerative joint disease increases.

Methods of diagnosis

History. When the disk is anteriorly displaced, the history may include a long recital of a series of events that started years before with the placement of a crown or a fixed bridge. It may have started when a dentist adjusted the occlusion and may have progressed through years of unsuccessful attempts to treat the TMJ. If one analyzes such histories, it will become apparent that the beginning of a very high percentage of such problems started with some alteration of the occlusion. From that point on the progression of symptoms often parallels the progressive stages of disk derangement.

If the history reveals the use of bite splints, the splints should be examined for accuracy. My experience is that very few occlusal splints are in correct harmony with a verified centric relation. Patients also frequently report with positioning devices that do not correctly relate the jaw to an acceptable joint alignment. It is important to evaluate each appliance to be able to understand the results reported in the patient's history.

A complete history should be encouraged, and every rational description should be evaluated to see if it can be explained and related to the current condition. Knowing that disk displacement is at the end of a sequence of progressively deformative derangements, the history can provide many helpful clues regarding the course of the disorder and its effect on the patient.

Clinical observations. On opening, the jaw will normally deviate toward the side of the displacement, sometimes very sharply. If the displacement is reducible, the reducing condyle may suddenly jump forward, bringing the mandible back to a more centered relationship after reduction. If it is nonreducing, the mandible will stay deviated on opening.

It is often difficult or impossible to move the jaw laterally away from the displaced side, but it moves easily toward the displaced side.

If reduction occurs immediately on opening, the posterior attachments to the disk are still reasonably intact. If reduction does not occur before the condyle has translated forward about 3 mm (about two finger widths of opening), the posterior attachment is probably damaged too badly to recapture the disk and have it stay recaptured during function.

Manipulative testing. If the condyle is loaded with upward pressure against vascular innervated tissue, there will be some response of tenderness or tension. With newly displaced disks, pressure may cause sharp pain. The discomfort must be distinguished from that caused by applied tension against the contracted lateral pterygoid muscle or from pathosis, but any sign of discomfort should alert us to the possibility of disk displacement. Use of other diagnostic tests may be necessary to distinguish between the other possibilities of pathosis, or muscle bracing.

If a disk displacement is confirmed but loading of the joint does not cause discomfort, it is an indication that adaptive remodeling may have altered the retrodiskal tissues to form a new bearing-pad extension of the displaced disk. Even though the disk may be displaced, the new alignment may be acceptable if it permits medial-pole bracing of the condyle. The same may be true in some bone-to-bone relationships if the articulating surfaces of the condyle and eminence have remodeled to hard eburnated surfaces.

Manipulative loading of the joints is an extremely valuable test to determine whether an acceptable level of comfort can be achieved with whatever conditions are present.

Palpation. Finger pressure through the skin depression behind the condyle when the jaw is open will usually provoke tenderness in varying degrees depending on the condition of the posterior attachment. Palpation of masticatory muscles is almost certain to cause a tenderness response in the incoordinated muscles that are involved in the jaw displacement.

Auscultation. TMJ Doppler auscultation is an almost foolproof method for determining whether the condyle is or is not on the disk. It is also very reliable for determining the precise point of recapture and displacement when the disk is reducible because the reciprocal clicks are audible even when they cannot be heard through a stethoscope.

The character of the amplified crepitus sounds are also diagnostic: The more coarse

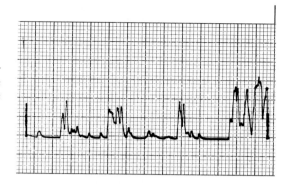

Fig. 10-10. Dopplergram showing coarse crepitus similar to what is commonly seen when there is damage to the retrodiskal structures that permits some bone-to-bone contact.

the crepitus, the more there is breakdown of the posterior ligament. Chirping sounds indicate perforation of the ligament. If the chirping is mixed with very coarse crepitus, there is a probability that the posterior ligament has been severely damaged or lost and there is a bone-to-bone articulation (Fig. 10-10).

Ankylosis of the disk would produce opening and closing clicks at the same protrusive position of the condyle. If the disk is not ankylosed but is still reducible, the opening click usually occurs at a more open relationship than the closing click. If the disk is not recapturable, crepitus will be heard for all jaw movements and there will be no click.

Radiographic findings. If the disk is completely displaced, lateral transcranial films usually show the condyle distal to a centralized position in the fossa. The space above the condyle is often diminished also, but the diagnosis cannot be based solely on transcranial radiographs because variations in condyle-fossa contour can cause an appearance of displacement when one does not exist. Variations in beam angulation can also distort the apparent condyle position, and so transcranial films should always be used in combination with other diagnostic tests. Nevertheless, transcranial films have great value in many instances, often disclosing important information about the condition of the condyle or eminence such as remodeling changes at the bony surfaces, degenerative joint disease, or other forms of pathosis (Fig. 10-11).

CT scan imagery using blink mode can show any part of the articulation including the disk, but images are recorded in a static relationship only. It is critical in patients with TMJ disorders to learn how the disk behaves in function.

Arthrography enables us to see the movement pattern of the disk as the condyle translates forward and backward on the eminence (Fig. 10-12). The action can be viewed through combining arthrography with fluoroscopy. In some patients an accurate profile of the disk that shows the flexure pattern can be captured, but profile accuracy cannot be relied on completely. Nevertheless the condition, position, and movement patterns of disk function can be determined more practically through arthrographic methods than by other methods available at this writing. *Differential arthrography* can be used to assess the influence of muscle incoordination versus ankylosis or adhesions, when the displaced disk is nonreducible.

Perforations in the disk or its attachments can also be detected with arthrography (Fig. 10-13).

Axiographic findings. Axiography is a valuable diagnostic modality for complete disk displacement because it can clearly identify the instant of recapture if it occurs. By graphically comparing the point of recapture on opening, with the point of displacement on closing, you can determine whether the disk is ankylosed and you can measure the distance the condyle travels forward before recapture occurs (Fig. 10-14). If it is more than 3 mm, functional disk reduction probably cannot be achieved without reparative surgery.

Combining input from axiography with TMJ Doppler auscultation, we can determine not only the condylar path, but also the character of the articulating surfaces along that path for a very reliable noninvasive diagnosis. This combination has greatly reduced the need for arthrography except when the probability for surgery is indicated.

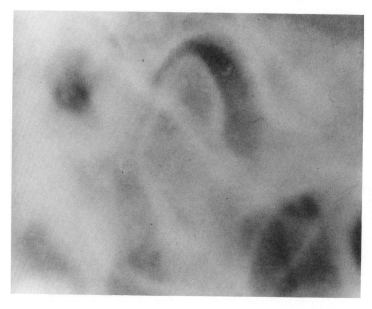

Fig. 10-11. Transcranial radiograph of TMJ with complete anterior displacement of the disk. Notice that the condyle is posteriorly and superiorly displaced in the fossa.

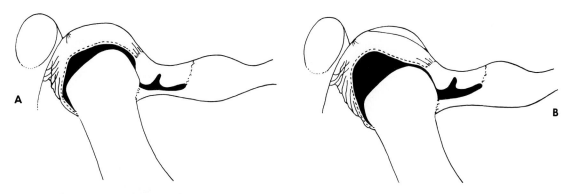

Fig. 10-12. Arthrography combined with fluoroscopy shows the action of the disk during function. This illustration shows the dye pattern in retruded position, **A**. Notice that the dye extends well forward of the condyle in the inferior joint space and outlines the underside of the disk. The posterior band has been pushed forward, nearly obliterating the normal seating area for the condyle. In **B**, the disk has been shoved ahead of the protruding condyle without reduction. Diagnosis: nonreducible disk derangement. Disk is not bound down and is most likely repairable.

Fig. 10-13. Arthrogram pattern when there is a perforation in the retrodiskal tissues. Notice how dye leaks through from the inferior joint space into the superior joint space. In this illustration, the disk is folded in front of the protruding condyle. **A,** Orientation of tissues: posterior band of disk, *a;* anterior band of disk, *b;* superior lateral pterygoid muscle, *c;* inferior lateral pterygoid muscle, *d;* posterior ligaments and retrodiskal tissues, *e;* condyle, *f;* inferior joint space, *g;* superior joint space, *h;* perforation through posterior ligament, *i.* **B,** Dye in inferior joint space only. **C,** Leakage of dye through a perforation, *arrow,* in the posterior ligament. Notice how dye then spreads into superior joint space.

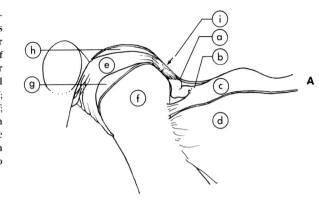

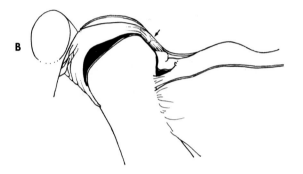

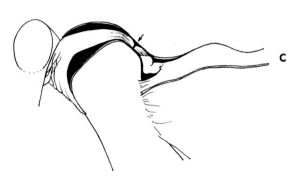

Fig. 10-14. Axiograph of protrusive path from lateral viewpoint shows point of reduction on opening is different from point at which condyle clicks off disk during closing. This indicates that the disk is not ankylosed or bound down to the bony surface.

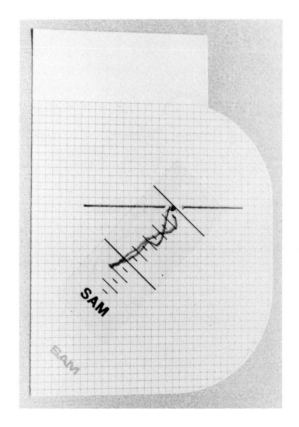

Mounted casts. If the disk can be recaptured and can travel with the condyle back to a verifiable centric relation, a bite record can be taken at that relationship and the casts mounted with reasonable accuracy for diagnosing occlusal disharmony. In patients with complete disk derangement the centric relation position, when capturable, should be considered a tentative treatment position because some changes in joint position can occur as the disk alters its shape after being distorted by the displacement and then being returned to a loaded position.

In nonreducible joints that have undergone adaptive remodeling of a disk extension, manipulative testing may show the new condyle-disk relationship to be acceptable. If the position is comfortable when loaded and functional excursions are acceptable, that verified position can be used as the correct jaw-to-jaw relationship for mounting the casts.

If a nonreducible disk displacement results in an uncomfortable condyle position that cannot be rectified, mounting of casts to that uncomfortable relationship has limited value. The purpose of mounted casts is to study the occlusal relationship at the *comfortable* position of the condyles so that harmony between the occlusion and the TMJs can be achieved. If centric relation cannot be achieved, a treatment position based on axiographs, radiographs, and other guidelines for determining the most physiologic relationship may be selected. Casts mounted in that relationship may be used for fabrication of occlusal splints made to the tentative treatment position, but final occlusal correction cannot be achieved until adaptation or corrective therapy has repositioned the condyles to an acceptably stable and comfortable relationship. A superior repositioning splint is the appliance of choice when a tentative treatment position is used, the SAM MPI or Dénar CMP system can be used to monitor the changes that occur in the joint, or the casts can simply be remounted as the position changes.

Diagnostic occlusal therapy. Occlusal therapy should always have a specific purpose in mind. Diagnostic occlusal therapy should be designed to test a definitive premise that is related to a suspected or diagnosed condition. In complete anterior disk displacements the following determinations must be made before a final treatment plan can be selected:

1. Can the disk be recaptured?
2. Will the disk translate with the condyle to centric relation?
3. Will the recaptured disk stay aligned in function?

On disks that can be recaptured and returned to centric relation without losing alignment, an anterior bite plane can be used diagnostically to see if the disk will stay aligned in function. If the displacement is intercepted early enough before the posterior attachment has been damaged too badly, it is not uncommon at all to be able to recapture the disk and have it stay aligned in function. When this occurs with the use of an anterior bite plane, a diagnosis of mandibular displacement from occlusion is confirmed as the cause of the disk displacement. If the joint is more *un*comfortable with the anterior bite plane, the diagnosis is clear that even though the disk is reducible it will not stay aligned in function. It should then be treated accordingly.

If the disk is irreducibly displaced but manipulative testing shows an acceptable comfort level when the joint is loaded, suspect that remodeling of the vascular retrodiskal tissues has occurred to provide an avascular, fibrous extension of the disk. If the joint is comfortable with an anterior bite plane when the disk is known to be anteriorly displaced, the beneficial adaptive response is confirmed and you may proceed with final occlusal treatment as soon as positional stability has been assured (usually through the use of a full occlusal bite plane).

If TMJ Doppler analysis has shown a bone-to-bone articulation, confirmed with radiographs and other tests, you may use full occlusal splints diagnostically to see if reasonable joint stability can be achieved by a reduction in muscle hyperactivity. If degenerative joint disease is active from excessive muscular loading, it may be possible to reverse the regressive remodeling with a more peaceful neuromuscular system that reduces the force against the articular surfaces and allows adaptive repair.

If a dentition requires extensive restoration of the occlusal surfaces, equilibration may be used directly rather than using full occlusal splints because any adjustments to natural teeth can be refined if needed in the final restorations.

If the disk is anteriorly displaced but can be

recaptured with no more than 3 mm of protrusion and it will not stay aligned with the condyle when translating back to centric relation, or will not stay aligned in function, you may fabricate a diagnostic occlusal splint to see if the alignment can be maintained in a forward jaw position. If alignment of the disk can be maintained in function at the forward jaw position, you can alter the same appliance to see if the condyle and disk can be slowly moved back to centric relation without loss of disk alignment. Anterior positioning splints have no value if the disk is ankylosed or is nonreducible, and so determination should always be made before any anterior positioning devices are prescribed.

TREATING COMPLETE DISK DISPLACEMENTS
Treatment categories

For treatment purposes, the various conditions of complete disk displacement can be categorized into treatment groups:
1. Complete anterior disk displacement
   a. Reducible to function
   b. Segmentally reducible to function
   c. Reducible but not maintainable in function
   d. Nonreducible, repairable
   e. Nonreducible, nonrepairable
2. Posterior disk displacement

By extending the diagnosis to further define the various conditions that exist within the broad group of anteriorly displaced disks, you can target treatment toward specific conditions rather than using a broad-spectrum nonspecific treatment for all displaced disks. The need for this type of specificity becomes apparent in a practice that sees a large number of patients with TMJ disorders. It is not uncommon to see patients wearing anterior repositioning splints for the purpose of capturing ankylosed, nonrepairable, or even nonexistent disks. Such erroneous, empiric treatment has no chance for success. If the exact purpose of the prescribed treatment is not targeted at a clearly defined condition, the diagnosis is incomplete.

Complete anterior disk displacement, reducible to function

Treatment for displaced disks that are reducible to function, should have three objectives that must be fulfilled:

1. Recapture of the disk in correct alignment
2. Translation of the condyle to centric relation without loss of the recaptured disk
3. Maintenance of correct disk alignment in function

Since these three goals cannot be achieved out of sequence, the starting point for treatment is always directed toward recapturing the correct alignment of the disk. Complete displacements of the type that are reducible can present two distinctly different conditions that require different treatment formats. From a treatment perspective, functionally reducible disk displacements should be divided into those displacements that are self-reducing versus those that require some form of manipulation or therapeutic intervention to achieve disk recapture.

Self-reducing disk displacements compose the large group of reciprocally clicking joints that click onto the disk on opening and click off the disk on closure. But self-reduction of the disk alignment does not automatically mean the alignment can be maintained in function. After reduction is achieved, you still must determine if the disk and its attachments are intact enough to travel with the moving condyle through the full range of function. To test that, you must disengage all occlusal interferences to rule out mechanical displacement. There are four effective ways to quickly determine if the recaptured disk will function in correct alignment:
1. Through cotton roll separation of the teeth
2. Through the use of a central bearing point
3. Through use of a flat, anterior bite plane
4. Through methods that equalize occlusal pressures while eliminating all incline contacts

The reduction of a disk displacement to function can sometimes be verified on the spot by use of a long cotton roll laid across the arch approximately in line with the premolar area on each side. Sometimes just the separation of the teeth eliminates the muscle incoordination and allows the disk to reduce spontaneously. More likely, it will be necessary to recapture the disk with judicious manipulation and then load the joint with bilateral pressure to verify the position. Pressure is maintained while you hinge the jaw a few times before closing into

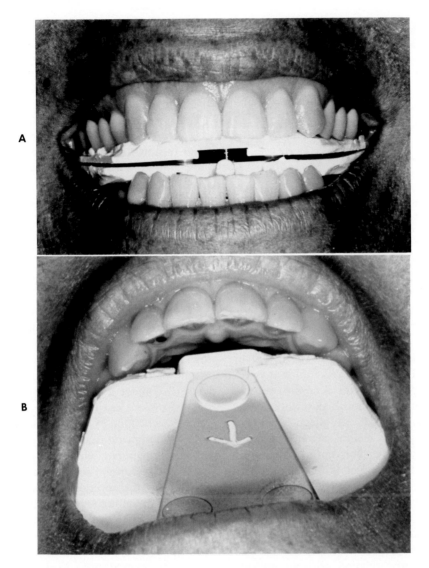

Fig. 10-15. Central bearing point device used for stereographic recordings, **A**, can also be used as muscle deprogrammers. Single bearing point permits the condyles to travel in any direction without influence from occlusal contacts so that the muscles have no programming for deviation. Their own coordinated function is the only control. The central bearing point can also provide a visual gothic arch record of jaw movement to aid in determining whether centric relation was reached. A sharp point on the tracing indicates centric relation, **B**.

contact with the cotton roll. If disk alignment is not lost while you are manipulating, release the hands and have the patient close into the cotton. If clenching into the cotton roll does not cause the disk to be displaced, the prognosis is good for treatment with occlusal correction.

A central bearing point works the same way the cotton roll works, that is, by disengagement of occlusal-incline interferences, but a central bearing point device provides perhaps the surest freedom for the condyles to move without restriction (Fig. 10-15). Muscle inco-

ordination can be eliminated quickly if occlusal displacement is the cause. If condyle-disk alignment is maintained while the central bearing point is in place, it is almost a sure sign that the anterior displacement of the disk can be effectively resolved by correction of the occlusion.

The anterior bite plane can be used, as already described, to test the functional stability of the disk alignment for a day or two. Pressure-equalizing devices, such as the Aqualizer (Fig. 10-16), also permit unrestricted access to

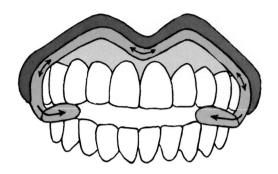

Fig. 10-16. Aqualizer device is illustrative of a method for muscle deprogramming. Water-filled pads connected for equalization of pressure separate the teeth and thereby eliminate influence from tooth inclines that displace the mandible. The muscles are free to position the condyle in a seated position without interference.

centric relation, and so they are useful for testing as well as for reduction of muscle hyperactivity.

If the disk is capable of staying aligned in function, it will generally do so once it is recaptured and permitted free access to centric relation. Any of the previously described methods will work to make that diagnosis. However, that diagnosis cannot always be confirmed so easily in the short time a cotton roll or a central bearing point is in place. Minor changes in the newly reloaded disk may help to stabilize the alignment if given more time. If the disk stays reasonably stable but displaces only with rapid or extreme jaw movements, a full occlusal bite plane can be helpful, adjusted precisely to centric relation, with an anterior ramp for posterior disclusion in all eccentric positions.

The patient should also be instructed to make no unnecessary or extreme jaw movements and to wear the splint continuously, even when eating (a soft diet). Stability is usually improved as the disk recontours itself in the improved relationship.

Recapture of the disk to function is often spontaneous once the mechanical reasons for mandibular deviation are corrected or disengaged, but recapturing the disk in some patients is more complex. If the disk displacement has resulted in a closed lock that is held tightly by hypercontracted or spastic musculature, the disk may be prevented from reduction because of the tight loading against its posterior band. In such cases, reduction may be facilitated by distraction of the condyle

away from the eminence to make room for the disk to be pulled back between the two articular surfaces. If enough elastic fibers are still intact to pull the unlocked disk back, the downward distraction of the condyle may be effective. An excellent method for accomplishing this is illustrated in Fig. 10-17.

The effectiveness of this procedure is related to how soon it is done after the closed-lock condition began. The sooner the treatment, the better is the chance of reduction to function. The procedure works well on jaws that have suddenly luxated. It is rarely effective on closed locks that have been displaced for extended periods. It should nevertheless be tried on any closed-lock situation because it occasionally will result in reduction of the disk when least expected.

If reduction occurs after an extended period of closed-lock displacement, there will be a separation of the posterior teeth because the thickness of the disk will be added to the height of the condyle. The teeth will erupt back to contact if the disk stays aligned, but the first priority is to make sure disk alignment can be maintained in function. Sometimes a flat anterior bite plane is all that is needed to keep the disk alignment while the posterior teeth erupt. If so, eruption must be monitored carefully so that the anterior appliance can be discarded when enough eruption has occurred to occlude the posterior teeth.

When a full occlusion is possible, it should be equilibrated as needed to prevent a recurrence of mandibular displacement, which could retrigger the disk displacement. If orthodontics or restorative procedures will be required to correct the occlusal disharmony, it will be an advantage to use a full occlusal bite plane to stabilize the joints first (superior repositioning splint). Occlusal treatment cannot be finalized until the joints are stabilized.

A large number of anteriorly displaced disk problems are caused by distalization of the condyle. The causes of distal displacement are discussed in Chapter 9. Treatment consists in correcting the position or contour of any contacting surfaces that force the condyle distally during maximum jaw closure. It is not unusual to find that a distalized mandible can be manipulated rather easily into a verifiable centric relation. Often the jaw must first be brought forward a little bit with no pressure being applied, to recapture the disk. Then after the

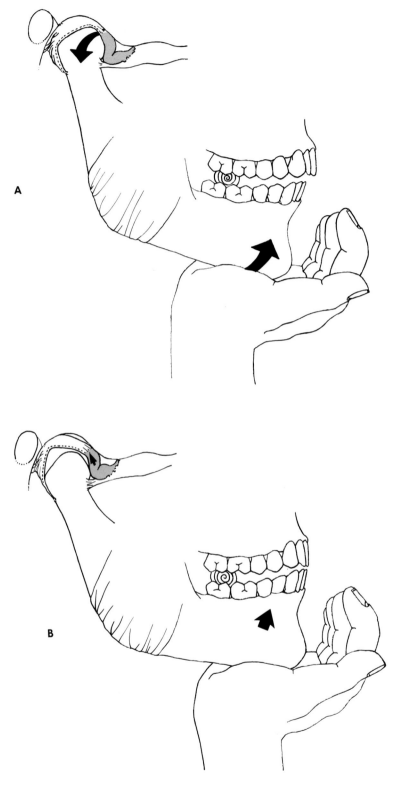

Fig. 10-17. A, Distraction of condyle from a muscle-loaded, closed lock requires a pivot between the molar teeth and external pressure up at the chin point. This pivots the condyle away from the eminence and provides room for the disk to move back. **B,** When enough space is created, the disk can then be pulled back between the condyle and the eminentia if there is enough tension left in the posterior elastic ligament and if the muscle can release it. Several minutes of distraction may be required. The process will not work if the disk is ankylosed or adhesed.   *Continued.*

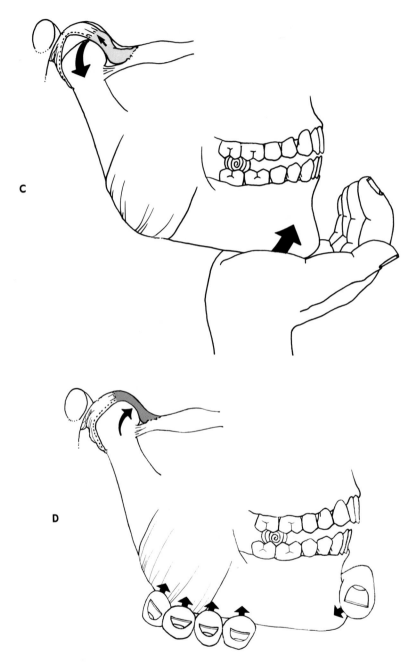

Fig. 10-17, cont'd. C, The disk may snap back into place or it may slowly extend back. The distraction should be maintained without interruption for best results. **D,** If the disk returns to correct alignment, release of the distraction will not cause discomfort. At that point manipulation should be used to test for centric relation and also to load the condyles forward toward the eminentiae to help hold the alignment in the concavity of the disk. Teeth should be separated so that displacement is not retriggered. An anterior bite plane can then be used to see if the disk will stay aligned in function.

condyle-disk alignment has been achieved in a slightly protruded position, upward pressure can be used to keep the condyle loaded in the center of the disk while slowly easing both condyle and disk back to centric relation. Now, while maintaining the upward pressure with bilateral manipulation, hinge the jaw a few times but stop short of tooth contact. If the joints are completely comfortable while loaded, maintain the pressure and hinge the jaw delicately to the first point of occlusal contact. Tap lightly a few times against the contact to get the patient used to that position. Then hold the jaw at the first point of contact. Now observe very carefully the direction the mandible slides from first point of contact to maximum intercuspation when the patient squeezes.

If the shift tends to distalize either condyle, see if the disk displaces as the tooth-directed distalization occurs. If it does, you are dealing with a true mechanical displacement as the cause of the disk problem. Disks that do not displace until tooth contact occurs have an excellent prognosis for a quick return to function. Treatment must be directed at freeing up the occlusion to allow the mandible a more forward intercuspated position that is coincident with the verified centric relation. This may be accomplished directly with occlusal equilibration, or provisionally with the use of a bite plane corrected to centric relation.

Forward displacement of the condyle. Because the role of muscle incoordination as a cause of disk derangements has been ignored by so many clinicians, the concept of forward displacement of the mandible being related to anterior disk displacement has also been missed. The observant diagnostician, however, will find that the majority of disk derangements do in fact occur with no evidence whatsoever of any distalization of the condyle. When the displaced disk is recaptured and the aligned condyle-disk assembly is moved to a verified centric relation position with the teeth apart, it is not unusual to find, on tooth contact, that the mandibular shift from centric relation to maximum intercuspation is *forward.* Furthermore, when the mechanical cause of forward displacement is corrected, the disk alignment stabilizes and the tendency for disk displacement is eliminated almost immediately in many of these patients.

When a disk displacement can be reduced to alignment that is retained in function, the patient should be advised to avoid hard foods or wide opening for a few weeks as a precaution against recurrent displacement of the disk because the posterior attachments and the collateral ligaments are obviously stretched to some degree and thus not as protective of the disk alignment as they would normally be. Apparently the changes in the disk attachments are reversible in most patients because maintenance of the alignment is not generally a problem if the occlusal harmony is monitored.

With any recaptured disk that has been in a closed-lock relationship, there is the possibility of some changes in the disk after the condyle is realigned into its center bearing area. These adaptive changes may be no more than minor realignment of fiber patterns or they may involve some adaptive remodeling, but any changes in the disk will probably result in some slight changes in the centric relation position of the condyles. For that reason, final occlusal treatment should be delayed until the centric relation position appears to be stable. Provisional occlusal correction can be made on a full occlusal splint that is precisely adjusted to centric relation and checked at intervals of 2 to 4 weeks. When the need for further adjustment to the bite plane is reduced to minute corrections, or none at all, that is evidence that the condyle-disk alignment has become stabilized. Tooth mobility must also be considered as a factor here, and that also should be as stable as possible before final occlusal treatment is completed. If extensive restorative procedures are needed, provisional occlusal correction can be accomplished directly through equilibration of the teeth or on cemented provisional splints.

The earlier a complete disk displacement can be treated, the better will be the prognosis for maintaining correct alignment. The longer the displacement goes untreated, the greater the chance for irreversible damage to the disk or its attachments. Preserving the integrity of the disk preserves also the synovial lubrication and nutrition that is important to the health of the joint structures.

Complete anterior disk displacement, segmentally reducible to function

A complete disk displacement that can be reduced only to a partial recapture of the disk will almost always be nonreducible at the lateral pole. Treatment will be related to the reasons for nonrecapturability of the lateral part of the disk. These reasons necessarily involve stretching or tearing of the lateral diskal ligament and at least part of the posterior attachments to the disk, and they usually but not always include some changes in the disk itself. The most commonly found deformities are related to flexure of the disk with resultant remodeling, which is related to how long the flexure has been occurring and how the posterior band is loaded as a result of the flexure.

If the medial pole can recapture its part of the central bearing area of the disk and then maintain that alignment back to centric relation, it may be possible to achieve a functional maintainability of the alignment by elimination of all causes of muscle incoordination. Treatment would consist in a muscle relaxation splint made to perfectly coincide with the treatment position at centric relation. The centric relation would have to be considered a tentative position because it would not include proper alignment of the complete disk, but the most important requirement of medial-pole bracing could be accomplished, and this is the essential requirement for achieving a peaceful neuromusculature.

If the medial pole part of the condyle-disk assembly can brace against the uppermost medial part of the fossa, the lateral pterygoid muscle can release its contraction against the elevator muscles. When this can occur, there is no trigger for antagonistic incoordinated muscle contraction.

It appears from our clinical observations that a partially deranged disk has a reasonable chance of remodeling into an acceptable functioning pad for the condyle if we can achieve a coordinated muscle function. If the disk is aligned with the medial pole and is not overloaded by muscle hypercontraction, it serves as a pad to prevent overload on the retrodiskal tissues that are between the lateral part of the condyle and the eminentia. This is sometimes a relationship that stimulates an adaptive response of fibrous remodeling of the retrodiskal tissues combined with a disappearance of blood vessels and nerves from the newly formed pad.

To accomplish the above results, the muscle relaxation splint must be kept in near-perfect harmony with the centric relation of the moment. As joint changes occur, the splint must be adjusted to preserve the harmony between the occlusion and the braced position of the

aligned condyle-disk assembly at the medial pole. The muscle relaxation splint must be fabricated so that it fits comfortably and securely. It should have an anterior guidance ramp that discludes all posterior teeth in all jaw positions except centric relation. It should be worn at all times. It is effectively a superior repositioning splint.

The criteria for using this treatment approach are two:

1. Medial pole alignment with the disk must be maintainable in function.
2. The level of comfort and function must be tolerable to the patient while wearing the splint.

The patient should be counseled to understand that changes in the joint occur slowly and that patience will be required because many adjustments to the splint may be necessary before the joint returns to a stable relationship. At that point, the splint can be discarded, and whatever occlusal therapy is needed can be accomplished in final form.

If the disk can be partially recaptured but a tolerable level of comfort or function is not achievable, the derangement should be treated as a stage 5 lateral pole disk displacement.

Complete anterior disk displacement, reducible but not maintainable in function

Being able to recapture a displaced disk does not necessarily mean it will stay recaptured during function. There are three types of disk problems that may prevent maintaining alignment through the functional range of condylar movement:

1. *Hyper*mobility of the disk
2. *Hypo*mobility of the disk
3. Deformity of the disk

Disk hypermobility results from the disk being too loosely connected to the condyle and the temporal bone attachment. Even though the disk may be recapturable at some point along the protrusive path, damage to the elastic fibers or the ligamentous attachments to the disk allows it to slip out of position as the condyle travels forward and back on the eminentia.

Disk hypomobility results from the disk being immobilized by adhesions, ankylosis, or muscle spasm. The condyle may move on and off the disk, but the disk cannot move to travel with the condyle.

Deformity of the disk results from *either* overloading *or* underloading parts of the disk. Although a prolonged overload or misdirection of forces can cause changes in the shape of the disk, a common factor in disk derangement results from unloading the medial pole. A forward displacement of the condyle during intercuspation leaves a void where the medial pole normally fits into a thin concavity of the disk. A correctly aligned condyle-disk assembly, in turn, loads against the reinforced, medial concavity of the bony fossa. When the condyle is held forward down the eminence, the thin, concave bearing area of the disk begins to thicken to fill the space left by the vacated condyle.

The medial pole–bearing area of the disk is normally one of the thinnest parts of the disk but it can become thickened by several millimeters to a convex shape over a period of time if the condyle is anteriorly displaced by occlusal inclines. The medial thickening can also be encouraged by the medioanterior rotation of the disk as the lateral diskal ligament breaks down.

If the medial part of a thickened, nonreducible disk can be observed through a surgical microscope, it will be evident why it cannot stay aligned with the condyle in function. Surgical thinning of the medial pole–bearing surface of the disk regains a stable concave seat for the medial pole and permits function without displacement.

It is probable that any hypermobile disk that will not stay captured in function will eventually become nonreducible unless treated. We have three treatment choices:

1. Mandibular repositioning
2. Surgical correction
3. Using the patient's adaptive response

Mandibular repositioning splints have one basic purpose—to move the mandible to a position that aligns the condyle with the displaced disk. Mandibular alignment is achieved by relating steeply inclined occlusal surfaces on the splint, so that maximum intercuspation occurs at the position that aligns the condyle with the forwardly displaced disk. The intended effect of this forward repositioning of the condyle is to relieve the retrodiskal tissues from being compressed by the condyle. If the condyle-disk assembly is held in a forward position, it allows the retrodiskal tissues to heal and regain elasticity. As the posterior ligament

heals, its ability to pull the disk back with the condyle improves, and so the condyle can be allowed to move back to centric relation as the elastic traction improves to keep the disk aligned. This is managed by adjustment of the inclines of the respositioning splint in incements until the condyle and disk are articulated at centric relation.

When function can occur comfortably in a verifiable centric relation without displacement of the disk, final treatment of the occlusion can be achieved. No interferences to centric relation should be allowed to remain in the final occlusal treatment. If centric occlusion is not made to coincide with centric relation, the realignment of the disk will not hold.

Corrective surgery can be used to preserve the disk if damage has not progressed too far. Preserving the disk has the advantage of also preserving the nutritional and lubricating effects from the synovial fluids, both of which are preventive for degenerative joint disease.

Surgical correction procedures include the following:

1. Meniscoplasty, to reshape deformed disks
2. Release of superior pterygoid muscle contracture
3. Plication, to shorten the posterior attachments, which help to hold the disk in place on the condyle
4. Release of an adhesed or ankylosed disk
5. Removal of bony spicules on articular surfaces
6. Correction of pathologic deformities or growth abnormalities
7. Repair of perforations or tears in the posterior and collateral ligaments

Using the patient's adaptive response may be considered if the disk will not stay aligned in function and the posterior ligament is too badly damaged to respond to anterior repositioning. If surgical intervention is ruled out, an attempt can be made to get an adaptive response in the retrodiskal tissues by reducing muscle incoordination to the minimum. A full occlusal splint harmonized to the most comfortable joint position may produce an acceptable result. The patient should be aware in advance that the adaptive response occurs slowly; so patience is required. Repeated adjustment of the splint is required as changes in the joint occur.

The prognosis for adaptive remodeling of

the retrodiskal tissues may be more acceptable than one might expect. Before we had a better understanding of the function of the disk, most TMJ disorders were treated without regard for the disk when attempts were made to reduce muscular overload. If the occlusion was maintained in meticulous adjustment long enough, even patients with disk displacements generally improved. There were exceptions, but fortunately they composed a very small percentage of patients. Because of the high success rate enjoyed by some dentists who were extremely proficient at occlusal therapy, there may be some reluctance to consider a surgical approach. New and vastly improved microsurgical techniques enable the specially trained surgeon to repair defects in many joints more directly and with, I suspect, a better long-term prognosis than what can be achieved by adaptation of a misaligned disk. The criteria for advocating surgical correction over more "conservative" occlusal therapy are based on three decisions:

1. Is the level of discomfort intolerable to the patient?
2. Is the discomfort unrelieved by noninvasive treatment?
3. Is the potential for further pathosis unfavorable without surgical correction?

Unless there is a probability of intolerable discomfort or imminent pathosis without surgical intervention, the conservative treatment of displaced disks is the preferred approach. The reduction of muscle hyperactivity is essential to the success of the surgical approach anyway, and so occlusal therapy, usually with full occlusal muscle relaxation splints, should be attempted before the final decision for surgery is made.

Complete anterior disk displacement, nonreducible but repairable

The options for nonreducible disk displacements are narrowed down to two:

1. Surgical correction or repair
2. Using the patients adaptive response

Anterior repositioning devices have no value for a noncapturable disk. In fact they are contraindicated. The purpose of anterior repositioning is to unload the retrodiskal tissues so that they can heal and regain the elastic traction necessary for pulling the disk back with the condyle. We pay a price for anterior repositioning because it produces muscle incoordi-

nation. Whenever the mandible is displaced forward of centric relation (even when it is intentional) the combination of lateral pterygoid bracing against elevator muscle contraction occurs. Incoordinated antagonistic muscle contraction has a tendency to develop into muscle *hyper*contraction. So unless that hypercontraction is directed through the disk, the loading is applied onto the very tissues we are trying to heal. If beneficial adaptive changes are to be encouraged in the retrodiskal tissues, they will occur more readily with the decreased muscle loading of a peaceful neuromuscular harmony. We do not achieve a peaceful neuromusculature with anterior repositioning forward of medial-pole bracing by bone.

Recapture and repair of a nonreducible disk displacement requires three conditions:

1. The disk must be intact enough to be correctable to a functional state.
2. The disk must be capable of translation (with treatment if necessary).
3. Damage to the posterior ligamentous attachments must be within limits that permit repair.

If the disk is nonreducible, the first treatment decision is whether recapture of the disk is essential for an acceptable level of comfort and function. In some situations, even though a displaced disk could be surgically reduced, adaptive changes that have already occurred make invasive treatment unnecessary. The decision for invasive versus noninvasive treatment should not be based on an "always" or "never" mentality. Both choices should be considered for each patient, and the decision should be made on the basis of which type of therapy will have the best chance of restoring the joint to an acceptable level of comfort without sacrificing functional stability.

Using the level of comfort or discomfort as a criterion for determining treatment has validity only if the *cause* of the discomfort has been clearly determined. Without question, the cause of discomfort is far more likely to be related to muscle incoordination than it is to intra-articular sources. This point is proved to us repeatedly by the routine success of muscle-relaxation splints, even on patients with displaced disks. More study is necessary, but it appears probable that if we can achieve a level of comfort that is acceptable to the patient, coincidental with a peaceful neuromusculature, we will also achieve adaptive remodeling of the articular structures if treatment is initiated early enough.

Although adaptive remodeling of either hard or soft tissues may make the joint more comfortable, the stability of those remodeled tissues may be tenuous. It does appear that such patients require more frequent refinement of their occlusions in order to maintain comfort because even slight positional changes in the joint create disharmony with the intercuspal relationship. If, however, the treatment is initiated in time to salvage enough of the retrodiskal tissues to prevent a bone-to-bone articulation, the prognosis for long term stability seems to be quite good.

There are patients with displaced disks who do *not* respond to muscle-relaxation therapy. Their level of pain in the joint is intolerable, and the source of pain is related to compression of the retrodiskal tissues that are still reasonably intact. If diagnostic analysis clearly depicts a condition that is correctable only by invasion of the joint space, corrective surgery can be accomplished to reposition the disk and repair the ligamentous attachments. This preserves the valuable synovial tissues as well as the disk and the protective fibrocartilage on the articular surfaces.

In addition to the need for meticulous surgical procedures, there is one major requirement for an acceptable success rate in reparative TMJ surgery, that is, the reduction of muscle hyperactivity both preoperatively and postoperatively. Occlusally caused displacement of the mandible must be corrected so that there is harmony between the position of the repaired joint and maximum intercuspation. This is usually accomplished by fabrication of an occlusal splint to harmonize with the tentative treatment position for the joint and then refining of the occlusion on the splint to precisely relate to the repaired joint position. Occlusal equilibration on the appliance should be done immediately after surgery to reduce the tendency for muscle incoordination. This procedure reduces the potential for muscle hypercontraction and its consequent overload on the newly repaired joint structures.

The use of an anterior bite plane is a practical and effective muscle-relaxation splint to use in combination with TMJ surgery for correction of a displaced disk. Eliminating all posterior occlusal stops may seem like an odd way to reduce the load on the joint, but it works very effectively because of the effect of posterior disclusion on elevator muscle contraction. Posterior disclusion causes two of the three elevator muscles to release and thus reduces muscular loading of the joint. The procedure has the added advantage of being easier to fabricate before surgery. Postoperative adjustment is simplified because only the anterior teeth contact. As soon as reasonable joint stability is confirmed, the appliance should be converted to a full occlusal splint to prevent supraeruption of the posterior teeth. Periodic adjustment of the splint should continue until minimal or no adjustment is needed. At that point, final occlusal treatment can be completed if needed.

Complete anterior disk displacement, nonreducible and nonrepairable

The disk may become irreparably displaced because of damage to either the disk itself or the ligaments that attach it to the condyle and the temporal bone.

Destruction of the disk can occur when it is folded, bunched up, or torn so that subsequent loading leads to disintegration or noncorrectible misshaping. Destruction of the diskal ligaments results from tearing or perforations that destroy too much of the ligament to permit repair.

Microsurgical reparative techniques continue to improve, and today there are very few damaged disks that cannot be reshaped and repaired, but there are some that are unquestionably unsalvagable. Most nonrepairable disks are found in older patients, and in many cases, the adaptive process will have already changed the contours of the articular surfaces before you see the patient for examination.

How the bony articular surfaces respond to the loss of the disk is the primary determinant for selection of treatment. Examination may reveal any of the three following conditions:

Adaptive remodeling. If the articular cartilage stays intact, the condyle and eminentia can remodel to reshape the articular surfaces so that they conform to functional loading without the disk.

Noninflammatory degenerative joint disease. If the articular cartilage is damaged, the bony surfaces start to break down. There is some evidence that early or slowly progressing degenerative joint disease is noninflammatory and is reversible, or at least self-limiting if the overload is reduced.

Inflammatory degenerative joint disease (osteoarthritis). Inflammation appears to be a secondary sequel to unstabilized remodeling of bony surfaces that are overloaded.

Gross changes in the articular surfaces can be expected to match the meniscus displacement and its altered shape. If the primary soft tissues change shape, the secondary (bone) tissues adapt. If the primary tissues can be corrected in time, corrective reshaping of secondary tissues can occur as a normal process of adaptive remodeling. If the displaced soft tissues cannot be repaired, the remodeling process continues to adapt the shape of the articular surfaces to conform to the surfaces they load against. The process progresses continuously after the onset of disk displacement. Whether the remodeling process remains a reparative adaptive response or becomes a degenerative disease depends on the combined factors of host resistance and the degree of bruxing or clenching that determines the intensity of load that the bony surfaces must resist. Severe bruxing or clenching when the disk is displaced will most certainly lead to flattening of the condyle and often the eminentia. If the load is greater than the adaptive capacity to conformative remodeling, inflammatory degenerative changes start to occur. Degenerative joint disease varies from patient to patient and is affected by general factors of health, nutrition, and body chemistry changes such as those occurring with hormonal imbalances.

Even in severely flattened condyle and eminentia contours however it is possible to have a reasonable degree of stability and an acceptable level of comfort. This depends on the character of the remodeled bone surfaces, which in some instances form very hard smooth surfaces referred to as eburnated bone.

Radiographically, the trabeculas in eburnated bone are densely packed and the articular surfaces have the appearance of cortical bone. The severe flattening of the articular surfaces is evidence that the disk is absent. The bone-to-bone contact of the condyle against the eminentia is evidence on properly angulated transcranial films. Radiographs should be taken in both the superior hinge position and in opened (protrusive) position to observe the comparative condyle position in function (Fig. 10-18).

TMJ Doppler auscultation of bone-to-bone contact generates a chirping crepitus that often sounds like a gate swinging on rusty hinges. The crepitation can be rather coarse depending on the roughness of the surfaces that rub. If the fibrocartilage that covers the articular surfaces is still present, the Doppler sounds are less coarse, an indication of articular surfaces that are smoother. As those surfaces break down, the sounds generated are more gravelly.

Axiographic recordings present a protrusive path that is often much flatter and less an-

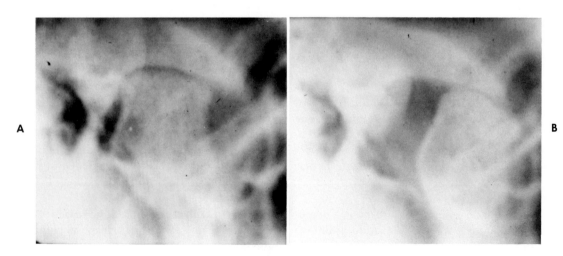

Fig. 10-18. Transcranial film of severely flattened condyle and eminentia, **A,** in retruded position. **B,** Protruded. When pathway is flattened, it indicates that the disk has been completely displaced.

gulated than the typical convex path (Fig. 10-19). This is an important observation because an abnormally flat condylar path may not be able to disclude the posterior teeth in protrusive excursion. Alteration of the anterior guidance may be necessary to prevent posterior occlusal interferences in the functional ranges.

Clinical observations. The complete displacement of the disk almost invariably leads to progressive flattening of the condyle unless the retrodiskal tissues adapt to form a new pad of fibrous tissue. Flattening occurs as a result of loading the condyle against the eminentia without the biconcave disk interposed to maintain the rounded shape of the condyle. If both the condyle and the eminentia are flattened, that is a sign that the overload on the joint occurs through its range of function. Such a functional overload is particularly damaging to the articular surfaces because without the disk present, the lubrication and nutrition from synovial fluids is also lost. Thus the surfaces of the articulating bones gradually break down, causing a loss of height of the condyle. This loss of height appears to be progressive whenever the disk is lost, and it leads to a further progressive problem of maintaining occlusal harmony.

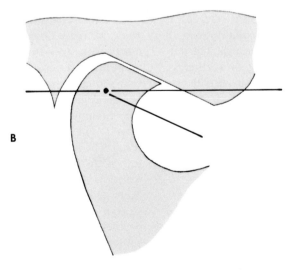

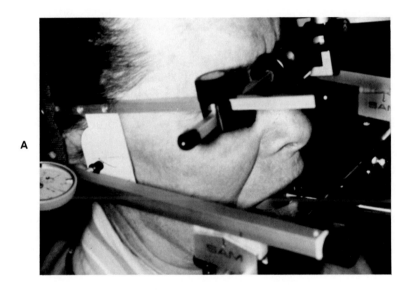

Fig. 10-19. A, Axiograph of flattened condyles shown in Fig. 10-18. **B,** Drawing of condyle shape and path on flattened eminentia.

Because all elevator muscles are behind the teeth, any loss of condylar height causes the upward migration of the condyle to load the most posterior tooth. The damaging effect of such a posterior occlusal pivot is compounded because it separates the anterior teeth and prevents them from fulfilling their job of discluding the posterior teeth in eccentric movements. The result is muscle hypercontraction that overloads both the TMJs and the occlusion. So the joint that is already compromised by loss of its disk is also subjected to the increased loading from the musculature. The problem is progressive because the more the condyle flattens, the more the load is applied to the occlusion.

Perhaps the most dramatic clinical evidence that TMJ problems cannot be separated from occlusal problems can be verified by a consistent observation: Severe wear of upper molar lingual cusps is virtually never seen without also finding commensurate changes in the shape of the condyles or the eminentiae, or both. Nor is severe flattening of the condyle and eminentia observed without directly related occlusal wear. Mongini has shown that changes in condylar shape are directly related to wear patterns in the occlusion and vice versa. If one remembers that maximum muscle contraction does not occur until the teeth are together, it will be obvious that loading of the condyles occurs at that jaw position that relates to maximum intercuspal contact.

Treatment

Because loss of the disk also reduces the nutrition and lubrication to the joint surfaces, it does not seem possible to completely stop all degenerative breakdown on the articular surfaces when the disk is missing. Nevertheless, an acceptable comfort level can usually be achieved with a manageable degree of stability if muscle incoordination can be corrected. The adaptive process can favorably alter even a bone-to-bone relationship in most patients if the nearly continuous loading on the joint can be reduced to intermittent loading with reduced intensity. That is the goal of treatment, and it can usually be achieved by correction of the occlusion to make it noninterfering to the superior hinge position of the condyles.

When the disk is missing, the superior hinge position is determined by bone-to-bone bracing at the medial pole simultaneous with contact against the eminentia. Even in severely flattened condyles, the medial pole of the condyle is still capable of stopping the upward translation of the condyle against the eminentiae. At the bone-braced superior position, the lateral pterygoid muscles can release contraction and allow the elevator muscles to seat the condyles without antagonistic muscle bracing. Even though the disk is missing, muscle coordination can still be achieved if the condyle is free to slide to the superior position without interference from the teeth. The position should be tested for comfort while loading occurs with bilateral pressure. If multiple centric relation stops of equal intensity can be achieved along with immediate disclusion of all posterior contacts in eccentric movement, muscle coordination can be established. Of course, centric relation must be defined differently if there is no disk present. It becomes simply "the most superior position of the condyles against the eminentiae." All aspects of centric relation remain the same except for the alignment of the disk.

Harmonization of the occlusion may be accomplished provisionally on a full occlusal bite splint, or it may be accomplished directly through equilibration. It is a common misconception that when dentitions have been worn flat, there are no occlusal interferences. If both condyles are positioned on their most superior axis against the eminentiae, there will invariably be premature contacts as well as posterior interferences in eccentric pathways (in untreated patients).

If the condylar path has become too flat to work out lateral or protrusive disclusion of the posterior teeth by equilibration, it may be necessary to restore the anterior teeth to provide a disclusive anterior guidance angle. Equilibration should be completed first to eliminate all centric-relation interferences and then eccentric excursions should be adjusted as far as possible before the anterior guidance is altered. The steeper anterior guidance will interfere with the extremely flattened envelope of function that the patient has developed, and so there will be a tendency to brux against the steeper inclines. This does not create any problems of discomfort as a rule, but it does subject the anterior teeth to lateral forces that could be damaging. The best rule is to steepen the anterior guidance only as much as necessary to adequately disclude the posterior teeth in all excursions, allowing for some eventual wear of the anterior inclines.

The most important occlusal change to make when the disk is irreparably displaced is to provide disclusion of all posterior teeth in all mandibular positions except centric relation. This always involves the anterior guidance as a disclusive factor. The main purpose of this occlusal relationship is the reduction of elevator muscle loading on the condyles. This reduction occurs when posterior teeth disclude. I have found that providing this type of occlusal function noticeably reduces the amount and frequency of postoperative occlusal corrections needed for patients with no disks.

Patients should be made aware that periodic correction of the occlusion will be necessary to keep the neuromuscular system as peaceful as possible. When the disk has been lost, some degenerative changes seem to occur continuously on the articular surfaces regardless of treatment. Maintaining occlusal harmony reduces the changes to a manageable level. An occlusal splint, processed in acrylic resin, is often helpful in reducing the amount of wear on the teeth. It should be adjusted for simultaneous, equal-intensity stops on all teeth in centric relation and for disclusion of posterior teeth in all eccentric positions. Most patients are able to maintain the occlusal surfaces reasonably free of extensive wear just by wearing the appliance at night.

Inflammatory degenerative joint disease, osteoarthritis. When the load applied through the condyle is greater than the patient's adaptive capacity for remodeling to occur without inflammation, the articular cartilage breaks down, and soft, vascular tissue invades the articular surfaces. All bearing surfaces may be involved, including the disk if it is still present. The joint may become painful as the loss of the articular cartilage exposes the sensory nerves of the periosteum. Condylar height may be lost, sometimes rather suddenly, thereby intensifying occlusal disharmony and its resultant muscle incoordination. I have not seen a single patient with active osteoarthritis of the TMJ who did not present with concomitant masticatory muscle tenderness when palpated.

Bilateral loading of the joints produces a range of discomfort from tenderness to sharp pain. It is usually this response to routine test-

ing of the joints that first alerts us to the possibility of intra-articular pathosis, which then must be confirmed by radiographic methods.

Lesions in the articular surfaces can usually be seen on transcranial films, but a panoramic radiograph sometimes gives a better image. If a lesion cannot be confirmed by either method in a suspected osteoarthritic joint, a submental vertex view may be used to locate it in some instances. The most reliable method, however, for a laminar assessment of the joint surfaces is tomography. A TMJ that cannot resist loading without discomfort should be analyzed with progressively more specific methods until the source of discomfort is determined. Arthrography, computerized tomography, and nuclear magnetic resonance all have value in the search for a verified diagnosis in certain cases and may be selected on the basis of specific need.

The onset of osteoarthritis in the TMJ is apparently more complex than can be explained solely by muscular overload. There appears to be a greater tendency for the disease in females, but at least clinically there also appears to be an increased predisposition for symptoms related to muscle incoordination in women. The role that hormonal imbalance plays could be directed toward disturbances in calcium metabolism that affects both bone and muscle function so that too could be a factor. The common finding of osteoarthritis occurring unilaterally raises some doubts about a generalized metabolic factor as the principal cause and seems to indicate that host resistance is more of a *contributing* factor. Despite the role that various contributing factors appear to play in the onset of the inflammatory stage, osteoarthritis does not appear to be initiated in the absence of an overload. Furthermore, the reduction of the load on the damaged joint seems to stop the pathosis and stimulate regenerative remodeling. If the disk is intact enough to be repaired or repositioned, the remodeling occurs more rapidly and may even recontour the condyle back to a normal convex shape. The remodeled joint contour depends on the contour of the surface that it functions against; so if the disk is absent, the condyle may adapt itself to a flattened surface, but functional harmony can still be achieved in most instances if muscular overload can be reduced sufficiently.

When active osteoarthritis is observed, the

finalization of occlusal surfaces should not be attempted. Until the pathosis is stopped and the defect repaired, the superior axis position cannot be determined with certainty. It then becomes necessary to work with a tentative treatment position. Full occlusal splints offer the best choice for the progressive adjustment of the occlusion as the condyle's position changes during its adaptive remodeling. After the joint stabilizes to a point that requires only minimal occlusal adjustment, occlusal surfaces can be restored. If the disk is absent, the best result that can be achieved will not completely stop all degeneration at the articular surfaces, but it can usually be slowed to a level that allows occluso-muscle harmony to be maintained with minimal periodic occlusal adjustment. Nighttime use of a full occlusal splint can help in this maintenance effort.

11

Occlusal splints

The purpose of occlusal treatment is to make the teeth conform to a correct skeleton-related position of the *condylar axis.*

The purpose of occlusal splints is to provide an *indirect* method for altering the occlusion until the correctness of the condylar axis position can be determined and confirmed.

The most common cause of masticatory muscle pain is displacement of the mandible to a position dictated by maximum intercuspation of the teeth. Displacement of the mandible always results in displacement of the condyle-disk assemblies, which in turn can lead to progressive changes in condyle-disk alignment. The misalignment, along with connective-tissue changes that can occur within the articular components, may make it difficult to determine the correct position for the condylar axis. Injury to intracapsular tissues may also make it difficult to ascertain the physiologic seated position for the condyle.

There are exceptions, but it is generally improper treatment to directly alter an occlusion until it can be altered to conform to a condylar axis that has been verified as correct. Occlusal splints provide an acceptable surface for reversible occlusal treatment that can be altered as needed, to conform with tentative treatment positions for the condylar axis. Occlusal splints may be used to help determine what is wrong or to help treat a specific malrelationship that has been diagnosed, but there is no reason for using an occlusal splint empirically. The spe-

cific purpose of the splint should be determined before it is designed.

The purpose of the occlusal splint may be for verification that the correct position and alignment of the condyle-disk assemblies has been achieved. If verification is the intended purpose, however, use of the splint must be combined with knowledge of how the articular components function because the relief of symptoms is not in itself acceptable evidence of correct splint design. Certain types of splints may temporarily reduce symptoms while simultaneously provoking long-term instability.

A common fallacy regarding occlusal splints is that the relief of symptoms is the result of the increased vertical dimension.

The relief of symptoms from an occlusal splint is unrelated to the altered vertical dimension that occurs when the splint is in place. Occlusal coverage splints always involve some increase of vertical dimension, but changes in vertical dimension do not affect the position of the condylar axis in centric relation. That axis can stay in a fixed position during a jaw opening of 15 or more millimeters (Fig. 11-1). The correct axis must necessarily be located at an increased vertical to separate the occlusal inclines that cause the condylar displacement. But as soon as a stable centric relation axis can be confirmed, changes can be made directly to the dentition and the occlusal splint can be discarded.

Even though a corrected occlusion intercus-

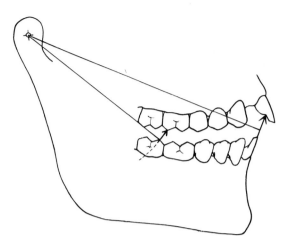

Fig. 11-1. Condylar rotation can stay on a fixed axis in centric relation for 15 mm or more of opening before translating forward. Up to the point of translation, changes in vertical have no effect on the position of the condylar axis.

pates at a lesser vertical dimension than the jaw-to-jaw relationship with the splint in place, neither the position of the condylar axis, nor the musculo-skeletal harmony will be adversely affected by the removal of the splint. The vertical dimension established by the splint does not have to be maintained in the final treatment.

WHAT OCCLUSAL SPLINTS *CAN* DO

Occlusal splints can perform one basic function. They can prevent the existing occlusion from controlling the jaw-to-jaw relationship at maximum intercuspation.

When the occlusal surfaces are covered, either partially or completely, the splint material becomes the occluding surface. How that occluding surface is contoured determines how the mandible must be positioned to occlude the teeth with the splint. Since the condyles must move as the mandible moves, the ultimate effect of the occlusal splint is accommodation of the condylar axis to the splint-dictated jaw relationship. This may be beneficial or detrimental depending on where the condyle-disk assemblies must move to conform to the occlusion established on the splint.

Although all other effects of occlusal splints are secondary to the control of jaw-to-jaw relationships, there are several side benefits that can result from occlusal coverage by a removable splint, as follows:

1. *Stabilization of weak teeth.* An occlusal splint can effectively stabilize weak or hypermobile teeth by the adaptation of the splint material around the axial surfaces. It can serve, in effect, as a retainer.
2. *Distribution of occlusal forces.* Reduction of stress on individual teeth can be effected by provision of more contacts of equal intensity against the corrected occlusal surface of the splint. This change also affects the proprioceptive input to the neuromuscular system.
3. *Reduction of wear.* Wear occurs against the splint rather than against the opposing teeth.
4. *Stabilization of unopposed teeth.* Providing occlusal contacts for unopposed teeth stops them from erupting. An occlusal splint is often an effective compromise when a patient is not ready for a more permanent prosthesis.

WHAT OCCLUSAL SPLINTS *CANNOT* DO

Occlusal splints cannot cause effects that are in violation of mechanical laws. Thus an occlusal splint does not unload the condyles. The popular claim that a posterior occlusal splint serves as a pivot for distraction of the condyles is in violation of facts of anatomy, laws of physics, and clinical data.[1,2]

Even if occlusal pivots are placed at the last molar on each side, the elevator muscles are behind the teeth and will effectively load the condyles against the eminentiae.

The concept that posterior splints distract the condyles has persisted in the literature for some time. It is often based on the erroneous belief that the forward pull of the masseter and internal pterygoid muscles produces an elevation of the *anterior* part of the mandible and thus rotates the condyles down. But regardless of the angulation of the elevator muscles, they attach at a considerable distance behind the last tooth. Even if the origin of the muscles were moved more forward, they would still not distract the condyles (Fig. 11-2).

UNSUBSTANTIATED CLAIMS FOR OCCLUSAL SPLINT THERAPY

A variety of unsubstantiated claims have been attributed to the use of occlusal splints. Some patients do respond to splint therapy with unexplained remissions of apparently unrelated symptoms. It is difficult to know

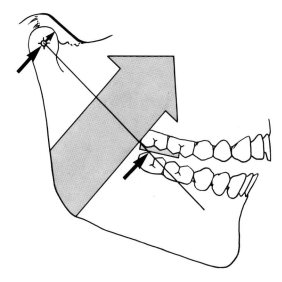

Fig. 11-2. Mechanics of muscle contraction. The elevator muscles are between the posterior teeth and the joints. Thus, even with a posterior bite-raising appliance, muscle contraction elevates the condyle and loads it against the eminentia. The posterior point of contact on the splint becomes a pivot point that is also loaded.

whether such occurrences are the result of some neurologic or biochemical response that is not yet understood or whether it is a result of psychologic factors. Some things are evident: Such responses are rare, and they are completely unpredictable. Furthermore, they are reported most often by therapists who combine splint therapy with strong suggestion that the symptoms will disappear. In some instances the methods are not unlike the snake oil salesmen of the past.

Analyzing unexplainable claims. If a therapeutic claim has no recognizable explanation that is consistent with known and proved biologic facts, such claims are highly suspect unless they can pass three tests for reasonable verification:

1. The test results are repeatable by other investigators.
2. The claimed results are verifiable when compared to a control group in double-blind studies.
3. Proper scientific protocol is used to collect all data and record results.

Some of the claims for occlusal splint therapy that have neither a verifiable explanation nor an acceptable substantiation are as follows.

1. *"Occlusal splints increase the wearer's strength."* There is no known biologic relationship that probably relates mandibular position

to total body strength or the strength of other anatomic functional units. Nor are there any acceptably scientific data that support such claims. In numerous double-blind studies, claims of increased strength have not been reproducible when proper scientific protocol was used in the collection of data.[3-5] The same can be said for claims of increased endurance because of wearing an occlusal splint.

2. *"Occlusal splints cause remission of unrelated diseases."* There have been numerous claims that the use of occlusal splints at an increased vertical have caused the remission of muscular dystrophy symptoms. Such claims have not been verified by supportable data. Spontaneous remission of several diseases can occur. If such a remission fortuitously occurs during occlusal splint therapy, the splint may be given the credit but there does not appear to be any consistency or predictability in such treatment, nor is there, up to now, any explainable theory that has scientific validity to give credibility to the concept.

3. Occlusal splints can cause a *"purging of system poisons."* Such claims were used by some of the early pioneers in occlusal splint therapy. Strong suggestion was used to convince patients that phenomenal body changes would occur when dental stress was eliminated. The effects, whether real or imagined, were probably related to hypnotic suggestion by intensely authoritative clinicians. Such effects were most likely intensified by the actual relief of masticatory muscle spasms, a benefit that could rightly be attributed to the occlusal splint.

4. Occlusal splints cause a *"regulation of multiple bodily functions."* Claims of correcting every type of biologic imbalance have been atrributed to occlusal splints. Some clinicians have reported success in the 90-percentile range for correcting problems such as irritated bowel, itchy scalp, dysmenorrhea, and vision problems. There are no acceptable data to support such findings, and it is not consistent with the findings of authorities in the field.

Patients do feel better if an occlusal splint results in reduction of masticatory muscle pain, and there can undoubtedly be autonomic responses to the relief of the pain.

The autonomic system can have a powerful effect on many bodily functions, but it is a dangerous assumption to suggest that splint therapy will cure specific problems without the relationship of the ailment to other causes being known.

In my own patients I have witnessed some extraordinary effects that occurred when the occlusion was corrected. In almost every instance the effect took place in a patient who was extremely concerned that the occluso-muscle discomfort was a more serious ailment than it was in actuality. Thus I would expect that both the cause of the problems and the relief of its symptoms were the result of autonomic nervous system phenomena. Those who claim that *routine* relief is achievable through occlusal splint therapy fail to consider the variety of other causative factors for disorders that may be more directly related than the masticatory system.

The arbitrary, empiric use of occlusal splints as a treatment for problems that are not definitively related to mandibular displacement is unscientific. At this stage there does not seem to be any supportable rationale for using an occlusal splint in the absence of a specific diagnosis of an occlusal disorder.

TYPES OF OCCLUSAL SPLINTS

There are only two types of occlusal splints (Fig. 11-3). Regardless of the many different splint designs, every occlusal splint can be classified as either

1. a permissive splint or
2. a directive splint

Permissive splints are designed to unlock the occlusion to remove deviating tooth inclines from contact. When this is accomplished, the neuromuscular reflex that controls closure into maximum intercuspation is lost. The condyles are then allowed to return to their correct seated position in centric relation if the condition of the articular components permits.

Because all corrective tooth inclines are either separated or covered with smooth plastic, permissive splints allow the muscles to function according to their own coordinated interactions, thus eliminating the cause and the effects of muscle incoordination. For this reason permissive splints are often referred to as *muscle deprogrammers.*

Any splint design is permissive if it unlocks occlusal incline contacts and provides a smooth gliding surface that permits uninhibited muscle positioning of the mandible. Per-

missive splints can be made for either anterior or posterior teeth, or for upper or lower (Fig. 11-4).

A properly made *centric relation occlusal splint* is a permissive splint. If centric relation can be clearly verified, an occlusal splint can be fabricated with multiple, equal-intensity occlusal contacts of the cusp tips on the opposing arch against the occlusal surface of the splint.

Such a splint is permissive because it provides no contraints on positioning of the condyles. They are free to travel up and down the eminentiae to the most superior seated position with no limitation of movement. Remember that the condyles are free to rotate as they travel along their unrestricted pathways, so vertical dimension is not a factor that relates to permissiveness of translatory movement.

If a centric relation splint is made with deep fossae and inclines that are too steep, it can be turned into a directive splint that limits condylar access to centric relation only. If the condyle-disk assemblies are capable of functioning in a stable centric relation, there would rarely be a reason for limiting them to that position only. It is *access* to centric relation that is desired, not restriction.

Centric relation occlusal splints should be fabricated with anterior guidance inclines that disclude posterior contact in all eccentric jaw positions (Fig. 11-5).

Directive splints are designed to position the mandible in a specific relationship to the maxilla. Any splint with occlusal fossae that intercuspate is a directive splint because the mandible is directed into the specific jaw-to-jaw relationship at which the intercuspation of the teeth occurs (Fig. 11-6). The positioning of the mandible may also be accomplished by contacting inclines against anterior teeth that direct the mandible to a particular position of closure.

The sole purpose of a directive splint is to position or align the *condyle-disk assemblies.* The jaw-to-jaw relationship that results from maximum intercuspation with the splint determines where the condyles must be at the intercuspated position. Thus directive splints should be used only when a specifically *directed* position of the condyles is required.

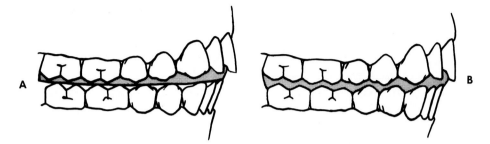

Fig. 11-3. There are only two basic types of splints. Permissive splints, **A**, permit the teeth to slide on a smooth surface so that condyles can move freely with no direction from intercuspal seating contours. Directive splints, **B**, require the mandible to be directed to a specific position in order for definite intercuspation to occur at the teeth.

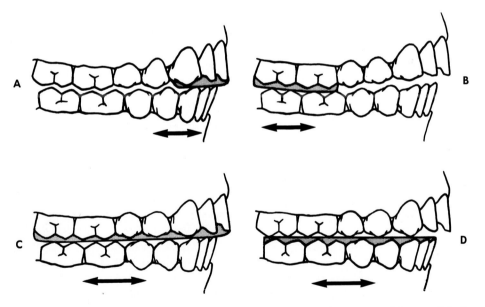

Fig. 11-4. Four types of permissive splints. All permit free horizontal movement of the mandible. Remember that while the anterior part of the mandible is moving horizontally the condyles must travel down and up the eminentia to move the jaw horizontally. Keep that in mind for any splint design. Permissive splints must have one side smooth. **A**, Anterior bite plane—flat surface separates all posterior teeth. **B**, Posterior bite plane—splint permits horizontal movement but becomes a pivot point for last tooth as condyles move upwardly. **C**, Full occlusal splint on the upper works the same as full lower splint, **D**. Both have some pivotal effect on most posterior teeth as condyles move back and up.

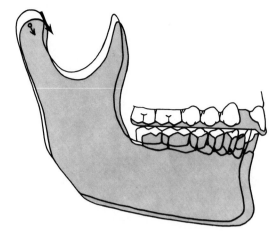

Fig. 11-5. Centric relation splint should have equal-intensity contact for each buccal cusp tip against a smooth surface. Posterior teeth should instantly separate from contact when any excursive movement is made. This can be acomplished by an anterior guidance ramp or the downward movement of condyles when the mandible leaves centric relation, or by use of both methods.

Fig. 11-6. Whenever a splint is made with occlusal fossae, the mandible is directed to the position of intercuspation. Where the mandible goes, the condyles must follow. However, the condyle will not stay in a distracted position, even if the intercuspation directs it there because the elevator muscles will load the condyle and the most posterior tooth contact. The desired condyle position should always be determined first before a directive splint is made.

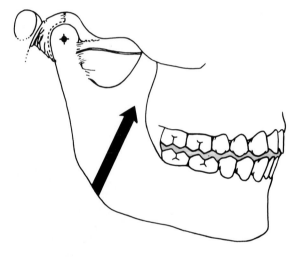

CONTRAINDICATIONS FOR DIRECTIVE SPLINTS

A directive splint is *contraindicated* if three conditions can be met:

1. The condyle and the disk can be aligned correctly.
2. The correctly aligned condyle-disk assemblies can move to the most superior position against the eminentiae without derangement.
3. The disks can maintain their alignment with the condyles during function.

If the above conditions can be verified, it is an indication that the joints are functioning in a physiologically acceptable relationship. There would be no need to alter that relationship, and so there would be no reason for using any appliance that directs the mandible away from that condylar axis.

Verification that the condyle-disk assemblies

are capable of normal function in the most superior position can be achieved on a tentative basis by testing in the following manner:

1. *Load testing the joints with bilateral pressure* (as outlined in Chapter 4). The absence of *any sign* of tension or tenderness in either joint during loaded hinging of the jaw is an indication that the condyle and the disk are acceptably aligned and are not braced down the slope of the eminentia by muscle. If this test is competently applied, it has been my consistent experience that there is no need or advantage gained by the use of any type of directive splint before occlusal treatment. If the disk is displaced, bone-to-bone contact may produce no discomfort when loaded, but the condition should be signaled by a screening history, Doppler analysis, or radiographs.

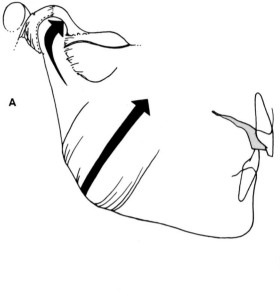

A

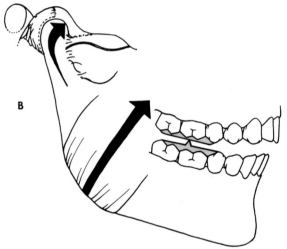

B

Fig. 11-7. A, *Anterior stop* with all posterior teeth separated allows the elevator muscles to seat the condyles at any position to which the mandible slides. Clench testing can be used to verify centric relation. Any sign of tenderness or tension in the joint area is an indication that the condyles are not in centric relation. **B,** *Central bearing point* frees the mandible to move wherever the muscles want to position it horizontally. Condyle position can be tested with the clench test.

The above manipulative test must be applied with the teeth apart. If the teeth are allowed to contact, deviating inclines can displace the condyles from the centric relation axis and cause activation of incoordinated muscle activity.

2. *Clench testing with the teeth separated.* If deviating tooth inclines can be separated by a cotton roll or any nondeviating device that keeps the teeth apart, the patient can apply strong muscle pressure to load the joints. The jaw should be tested for centric relation and then held on that closing axis for the first few clenches before the hands release it. The patient can then alternately clench and open to see if any discomfort can be noticed in either joint when loaded by the muscles.

This type of testing can also be accomplished with a central bearing point device or with a verified centric relation bite record made from a hard material or with a nondeviating anterior stop (Fig. 11-7).

3. *Doppler auscultation.* If Doppler auscultation reveals no crepitus or clicking during opening or closing and load testing of the joints is negative, there is no reason for using a directive splint.

The above methods can be used, even at the original examination appointment with a high degree of accuracy. If there is any question about the verification of position, alignment, or functional stability, further testing is indicated. A more comprehensive test during function can be used with minimal inconvenience to the patient.

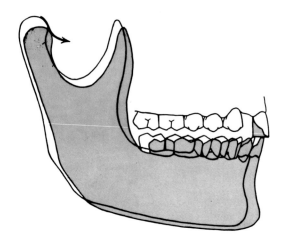

Fig. 11-8. The anterior bite plane permits vertical as well as horizontal movement of the condyles with no posterior tooth contact, a distinct advantage over posterior splints.

Comprehensive testing to rule out the need for a directive splint

The only reason for using a directive splint is an inability of the articulation to function physiologically in its seated relationship. A healthy joint does not need to be directed to that position. It will move in and out of centric relation as long as there are no mechanical barriers from interfering tooth inclines. Thus functional harmony can be tested by short-term use of a permissive splint to see if the joints stay comfortable and properly aligned in the *absence* of any directive inclines.

The ideal occlusal splint for testing the condition of the TMJs is a flat, smooth anterior bite plane. There are at least five reasons for selecting an *anterior* bite plane over other types of occlusal splints:

1. Separation of the posterior teeth permits vertical as well as horizontal movement of the condyles without interference (Fig. 11-8).
2. Separation of the posterior teeth substantially reduces the contractile strength and activity of the elevator muscles; thus the loading pressure against the joints is lessened.
3. The flat surface against the lower anterior teeth is easily fabricated because at that location there is no need to deal with the vertical aspects of the condylar path.
4. It is simple to provide an anterior lifting incline for posterior disclusion when needed.
5. If extended use is desired, it is readily converted into a full occlusal splint when

centric relation stability has been confirmed. Or it can be altered into a superior repositioning splint if the seated position cannot be verified.

Methods for fabricating an anterior bite plane

Anterior bite planes can be fabricated either directly in the mouth or indirectly on mounted diagnostic casts. Although direct fabrication has the advantage of requiring less time to make the appliance, it is not an acceptable method if the appliance is to be converted to a full occlusal splint. It is, however, a practical procedure to use it overnight as a muscle deprogrammer or to determine whether condyle-disk alignment can be maintained during function. Anterior bite planes should not be worn for extended periods.

Direct method

Indirect method. Any occlusal splint that is to be worn for an extended period should be fabricated on mounted diagnostic casts. Indirect fabrication permits processing of the acrylic resin for a denser finish that is more suitable for longer term use, as well as a more accurate fit. By extending the base to cover all teeth, you can first fabricate the anterior bite plane and then add the posterior occlusal contacts directly after centric relation has been verified.

There are two excellent methods for indirect fabrication. One can be made with acrylic resin for both the base and the occlusal table. The other utilizes a pressure molding system for the base (Biostar).

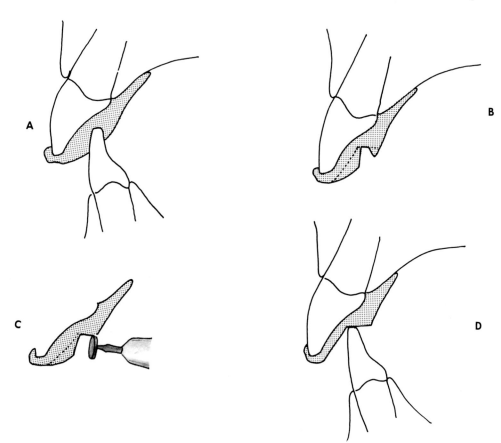

Steps in direct fabrication of an anterior bite plane. **A**, A doughy-stage mix of self-curing acrylic resin is adapted to the upper incisor teeth. The mandible is manipulated as nearly as possible into a pain-free terminal hinge axis and closed on the arc into the acrylic resin. The closure must stop short of posterior contact. **B**, When the setting acrylic starts to warm from the polymerization, the patient should open his mouth, the acrylic should be removed, and it should finish setting in cold water. *Dotted lines* show how the plane is trimmed to align with the lower incisal edges. **C**, The acrylic is trimmed and polished. **D**, The appliance should fit in the mouth and be held in place by the frictional grip over the incisal edges. It is then equilibrated to centric relation. Both condyles should be free to go to the terminal hinge position when the appliance is in place. When this bite plane is properly made, it should relieve most muscle spasm within minutes. Wearing it for several hours is usually the maximum required to eliminate any muscle spasticity that is related to occlusal interferences.

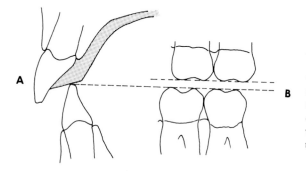

A, Anterior bite plane in place. Notice the relationship of the lower anterior teeth to the bite plane surface. The contacting surface should guide the lower incisors slightly downward during protrusion. **B**, Interocclusal space should be ample to prevent all posterior contact in centric or any excursion. The condyles should be free to seat upward with no interference of any kind from the posterior teeth.

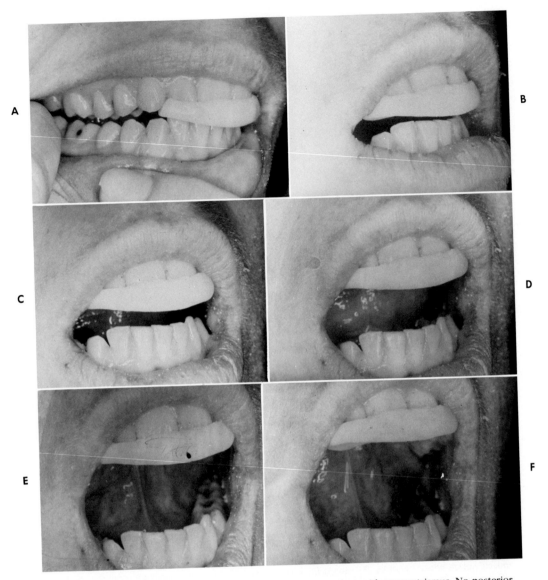

A, Directly fabricated acrylic anterior bite plane in place in a patient with severe trismus. No posterior teeth are allowed to contact. **B,** Patient is asked to open as wide as possible. This shows maximum opening possible immediately after placement of the anterior bite plane. **C,** Maximum opening 5 minutes after insertion of appliance. **D,** Maximum opening after 8 minutes. **E,** Maximum opening after 12 minutes of wearing bite plane. **F,** Maximum opening after 15 minutes. Anterior bite plane prevented interfering tooth inclines from contacting. With no proprioceptive stimulus to the muscles, the condyles are free to move up until braced by bone and ligament. The muscles are then free to relax and lose their spasticity.

Processed acrylic method (Fig. 11-9). An excellent acrylic bite splint can be processed with relative simplicity in the dental office laboratory.

1. Maxillary and mandibular casts are mounted with a facebow in centric relation. An extra maxillary impression provides a second cast for final fitting.
2. The vertical pin is set so that there is approximately 1 mm of space between the teeth that contact first.

3. Two thicknesses of baseplate wax are heated and pressed together and then adapted to the palate. While the wax is still soft, it is pressed into the lingual surfaces and rolled over the occlusal surfaces. Excess wax is trimmed away flush with the buccal and labial surfaces.
4. The wax on the occlusal surfaces is then softened a bit with a flame, and the articulator is closed to the vertical established by the incisal pin. The wax

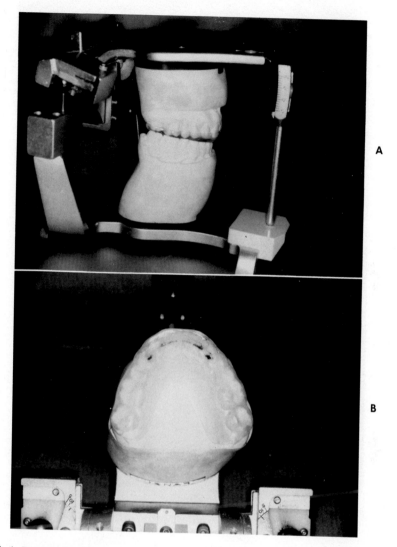

Fig. 11-9. A, Processed splint on articulator set at predetermined vertical. **B,** Splint is adjusted on articulator for anterior contact only.

Continued.

should be slightly indented by all the lower anterior teeth and by each buccal cusp tip.

5. The wax on the occlusal surface is then trimmed back so that the indentations are eliminated. The anterior bite plane is flattened so that the lower incisal edges equally contact a flat surface. Extend the flat surface about 1 mm in protrusive and lateral excursions. Then provide a ramp to the upper incisal edges.

6. Smooth wax and reduce any unnecessary bulk (Fig. 11-9, *A*).

7. Pour a counter model into the wax, using plaster. Make sure there are stops against part of the stone cast to provide a stable index for all four sides (Fig. 11-9, *B*). The cast should be lubricated with petroleum jelly or separating medium before the counter model is poured.

8. After setting, separate the counter model and remove the wax from the maxillary cast.

9. Block out interproximal undercuts on the lingual. Paint the maxillary cast and the counter model with separating medium.

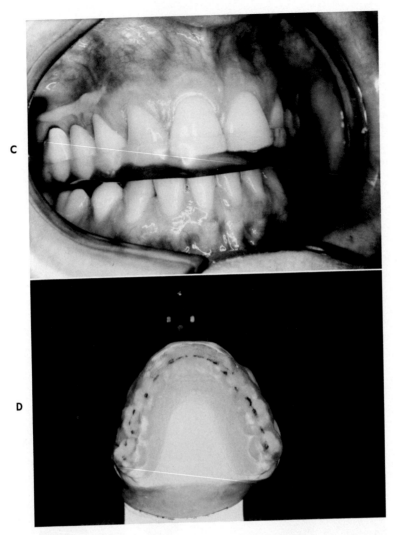

Fig. 11-9, cont'd. C, Note separation of posterior teeth. **D,** If extended use of splint is needed, contacts should be added later for all posterior teeth.

10. Make a mix of clear self-curing acrylic resin. When it reaches the doughy stage, adapt it against the maxillary cast so that it can flow freely over the palate and the occlusal surfaces. Immediately seat the counter model in place, and squeeze it against the maxillary cast until all the index points contact.
11. Trim away excess acrylic dough.
12. Immediately wrap the cast and counter model with heavy rubber bands to hold them firmly together and place them in a pressure pot.
13. After curing it, remove the counter model and replace the maxillary cast back on the articulator (Fig. 11-9, *A*). Do not remove the splint from the cast

until after occlusal adjustments have been made, if needed.
14. Refine anterior contacts so that there is uniform contact against a smooth flat surface. Use thin articulating ribbon. Be sure there are no posterior contacts. See Fig. 11-9, *B.*
15. Remove the splint from the cast. Smooth and polish the edges.
16. Fit the splint against the second maxillary cast to make sure it seats fully. The palate can be cut out at this time if a horseshoe shape is desired. All cutting or trimming should be done slowly enough to avoid warpage from generated heat.

17. Insert the splint and check with thin articulating ribbon to make sure all anterior teeth contact simultaneously in a verified centric relation closure. If not, make adjustments as needed. See Fig. 11-9, *C*.
18. Check with marking ribbon to make sure no posterior teeth contact in any excursion.

This is a diagnostic splint. It is only worn for a day or two to verify that the temporomandibular joints are comfortable and the disks stay aligned in function.

Some adjustments may be necessary on the anterior bite plane before the condyles become fully seated and the muscles are completely comfortable. There is no problem in wearing the anterior bite plane for a few days if comfort is improving, but if the patient becomes more uncomfortable, it should be removed and a more complete diagnosis should be made to determine the cause of the discomfort. If extended use of the splint is desired, it should be converted to a full occlusal splint (as described later in this chapter). See Fig. 11-9, *D*.

If centric relation can be verified and the patient is totally comfortable with the anterior bite plane, it can be discarded and the occlusion can be corrected to conform with the seated condyle position.

It is also possible to adapt a doughy mix of acrylic resin directly against the maxillary cast and fabricate the appliance without a waxup and counter model. This method may be faster, but the density of the acrylic is compromised and the splint will often require relining. The method is acceptable for an overnight splint but is not ideal for splints that may require extended wear.

Pressure-molded base method for anterior bite plane

1. Make two maxillary and one mandibular impressions. Pour immediately in hard stone.
2. Mount the maxillary casts using a facebow transfer.
3. Articulate the lower cast with a verified centric relation bite record. If the centric relation bite record cannot be verified but the position is reasonably comfortable when loaded, the mounting will be considered to be related to a tentative condylar axis position. The procedure for splint fabrication will be the same.
4. Set the incisal pin at a vertical so that there is approximately 1 mm of clearance between the teeth making first contact (Fig. 11-10, *A*).
5. Unscrew the upper cast and draw a line around the buccal and labial surfaces to indicate where the template will cover (about 2 to 3 mm on the buccal). Paint the cast with separating medium.
6. Place the cast, with mounting ring attached into the Biostar pot and fill the pot with pellets up to the line around the buccal and labial surfaces (Fig 11-10, *B*).

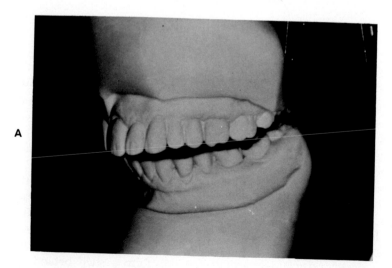

Fig. 11-10. A, Casts are separated on articulator for approximately 1 mm clearance.
Continued.

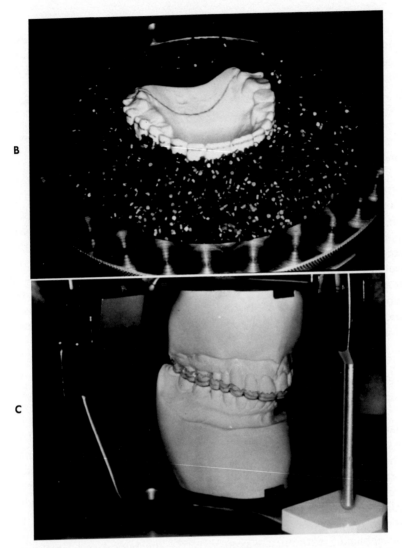

Fig. 11-10, cont'd. B, Cast is placed in pot and covered up to line with metal pellets. **C,** Excess template material is trimmed without cast being removed, and cast is put back on articulator with template in place. Occlusal thickness may need to be reduced to preset vertical.

7. Process a template using 2 mm thick material.
8. Remove the cast, and with adapted template material still attached, trim away the excess material using a sharp bur or Econo-Cut disk (Fig. 11-10, *C*). Do not remove the template from the cast until the occlusal contacts are completed.
9. Place the cast and template back on the articulator. It will be necessary to reduce the thickness of the template over the molars in order to close the articulator to the preset vertical. Use articulating ribbon and grind the marks until there is no contact on any posterior tooth. It may be necessary to open the vertical slightly to avoid contact.
10. Roughen the surface where the anterior bite plane material will be added. Moisten the roughened surface with monomer.
11. Mix clear orthodontic acrylic resin (self-curing) and knead it under cool running water until it is at a doughy consistency. Adapt it to the lingual surfaces of the upper anterior teeth to form a shelf behind the incisal edges (Fig. 11-10, *D*).

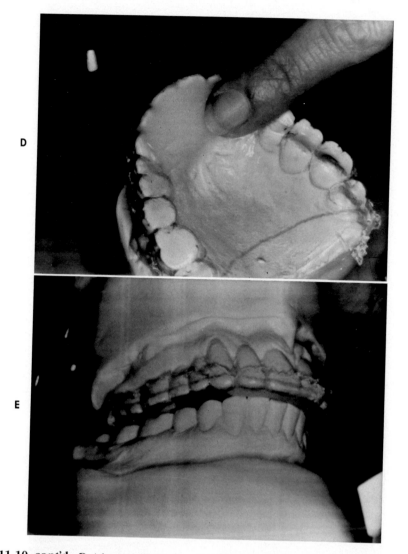

Fig. 11-10, cont'd. **D,** Adapt acrylic dough to form anterior shelf for bite plane. **E,** Close articulator to preset vertical, making sure that all lower incisors indent the acrylic dough. *Continued.*

12. Close the articulator, making sure that all lower anterior teeth slightly indent the acrylic dough. The lower cast should be lubricated with petroleum jelly so that it does not stick to the acrylic. Open and close the articulator several times to ensure solid contact plus enough acrylic to make a smooth protrusive path. See Fig. 11-10, *E.*

13. Smooth the acrylic dough where it joins the template by shaping it with extra monomer on the fingertip. Cut away any excess material and smooth again with monomer. Make sure only anterior teeth contact.

14. Let the acrylic dough set up.

15. Mark the base of the indentations, and remove all material around them to form a smooth flat surface for lower anterior contact. Taper the acrylic from those contacts to form a smooth anterior guidance.

16. When all anterior contours are completed and posterior disclusion is assured on the articulator, the splint can then be removed from the cast.

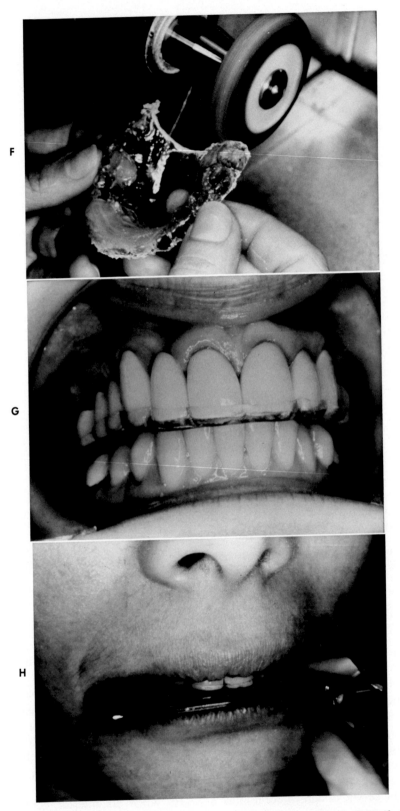

Fig. 11-10, cont'd. **F**, Shape edges of the splint and polish. **G**, Splint in mouth. **H**, Verify equal contact on anterior teeth only. Posterior contact can be added later if splint is to be worn for an extended period.

17. Using a large acrylic cutting wheel or an arbor band, shape the periphery of the splint. The palate can be removed, if desired. Undercuts into interproximal spaces can be relieved. See Fig. 11-10, *F*.
18. All rough areas can be polished.
19. The finished splint can then be tried on the second maxillary cast to make sure there are no undercuts that would prevent insertion.
20. Place the appliance in the mouth (Fig. 11-10, *G*). Check for any posterior contact using thin articulating ribbon. Verify that all lower anterior teeth contact with equal intensity and slide smoothly on the anterior ramp. Posterior teeth should not contact in any jaw position.

INSTRUCTIONS TO THE PATIENT. The patient should have a clear understanding of the following.

The anterior bite plane serves two purposes:

1. It is a diagnostic splint to be worn for a day or two to ascertain that the temporomandibular joints are comfortable and will stay aligned with their disks during function.
2. It is a muscle deprogrammer. By separating the posterior teeth it permits complete muscle freedom to position the mandible where the muscles function physiologically. If there are no intracapsular problems to prevent proper seating of the condyles, the joints should become completely comfortable while wearing the anterior bite plane. This normally occurs within a few hours.

The splint should be worn at all times and should be removed only for cleaning.

The patient should return within a day or two for verification that the joints are comfortable. If muscle release occurs and the condyle seats farther up the eminence, the anterior plane may need to be adjusted. As long as such adjustments lead to improved comfort, it indicates no serious intracapsular problem.

If the anterior bite plane causes increased discomfort, it indicates that an intracapsular problem exists. Further diagnostic steps are needed to determine the specific nature of the problem. The anterior bite plane use should be discontinued.

If the condyles can function with no discomfort, it will be evident in a short time. The anterior bite plane should then within a few days either be converted to a centric relation splint or a superior repositioning splint. Or it can be removed, and occlusal corrections can be made directly on the teeth.

Extended use of an anterior bite plane is contraindicated. Any splint that covers only part of the dentition results in intrusion of the covered teeth and supraeruption of the uncovered teeth.

This design for the anterior bite plane permits easy conversion to a full occlusal splint.

Methods for converting an anterior bite plane to a full occlusal centric relation splint

As soon as you can ascertain that the temporomandibular joints can function comfortably with the anterior bite plane, it should be converted to a full occlusal splint if it is to be worn for an extended period.

1. Remove the splint from the mouth, and roughen the surface of the template where it covers the occlusal surfaces of the posterior teeth.
2. Dry the roughened surface, and moisten it with acrylic monomer.
3. Mix some clear, self-curing, orthodontic acrylic resin, and adapt it to the template on the posterior segments. Check the amount of clearance first so that the thickness of acrylic dough needed can be judged better.
4. When the acrylic is at a doughy stage, smooth it into the template with monomer on the finger. Place the splint back into the mouth.
5. Using bilateral manipulation, verify centric relation and then have the patient close on that axis. Make sure that all posterior teeth indent the acrylic dough.
6. Have the patient slide forward, left, and right, maintaining firm contact of the lower anterior teeth against the anterior guide ramp on the splint. Ask the patient to move the jaw in all directions to generate border paths for all posterior teeth. Continue this until the

acrylic dough starts to set. Then remove the splint and let the acrylic complete its set.

7. With a pencil, mark the deepest part of each cusp indentation.

8. Grind away all excess acrylic on the occlusal surface. Leave the pencil dots representing the cusp-tip position.

9. Smooth any rough surfaces and polish.

10. Place the splint back in the mouth, and check all occlusal contacts with a thin marking ribbon. It is essential that all contacts touch simultaneously in centric relation.

11. With marking ribbon in place have the patient slide the jaw in all directions. Clear all contacts of posterior teeth except centric relation. The anterior teeth should maintain contact against the ramp through excursions.

INSTRUCTIONS TO PATIENT. The patient should be completely comfortable with the centric relation splint in place. If clenching against the splint produces any discomfort in any tooth or in either joint, the patient should call for an appointment. Equilibration of the splint should result in complete return to comfortable function.

The splint should be worn at all times.

If the centric relation position is stable, the splint can be removed and the occlusion can be corrected directly in the most noninvasive way. This should be done as soon as practical.

If direct correction of the occlusion must be delayed for any reason, the centric relation splint may be worn for an extended period without causing harm.

If habitual bruxing is a persistent problem, the centric relation splint may be worn at night to reduce wear on the natural teeth.

REPOSITIONING SPLINTS

There is never a need to reposition the mandible if correct condyle-disk alignment can be achieved in centric relation and maintained during function.

Anterior repositioning splints

The purpose of anterior repositioning splint therapy is to direct the condyle to function on the disk and prevent it from loading the retrodiskal tissues. Accomplish this by holding the mandible forward in a protruded position that aligns the condyle onto an anteriorly displaced disk. The reduction of pressure behind the disk allows the synovial fluid to circulate better through the joint spaces and aids the healing process.

The practicality of anterior repositioning splints is limited to those joints that have not been damaged beyond their capacity for adaptive repair of connective tissues. It is very unlikely that adaptive repair can be successfully achieved by anterior repositioning therapy if subluxation of the disk occurs before the jaw closes 5 mm from the reduced position, or unless reduction occurs before it protrudes 3 mm or less from the retruded position. Disk recapture at dimensions greater than these are indicative of connective tissue damage that is too extensive for adaptive self-repair. Even though the disk may be recaptured, it is unlikely that the realignment can be maintained in function.

Anterior repositioning splints should not be considered unless reduction of the disk can be verified. The disk must also be capable of sliding movement. An ankylosed disk will not respond to anterior repositioning splint therapy, nor will a disk that is too badly deformed.

If anterior repositioning is indicated, a reduction in discomfort should be noticed in a short time. If the discomfort remains after 2 to 3 weeks, it is an indication that condyle-disk alignment has not been achieved and the prognosis with this type of splint therapy is poor. At that point, arthrograms are usually indicated to determine why disk alignment is not being achieved. An explanation is in order so that the patient can determine whether to proceed with arthrographic analysis and possible surgical correction.

Because of the potential for discomfort and delay involved in unsuccessful or unneeded anterior repositioning splint therapy, it has been the practice in my office to complete the diagnosis *before* such a splint is made, even if it requires arthrograms. In most instances the diagnosis can be made quite accurately without arthrograms, by use of Doppler auscultation, clinical observation, films, and sometimes axiography. If it can be determined that the disk is reducible and can move within an acceptable range with the condyle, the splint therapy can be designed with a more predictable prognosis. If there are uncertainties about the diagnosis, it is almost always an advantage to resolve them as early as possible before a treatment plan is determined.

Fabricating anterior repositioning splints

There are three basic requirements for an anterior repositioning splint:

1. The mandible must be directed by the splint to a position that aligns the condyle with the disk.
2. The mandible must be prevented from closing or clenching distally to the position of disk alignment.
3. Both anterior and posterior segments should share anchorage for directing the mandible forward.

Procedure for maxillary anterior repositioning splint

1. Upper and lower impressions should be made and casts poured.
2. The upper cast should be mounted with a facebow transfer.
3. The lower cast should be articulated with a bite record made in the following manner.
   a. Adapt three thicknesses of softened baseplate wax to the upper arch (either Delar wax or Moyco Beauty Pink extra-hard wax). Trim excess wax back to the buccal surface.
   b. Have patient protrude the mandible until the displaced disk is reduced. This may involve lateral or opening movements to achieve reduction.
   c. After the disk is recaptured, close to light contact with the wax then gently slide back along the wax until the disk is displaced. Note the point at which displacement occurs, and then repeat the process but stop the retrusion just before the disk is displaced. At that point have the patient close into the wax just enough to indent the underside. At this stage the wax should be firm enough to prevent a deep indentation. Make a mark in the wax to indicate the position of a specific cusp tip on both sides. Line it up with a mark on the tooth (Fig. 11-11).
   d. Remove the bite record. With a flame, slightly soften the underside where the indentations were made and refit it against the upper teeth.
   e. Using the mark in the wax, guide the related cusp tips to that alignment on both sides. The condyle and disk

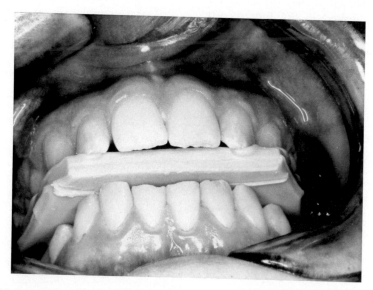

Fig. 11-11. Bite records for anterior repositioning splint. Hard wax is softened and adapted to the upper arch. At least three thicknesses should be used. After trimming find the position of the jaw just before it clicks off the disk. Slightly indent the wax at that position and then mark both the tooth and the wax so that the alignment can be copied. Then soften the underside of the wax and close into it at the marked position. This is the correct jaw relationship to which the anterior repositioning device should be fabricated.

should be aligned in that relationship. Have the patient close little by little into the wax to a point just short of tooth contact. Be sure that the posterior teeth indent the wax record. Chill the wax with air.

f. Remove the bite record and chill it in ice water. If needed, trim away any soft-tissue impingements or undercuts.

g. Refit the bite record against the upper teeth, and then have the patient move the jaw gently into the indentations. The condyle should click onto the disk and stay reduced during closure into the bite record. If it doesn't, the record is not acceptable for fabrication of the anterior repositioning splint.

NOTE: The reason for using a hard wax such as Delar is that one can check the jaw position repeatedly if need be without distorting the record. Thus the effectiveness of the selected jaw relationship can be verified before the splint is fabricated. At that jaw position the disk should be reduced, and the patient should be reasonably comfortable.

4. The mounted casts, articulated with the above bite record should be set at the vertical established in the bite record. This is the exact relationship that will be used to fabricate the anterior repositioning splint.

5. The template for the upper arch should be fabricated in the same manner as a centric relation splint or a superior repositioning splint. For stability and retention, the template should extend 2 to 3 mm up the buccal surfaces of all the posterior teeth. On the lingual, full palatal coverage seems to be acceptable though most clinicians advocate removing the palatal part of the template except for several millimeters of coverage apical to the gingival crest. If the template is made on a Biostar, final trimming is not completed until after the acrylic ramp has been added. All occlusal contours are completed before removal of the splint from the cast. Then the edges are shaped and polished.

6. Clear self-curing acrylic resin is added to the template to form definite occlusal indentations from the lower posterior teeth. The opposing model should be lubricated to prevent sticking. In the anterior part, a reverse ramp is shaped so that it is long enough to extend behind the lower incisors when the jaw is at rest. This ramp should engage all lower anterior teeth including the canines (Fig. 11-12). Close the articulator to the preset vertical and allow the acrylic dough to start its initial set. At that point, remove the upper cast with ring still on it and place it in a pressure pot for curing.

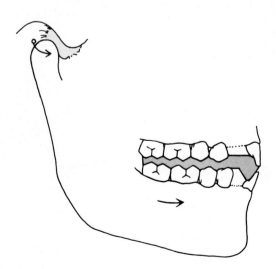

Fig. 11-12. Anterior repositioning splint should engage the lingual surfaces of the lower anterior teeth *and* the inclines of the posterior teeth so that all teeth share the directive forces.

7. After curing, replace the upper cast back on the articulator and make whatever adjustments are needed to the occlusion to ensure equal-intensity contact and multiple incline contacts on both the anterior and posterior teeth so that the mandible is guided into the protruded relationship and stabilized there during closure.

8. After all occlusal adjustments have been made, remove the splint from the upper cast and finish all margins. Shape the periphery of the splint and smooth out the labial margin from canine to canine so that it just barely laps over the incisal edges. Taper the anterior margin so that there is no thick roll at that point.

9. Insert the splint. With thin articulating ribbon, check for and remove any premature contacts. Preserve all forward directing inclines, but be sure they work together.

Procedure for mandibular anterior repositioning splint. The same procedures apply for the mandibular splint except that the anterior ramp is left off. Indentations for the upper posterior teeth should be deep enough to firmly stabilize the mandible forward. About a 2 mm extension down the labial and lingual surfaces is recommended.

If a lower splint is to be fabricated, an extra set of impressions should be made and both sets should be poured and the casts mounted. The casts are usually damaged when the splint is removed, but there will still be both an upper and lower opposing cast that is not damaged. Since the original mountings are made in a protruded relationship for the reduction of the disk, this mounting can serve as a reference point to compare with, if desired.

INSTRUCTIONS TO THE PATIENT. Whether a single appliance can be used depends on the type of jaw-to-jaw relationship. In most cases the maxillary appliance should be worn at night or whenever the patient can wear it without creating a problem for speaking or eating. It is the most effective splint because of the anterior ramp. Whenever the upper splint cannot be used, the mandibular appliance must be worn. Either the upper or the lower appliance must be worn at all times, with removal only for cleaning.

The patient should be on a soft diet. *The Non-chew Cookbook* by Randy Wilson is an excellent source of recipes for patients during this period.

Based on a study by Williamson of 300 patients,[6] the average time for treatment with anterior repositioning is 3 months. However, it is extremely important that after anterior repositioning, a superior repositioning splint should be worn to allow complete reseating of the condyle-disk assembly up the eminence to the superior centric relation axis.

The superior repositioning splint should be worn until no further adjustments are required, an indication that a stable relationship has been achieved. It is not acceptable to alter an occlusion to conform to a forwardly positioned condyle. Unless the superior position is achieved and confirmed, the long-term stability will be compromised.

Indirect fabrication of anterior repositioning splints can be achieved with great accuracy and considerably reduced chair time. After the condyle-disk alignment and position have been determined, casts should be remounted in a verified centric relation. Then a determination can be made regarding the choice of treatment for occlusal disharmony.

Potential side effects from anterior repositioning splints

The most avoidable side effect from anterior repositioning splints is the expense and discomfort of wearing an appliance when it is not needed or when it has no chance of success. If an anterior repositioning splint directs the condyles to a joint position that does not align with the recaptured disk, it will increase the damage to the connective tissues and do intensified harm to the vascular retrodiskal tissues.

Any anterior repositioning device is an automatic stimulus for muscle incoordination. The protruded relationship of the mandible *requires* lateral pterygoid activity during elevator muscle contraction into the intercuspal position. It is probable that this is also a trigger for hypercontraction of the masticatory muscles, which effectively increases the load applied through the condyles. This is a necessary price to pay *if* it occurs through a correctly aligned disk, but it is a damaging penalty to pay when it results in overloading tissues that are already damaged. Improperly made anterior repositioning splints can cause undesired movement of an entire segment of the dentoalveolar process. If lower incisors are used to hold the mandible forward by contact against an upper acrylic incline, the lower teeth may be moved forward as the mandible is pulled back to its seated position. A single segment of the dentition should not be used for an extended time to cause anterior repositioning, unless the segment is stabilized to the rest of the arch.

Remember that anterior repositioning is for a treatment position only. The treatment is not complete until the aligned condyle-disk assemblies are capable of functioning comfortably at the superior position against the eminentiae. This requires a splint of different design.

Superior repositioning splints

The purpose of anterior repositioning therapy is fulfilled when the retrodiskal tissues have healed sufficiently to regain a backward pull on the disk. However, either the condyle or the disk may have difficulty moving back to centric relation after being held forward. There is reason to suspect that the inferior lateral pterygoid muscle is shortened by long-term use of anterior repositioning devices. This makes it more difficult for the muscles to release the condyles to their most superior position. Deformity of the displaced disk may also require time to adaptively remodel to a stable contour.

The purpose of a superior repositioning splint is to eliminate the effect of the neuromuscular reflex that directs the mandible to close repetitively into the maximum intercuspation position. By covering the occlusal surfaces with plastic to provide a smooth surface, you can eliminate the reflex and the mandible can have free access to the seated position.

The goal is a true skeletal relationship of the mandible to the maxilla and not one that is influenced by the maximum intercuspation of the teeth. The purpose of the superior repositioning splint is to establish the correct skeletal relationship before the correct occlusal relationship is determined.

The fabrication of a superior repositioning splint is identical to the centric relation splint described in this chapter. It is especially important that the anterior guidance on the splint must disclude all posterior teeth in all jaw positions except centric relation. This is to prevent muscle hyperactivity and increased loading of the joints. As the condyle migrates up the slope, the anterior disclusive effect is lost and a fulcrum developes on the most posterior tooth, reactivating the muscle incoordination.

It is essential that the splint be adjusted repeatedly as needed, to maintain equal intensity contacts on all the posterior teeth and to reestablish anterior guidance for posterior disclusion. These adjustments must continue until the condyle is stabilized in its most superior position against the articular eminence. When this occurs, it will be obvious because the need for repeated occlusal adjustments to the splint will cease.

The time required to achieve superior positioning of the condyle-disk assembly varies from patient to patient. It may occur in a few days, or it may take several months. The determining factors appear to be related to the amount of deformity of the recaptured disk, and the condition of the inferior and superior bellies of the lateral pterygoid muscles.

Failure of the inferior lateral pterygoid to release the condyle is rare though in some patients it comes slowly. Whether the disk stays aligned as the condyle is released up the slope depends in part on the condition of the superior lateral pterygoid muscle.

Prolonged anterior disk displacement often results in shortening of the superior lateral pterygoid muscle, which controls the alignment of the disk. The same effect can occur from unnecessary anterior repositioning that holds the mandible further forward than is necessary. This side effect can make it more difficult for the disk to be released to its centric relation alignment. Either anterior disk displacement or prolonged use of anterior repositioning devices may result in fibrous contracture of the muscles at the shortened dimension. This is a common finding for nonreducible disk derangements. Through a surgical microscope it can be clearly seen that some disks cannot be pulled back into place until at least part of the fibrous restrictions are released to allow the muscle to stretch out to its original length. It is sometimes necessary to cut through enough of the fibrous contracture to permit the muscle to release the disk.

The disk can then be pulled back into place and be plicated into an unstrained normal relationship. If the fibrous infiltration is not too severe, it may be possible to release the contraction slowly through the progressive repositioning toward a centric relation axis.

Even when the disk will not be released all the way to centric relation, the superior repositioning splint may be beneficial. It offers an alternative when the disk cannot stay aligned and the patient elects against reparative surgery. A slow, controlled migration up the slope of the eminence may stimulate scar tissue formation or conversion of retrodiskal tissues into an avascular, fibrous substitute for the displaced disk. This pseudodisk may be an adequate functional surface for the condyle to load against without producing discomfort. This is a compromise treatment however, and there is no assurance that formation of the disk extension will occur.

Regardless of whether the disk can or cannot move up the eminence to the superior position with the condyle, it is still important to achieve superior positioning for the condyles because only at that position of medial-pole bracing can masticatory muscle coordination be achieved. A coordinated, peaceful neuromuscular system is all the more important in permanently displaced disks because it reduces the load against articular surfaces that lack the benefit of synovial fluid lubrication or nourishment. Breakdown of bone-to-bone articular surfaces appears to be substantially reduced if muscle coordination is maintained.

REFERENCES

1. Sears, V.H.: Occlusal pivots, J. Prosthet. Dent. **6**:332, 1956.
2. Ito, T., Gibbs, C.H., Marquelles-Bonnet, R., et al.: Loading on the temporomandibular joints with five occlusal conditions, J. Prosthet. Dent. **56**:25-31, 1987.
3. Bates, R.E., Jr., and Atkinson, W.B.: The effect of maxillary MORA's on strength and muscle efficiency tests, J. Craniomandibular Pract. **1**(4):37, 1983.
4. Yates, J.W., Koen, T.J., Semenick, D.M., et al.: Effect of a mandibular orthopedic repositioning device on muscular strength, J. Am. Dent. Assoc. **108**(3):331, 1984.
5. Parker, M.W., Pelleu, G.B., Jr., Blank, L.W., et al.: Muscle strength related to use of interocclusal splints, Gen. Dent. **32**(2):105, 1984.
6. Williamson, E.H., and Sheffield, J.W.: The non-surgical treatment of internal derangement of the temporomandibular joint: a survey of 300 cases, Facial Orthop. Temporomandibular Arthrol. **2**(10):18-21, 1985.

12

Selecting instruments for occlusal diagnosis and treatment

The single most important purpose of an articulator is to relate the lower cast to the upper cast in centric relation. To accomplish this relationship and maintain it during any change of vertical dimension, both casts must have the same relationship to the horizontal axis on the articulator that the dental arches have to the condylar axis on the cranium (Fig. 12-1). So the first requirement for acceptability of an articulator is that it must accept a facebow mounting.

Reproducing the horizontal axis is the essential first requirement because the accuracy of all other relationships depends on a correct starting point. If the condyles rotate the mandible open on one axis (for the bite record) and the articulator condyles rotate to close on a different axis, the casts will follow a completely different arc of closure and a serious error will result in the relationship of the lower cast to the upper cast (Fig. 12-2).

The common use of inadequate articulators is a baffling inconsistency, since the basic geometry that it violates is so simple to understand and the error it produces is so substantial. It is obvious that we cannot open on one axis and then close on a different axis and still return to the same position. Since it is most of-

ten necessary to record centric relation at an opened vertical to avoid interfering tooth inclines, the articulated casts must be able to close on that same arc to determine correct tooth-to-tooth relationships in centric relation at the most closed position.

It is not enough to determine just the first point of contact. We must analyze the centric relation path of each tooth from that first contact all the way to the most closed position. For diagnosis, this most often requires some equilibration of the casts to eliminate interferences to the centric relation path of closure. Correct tooth-to-tooth relationships can be accurately analyzed only at the same vertical as the intended final intercuspal contact.

The upper cast is related to the condylar axis and the Frankfort plane through the use of a facebow transfer. The lower cast is related to the upper cast by a centric relation bite record. If the condylar axis is in correct relationship to both casts, the articulator can hinge open or close and still maintain the casts in centric relation. Only if casts are mounted with a facebow, do changes in vertical dimension not affect the accuracy of the arch-to-arch relationships.

Centric relation is the starting point of oc-

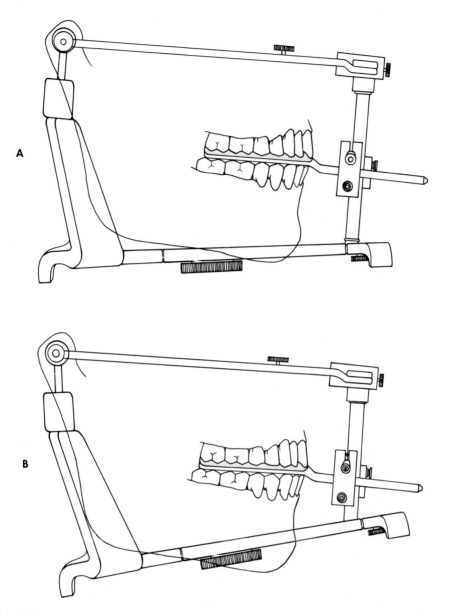

Fig. 12-1. **A,** The facebow relates the upper cast to the same axis position on the articulator as the condyle axis on the patient. When the lower cast is correctly related to the upper cast, the opening and closing arc will follow the same pathway on the articulator as it does on the patient. **B,** As long as the casts are directly related to the horizontal axis, changing the height of the casts does not change the opening-closing arc or the accuracy of the mounting. When the upper cast is seated in the facebow fork, any change of elevation rotates around the condyle balls and thus maintains a correct relationship with the horizontal axis.

clusion. It is the arch-to-arch relationship to which all the stable holding contacts must be coordinated. This static relationship in centric relation must be established first, before the dynamics of function can be analyzed or determined. After the casts have been related in centric relation, the second most important purpose of an articulator is to reproduce the paths that the lower teeth travel in relation to the upper teeth during function. You may do this by reproducing the border movements of the condyles and combining those condylar pathways with correct anterior guidance paths, or you may do it by recording the *results* of anterior and posterior determinant pathways at the site of the teeth themselves.

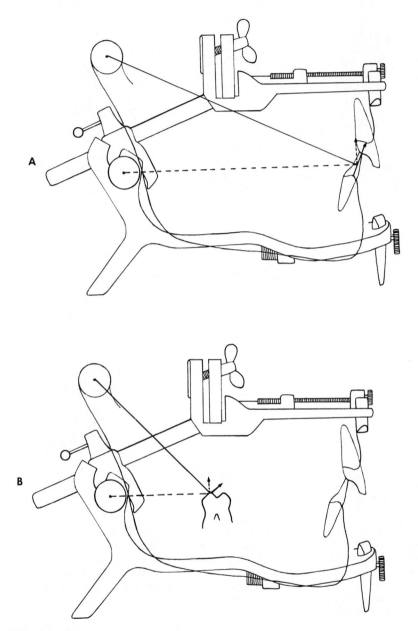

Fig. 12-2. The more the horizontal axis is missed on the articulator, the greater the error will be in the closing arc for the casts. The *solid line* represents the correct arc of closure that results from condylar rotation. The *dotted line* represents the closing arc for casts mounted on a Galetti articulator when the horizontal axis is nearly level with the occlusal plane. **A** illustrates the severe error that occurs at the anterior teeth if there is any change in vertical from the relationship with the bite record in place. **B** shows how the error increases in the posterior segments, so much so that for each millimeter of thickness in a bite record there can be a millimeter of error in the closure to centric relation.

CONDYLAR GUIDANCE

The major difference in the various types of articulators is related to variations in how the articulator duplicates the patient's condylar pathways. In evaluating any articulator, you should understand that no matter how sophisticated the instrument it can still do no more than the following regarding condylar movements:

1. Reproduce the horizontal axis of condylar rotation (Fig. 12-3).
2. Reproduce the vertical axis of condylar rotation (Fig. 12-4).
3. Reproduce the sagittal axis of condylar rotation (Fig. 12-5).
4. Permit simultaneous multiple axes of rotation during condylar translation.
5. Reproduce straight protrusive pathways of each condyle (Fig. 12-6).
6. Reproduce the pathways of each condyle during straight lateral excursions of the mandible (Fig. 12-7).

7. Reproduce the multiple pathways of each condyle during all possible excursions of the mandible between straight lateral and straight protrusion (Fig. 12-8).

Although there are many claims made regarding complete adjustability of condylar paths, very few instruments are actually capable of reproducing all seven of the above condylar movements without some interpolation.

The first six listed movements can be accurately reproduced on most quality gnathologic instruments, but the seventh requirement, recording all the paths *between* straight protrusive and straight lateral, must be interpolated.

Regardless of how precisely the various condylar movements may be copied on an articulator, condylar movements alone do not give enough information to determine complete occlusal contours. The anterior guidance must also be incorporated into the border movements that are copied by the articulator.

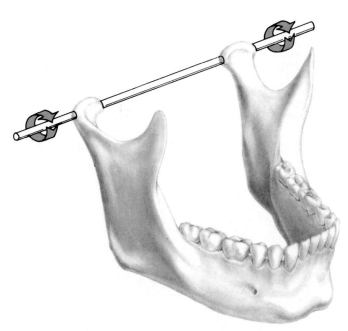

Fig. 12-3. The horizontal axis of condylar rotation is the most critical of all mandibular movements. The jaw can open and close on this axis without any change of position of the axis (a fixed axis). Thus, if it is duplicated on the articulator, changes in vertical can be made without any error being created.

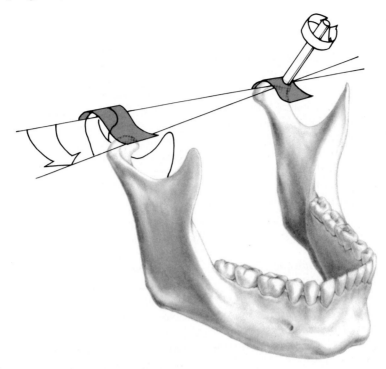

Fig. 12-4. The vertical axis of rotation can be better visualized when one looks at a composite of rotation because lateral rotation actually occurs around the lateral pole of the rotating condyle. As rotation occurs, the orbiting condyle must travel *down* the slope of the eminence. The medial pole on the rotating side must also travel down its slope but for a lesser distance. Because the condyles load against inclines, a pure vertical rotation is not possible without being combined with a sagittal rotation of the working-side condyle.

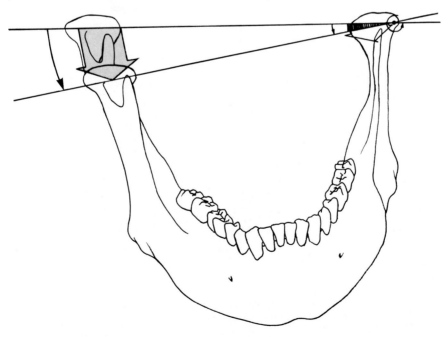

Fig. 12-5. The sagittal axis of rotation is essential for lateral movement to occur. This is so because the orbiting condyle must move down to enable the working-side condyle to rotate. This results from the design requirement of preventing the lower posterior teeth from moving horizontally toward the midline because to do so would clash with the upper lingual cusps and make the functional purpose of the curve of Wilson not work.

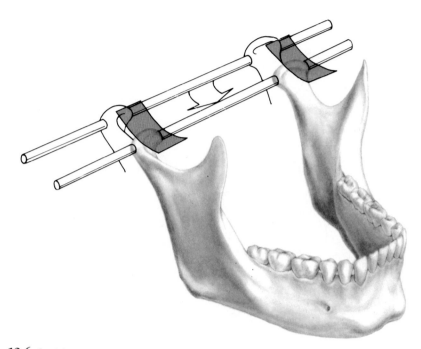

Fig. 12-6. Straight protrusion can occur only with simultaneous downward movement of the condyles. The condyles are free to rotate at any point on this forward path; so visualize this movement as translation of the horizontal rotational axis.

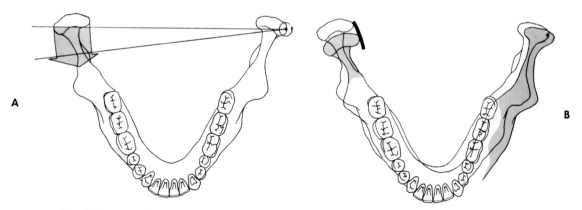

Fig. 12-7. The *broad arrow* represents the pathway of the orbiting condyle if all movement were confined to a *fixed* vertical rotation of the working-side condyle, **A**. The progressive side shift that occurs as the orbiting condyle is pulled inwardly along the medial fossa wall is at a greater angle than what would result from an arc around a fixed axis. This results in a side shift of the working condyle that occurs simultaneously with its rotation, **B**. It is important to realize that this side shift cannot occur until rotation has moved the orbiting condyle forward and downward to disengage its medial pole from its bony stop.

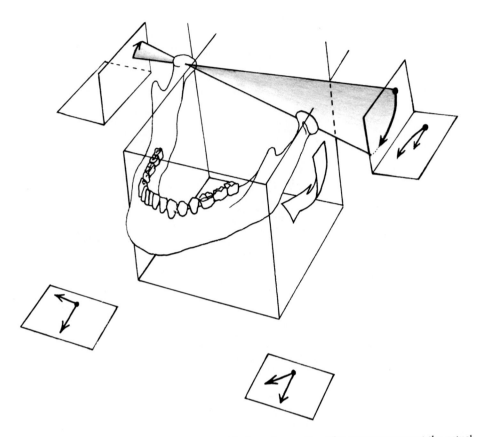

Fig. 12-8. Multiple pathways represented in a right lateral excursion. The *arrows* represent the actual paths of moving markers on fixed position recording plates if the marking styli are attached to the mandible. Notice that the distally directed path recorded for the rotating condyle is not representative of the actual movement of the condyle. It is rather the path that the stylus would travel outside the rotational axis. Misinterpretation of recordings often leads to an erroneous assumption that the condyle itself is moving distally and upwardly.

ANTERIOR GUIDANCE

In using any articulator, remember that anterior guidance is a product of functional movements that fall *within* the outer limits of possible jaw pathways. Recording only condylar paths does not furnish enough information for the instrument to reproduce jaw movements that are the same as the patient makes in function. The anterior guidance is a separate determinant that must be recorded in addition to condylar pathways. It is the combination of anterior guidance and condylar guidance that determines the border path of each lower posterior tooth.

If the anterior guidance is correct in the mouth, the anterior teeth on the articulated casts can dictate the movements at the front of

the articulator or can be used to fabricate a customized anterior guide table. But if the anterior guidance is not known, it cannot be determined on the articulator, regardless of how precisely the condylar paths are reproduced.

Anterior guidance must be determined in the mouth before it can be copied at the front of the articulator, just as condylar guidance must be determined on the patient before it can be copied at the back of the articulator. If both the front and rear pathways are correctly copied, the path of each tooth between those two determinants will also follow correct paths (Fig. 12-9).

Instruments that duplicate the exact path of the patients condyles are referred to as *fully adjustable instruments.* Precise recording of

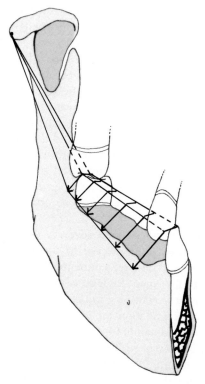

Fig. 12-9. The path of the lower posterior teeth in working-side function is dictated by both the anterior guidance and the condylar guidance. The anterior guidance is by far the dominant determinant. The pathways of the lateral anterior guidance are reproduced by each posterior tooth except that the length of the stroke becomes progressively shorter the closer the tooth is to the condyle. The effect of any condylar side shift is lost because the separation effect from the anterior guidance and the orbiting condylar path occurs first.

condylar paths was believed to be essential for conformity with some of the early concepts of gnathology. When it was believed that the condylar paths were the sole determinants of anterior guidance, it was a logical assumption that condylar paths must be precisely recorded. This concept was further enhanced by a belief that occlusal stops should be on the sides of cusps and the walls of fossae to form a tripod of contact around each stamp cusp. The earliest concepts also included a need for bilaterally balanced function on all posterior teeth, and the entire concept was further complicated by an almost religious fervor that insisted the mouth was an unacceptable articulator. Thus all occlusal restorations were to be designed and fabricated according to the pre-

cise dictates of the fully adjustable instrument. No corrections were allowed unless they were made on the articulator.

If all the dogmas of early gnathology had been correct, we would indeed need to use fully adjustable instrumentation on all occlusal restorations. But as many of the original beliefs have been proved inaccurate, the exclusive dependence on the condylar path has been diminished to a more realistic use of completely adjustable instrumentation when the precise condylar path is needed, and the use of simpler instrumentation when the condylar path is not a controlling factor.

The principle changes that have eliminated the original complete dependency on fully adjustable instrumentation include the following.

The realization that bilaterally balanced occlusion is traumatogenic. Because of a normal flexibility of the mandible, there is no way to harmonize the posterior contacts on the balancing side for all degrees of muscle contraction. Thus balancing-side function usually results in unacceptable stress or wear. Because of so many problems of tooth hypermobility, bilateral balancing of occlusions was abandoned many years ago, except for dentures.

The realization that condylar guidance does not dictate anterior guidance. Anterior guidance actually influences occlusal contours more than condylar guidance because it is the principle discluder of posterior teeth in working excursions. Since it must be determined as a separate entity, unrelated to condylar paths, the importance of condylar guidance diminishes whenever the anterior guidance is steep enough to effectively disclude the posterior teeth.

The realization that tripod contact is no more stable than cusp tip–to–fossa contact. The difficulty of making tripod contacts on the sides of cusps created a need for precise excursive reproduction to align with the fossa walls and to prevent collisions of cusps. As the contacts were moved from the sides of the cusps and the walls of the fossae to the tops of the cusps and the brims of the fossae, the occlusal morphology became arbitrarily flatter and less dependent on precise pathways through grooves. Early claims that tripod contacts never needed adjustment were abandoned as it became apparent that tripod contact was not a guarantee of stability.

The realization that complete posterior disclusion by the anterior guidance is the most desirable occlusion. Because of its proved effect on elevator muscle activity, posterior disclusion is the goal of occlusal treatment whenever it can be achieved. This eliminates some major concerns regarding incline pathways and ridge and groove directions.

Realization that an immediate side shift cannot occur from a correct centric relation. With changes in our understanding of centric relation, the concept of "most retruded" was replaced by "most superior." At the most superior position, the condyles are braced medially, and so they cannot travel horizontally toward the midline. This eliminates the concern about immediate side shift and simplifies requirements for instrumentation because without an immediate side shift the lateral anterior guidance is the dominant controlling factor in working-side jaw pathways. If fossa-wall angulation on the teeth is related to the lateral anterior guidance, the downward condylar guidance on the balancing side will only *add* to the disclusive effect.

If the working-side fossa inclines are flatter than the lateral anterior guidance, the posterior teeth will be separated in lateral working excursions before any side shift can take place.

SIMPLIFYING INSTRUMENTATION

Eliminating the need of excursive contacts on the posterior teeth is not a license to *ignore* condylar guidance. It just makes it possible to simplify instrumentation for most patients because *any* condylar path that is flatter on the articulator than the path on the patient will result in posterior restorations that disclude the moment the condyle starts down a steeper eminentia in the patient.

Setting the condylar paths flatter on the articulator has neither an effect on centric relation contacts nor any effect on correct anterior relationships as long as it is not changed after the anterior guidance is properly recorded on the instrument.

With new data showing the advantages of posterior disclusion, the goal of most occlusal treatment is to make sure the *combination* of condylar guidance and anterior guidance can separate the posterior teeth when the mandible moves forward or sideward from centric

relation. This treatment goal is further simplified by three different studies involving several hundred patients that showed that for all the patients tested, the *minimum* horizontal condylar path was 25 degrees. At the beginning of the protrusive path, the average incline is close to 60 degrees. This means that occlusal restorations fabricated on an articulator with 20-degree condylar paths would automatically separate if placed in a mouth with steeper condylar paths. Since almost all patients have condylar paths that are steeper than 20 degrees, this procedure is not so arbitrary as it may seem.

If the joint has been severely damaged by degenerative joint disease to the extent that the normally convex eminentia has been flattened to less than 20 degrees, it would be evident from a routine examination, that is, if a routine examination includes an evaluation of the temporomandibular joints and an analysis of wear patterns on the teeth. When upper lingual cusps are worn flat, it is almost a certainty that both the condyle and the eminence are also worn flat. This is an indication to record the condylar path accurately rather than to use an arbitrary setting. This is especially important if the anterior guidance is also worn flat. If one chooses not to record the condylar paths in such patients, the *effect* of the flattened path must be accounted for by other methods such as a functionally generated path.

When the anterior guidance is relatively steep, the protrusive or lateral condylar path loses its importance because almost no horizontal function can occur without separation of the posterior teeth by the anterior guidance.

If the anterior guidance is fairly flat, posterior restorations will still be discluded if they are fabricated at the 20-degree condylar setting on the articulator for any patient that has a condylar guidance that is within the normal range of 25 degrees or steeper, as long as the fossa walls on the posterior teeth are no steeper than the lateral anterior guidance and the occlusal plane is correct.

In the determination of what an instrument must do, a proper understanding of the role of the anterior guidance is necessary. In the past, importance was placed on precise recording of the condylar guidance: the anterior guidance was determined arbitrarily. The reverse of this is more logical for the following reasons:

1. Anterior teeth *maintain* contact from centric relation to the end point of function in all excursions. (All functional excursions do not maintain tooth contact, but the anterior guidance must be able to separate posterior contact through all functional excursions.)
2. The anterior guidance must be in harmony with the envelope of function, or tooth contact can create stress or wear. Thus it is important to record anterior guidance correctly. It is also directly related to the neutral-zone stability of the anterior teeth, and so an arbitrary anterior relationship will usually conflict with either the neutral zone or the envelope of function.
3. Posterior teeth ideally contact only in centric relation. They are in space for all other jaw positions.
4. The amount of separation by the posterior teeth in excursions does not seem to matter. Whether the lower posterior teeth just barely miss the upper inclines in function or they open and close on a near-vertical path has no discernable effect on function, comfort, or stability.
5. Since the only requirement for posterior tooth pathways is that they *miss* upper tooth inclines, the condylar path can be set arbitrarily flat enough on the instrument to cause posterior disclusion in the mouth. A 20-degree condylar path will accomplish the necessary disclusion on most patients.

How to tell when an arbitrary condylar path setting is or is not acceptable

Although the use of an arbitrary 20-degree condylar path is practical for most restorative cases, the decision to use a set 20-degree path should never be an arbitrary decision.

First of all, the requirements for instrumentation may vary, depending on whether the articulator is to be used for diagnosis or for fabrication of restorations. If all upper and lower posterior teeth are to be restored, instrumentation can be kept simpler because we can control the occlusal plane and the occlusal fossae contours in the restorative process.

Occlusal diagnosis becomes more complex on patients who do not need restorations but who have occlusal plane problems or gross interferences to the excursive pathways. On these patients we need to know how steep the condylar paths are so that we can determine how much occlusal reshaping is required to eliminate the occlusal interferences to excursive pathways. If restorations or orthodontics will be required, it should be determined before treatment is started.

Some occlusions must depend almost solely on the condylar path for disclusion of the posterior teeth. An examination of the patient should reveal when a set 20-degree path is not acceptable. More accuracy of condylar path is required when either of the following conditions are noted:

1. The anterior guidance cannot disclude the posterior teeth in protrusive or balancing excursions.
2. Severe wear has resulted in loss of upper lingual cusps. This is an indication of an abnormally flattened condylar path.

The condylar path is a critical determinant of posterior occlusal contours in each of the above situations. When the goal of posterior disclusion cannot be accomplished by the anterior guidance, you must rely on the downward path of the condyles to separate the back teeth in excursions. This can occur even with a flat anterior guidance as long as the occlusal plane is acceptable because the occlusal fossae can then be designed with fossa walls that are flat enough to be discluded by the combination of anterior guidance and the actual condylar guidance.

There are several instrument choices for diagnosis and treatment planning of such problem cases. Choices for the restorative phase are more inclusive because when the posterior teeth have been prepared out of all contact, the *effects* of condylar guidance and anterior guidance can be recorded at the teeth, eliminating the need for reproduction of the condylar path itself.

Instruments that can be used effectively for either diagnosis or treatment include the following types:

1. Fully adjustable articulators
2. Semiadjustable articulators
3. Combination (set condylar path *or* fully adjustable articulators)

Any of the above types of instruments can be used with great success if the operator understands the goals of occlusal diagnosis or therapy. It is strongly recommended that all three types be understood because the selection of an instrument is a very important decision that relates to practicality as well as effectiveness.

FULLY ADJUSTABLE INSTRUMENTS

The term "fully adjustable" refers to the reproducibility of the patient's condylar paths. Any variation from one type of fully adjustable articulator to another will be limited to mechanical variations that affect the ease of reproducing the condylar paths. Instruments may also vary in their quality of materials and workmanship.

Only instruments that can reproduce all condylar border movements including protrusive-lateral paths can be truly said to be fully adjustable. Very few can make that claim, and even then there is divergent opinion among instrument buffs about either the importance or the validity of the claims of complete adjustability.

There are two basic methods for recording the condylar paths: pantographic tracings and stereographics. Actually, neither method records the true anatomic contours of the temporomandibular joint, and the articulator does not reproduce the anatomy of the joint. It is merely a mechanical equivalent that makes the back end of the articulator capable of going through the same movements that the back end of the mandible follows in function. The condyles on the articulator are not shaped like the irregular condyles in the skull, but they can be made to duplicate the movements of the real condyles. How the *paths* of the condyles are recorded and mechanically duplicated determines the type of instrument.

PANTOGRAPHIC INSTRUMENTS

The use of pantographics has become far more practical since the introduction of the Dénar Pantograph. Because of a simplified procedure of using vinyl clutch formers, a central bearing point set of clutches can be fabricated in a matter of a few minutes. The clutches are then adapted to the Dénar Pantograph, which traces mandibular movements on tracing plates. The stylus that draws the pathway lines on the tracing plates is held against the plates by rubber bands, but it can easily be disengaged from the plate when one presses a button that permits air pressure to deactivate each stylus from contact. With practice, a pantographic tracing can usually be achieved within a reasonable chair time of 30 to 45 minutes. Some experts can cut that time considerably. If the procedures outlined in Figs. 12-10 to 12-17 are used, total chair time needed is reduced to about 10 minutes.

The pantographic technique does have the advantage that goes with the use of a central bearing point. With a properly located central bearing point, all occlusal interferences are disengaged when the condylar pathways are recorded. There is no tooth contact during the tracing procedures. Manipulation of the mandible is simpler because of the complete absence of any occlusal interferences at the opened vertical.

Complete preoperative occlusal analysis is possible on models to a more refined degree than is possible with semiadjustable articulators. The improvement in accuracy, however, is limited to the difference between straight-line versus curved pathways plus the differences of timing of the Bennett shift. It is doubtful whether such factors produce any real clinical advantages at the preoperative stage, since the analysis of centric contacts, arch relationships, and generalized excursive pathways can be accomplished on a semiadjustable instrument with a degree of accuracy that is usually acceptable for preoperative planning.

If the articulator is to serve as the mechanical equivalent of mandibular movement for fabrication of the finished restorations, then the improved accuracy does have clinical practicality. If the instrument is to be programmed to the pantographic tracings, it might just as well be done for the preoperative study and then be used for the entire case.

If pantographic tracings are to be used to program the articulator, it is necessary for the pantograph to be correct. Unfortunately, the pantograph can be no better than the operator's ability to manipulate the mandible with the pantograph attached. Allowing the patient to record border movements without expert assistance from the operator will result in incorrect tracings. They will generally fall short of the outer border limits. The mandible must be manipulated to correctly capture the outer limits of movement.

Text continued on p. 221.

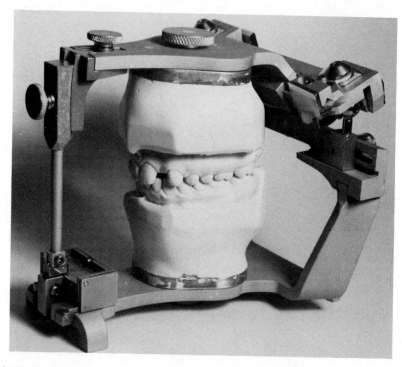

Fig. 12-10. The Dénar Articulator. A centric relation bite and a facebow record made at the first examination appointment were used to mount the diagnostic models. The easily mounted models can then be used by the assistant to set up the pantograph in the laboratory.

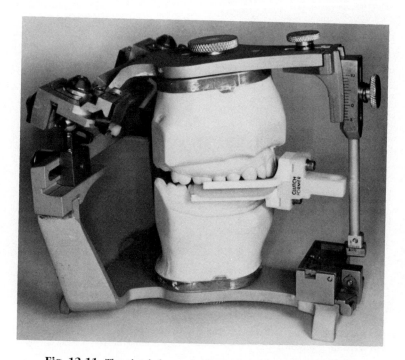

Fig. 12-11. The clutch former is checked on the mounted models.

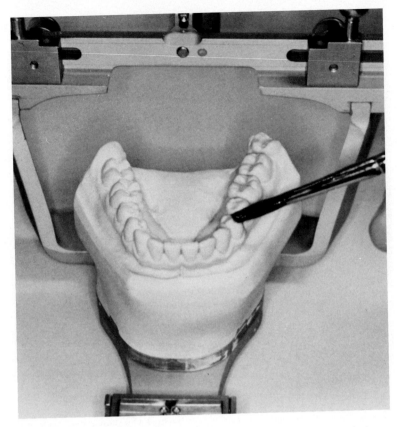

Fig. 12-12. The upper and lower models are painted with a heavy coat of tinfoil-substitute separating solution so that the acrylic resin will not stick.

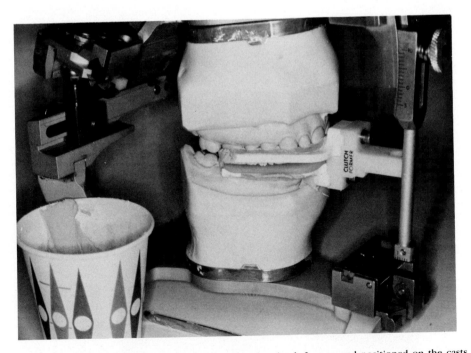

Fig. 12-13. The acrylic material is mixed, placed in the clutch former, and positioned on the casts. The casts are kept on a terminal axis arc of closure. Care should be taken to keep the acrylic from engaging undercuts. One must not use too much acrylic.

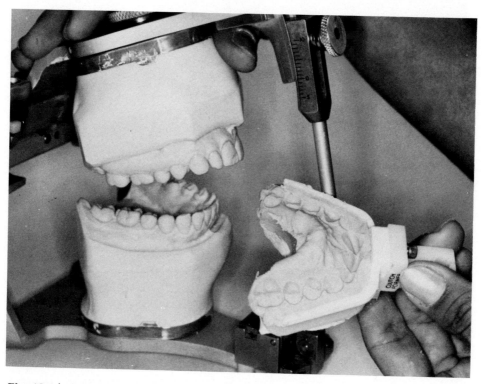

Fig. 12-14. When the acrylic resin begins to become warm, the articulator is opened and the clutch former removed. The acrylic should be allowed to complete its set.

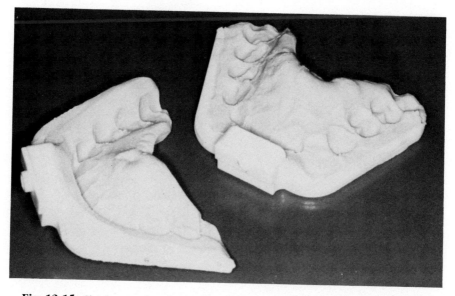

Fig. 12-15. Clutches are shaped up, any undercuts are relieved, and edges are smoothed.

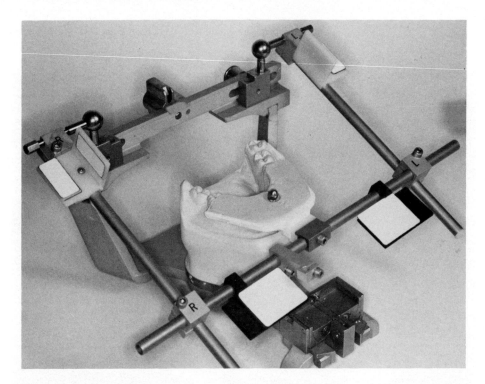

Fig. 12-16. The lower clutch is seated back on the model and checked to make certain it fits solidly, and the lower half of the pantograph is set up. The tracing plates can be easily positioned in correct relation to the condyles, which have been related to the casts by the facebow record.

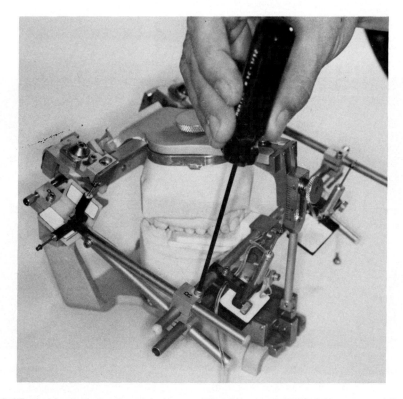

Fig. 12-17. The clutch is placed on the upper model and the second half of the pantograph is set up. The pantograph is now ready to be placed on the patient at the next appointment. No chair time has been lost making the clutches or setting up the pantograph. The tracings can be completed in a minimal amount of time (easily under 5 minutes). Besides the saving in chair time, a big advantage to this approach is that the clutches fit the diagnostic models so perfectly that they can be repositioned on the same models to set the condylar paths on the instrument.

Manipulation should start with the recording of the terminal hinge position and all lateral tracings should emanate from it. Failure to do so will result in restorations with interferences in the extreme border positions just lateral to centric relation.

When manipulating the mandible for a correct pantographic tracing, it is extremely important that the condyles be in their most superior position for the centric relation part of the tracing. *The central bearing point permits easy positioning of the condyles into this superior position, but it also permits a very common error to occur if correct manipulation is not used.* If upward pressure is exerted at the symphysis, the condyles will have a tendency to arc down and back from centric relation. The central bearing point serves as a fulcrum when the teeth are separated, and even slight upward pressure on the chin has the effect of dropping the condyles on a right-angled path from the eminentia.

If the condyles are not in their most superior position when lateral movements are started, they will not be braced medially as they should be in centric relation. An immediate side shift before any working-side rotation occurs is the result of improper manipulation. If the orbiting condyle starts its movement *from the superior position,* it will not move medially until it starts its forward movement. In other words, the orbiting condyle should always have a *gradual* side shift if movement starts from a correct centric relation.

Some form of two-handed technique (Fig. 12-18) is preferable to achieve correct border recordings when a pantograph is used. The same method described for recording centric relation (Chapter 4) can be used effectively with the pantograph in place with very little modification.

It is very difficult to record correct centric and border movements with the patient sitting up straight. The supine position makes manipulation much simpler.

If a one-handed technique is used to position the mandible in centric relation with the central bearing point in place, the dentist must be certain to exert a *downward* force on the chin as the mandible is retruded. This has the effect of seating the condyles upward. It is not, however, as dependable as a two-handed technique, and it lacks the control afforded by two hands.

The companion articulator for use with the Dénar Pantograph is the Dénar Articulator. It is matched to the pantograph and is easily programmed to duplicate the tracings. The Dénar is well made, is reasonably priced, and can be used effectively in any situation that requires the use of an articulator.

There are several other articulators that will also adjust to pantographic tracings. The selection of which instrument to use is purely a matter of personal preference.

It is believed by some that fully adjustable instruments can be used to produce "balanced" occlusions that can function without stress in all excursions, but the concept of a balanced occlusion is not a practical goal, regardless of how precisely the articulator reproduces lateral movement. In lateral movement, the orbiting condyle is unbraced and the mandible is subject to flexing. The degree of flexing of the mandible depends on the intensity of the muscle contraction. No matter how precise the recording device, it would be impossible to harmonize any occlusion to all the variations of muscle contraction on the unbraced condyle side.

Furthermore, it has been repeatedly shown clinically that there is no disadvantage to balancing-side disclusion. Since the harmful effect of balancing-side interference is so great and the benefits of "balanced" occlusion are so elusive, there does not seem to be a single practical reason for attempting to achieve it.

The reproducibility of correct lateral-protrusive paths could be used to possible advantage if an instrument approach is desired for providing working-side group function. Again, it is a matter of preference. The fully adjustable instrument has the capabilities if the operator wishes to select it. If it is to be programmed to reproduce lateral protrusive pathways, those paths must be recorded additionally on the pantograph or the articulator paths would be no more than interpolations.

A disadvantage of pantographic devices is that the tracings must be made at a considerably opened vertical dimension to make room for the clutches. It is essential that the terminal hinge axis must be recorded precisely or the incorrect axis of closure will introduce errors.

It is also probable that in some mouths, at least, the border movements are different at the opened position from what they are at the correct vertical.

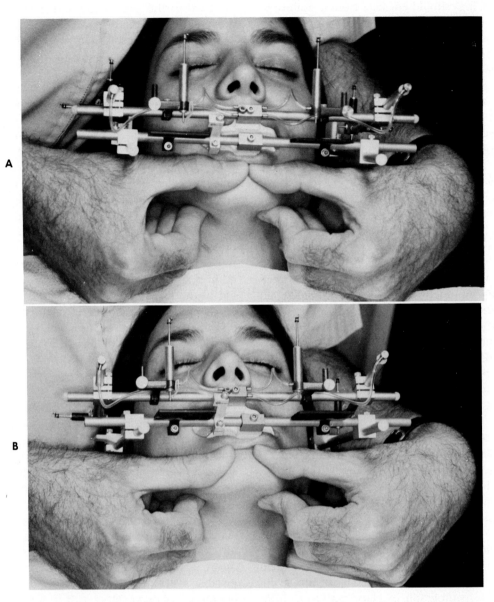

Fig. 12-18. A, For accuracy in recording the border movements, *the mandible must be manipulated with the pantograph in place.* Notice the stabilized head position between the forearm and ribs and the correct position of the thumbs (touching each other). Placed in the notch over the symphysis, they are in position to exert a downward-backward pressure during manipulation. Notice the fingers placed to exert upward pressure on the condyles during manipulation for verifying centric relation position of the condyles. Even with the pantograph in place, the mandible can be manipulated with extremely good control. The pantographic tracings can be no more accurate than the paths of movement that the operator records. Many pantographic errors result from failure to achieve a true terminal hinge condyle position during any part of the tracing. **B,** Lateral excursions are recorded after the terminal hinge position has been achieved. Firm upward pressure should be maintained on the working-side condyle. In this left lateral excursion, the right hand is moved slightly to apply pressure up and in on the orbiting condyle. With this kind of firm control, it is permissible for the patient to help without fear of recording a protrusive lateral path instead of the straight lateral border path that is so important.

Errors in mounting are common and easy to make. The slightest movement of either clutch produces a magnified error at the tracing plate. Studies done by Helsing have shown that reproducibility of pantographic tracing is seldom achieved. Nevertheless, the pantographic procedure can be used as a practical approach to minimize postplacement adjustments if used with a correct anterior guidance. Any dentist who operates under the illusion that any pantographic instrument is capable of uniform perfection, however, is probably accepting less than optimum occlusal refinement as a finished result. The same may be said for all other techniques.

MISINTERPRETATION OF PANTOGRAPHIC TRACINGS

There are two common misinterpretations regarding pantographic tracings. The first misconception is that the tracings represent the actual path of the condyles. Actually, the path that is drawn on the tracing is a mirror image of the condylar path and not the path that the condyle travels. The writing point is fixed to the upper clutch and stays stationary as the recording plate moves with the lower jaw, producing a reversal of the jaw path. Thus a convex eminence is recorded as a concave path (Fig. 12-19).

The second misconception is in the interpretation of what appears to be an immediate side shift. This part of the tracing does not relate to a side shift at all. It is the result of the *downward* movement of the recording plate as the orbiting (balancing) side condyle travels down the steepest part of the eminence. As the tracing plate moves down, it arcs in a curve around the rotating condyle, but the writing point extends straight down to draw a sideways line (Fig. 12-20). The steeper the condylar path, the more the false "side shift" will appear. This supposed shift of the condyle cannot happen if the condyles are in the uppermost position that is medially braced. Furthermore, even severe "side shift" recordings do not show up in a gothic arch tracing done intraorally.

If the recording plate on the pantograph is aligned parallel with the protrusive path, the extension of the writing point will be eliminated and the "side shift" will disappear. Medial-pole bracing is an essential part of ana-

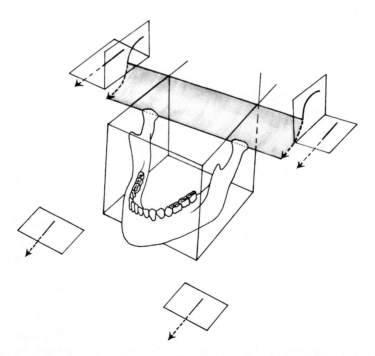

Fig. 12-19. Typical pantograph results in recordings that are mirror images of the actual path because the recording plate moves with the mandible while the stylus is fixed. The protrusive path of the recording plate is illustrated by the *dotted lines.*The recording by the fixed position of the stylus against the moving plate is shown as the *solid lines.* A pantographic recording must be interpreted. It does not represent the actual jaw movement.

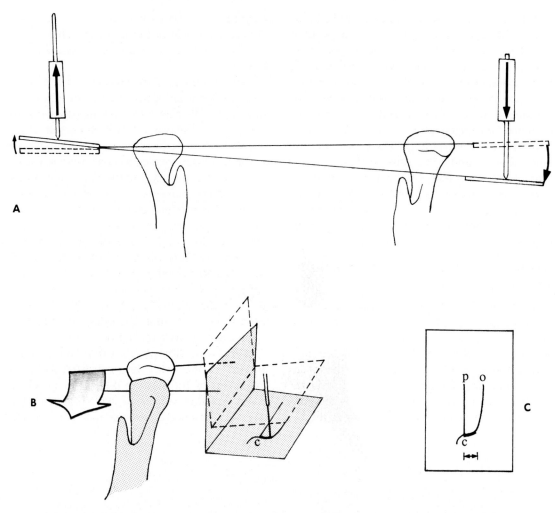

Fig. 12-20. False recording of an "immediate" side shift can result from the downward movement of the orbiting condyle, which moves the recording plate to an angled position, **A.** As the stylus extends straight down to follow the plate, it draws a sideways line from centric relation, *c,* **B.** The forward movement increases as a condylar path flattens to cause the completion of the pantographic recording. In **C,** the recording shows the protrusive path, *p,* the orbiting path, *o,* and the centric relation, *c.* The little tail that extends forward of the centric relation dot is the back line that occurs during working-side rotation. The *arrow* represents the amount of "immediate" side shift that is recorded but does not actually exist if the recording is started at centric relation.

tomic design that is responsible for the "mid-most" position of the mandible in centric relation.

It is a mystery why such an easily explained error in pantographic interpretation has been so difficult to dispel.

STEREOGRAPHIC INSTRUMENTS

One of the simplest "fully adjustable" instruments to use is the TMJ Articulator (Fig. 12-21). All border movements can be accurately recorded in three dimensions by means of simple intraoral clutches that are stabilized by a central bearing point.

The recordings are made by indenting three or four points into doughy self-curing acrylic resin on the surface of the opposite clutch and then moving the mandible through all border movements. Protrusive lateral movements can be included. When the stereographic recording is completed, the acrylic guide paths are allowed to set hard. The condyle paths on the instrument are then made in self-curing acrylic as dictated by the points of one clutch sliding in the indented recordings of the other. Since the three-dimensional recordings were made in the mouth by the paths of the condyles, the procedure can be reversed and the paths in

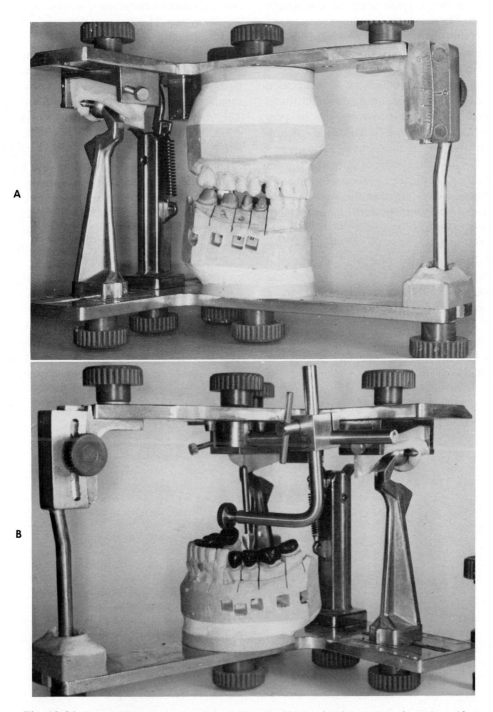

Fig. 12-21. A, The TMJ Articulator with condylar paths fabricated and a customized anterior guidance comes as close to being a fully adjustable instrument as can be achieved. **B,** The *Fillastre Carver* in position on the TMJ Articulator. If the condylar paths and the customized anterior guide table are both correct, this carver can be used to trace the exact ridge and groove direction and fossae contours on the lower occlusal surfaces. It can be moved from tooth to tooth to the position of each upper lingual cusp.

the clutch can dictate the mechanical equivalent of condyle movement on the articulator.

The procedure is quite practical and simple to execute. The intraoral clutches are very stable, since they have no extraoral appendages. The TMJ instrument is sturdy and easy to program.

Stereographic techniques have a decided advantage in the use of the three-dimensional recordings. *All* border pathways can be programmed into the condylar guidance, including protrusive-lateral movements. The instrument can be used in combination with customized anterior guidance procedures and all other procedures outlined in this text. It lends itself well to sophisticated Pankey-Mann-Schuyler procedures.

The TMJ instrument is an excellent articulator for fabricating dentures. The intraoral clutches are stabilized by the central bearing point and all recordings are made intraorally within the central area of the bases. This is a decided advantage over pantographic devices which frequently have a tendency to tilt the denture base with the weight of the external appendages.

SEMIADJUSTABLE INSTRUMENTS

What was once considered a shortcoming of semiadjustable articulators is now considered an advantage. The biggest difference between fully adjustable and semiadjustable articulators is that the condylar pathways are limited to straight lines for semiadjustable instrumentation. Because of this limitation, these instruments are referred to as *checkbite articulators*. This means that the horizontal condyle paths are set to align with a bite record made at centric relation and another bite record made in the protrusive position. This resultant path is a straight line between the two points. Lateral pathways are set from the centric bite record plus bite records made in left lateral and right lateral jaw positions. The resultant straight line sets the gradual side shift of the balancing condyle on the articulator.

The advantage offered by the straight-line pathway in protrusive movement is that it gives a built-in safety factor for the necessary disclusive effect. The condyles follow a *convex* path on any but the most damaged eminentiae. This convex curve will not be copied on the articulator. Only the two points of the check-

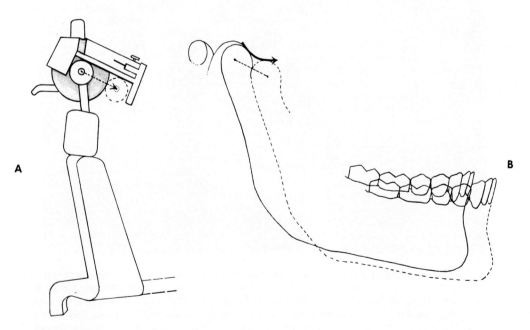

Fig. 12-22. Semiadjustable instruments generally follow a straight path, **A.** If the horizontal path is set by a check bite at the beginning and end of a convex path, **B,** the condylar path on the articulator will be flatter at the beginning of the protrusive path than it is in the patient, *dotted path.* This provides a safety factor because the patient's steeper path will disclude posterior teeth more than the articulator.

bite position will be correct (Fig. 12-22, *A*), but the path between the two points will be flatter than the actual convex path. This automatically produces a separation from any restorations made on the straight path when the condyles follow the convex path in the patient (Fig. 12-22, *B*).

The progressive side shift of the balancing-side condyle has often been portrayed as following a severe concave pathway, starting with an *immediate* side shift before any rotation occurs. This cannot happen if the starting point is at the medially braced centric relation. If one will observe numerous gothic arch tracings made by a central bearing point (Fig. 12-23), it will be obvious that the balancing-side condyle follows an arc around the rotating condyle. Rarely if ever will any side shift be noted on the lateral pathways of a gothic arch tracing. In fact, a gothic arch tracing is not even considered correct unless it has a point at the centric relation end.

Even if a concave path were followed by the orbiting condyle, straight pathways can still be set to follow a path that is angled inwardly more than the severest progressive side shift. A simple and completely practical procedure is to set all articulators to the maximum progressive side shift possible and leave them that way. This will automatically prevent balancing inclines from contacting for any occlusal schemes that are worked out on such a setting. Furthermore, there are no disadvantages to leaving all articulators at the maximum lateral setting because it takes away nothing that is needed and creates no problems.

For many years, all my articulators have been set only at the maximum progressive side-shift angulation of 15 degrees. I have seen no reason to alter that procedure. Balancing-side contact is *never* desirable (except for full dentures), and this practice helps to ensure disclusion of all balancing inclines.

For diagnostic studies, one can minimize errors of the checkbite technique by making the protrusive and lateral bite records fairly close to centric relation. The most important part of the condylar pathway is right after the condyle leaves centric relation, and so taking the eccentric bite records within about 5 mm from centric relation gives greater accuracy where it is needed most. The common practice of

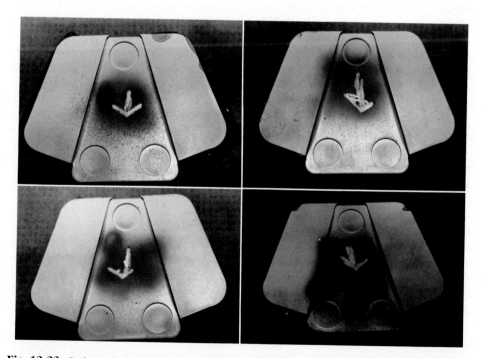

Fig. 12-23. Gothic arch tracings show no sign of any immediate side shift as evidenced by the pointed tracings. If a side shift were present, gothic arches would have a flat place instead of the point. Notice how some tracings show irregular jaw movements until muscle deprogramming and correct manipulation defines the border movements to centric relation.

taking the protrusive bite record at incisor end-to-end relationship can in some patients increase the error. In patients with severe overjet this may be too far protrusive. The checkbites should relate specifically to condyle paths for the first few millimeters of separation of the posterior teeth.

Semiadjustable instruments can often be set without the need for any checkbites. If the anterior teeth can maintain contact through the protrusive range in the patient, the condylar paths can be set on the articulator to permit the same protrusive contact. This is easily accomplished by mere steepening of the condylar path until the posterior teeth are just barely separated in protrusive excursions, allowing anterior contact.

If the patient's anterior teeth are separated by the posterior teeth in protrusion, this method cannot be used. That will be an indication for determining the condylar path by a more precise method.

If an arbitrary setting of 20 degrees for the condylar path is being used, it will not always disclude posterior teeth that do disclude in the mouth. If during examination of the patient you observe that the anterior teeth maintain contact through the protrusive range, the articulator paths are easily steepened until the posterior teeth just barely miss in protrusion. It is an advantage for the articulator to have adjustable condylar paths for this reason. The semiadjustable instrument thus provides the practicality of set 20-degree condylar paths, with the simplicity of easy correction when needed.

New understanding about the benefits of posterior disclusion has made the semiadjustable articulator the standard instrument for any type of occlusal treatment. You can even use the instrument with a pantograph or axiograph by observing the paths for the first 5 mm or so from centric relation and then setting the condylar path slightly flatter in protrusive relation and at a slightly increased angulation inward for the progressive side shift. The range can be very close to the actual patient pathways but with a slight safety margin that will only add beneficially to the desired disclusive effect.

Working-side excursions need be related only to the lateral anterior guidance because there is no clinically significant change in lateral angulation from the cuspid incline back, except for the progressive shortening of the stroke.

Semiadjustable instruments do not record the *precise* pathways of lateral and protrusive condylar movements, but by using any of the above methods, you can adjust the instrument to within a practical degree of accuracy for completely acceptable diagnostic uses. Its use as an instrument for *restorative* procedures can be more precise because even though the exact condylar pathways are not reproduced, the mechanical equivalent of jaw movements can be recorded with as much accuracy as is possible on any available instrument if the instrument's shortcomings are compensated for with the following:

1. Customized anterior guidance procedures (as outlined in Chapter 18). This is needed regardless of the adjustability of condylar guidances.
2. Simplified fossae contour technique to relate lower fossae form to the anterior guidance (described in Chapter 21).
3. Functionally generated path procedures to capture the precise border movements of each posterior tooth at the correct vertical dimension (see Chapter 23).

When recorded in this manner, the pathways of the posterior teeth reflect the precise influence of both the anterior guidance and the complete range of condylar border pathways. No interpolation of condylar border paths is necessary because the border movements are recorded directly at the site where the path of movement is important—at the posterior teeth themselves. The articulator is thus not used as a duplicator of jaw movements but rather as a device that relates the functional pathways to the cast of the prepared teeth. Since each of the above refinements can be used with advantage in *any* instrument approach, they do not constitute unnecessary, added work.

There are several semiadjustable articulators that fill all the requirements for quality instrumentation. The instrument of choice in my practice for many years has been the Dénar Mark II (Fig. 12-24). My reasons for selecting this instrument involve primarily the quality of workmanship and materials used. Because it has machined parts, it can be interchangeable with the other articulators in the Dénar system. The use of a field gage (Fig. 12-25) enables my staff to keep all instruments aligned the same for an extremely practical interchangeability from any Dénar articulator to another.

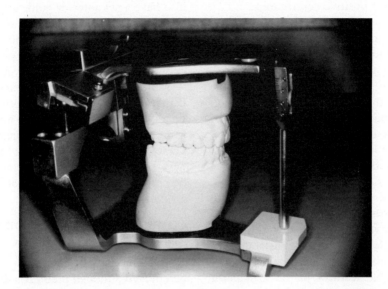

Fig. 12-24. Dénar Mark II articulator is a semiadjustable arcon instrument. It has all the capabilities that are needed for simple to complex procedures and is interchangeable with other Dénar articulators when aligned with a field gage.

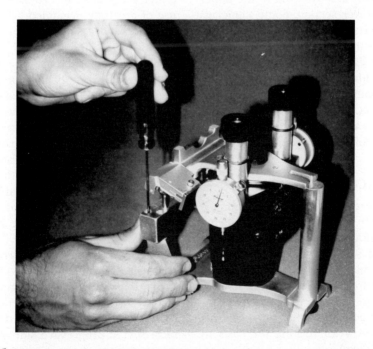

Fig. 12-25. The use of a field gage permits alignment of all the Dénar articulators so that they can be used interchangeably. Adjustments are made by lining up cross hairs in the gage to the same settings.

Other requirements for an acceptable semi-adjustable instrument include the following:

1. Must accept a facebow.
2. Must have a positive centric lock.
3. Must have an adjustable incisal guide pin that permits changes in vertical dimension without moving the position of the pin on the guide table.
4. Must have provisions for a transferable customized anterior guide table.
5. Must permit the casts to be secured by removable mounting rings.
6. Must have horizontal condylar paths that are adjustable from 0 degrees to at least 60 degrees.
7. Must have a progressive side-shift path up to at least 15 degrees.
8. Must have an intercondylar width of approximately 110 mm. Adjustability of this dimension is not a critical factor.

Other desirable features for an articulator are the following:

1. Reasonable visibility from the lingual.
2. Easy cleanability.
3. Does not come apart accidentally.
4. Arcon condylar guide.

A final feature that I find very desirable is a design that permits easy removal of the upper bow from the lower section. Some clinicians prefer that the articulator *not* come apart. My preference for being able to remove the upper bow is that it is easier to work with one arch for some procedures without the cumbersomeness of stabilizing an opened articulator. It also allows direct line removal of die models from bite records and makes it possible to verify the accuracy of the mounting with greater simplicity.

SET PATH ARTICULATORS

Because a 20-degree horizontal and 15-degree lateral path works so well for achieving posterior disclusion in the majority of patients, articulators with set condylar paths have become very popular. Such instruments may have all the features of an acceptable semiadjustable articulator except that the condylar paths cannot be adjusted. They *must* be able to accept a facebow for relating the casts to the correct horizontal axis.

The reason for the growing popularity of this type of instrument is solely related to cost. A set path instrument can be purchased for considerably less than an articulator with adjustable condylar paths because the machining of the movable paths is a costly process.

Unfortunately, most set path articulators also have a set anterior guide angle. This is unacceptable. Anterior guidance is never an arbitrary decision regardless of the type of articulator used; so there must be a provision for accepting a customized anterior guide table.

Although a set path instrument may be acceptable for a majority of restorative procedures, it will not be adequate for diagnosis on some patients with occlusal plane problems or inadequate anterior guidance. Many patients have needs that require the condylar paths to be considered, and for those patients a set path articulator is not acceptable.

COMBINATION SET PATH OR FULLY ADJUSTABLE INSTRUMENTS

The simplicity of a set path instrument can be enjoyed although it still has the capacity for complete adjustability when needed. This very practical combination can be found in a precisely machined instrument that, despite its much lower cost, fulfills all the requirements for quality instrumentation. The Dénar Combi articulator (Fig. 12-26) provides the option of either set path or full adjustment through the use of precisely machined inserts for condylar guidance and a simplified method for stereographic recording of condylar paths when needed. Through the use of a field gage, these instruments can also be kept aligned, and so they can be used interchangeably or even with other instruments in the Dénar system.

Because of its interchangeability, the Dénar Combi can be used with set paths as a standard instrument for most restorative needs, but when changes in condylar path are needed, the casts can either by transferred to a Mark II articulator or the condylar path inserts can be changed to accept a precise border path recording.

The *set condylar path insert* has a horizontal inclination of 20 degrees, which makes it flatter than the minimal angulation found in healthy articulations. The lateral path is curved to a more medially directed path than the most severe progressive side shift. Use of this insert permits direct fabrication of posterior restorations that will automatically be discluded by all but the most abnormally contoured condylar pathways as long as the correct anterior guidance is recorded.

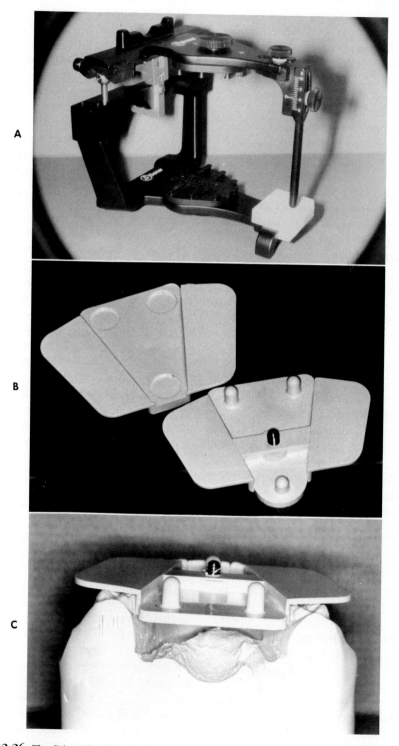

Fig. 12-26. The Dénar Combi Articulator, **A**, can be used as either a set path instrument or a fully adjustable articulator. Articulator is shown with 20-degree set path inserts in place. They are easily replaced with a zero-degree insert that can be used to record the condylar paths from a stereograph. The stereographic clutches, **B**, are offset so that the recording can be made at a minimal vertical opening, **C.**

The set condylar path insert can be used as the standard setting for the majority of restorative procedures. With the set path insert in place, the articulator can be used routinely *without modification* if the following two conditions are met:

1. If in the mouth the anterior teeth disclude the posterior teeth in excursions from maximum intercuspation.
2. The posterior teeth on the mounted casts are discluded by the anterior teeth in excursions from maximum intercuspation.

When the above two conditions are met, the instrument can be used for *either* treatment planning or restorative procedures without altering the set 20-degree path.

For *restorative patients,* minor alteration of the casts will sometimes be necessary to achieve posterior disclusion on a 20-degree set path articulator. If all posterior teeth are in need of restoration, this should not cause a problem for any patient whose anterior teeth maintain contact during protrusion.

Even if the anterior teeth are separated in the mouth during protrusion, it may not necessarily rule out the simplified approach of set path instrumentation. If anterior excursive contact can be achieved on the casts by occlusal plane corrections that do not require excessive posterior tooth reduction, there are no contraindications for using the set path articulator for patients who require restorations on all posterior teeth.

The adjustable path insert

For the analysis of some occlusal relationships, the set 20-degree path is not adequate. The safest rule for using the adjustable path insert for precise duplication of condylar paths is to use it for occlusal analysis whenever the anterior teeth are discluded by the posterior teeth. However, the following conditions specifically indicate the need for a nonarbitrary condylar path analysis:

1. Protrusive disclusion of anterior teeth when posterior teeth do not need restorations.
2. Restorative cases that would require severe changes to establish an "ideal" arbitrary occlusal plane.
3. Severely worn dentitions, especially when the upper lingual cusps have been worn flat.

Anterior disclusion and no need for posterior restorative dentistry

For posterior teeth that do not require restorations, the decision to drastically change their shape should not be an arbitrary one. A major purpose of occlusal analysis is to determine how best to achieve posterior disclusion. To accomplish that goal with the minimum amount of tooth reduction, we must take full advantage of the disclusive effect by the condyles. The steeper they move downwardly, the more they can help to separate the posterior teeth when the jaw protrudes, and the less reduction of tooth structure will be needed. The only way we can predetermine the amount of occlusal alteration required to achieve posterior disclusion is to know the actual condylar paths.

When posterior disclusion is lacking, it can be achieved either by lowering of the occlusal plane at the posterior teeth or steepening of the anterior guidance, or a combination of both. If disclusion is achieved by steepening of the anterior guidance, it is possible to create a damaging restriction of functional pathways. The determination of how much change is needed for the anterior guidance is dependent on how much disclusive help is possible from the condylar path and how much reduction is permitted for the posterior teeth without destroying too much enamel. *The adjustable condylar path should be used whenever formulation of a conservative treatment plan depends on a pretreatment determination of the precise amount of posterior tooth reduction required to achieve posterior disclusion.*

Severe occlusal plane problems

If all posterior teeth require restorations, it is generally no problem to determine an ideal occlusal plane and to restore to that ideal. In such cases the set 20-degree path can generally be used effectively. Some occlusal plane problems, however, are too severe to be corrected to an ideal curve without excessive reduction of teeth. *Even if the posterior teeth are to be restored, the adjustable condylar path should be used whenever it appears that an ideal arbitrary curve will require inappropriate tooth reduction.*

Severe wear

In patients with severe wear of upper lingual cusps, there is a probability that both the condyles and the eminentiae have been worn flat also. In such cases, the condylar path may actually be flatter than the 20-degree set path insert. Since this type of problem is also generally found with a flat anterior guidance, it can require special attention to both anterior guidance and condylar guidance. *In the restoration of severely worn dentitions the adjustable condylar guide should be used.*

METHOD FOR USING THE ADJUSTABLE CONDYLAR GUIDE INSERT

The decision to record and transfer the precise condylar guidance does not need to be made until after the diagnostic casts are mounted on the Dénar Combi articulator. The mounting is usually completed with the set 20-degree paths in place as a standard procedure, but since changing the inserts does not alter the centric relation position, either insert may be used for mounting. The zero-degree insert should be used whenever a customized condylar path is to be fabricated.

Fabrication of the customized condylar path is accomplished in two stages:

1. *The clinical stage* requires the use of a simple stereographic recording.
2. *The laboratory stage* requires the generation of condylar pathways in acrylic dough as programmed from the stereographic recording.

Neither of the above steps is difficult or time consuming and can be accomplished at any stage of diagnosis or treatment including at the time of tooth preparation.

Making the stereographic recording (clinical stage)

One of the simplest methods for recording all border movements in three dimensions is accomplished by a stereographic recording. This is done by means of intraoral clutches that are adapted to the occlusal surfaces with acrylic resin or compound (Fig. 12-26) and then stabilized in the mouth by a central bearing point (Fig. 12-27, *A*). The clutches can be adapted either directly in the mouth or to casts and then transferred to the mouth.

The recordings are made in self-curing acrylic resin by three recording points on the lower clutch. The self-curing acrylic dough is on the surface of the upper clutch. As the mandible moves through all border movements, the recording points follow a path dictated by the condylar movements. As the condyles travel down the eminentiae, the lower clutch moves down with them in the back while the front of the mandible slides on the central bearing point. This cuts a path into the acrylic dough that relates directly to the condylar paths. When the stereographic recording is completed, the acrylic guide paths are allowed to set hard (Fig. 12-27, *B* to *D*). This stereographic recording is then transferred to the mounted casts for the laboratory procedures.

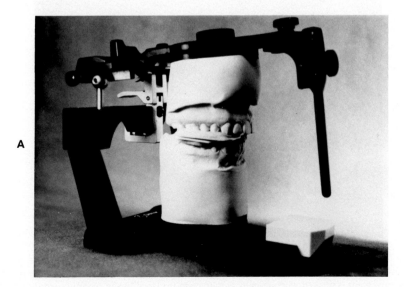

Fig. 12-27. A, Clutches adapted to casts with acrylic resin. This method saves chair time but is not necessary because clutches can also be adapted directly in the mouth.   *Continued.*

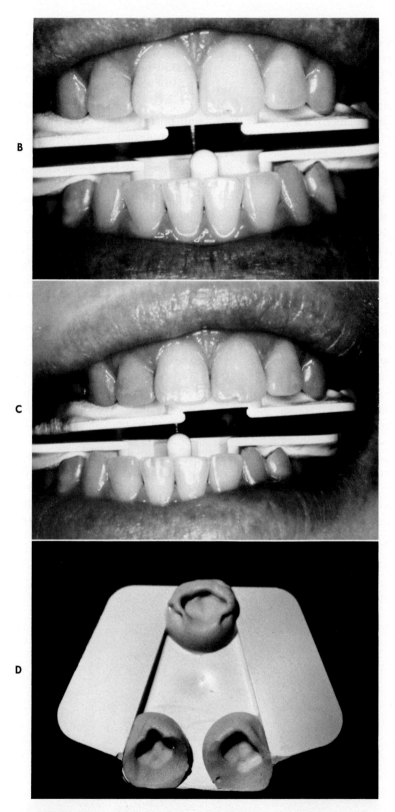

Fig. 12-27, cont'd. B, Clutches in mouth. Central bearing pin is screwed out so that clutches do not contact each other. **C,** Notice how the lower clutch travels down with the orbiting condyle on the left side. This movement is tracked when doughy acrylic resin is placed in the retention circles on the upper clutch. The jaw is guided through all excursions to record the paths in the acrylic dough. **D,** Completed recording.

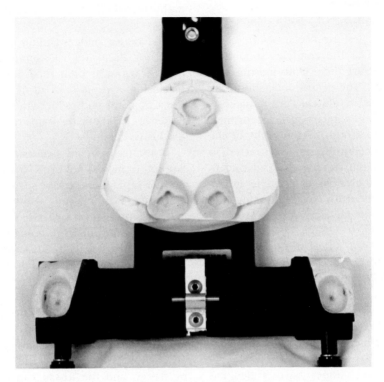

Fig. 12-28. Condylar paths generated directly into a doughy mix of acrylic resin when the articulator bows are moved through all excursions while the recording points on the lower clutch track in all three stereographic paths on the upper clutch.

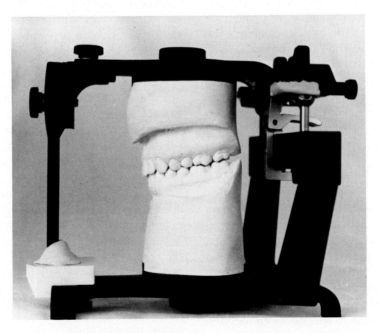

Fig. 12-29. Stereographic recording of condylar paths combined with customized anterior guidance provides complete range of functional movements.

Laboratory procedures

With the zero-degree condylar path insert in place, the clutches are placed on the casts. Their relationship to the condyles should be checked to make sure there is no interference to centric relation. The centric lock should be free to close when the clutches are in place.

Since the three-dimensional recordings were made in the mouth by the paths of the condyles, the procedure is simply reversed so that the paths in the stereograph can dictate the mechanical equivalent of condyle movement on the articulator by generating the condylar paths in doughy acrylic resin (Fig. 12-28).

The procedure is practical and simple to execute. The intraoral clutches are very stable because they have no extraoral appendages. The easy interchangeability of the condylar paths on the Dénar Combi articulator make it an excellent choice as an instrument for either diagnosis or treatment for any occlusal problem.

Stereographic techniques have a decided advantage in the use of three-dimensional recordings. *All* border pathways can be programmed into the condylar guidance, including protrusive lateral movements. The instrument can be used in combination with customized anterior guidance procedures (Fig. 12-29) and all other procedures outlined in this text.

The stereographic technique is excellent for denture fabrication. The intraoral clutches can be stabilized against the ridges by the central bearing point, and all recordings are made intraorally within the central area of the bases. This is a decided advantage over pantographic devices, which frequently have a tendency to tilt the denture base with the weight of the external appendages.

USING INSTRUMENTS TO ADVANTAGE (SUMMARY)

A great amount of time is often wasted on procedures that have little or no value on specific cases. The intelligent use of instrumentation can provide preciseness when it is needed and simplicity when simpler approaches are sufficient to satisfy the actual needs of a given case. By understanding the relationship of condylar movements to specific tooth inclines, you can use the articulator to serve the specific needs of *occlusal* contouring rather than an overriding concern for precise condylar

pathways whether they affect the outcome or not.

The better understanding of the effects of posterior disclusion has simplified demands for precise condylar path recordings. If posterior disclusion is desired in all excursions, setting the articulator with wider lateral pathways and flatter horizontal paths helps to accomplish the disclusive effect.

If disclusion in any excursion is desired, the amount of miss is not critical. Variations in disclusive separation do not seem to be discernable as far as function or stability is concerned.

If group function is desired on the working side, or if the anterior guidance cannot disclude the posterior teeth, and the occlusal contouring is to be achieved with a complete instrument approach, precise condylar path recording is necessary.

If functionally generated path procedures are used to record border movements, it is not necessary to also record them precisely on the articulator. Fossa walls on the lower teeth can be flatter, and the fossae can be opened out more because even in group function there is no necessity for fossa incline contact on lower posterior teeth.

There are many articulators from which to choose. A comfortable instrument that is a quality product should be selected. It is an advantage to determine the type of instrument you wish to work with and then stay with that same type as much as possible because this enables you to standardize your procedures at the chair and in the laboratory. Working with instruments that are interchangeable with each other and with other instruments in a system is a decided advantage.

The use of a combination set path or fully adjustable instruments can reduce the cost of instrumentation while still providing a complete range of programmability.

No articulator should be considered that does not accept a facebow orientation of the casts.

Simple hinge type of articulators are limited only to movements the patient cannot make. They are a cause of major errors in occlusal contouring and have no value for restorative procedures or occlusal analysis.

SUGGESTED READINGS

Bennett, N.G.: A contribution to the study of the movements of the mandible, Proc. Soc. Med. (Odontol.) **1**:79, 1908; reprinted in J. Prosthet. Dent. **8**:41, 1958.

Levinson, E.: The nature of the side shift in lateral mandibular movement and its implications in clinical practice, J. Prosthet. Dent. **52**:1, 1984.

Lundeen, H.: Condylar movement patterns engraved in plastic blocks, J. Prosthet. Dent. **30**(6):866-875, 1973.

Ricketts, R.M.: Orthodontic diagnosis and planning, their roles in preventative and rehabilitative dentistry, Denver, 1982, Rocky Mountain Orthodontic Publishers.

Solberg, W. K., and Clark, G. T.: Reproducibility of molded condylar controls with an intraoral registration method. Part I. Simulated movement, J. Prosthet. Dent. **32**:520, 1974; Part II. Human jaw movement, J. Prosthet. Dent. **33**:60, 1975.

Swanson, K.H.: A new method of recording gnathological movements, Northwest Dent. **45**:99-101, 1966

Swanson, Wipf Articulator Co. (TMJ) Articulator Manual, Thousand Oaks, Calif.

13

Mounting casts

Regardless of how perfectly a centric relation bite record is made, it is a rare dentist who maintains that accurate of a jaw relationship through the mounting of the casts. This is so because the slightest lapse of rigid quality control in mounting can lead to significant errors in the relationship of the casts on the articulator. It is my consistent observation that the most commonly used mounting procedures fail to achieve even a practical degree of accuracy in all but the most meticulous practices. Yet the time and effort wasted in correcting occlusal errors that result from improperly mounted casts is far greater than the time required to avoid the error.

There are four basic steps required for correct mounting of casts:

1. Relating the upper cast to the condylar axis
2. Relating the lower cast to the upper cast
3. Verifying the accuracy of the mounting
4. Setting the vertical dimension

RELATING THE UPPER CAST

The upper cast is always the first cast to be mounted. A facebow recording is one of the *essential* steps for proper mounting because after location of the condylar axis in the skull it provides a method of transferring that axis to the articulator and relating the upper cast to it.

The lower cast is likewise related to the condylar axis when it is positioned against the upper cast by means of a centric relation bite record. If a centric relation bite record is made at an opened vertical, the accuracy of the bite record will be maintained only if the closing axis is the same on the articulator as it is on the patient. This is the principle purpose of the facebow recording.

The upper cast must also be related to some point on the face so that the occlusal plane will be properly aligned. The point on the face can be arbitrary, but the usual landmark is the infraorbital foramen. Although an infraorbital pointer is often used to determine the vertical position of the upper cast, it is not a totally necessary procedure. If the labial surface of the upper incisors is aligned with the perpendicular, the cast position will generally be in an acceptable relationship. The relationship of the cast to the condylar axis will be maintained regardless of the height of the cast as long as a facebow is used. The vertical positioning of the cast always relates to the condylar axis as the casts move on an arc around the axis (Fig. 13-1), and so the vertical positioning is just a mat-

Fig. 13-1. With a facebow mounting, A, the casts are always related to the condylar axis regardless of the height of the cast, B and C. Thus the opening/closing arc is maintained correctly whether or not the casts are related to a vertical landmark on the face. Although the axis is constant, the angle of the condylar path is not. Condylar-path angulation always relates to the height of the cast, and so it becomes steeper as the upper cast is lowered, C.

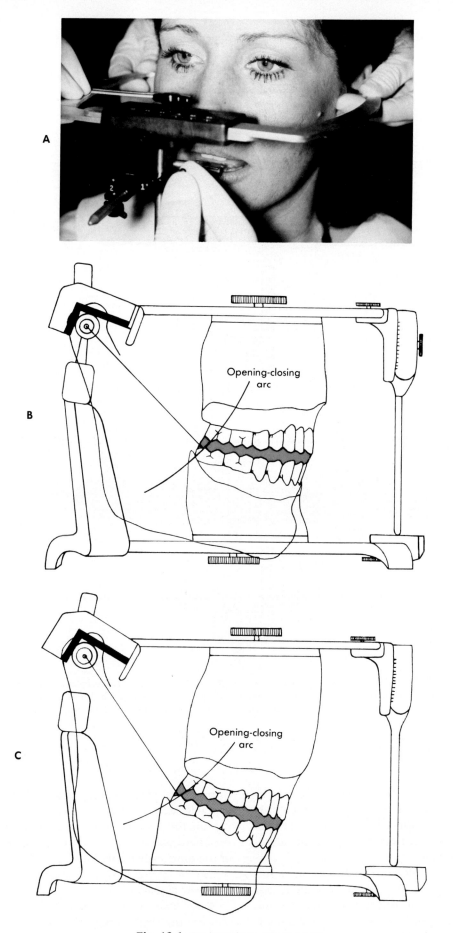

Fig. 13-1. For legend see opposite page.

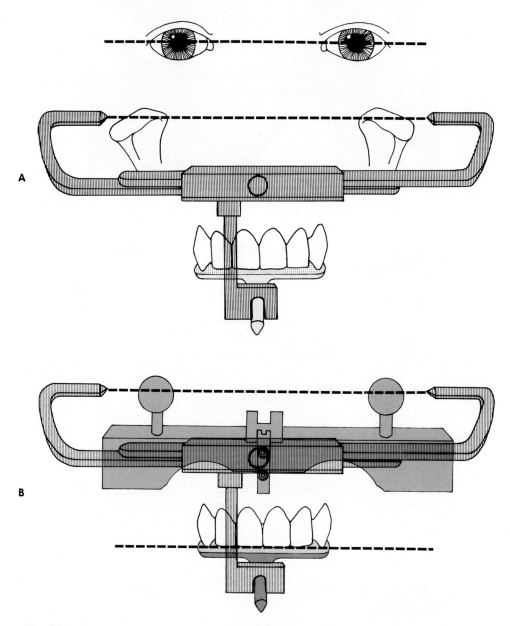

Fig. 13-2. The bow of the facebow should always be observed to make sure it is parallel to the eyes, **A**. If alignment is correct, the casts will align with the condyles on the articulator, **B**. The occlusal plane can then be aligned with the bench top in the lab to produce an esthetically pleasing plane in the patient.

ter of convenience. Repeatability of the mounting can be achieved by transfer bite records that are made on the articulator. It is not necessary to repeat a facebow record for subsequent mountings.

In addition to the correct slant of the posterior occlusal plane, the alignment of the incisal plane must also be oriented to the face, the lips, and the eyes. What is needed is a mounting that leaves no doubt about whether the ex-

isting incisal plane is acceptable and, if not acceptable, what corrections are needed to align it with the interpupillary line, in addition to the condylar axis. A slanted incisal plane is one of the most esthetically unacceptable mistakes. It can be avoided with proper attention to face-bow alignment.

When making the facebow record, always observe the relationship of the bow to the interpupillary line (Fig. 13-2). The condylar axis

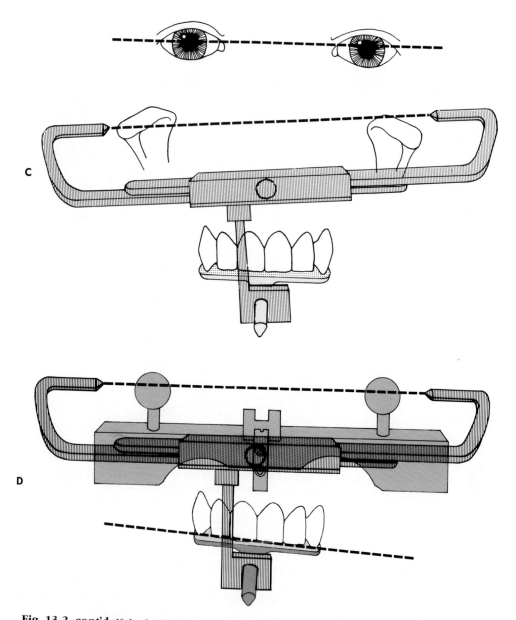

Fig. 13-2, cont'd. If the facebow is not aligned with the eyes, **C**, the casts will be set on the articulator at an angle when the bow is aligned with the articulator condyles, **D**. This gives an erroneous alignment of the casts. If the technician lines up incisal edges of any restorations parallel to the bench top, the incisal plane would be angled, a serious esthetic mistake.

is usually parallel to that line, and by observing the alignment from the front, you can see any discrepancies.

If the restorative procedures outlined in this text are followed, all bite records for the restorative phase will be made at the correct vertical or so close to it that a *slightly* missed condylar axis will have insignificant effect on the arc of closure from the vertical dimension of the bite record. But a misalignment with the interpupillary line can have a noticeable and unpleasant effect on the incisal plane. For that reason, if there is a slight discrepancy between the condylar axis and the interpupillary line, it is usually better to align the bow with the eyes, especially for restorative procedures involving anterior restorations. The same is true whether a conventional facebow or an earbow is used.

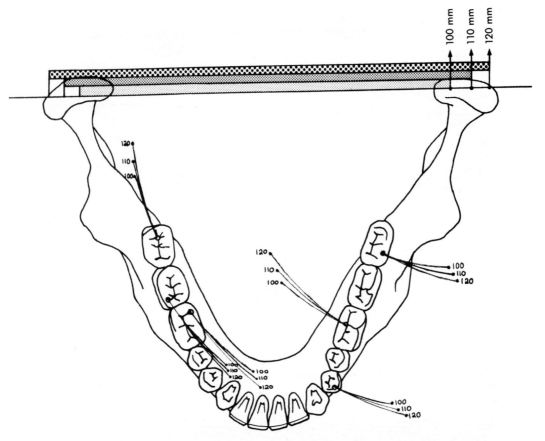

Fig. 13-3. Illustration showing that the difference in the path of cusp tips is indistinguishable through the pathways at the functional contact range. There is no advantage to a changeable intercondylar distance. If the set distance is 110 mm, it will be acceptable for all patients, especially in a disclusive posterior occlusion.

When casts are mounted without a facebow, they are invariably positioned to align the existing occlusal plane parallel with the bench top. If the occlusal plane is high on one side in the mouth, the cast will generally be tilted to straighten the occlusal plane on the articulator. This perpetuates the error and removes any visualization of correct relationship of the teeth to the eyes, lips, or face. If casts are mounted with a facebow related to the interpupillary line, the technician can align the incisal plane parallel with the bench top and it will be correct regardless of how misaligned the teeth are in the mouth.

Most facebows can be used with a variety of different articulators. The match is acceptable as long as the axis-locator rod on the facebow can be aligned with the axis of the articulator.

On articulators with *set* intercondylar distance, the axis-locator bars are released and set to the instrument, with both sides being made

sure that they are set the same. On instruments with *variable* intercondylar distance, the patient's measurements are transferred to the instrument, which is altered to the patient's intercondylar width.

There are several different articulators with variable intercondylar width, but there is really no advantage to be gained over an instrument with a set intercondylar width of 110 mm. The width of human faces is suprisingly consistent and very few patients will have an intercondylar width that varies more than 10 mm from the average 110 mm. From the narrowest to the widest intercondylar widths, any variance in the lateral path of a lower cusp tip will be indistinguishable from the average path for the first 3 to 4 mm at the occlusal level (Fig. 13-3).

The need for measuring and transferring intercondylar width precisely is further made unnecessary by posterior disclusion.

There is, however, an important relationship between the path of lower anterior teeth and the intercondylar width. If anterior guidance is determined and fabricated from articulator settings, differences in intercondylar width would result in significant enough difference in the path of the lower incisal edges to affect the lingual contours of the upper anterior teeth. However, determination of anterior guidance on any articulator is not recommended. Anterior guidance must be determined in the mouth and then copied on the articulator. Use of a customized anterior guidance as described in Chapters 16 and 18 will precisely copy the lingual contours just as well on an articulator with a set 110 mm intercondylar width as it will on a variable instrument. So even on articulators with variable intercondylar width, it is logical to set the width at 110 mm and use it that way unless there is a special need for analysis of an existing occlusion with a severe variation from normal intercondylar width.

USING THE FACEBOW

The facebow is simply a device that relates the upper cast to the same axis on the articulator that is present in the skull. A facebow is simple to use and, with practice, usually requires less than a minute of chair time. It involves two basic steps:

1. Locating the condylar axis
2. Relating the upper arch to the axis

Locating the axis. The principle difference between one type of facebow and another is basically a difference of preciseness. The most accurate method for recording the correct horizontal axis includes the use of some type of kinematic device for locating the exact terminal hinge axis (Fig. 13-4). The value of such devices, however, is often negated by failure to record the *most superior* axis. A hinge position can be recorded at any point along the protrusive pathway. Unless good manipulative technique is used to verify that the recording is made at the superiorly braced position, the recorded hinge axis may be incorrect. More important is the fact that even the most precisely recorded hinge axis cannot compensate for an inaccurate centric relation bite record.

A kinematic facebow recording is most meaningful if the centric bite record is made at an extremely opened jaw position. Bite records made with clutches in place fall into

this category. However, if the centric bite record can be made at or near the correct vertical dimension, the accuracy achieved by palpation to locate the axis will be indistinguishable at the occlusal level from a kinematic recording.

The simplest, fastest, and also most popular device for recording the condylar axis is the *earbow*. The earbow utilizes the ear hole on each side as a reference point because of its close relationship to the glenoid fossa. The earbow transfer to the articulator interpolates where the condylar axis is normally in relation to the ear hole. So when the casts are mounted, they are related to an anatomic average position of the condylar axis that simply uses the ear hole as a reference point. Although variations do occur in this relationship, the potential error is small enough to be insignificant at the occlusal level if the bite record is made at or near the correct vertical dimension.

The Dénar earbow is particularly practical because it also uses a reference point on the face that is a set dimension from the incisal edges of the upper anterior teeth. This permits the use of a transfer jig for the bite fork that frees up the facebow for use on other patients, while also serving as a very easily used mounting jig.

METHOD OF PALPATION FOR LOCATING CONDYLAR AXIS

From a position behind the patient, place the index fingertip over the joint area and ask the patient to open wide (Fig. 13-5). As the condyle translates forward, the fingertip will drop into a depression where the condyle was.

The patient should then close. As the condyle translates back into the centric relation position, its position can be located by the fingertip. By asking the patient to open and close, it will be possible in most patients to feel the rotation and locate the axis within an average accuracy of 2 mm or less. The axis generally occurs near the center of the depression felt by the fingertip, so when this point is located, it should be marked with a dot from a felt-tipped pen or marking pencil (Fig. 13-6).

It is not always possible to articulate casts of unequilibrated occlusions near the correct vertical dimension. The centric bite record must be made before the first tooth contacts. Gross interferences therefore require rather thick

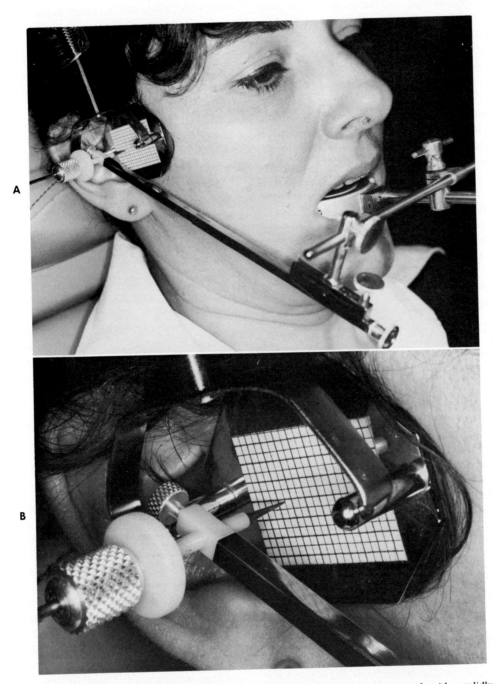

Fig. 13-4. A, A hinge axis locator (Lauritzen) is in place, attached to the lower teeth with a solidly secured clutch. The mandible is arced on its terminal axis, and the movement of the axis locator pin is observed to determine its relation to the pure rotational axis of the condyle. **B,** When the axis locator pin achieves a purely rotational movement, the location of the pin point is marked on the graph. The mark is often made directly on the skin, but this headgear device (Aderer) eliminates the error that sometimes results from the movement of the skin. When the terminal hinge axis is located, a facebow is used to relate the upper arch to the point of rotation.

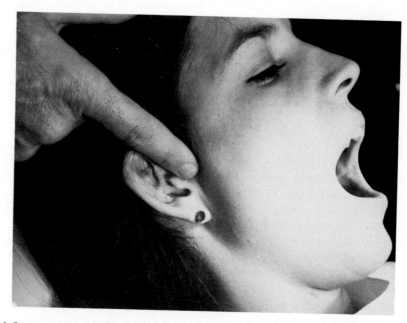

Fig. 13-5. Palpation for condylar axis. When the patient opens her mouth wide, the tip of the index finger drops into the depression left by the protruded condyle. When the jaw is arced open and closed, the condyle can be felt by the fingertip. The hinge axis can thus be located to within the dimensions of the condyle. Accuracy can be achieved within a general range of 1 to 3 mm error, which is insignificant if bite records are made close to the correct vertical dimension.

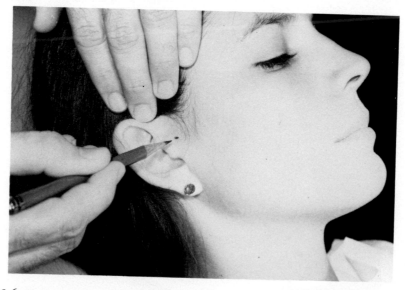

Fig. 13-6. The location of the axis is marked on the skin. Care should be taken not to move the skin when the mark is located.

bite records. If extreme preciseness is required at this stage for research purposes, the axis should be located kinematically. It would be rare however that such preciseness would be necessary for clinical purposes at the preliminary diagnostic state. During the restorative stages when preciseness is really needed, it is usually possible to record centric relation at or near the correct vertical, and so kinematic axis location is unnecessary.

USING THE FACEBOW

1. Softened base plate wax is wrapped around the bite fork and positioned against the upper teeth (Fig. 13-7). Indentations into the wax must be sufficient to stabilize the upper cast so that there will be no rocking of the cast.

    The indentations should not penetrate through to metal. For upper edentulous ridges, a stable base plate should be constructed and the bite fork should be attached to a bite rim on the base.

    The lower teeth can usually be closed into the wax on the underside of the bite fork to stabilize it, but if there is any movement of the bite fork or if it is possible to wiggle it while the teeth are closed into it, the fork should be held firmly against the upper teeth by the chairside assistant.

    It is not necessary to close into centric relation on the bite fork. Its purpose is for orientation of the upper cast only. Using the bite fork for a centric relation bite record creates unnecessary thickness and potential error if the axis location is not precise.

2. While the wax on the bite fork is being chilled by the assistant, the facebow is positioned and the intercondylar width is recorded (Fig. 13-8). The facebow is set according to the patient's facial width.

3. The bite fork is reinserted, and the facebow is positioned by the dentist so that the axis locators are positioned in line with the marks on the skin (Fig. 13-9).

4. While the dentist holds the axis locators in position, the assistant, without contacting the facebow at any other point (Fig. 13-10), tightens the set-screw mechanism that locks the bite fork into the correct relationship with the facebow.

5. The axis locators are loosened, and their relationship to the marks on the skin is checked. Both locators should be at the same setting and should lightly contact the skin directly over the marks. If the position is incorrect, the locking device on the bite fork should be loosened and the procedure repeated.

6. The bow should be observed from the front to make sure it is parallel with the eyes.

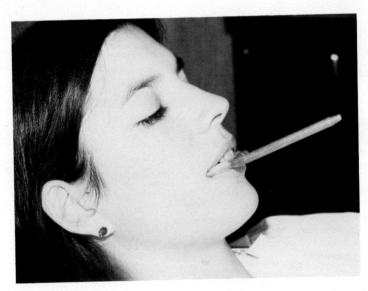

Fig. 13-7. The bite fork is placed. It should be solidly held by the teeth or the assistant should hold it in place. Indentations from the teeth should not penetrate the wax.

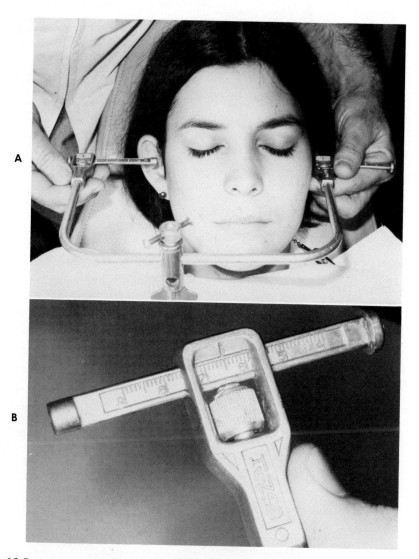

Fig. 13-8. A, Determining intercondylar distance. Measurements of the width are accomplished with the facebow. The axis locator rod on one side is moved all the way *out*, and the rod on the opposite side is moved *in* until it contacts the skin. Width is measured from the axis points on each side. **B,** All popular facebows are calibrated with a center reading of 6.5. This means that both sides would be set at 6.5 if one axis locator rod is all the way *out* and the other rod just touches the skin when it is all the way *in*. One can calibrate differences by adding to or subtracting from 6.5 reading. Notice in **A** that the rod that is *in* is about 1 cm from contacting the skin. This difference would be halved (0.5 cm) and subtracted from the 6.5 on each side. Thus both locator rods would be set at 6. If the face were wider and the *in* rod touched the skin 1 cm from the full *in* position, the amount would be halved and *added* to each side.

Fig. 13-9. The axis locator rods are set so that they just touch the skin on both sides at the same setting. The chilled bite fork is placed and the facebow is held in place at the axis marks.

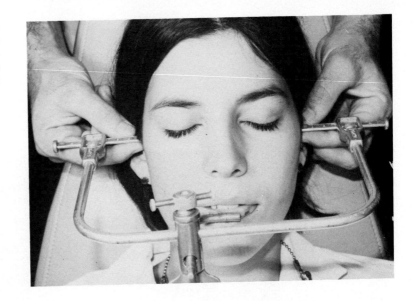

Fig. 13-10. A, While the dentist holds the axis locator rods in position, the assistant tightens the locking device. Notice that there is no contact with any other part of the facebow by the assistant while the locking device is being tightened. **B,** After the facebow is locked to the bite fork, the axis locator rod is released and its position is checked to make sure it has not been moved. It should then be reset at the correct-width calibration before the facebow is removed.

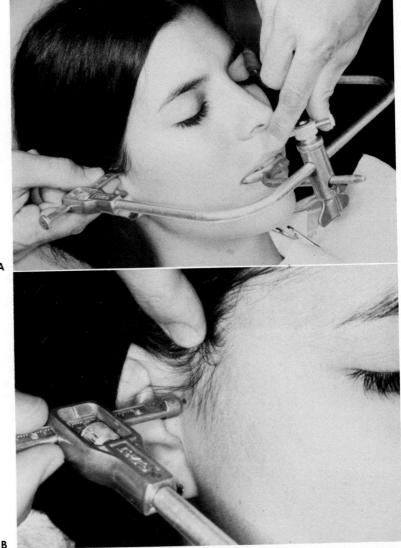

A

B

USING THE EARBOW

1. The bite fork is prepared the same as for use with the facebow. After indentation against the upper arch, it is removed and the wax is chilled.
2. The facial reference point is located and marked (Fig. 13-11).
3. The bite fork is reinserted, and the ear-bow is positioned to slide onto the fork while the locators are gently seated into the ear holes. At that point, the self-centering bow is locked (Fig. 13-12) to prevent it from slipping out of the ear holes.
4. The front of the bow is raised until the pointer lines up with the reference point on the face (Fig. 13-13).
5. While the assistant stabilizes the bow, it is checked to make sure that there is equal contact at each ear hole. The bow is checked from the front to make sure it is parallel with the eyes (Fig. 13-14).
6. When all alignments are correct, the locking screws are tightened (Fig. 13-15). All alignments are rechecked before removal of the bow.
7. The center lock is released so that the locator can be removed from the ear hole. The entire bow is then removed.
8. The transfer jig is then removed from the bow. The jig is all that is necessary for transferring the relationships to the articulator (Fig. 13-16).

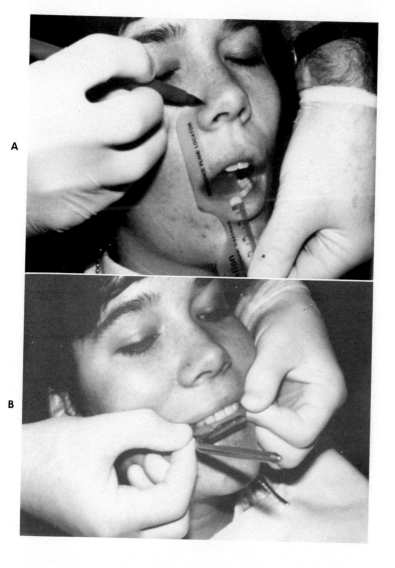

A

B

Fig. 13-11. A, The facial reference point is related to a set distance from the incisal edges of the teeth. The preciseness of the position is not critical, but it is nevertheless important if a transfer jig is to be used for the mounting. **B,** The bite fork is indexed to the upper arch. There must be no displacement when the lower teeth indent the wax on the underside to stabilize the bite fork in place.

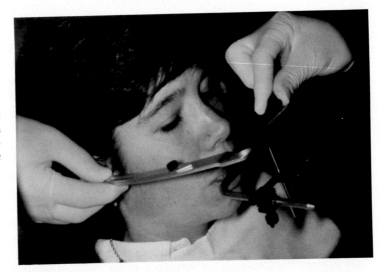

Fig. 13-12. The locking device is tightened when the earbow is aligned in the ear holes. This centers the bow and helps to stabilize it.

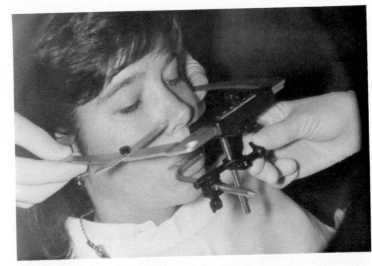

Fig. 13-13. The bow is aligned vertically with the facial reference point.

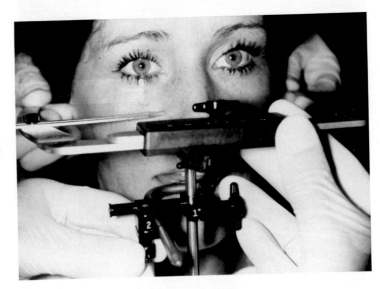

Fig. 13-14. The bow is checked to make sure it is aligned with the eyes.

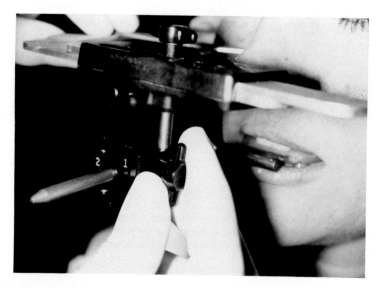

Fig. 13-15. When the bow is correctly aligned, the locking devices are tightened in proper sequence.

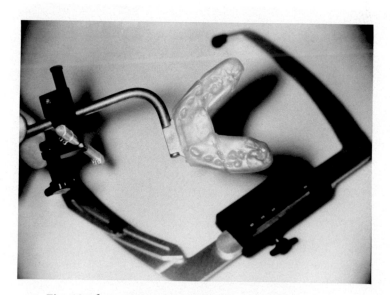

Fig. 13-16. The tightened transfer jig is removed from the bow.

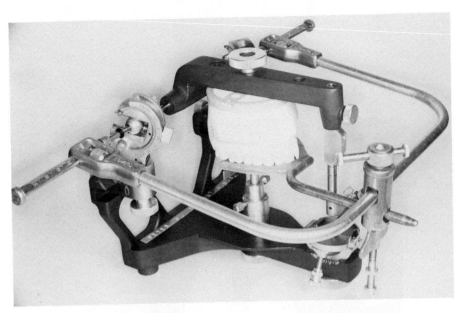

Fig. 13-17. The upper cast is seated in the bite fork index, and the fork is supported by a cast support directly under the cast. The support screw at the front of the facebow is also used. When the vertical positioning of the cast is determined, the cast is joined to the mounting ring.

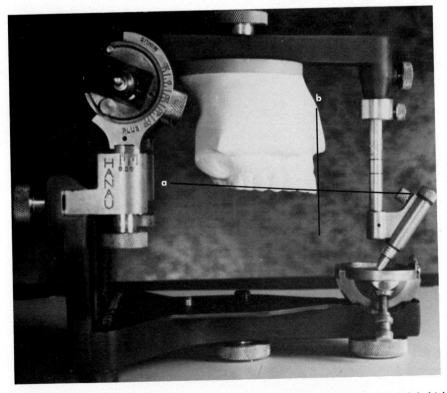

Fig. 13-18. Determine the vertical position by making certain that the occlusal plane is slightly higher in the back, *a*. The labial surface of the central incisors should be nearly vertical, *b*. The grooves on the guide pin should be ignored. They are not related to the incisal edge position.

MOUNTING WITH THE FACEBOW

1. Attach the cast support to the lower bow and lock the articulator in centric relation.
2. Align the axis locator of the facebow with the horizontal axle of the articulator.
3. When the facebow is positioned on the articulator's axle, place the upper cast in the indentations on the bite fork. The support screw in the front of the facebow is lowered to support the cast.
4. Adjust the support screw to position the cast at an acceptable height. It is important that the occlusal plane should be higher in the back. This will normally be achieved ideally when the labial surfaces of the upper incisors are vertical. When anterior teeth are excessively inclined, the slant of the occlusal plane should be the principle determinant of how high or low to position the upper cast.

If an infraorbital pointer is used, it will automatically result in an acceptable height for the cast.

5. When the case is positioned at the desired height, raise the cast support to contact the underside of the bite fork. The cast should be supported during the mounting procedure (Fig. 13-17).
6. When the upper cast is joined to the mounting ring on the articulator, the facebow can be removed (Fig. 13-18).

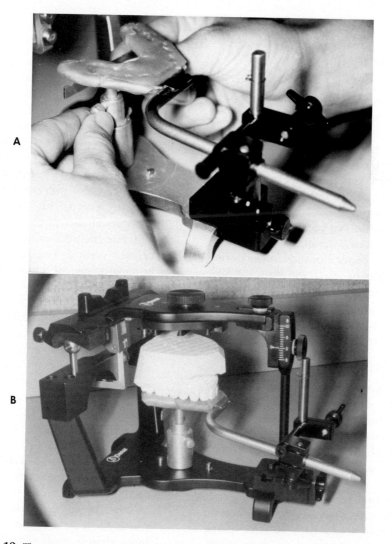

Fig. 13-19. The mounting jig is seated into a mounting block that replaces the incisal guide table. A cast support is used for stabilization, **A,** and the cast is seated into the bite fork index, **B**. This correctly relates it to the horizontal axis and determines its vertical position on the articulator.

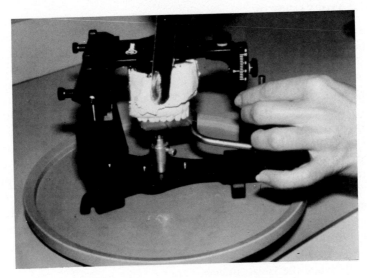

Fig. 13-20. The cast is joined to the upper bow.

MOUNTING WITH THE EARBOW

If the Dénar Slidematic earbow is used, the bite fork is attached to a mounting jig that can be removed from the earbow and placed in a mounting block on the articulator (Fig. 13-19). This simplified transfer system positions the upper cast at the correct height and relates it to the horizontal axis. It also eliminates the cumbersomeness of working around the face-bow in the mounting procedures. The mounting jig is very stable, but use of a cast support with it provides added stabilization of the cast and prevents any chance of movement during the laboratory phase.

Place soft stone on the upper cast and close the upper bow into it. Be sure the ring is properly engaged. Smooth the stone for a neat mounting (Fig. 13-20).

MOUNTING THE LOWER CAST

The articulator should remain locked in centric relation during this procedure. If the incisal guide pin is lengthened an amount equal to the thickness of the bite record, the upper bow of the articulator will be horizontal when the bite record is removed and the casts are in contact.

1. Test the bite record separately on both the upper and lower cast to make certain it seats completely with no rock. If the bite record is trimmed to show tooth-wax-tooth in the mouth and all soft tis-

sue impingement has been removed, there should be no problem in determining whether the bite record fits the casts as accurately as it fits the mouth.

2. Test the bite record now with both casts seated to make sure there are no parts of the casts that interfere with complete seating. If necessary, trim away any part of the cast that prevents full closure into the bite record. This should not involve any critical part of the cast. If it does, a new bite record should be taken at an increased vertical. Test also to see that the articulator can be closed without interference from the cast. Sometimes the casts must be reduced in thickness.

3. If the casts can both fully seat into the bite record, join them in this relationship with sturdy metal supports and sticky wax. Extreme care must be taken for this step to make sure the alignment with the bite record is perfect and the casts are securely stabilized. This step should be done with the upper cast attached to the articulator (Fig. 13-21).

4. Check again to make certain the articulator can close completely with no contact against the lower cast (Fig. 13-22). Also observe the amount of space between the lower cast and the ring. If there is more than a small space, two mixes of stone should be used to prevent an error

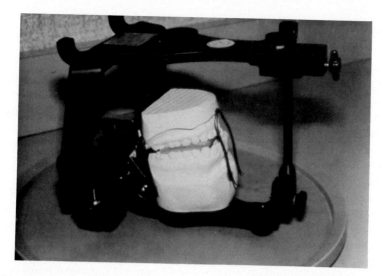

Fig. 13-21. The lower cast is anchored into place in the bite record. Sturdy supports should be used to prevent any slippage.

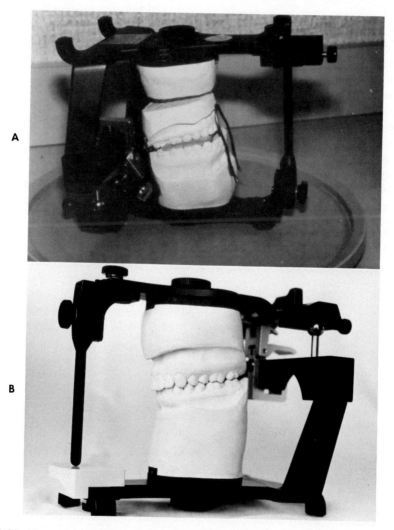

A

B

Fig. 13-22. Close the articulator to make sure there are no obstructions to the casts, **A**. If the distance between the cast and the mounting ring is more than a few millimeters, two mixes should be used to prevent distortion during setting of the stone. Join the lower cast to the articulator bow, **B**.

from dimensional changes that occur during setting of a large amount of stone or plaster.

5. Join the lower cast to the ring.
6. After the stone sets, remove the casts from the articulator and clean up the mountings. Smooth the stone using fine, wet-dry sandpaper under running water. Remove all excess stone from the articulator. Mountings should be neat and clean as well as accurate. Be certain that no debris gets into the threads of the mounting rings.
7. Return the casts to the articulator.

VERIFYING ACCURACY OF THE MOUNTING

The verification procedure is so important to the mounting process that it is reason enough to do all mountings under direct supervision in the dental office. This is a quality-control procedure that can be taught to a staff person. I have for years advocated the use of a lab assistant as one of the most important and cost-effective staff members. There does not appear to be a suitable substitute for this direct control if the errors of improper mountings are to be avoided. There are many quality-oriented dentists who insist on doing the mounting procedure themselves because of the importance of this step. There are two excellent

methods for verifying the accuracy of mountings. One is the split-cast technique (Fig. 13-23). The other is the stone-wax-stone method. Neither method will work without a meticulously made bite record in a hard material that will not be distorted by pressure from the casts. Proper trimming of the bite record is also critical.

The steps for verification using the stone-wax-stone method have stood the test of time in our office:

1. Verify that both casts are completely screwed down so that the rings are snug against the metal bows of the articulator.
2. Place the bite record between the casts.
3. Unlock the centric lock and raise the incisal guide pin. For this step, one of the advantages of a come-apart articulator will become evident.
4. Verify the fit of both casts into the bite record. There should be no cracks between the record and the cast. There should be a perfect stone-wax-stone adaptation (Fig. 13-24). With a hard-enough bite material, this is a counterpart of the split-cast method.
5. Now lift off the top bow with its upper cast attached. Have an assistant place a very thin Mylar strip or articulating ribbon (Accufilm) over the ball of one condyle. Reseat the upper bow and again

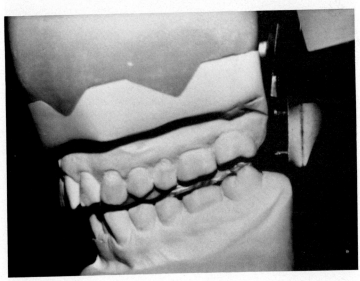

Fig. 13-23. The split-cast technique permits accurate verification of mounting accuracy. When the casts are seated precisely into the bite record, there should be no crack showing between the two halves of the split cast.

verify the stone-wax-stone relationship. Then observe whether or not the ribbon is being held by metal-to-metal contact of the condyle in its fossa (Fig. 13-25). Repeat the process for the opposite side.

If centric relation metal-to-metal contact does not occur at the fossae simultaneously with perfect stone-wax-stone contact at the casts, the mounting is defective. The ring should be removed from the lower cast, and the mounting should be redone.

It is important that the preceding test be used to verify all critical mountings. No matter how carefully the mounting may be performed, it is surprisingly easy for lab errors to creep in. In practices that are not definitively monitoring the accuracy of each mounting, the above test will be convincing because the average error found in most mountings is substantial.

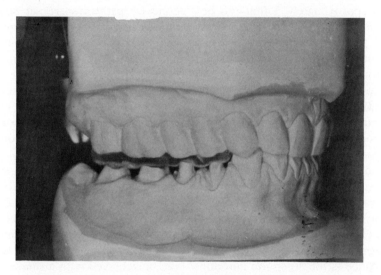

Fig. 13-24. A properly trimmed bite record pemits examination of the stone-wax-stone relationship. There should be no sign of any crack or space between the casts and the bite record.

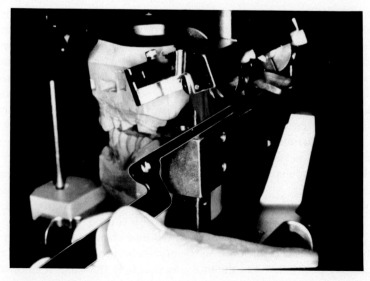

Fig. 13-25. With the centric lock opened and the incisal pin up, thin articulating ribbon should not slip through between the condyle ball against its fossa wall. The ribbon should be held tightly by the contact. If the ribbon is not held tightly, the mounting is inaccurate.

SETTING THE CONDYLAR GUIDANCE

As explained in Chapter 12, there are many factors to consider regarding the use of an arbitrary-set condylar guidance versus a guidance that duplicates or approximates the actual path in the patient. If the condylar paths are to be set by checkbites, the following procedures apply.

Horizontal condylar guidance

After the casts are mounted in centric relation, a second bite record made with the mandible protruded approximately 5 mm can be used to set the horizontal path. Extra-hard wax should be used for that record, the same as that used for centric relation bite records.

The wax protrusive checkbite should be trimmed back to the tips of each upper and lower cusp so that the adaptation of stone-wax-stone is clearly visible.

The centric lock is released, and the upper cast is moved back until it aligns with the indentations in the protrusive bite record. The condyle paths are now altered to varying degrees of steepness until the casts fit precisely into the protrusive bite record with no separation between the stone and the bite record. If there is separation at the distal part of the bite record, the guidance is too steep. An anterior separation between the cast and the bite record results from the condylar guidance being set too flat.

Lateral condylar guidance

Because there are no disadvantages to setting the lateral condylar guidance at a wider angle than is needed, an arbitrary setting of 15 degrees will work for almost everyone. However, if the lateral checkbite method is to be used, bite records are made for both a right and a left lateral excursion, ideally at a point where the upper and lower cuspid tips are aligned. The wax record is trimmed so that the juncture of tooth-wax-tooth is visible so that it can be compared with a stone-wax-stone relationship on the casts.

The centric lock is released, and the lateral adjustment lock screw is loosened on each side. The lateral paths are opened to the widest position. The left lateral checkbite is placed, and the casts are positioned into the indentations. The balancing-side condyle path on the right side of the articulator is rotated to contact the condyle ball. The process is then repeated for the opposite side.

For track instruments, the balancing-side condyle path is rotated in until it contacts the lateral stop on the axle.

The protrusive checkbite should be rechecked after the lateral paths are set.

USING TRANSFER BITE RECORDS TO ELIMINATE THE INFRAORBITAL POINTER PROCEDURE

The infraorbital pointer provides a uniform method of establishing the vertical position of the upper cast on the articulator. Once the condylar pathways are set (either by checkbite, pantograph, or stereograph), there will be no need to reset them if the original upper model and all subsequent models are all at the same position. As a restorative case progresses, teeth are equilibrated, prepared, and restored. New models are required at each step of the restorative procedure. The usual procedure is to mount each new set of models with a new facebow recording that also employs an infraorbital pointer repeatedly set to the same spot on the patient's face. Condyle-axis location is often tattooed on the skin to assure accuracy of that part of the facebow recording. Although the procedure is effective, it requires an unnecessary waste of time. The same results can be achieved with a simple laboratory step.

As already discussed, the vertical position of the upper cast can be set by raising or lowering the front of the facebow until the labial surfaces of the central incisors are vertical. Some anterior teeth are tilted inward, and some are near horizontal. If the central teeth are not in a normal relationship, the occlusal plane can be used as a guide for positioning the upper cast. The front of the occlusal plane should be set slightly lower than the back. This may seem arbitrary, but regardless of the position of the casts vertically, they will not lose their correct relationship with the terminal axis as long as the model is positioned on the bite fork and the axis locators are in position on the articulator. Condylar guidances are not set until the casts are mounted, and then these guidances are relative to whatever vertical cast position is used.

When changes are made in the mouth and new models are poured, they can be mounted in precisely the same relationship as the previous casts by use of a transfer bite. Let us use an example to explain the procedure. The original diagnostic models have been mounted and all condylar settings have been made. Equili-

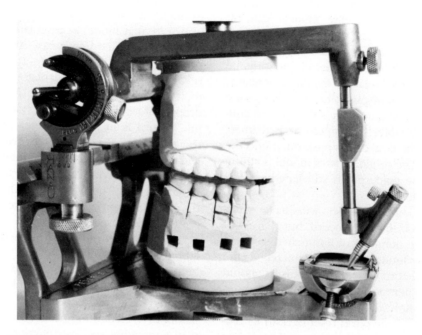

Fig. 13-26. Transfer checkbite. It is not necessary to take a new facebow record for each procedure if a transfer bite is used. Example here shows a completed fixed prosthesis on the cast. In preparation for the transfer bite, the incisal pin is lengthened and a wax record is made at that opened position.

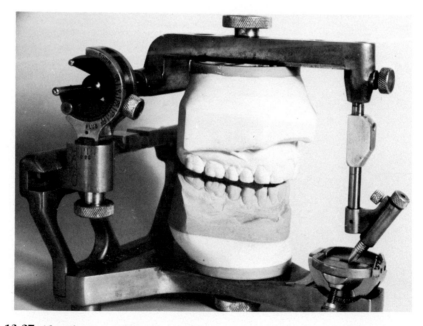

Fig. 13-27. After placement of the restorations, a new cast is made and then seated into the indentations in the transfer bite. This relates the new lower cast to the exact same relationship as the previous cast. The opposing cast is now mounted with a new centric relation bite record. This procedure works equally well on any type of articulator that accepts a facebow.

bration procedures that change the occlusal surfaces are then completed, and new impressions are made. The new models can be mounted in the same relationship to the condyles without a new facebow being taken. A simple wax bite is made on the original models in centric relation on the articulator. When the wax is in place, the bite is opened so that the incisal guide pin is dropped to contact the guide table. The upper cast is then removed, and the new cast is positioned into the bite record. The original lower model is still in place, and the guide pin is still lengthened at the same position.

The new upper model will have voids against the transfer bite record, but there will still be ample numbers of untouched stops so that the new model will be completely stable in the bite record despite the voids. It should be joined in that position to the upper mounting ring. After the new upper model is mounted, the guide pin is reset back to its regular position. The new lower model is then mounted by means of a new centric-relation bite record made on the patient.

This procedure can be repeated at each new step of the restorative treatment. As an example, when the lower posterior teeth are prepared, that model is articulated against the correctly mounted upper cast. After the lower restorations are completed, a transfer bite record is made on the articulator with the restorations in place (Fig. 13-26). The guide pin is dropped to contact the guide table when the bite record is in position. After placement of the restorations a lower impression is made and the new model is positioned into the transfer bite record and joined to the lower mounting ring. The guide pin is then reset and the new upper cast (which may be a die model of prepared upper teeth) is articulated against the lower model with a new centric relation bite record (Fig. 13-27).

This procedure is simple, yet very accurate. It eliminates the chair time required for taking repeated facebow records and simplifies the laboratory remounting procedures. It works as well on gnathologic instrumentation as it does on semiadjustable articulators.

14

Pankey-Mann-Schuyler philosophy of complete occlusal rehabilitation

One of the most practical philosophies for occlusal rehabilitation is the rationale of treatment that was originally organized into a workable concept by Dr. L.D. Pankey.

Utilizing the "principles of occlusion" espoused by Dr. Clyde Schuyler, Dr. Pankey integrated different aspects of several treatment approaches into an orderly plan for achieving an optimum occlusal result with minimum stress on the patient or the dentist.

Dr. Arvin Mann contributed to the concept by working with Dr. Pankey in the development of the first specialized instrument for developing the occlusal plane. The instrument became known as the Pankey-Mann instrument, and even though it has long ago been replaced by a simpler system, the overall concept of treatment is still referred to as the Pankey-Mann-Schuyler philosophy (abbreviated to PMS).

Contrary to some popular misconceptions, the PMS approach is not so much a technique as it is a *philosophy* of treatment that organizes the reconstruction of an occlusion into a sequence of goals that must be fulfilled. It is true that certain techniques have become closely associated with the PMS philosophy, but it is also true that there has been a contin-

uous trend toward improving and simplifying almost every aspect of treatment without noticeably changing the basic philosophy of treatment. Furthermore, the overall concept of treatment is not limited to any specific instrument or method. There is considerable flexibility of treatment within the PMS philosophy as long as its goals of optimum occlusions are not sacrificed.

Since its inception, the philosophy has had as its goal the fulfillment of the following principles of occlusions as advocated by Schuyler:

1. A static coordinated occlusal contact of the maximum number of teeth when the mandible is in centric relation
2. An anterior guidance that is in harmony with function in lateral eccentric positions on the working side
3. Disclusion by the anterior guidance of all posterior teeth in protrusion
4. Disclusion of all non−working side inclines in lateral excursions
5. Group function of the working-side inclines in lateral excursions

Most PMS advocates now vary the fifth goal of working-side group function to permit more flexibility in distributing lateral stress. This is discussed in detail in Chapter 19.

To accomplish these goals, the following sequence is advocated by the PMS philosophy:

PART 1. Examination, diagnosis, treatment planning, prognosis

PART 2. Harmonization of the anterior guidance for best possible esthetics, function, and comfort

PART 3. Selection of an acceptable occlusal plane and restoration of the lower posterior occlusion in harmony with the anterior guidance in a manner that will not interfere with condylar guidance

PART 4. Restoration of the upper posterior occlusion in harmony with the anterior guidance and condylar guidance. The functionally generated path technique is so closely allied with this part of the reconstruction that it may almost be considered part of the concept, though new understanding of the effect of posterior disclusion has made this unnecessary for most occlusal restorations (see Chapter 12).

Each one of these steps has undergone a continuous metamorphosis as techniques to accomplish the goals have been improved and modified with a wide choice of sophisticated options. One of the most impressive advantages of PMS is the latitude of sophistication it permits. Treatment modes within the concept can be varied from the simplest techniques for the beginning restorative dentist to the most precise details of the master reconstructionist.

Many men have contributed to the gradual improvement and simplification of PMS techniques. New manipulative techniques have improved the recording of centric relation (described in Chapter 4) and the more accurate recording of border movements when the functionally generated path technique is used (Chapter 23).

Our technique for customizing the anterior guidance (Chapter 16) and for recording the precise amount of needed "long centric" (Chapter 15) has enabled us to perfect each occlusion to an amazingly accurate degree. Our waxing technique for lower posterior teeth (Chapter 21) guarantees proper cusp-tip location, and our simplified technique for establishing the correct lower fossae contours (Chapter 21) has certainly made it easier for us and our technicians to achieve greater accuracy with simplicity.

The determination of an acceptable occlusal plane was first simplified by Fillastre and then further improved by Broadrick. The Broadrick Occlusal Plane Analyzer is so simple to use that it has become the standard method of analyzing the occlusal plane for posterior occlusal reconstructions (Chapter 20).

The PMS philosophy is not limited to any specific instrument. Swanson and Wipf adapted the Broadrick "flag" for their temporomandibular-joint stereographic articulator, and Fillastre developed a device for the same instrument that determines ridge and groove directions on the lower occlusal wax patterns.

Guichet adapted the PMS concept of establishing an acceptable occlusal plane by adding a "flag" device to the Dénar Gnathological Articulator.

Courtade developed the Verticulator device for accurate adaptation of the functionally generated path model against the die model.

Not all of these variations are in common use, but they are listed to illustrate the wide range of flexibility with the PMS philosophy. I hope improvements will continue to be made that will permit even greater simplicity with still better results.

The restorative methods outlined in this text explain many of the reasons for the order of sequence, as well as the rationale of each sequential step. Although many of the techniques vary from the original technique steps in PMS, I believe that they do not represent a departure from the overall concept of the PMS philosophy.

The advantages of the technique are many. Some of the major ones are as follows:

1. It is possible to diagnose and plan treatment for the entire rehabilitation before a single tooth is prepared.

2. It is a well-organized, logical procedure that progresses smoothly with less wear and tear on the patient, operator, and technician.

3. There is never a need for preparing or rebuilding more than eight teeth at a time.

4. It divides the rehabilitation into separate series of appointments. It is neither necessary nor desirable to do the entire case at one time.

5. There is no danger of "getting lost at sea"

and losing the patient's present vertical dimension. The operator knows exactly where he is at all times.

6. The functionally generated path and centric relation are taken on the occlusal surface of the teeth to be rebuilt at the exact vertical dimension to which the case will be constructed.

7. All posterior occlusal contours are programmed by and are in harmony with both condylar border movements and a perfected anterior guidance.

8. There is no need for time-consuming techniques and complicated equipment.

9. Laboratory procedures are simple and controlled to an extremely fine degree by the dentist.

The Pankey-Mann-Schuyler philosophy of occlusal rehabilitation can fulfill the most exacting and sophisticated demands, *if the oper-ator understands the goals of optimum occlusion.* And it can achieve these goals with great simplicity and orderliness of technique. It can be combined with other techniques, and it can be adapted to any occlusal problem. An understanding of the PMS philosophy is a tremendously valuable aspect of the complete dental education.

REFERENCES

1. Mann, A.W., and Pankey, L.D.: Oral rehabilitation, J. Prosthet. Dent. **10**:135-162, 1960.
2. Mann, A.W., and Pankey, L.D.: The P.M. philosophy of occlusal rehabilitation, Dent. Clin, North Am., pp. 621-638, 1963.
3. Mann, A.W., and Pankey, L.D.: Oral rehabilitation utilizing the Pankey-Mann instrument and functional bite technique, Dent. Clin. North Am., pp. 215, 1959.
4. Schuyler, C.H.: Correction of occlusal disharmony of natural dentition, N.Y. Dent. J. **13**:445, 1947.
5. Schuyler, C.H.: Factors in occlusion applicable to restorative dentistry, J. Prosthet. Dent. **3**:722-782, 1953.

15

Long centric

If the concept of centric relation is understood, it will be clear that it refers to a precise location of the condyle-disk assemblies. "Centric relation" refers to the exact point at which the *loaded* condyle-disk assembly is braced by bone at the most superior position possible against the eminentia. At this loaded position that occurs from firm contraction of the elevator muscles, the disk is compressed and the condylar axis reaches what we refer to as the apex of force position. It is this position that can be located repeatedly and recorded with needle-point accuracy. Consequently it is somewhat confusing to think of such a precise point as being "long."

The term "long centric" is misleading because there cannot be such a thing as a long precise point. It is even harder to accept the concept of a long centric, with the current understanding that the medial pole of the condyle-disk assembly is stopped by bone, which is unyielding, at least within the range of normal function. The original concept of long centric probably garnered some advocates for the wrong reason, because of clearly erroneous beliefs that the condyle either rested in a yielding mass of soft tissue or was simply suspended in space. Because both of those beliefs portrayed the condyle as resting on rather spongy articulations, it was postulated that a precise occlusal relationship was incompatible with an imprecise centric relation. Thus there must be created an "area" of

centric on the teeth to accommodate an "area" of centric at the condyle.

Because of similar misconceptions about the firmness of the medial-pole stops, the "midmost" concept of centric relation was also considered to be a spongy articulation. Thus long centric was also quite often combined with a lateral area of freedom that was referred to as a "wide centric."

On the opposite side of the "long centric" argument were those who believed that centric relation was such a precise point that occlusal contacts should be contoured to provide no horizontal freedom forward of centric relation. Advocates of this belief often contoured the occlusal surfaces to lock the teeth into this restricted relationship by tripod contacts on three sides of each cusp, relying on the downward movement of the condyles to unlock the centric relation contact. Great pains were taken to relate cusp inclines to precise condylar border pathways, and then the anterior guidance was arbitrarily steepened or flattened to conform to the condylar path angulation. This produced a very precise occlusal relationship with possible restrictions on horizontal freedom during functional jaw movements.

Since the downward movement of the condyles was in fact usually able to disclude the posterior tripod contacts, the effect of the restricted occlusion was more related to the arbitrary confinement by the lingual inclines of the upper *anterior* teeth. Patients often com-

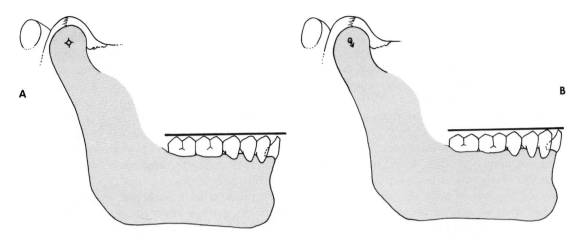

Fig. 15-1. A flat long centric area is not needed on the posterior teeth even if it is incorporated into anterior tooth contact. The condyles cannot move forward from centric relation, **A**, without moving down the eminentiae. This displacement prevents the lower posterior teeth from moving horizontally forward, **B**, even if the anterior guidance is flat.

plained that the front teeth hit hard or bumped, even though no interference could be shown in centric relation. Explanations that "my bite is different when I'm sitting up" were frequently ignored.

To recapitulate, the most common attitudes about the concept of "long centric" could be boiled down to two beliefs:

1. Horizontal freedom was needed in the entire occlusion to accommodate a resilient relationship at the articular surfaces.
2. Horizontal freedom was *not* needed in the occlusal relationship because there is no resilience of the articulation at the centric relation position.

Let's understand what the term "long centric" was *intended* to mean even if we disagree with the semantics. Perhaps then, some of the confusion can be eliminated. I will define the term "long centric" as *freedom to close the mandible either into centric relation or slightly anterior to it without varying the vertical dimension at the anterior teeth.*

Two points about long centric should be clarified to facilitate further understanding:

1. *Long centric involves primarily the anterior teeth.* In a healthy articulation of the condyles there can be no horizontal protrusive path of posterior teeth. Even with a zero-degree anterior guidance the condyles must move downwardly as the jaw moves forward. The lower posterior teeth must move downwardly with them

(Fig. 15-1). Thus a flat protrusive area is usually not necessary on posterior teeth, especially in the molar region.

2. *Long centric refers to freedom from centric, not freedom in centric.* The principle concern regarding long centric is the restrictive effect that can result from the lingual inclines of the upper anterior teeth. If the lower incisal edges are in contact with steep lingual inclines at the centric relation jaw position, those same inclines may interfere with postural closing patterns that do not conform to the centric relation axis. If no horizontal freedom is provided for a slightly protruded postural closure, the lower incisal edges will strike the lingual *inclines* of the upper anterior teeth. If those inclines are steep enough, they can provide a wedging effect at first contact, which, in varying degrees, may interfere with the normal pattern of postural jaw closure (Fig. 15-2).

The provision for long centric simply moves the lingual incline forward so that the jaw is free to close without restriction either in centric relation or in the slightly protruded relationship that occurs at various postural positions of the head (Fig. 15-3).

There is a basic rule for optimizing the comfort and stability of any occlusal relationship, as follows: *When the teeth come together in a postural closure, the lower incisors should not strike an incline before reaching full closure.*

There are anatomic and physiologic reasons for accepting the concept of "long centric." The fit of the condyle into its disk is not like the fit of a machined ball in a bearing. Rather, there is some front-back play permitted by the disk that allows the condyle to hinge freely anywhere within the limits of the anterior and posterior lips of the disk. When the mandible is closed firmly, the strong contraction of the muscles of closure pulls the condyle to the back of the disk against its posterior lip. Light

closure from the rest position may be of insufficient intensity to completely pull the condyle into such a terminal position, and there will consequently be a slight difference between the firm terminal hinge closure of centric relation and a light closure from the rest position.

A further difference between centric relation closure and a light closure from rest position could occur if the position of the mandible is influenced through a less intense closure by muscles of posture and facial expression. The postural position of the mandible during light closure can affect the position of the en-

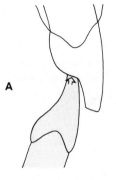

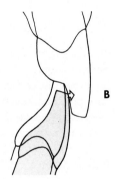

Fig. 15-2. A, Centric relation contact. **B,** Contact against the lingual incline when the jaw is closed lightly from a postural position. This patient should have the freedom of a long centric.

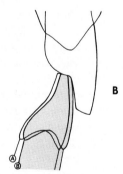

Fig. 15-3. A, Centric relation closure. **B,** Postural closure. Illustration *on right* shows how the lingual inclines of the upper incisors are reduced to allow for postural closure without wedging against a steep incline.

Fig. 15-4. The amount of long centric needed is equal to the difference between centric relation closure, *a,* versus postural closure, *b.*

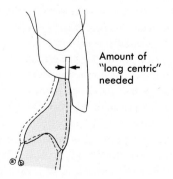

Amount of "long centric" needed

a. Centric relation closure
b. Light closure from postural rest

tire condyle-disk assembly as well as the position of the condyle in its disk.

Regardless of the cause, we do know from clinical studies that many patients exhibit a difference between centric closure and light closure from rest when they are in their postural position, and it is precisely this difference between the two positions that dictates the amount of "long centric" that any patient should have (Fig. 15-4).

In establishing the need for "long centric" in any given patient, it is absolutely essential that all interferences to terminal hinge closure be eliminated. If centric relation interferences are present, the path of closure will be dictated by the proprioceptors of the teeth instead of by the normal physiologic function of the muscles.

In the absence of any centric relation interferences, it has been our experience that the difference between centric closure and light closure from rest rarely exceeds 0.5 mm. The usual "long centric" would be close to 0.2 mm, and there are many patients who require no "long centric" at all because their light closure from rest is identical to their firm closure into centric relation.

It might be difficult to understand how such minute differences in the paths of closure can be significant, but it is just such minutiae that make the difference between just acceptability and complete predictable comfort. The dentist will only have to provide a needed "long centric" for one patient who has been "locked in" to centric relation (even a perfect centric relation) to get an idea of the usual reaction of patients to their new freedom.

If the vertical dimension is *less* when the teeth contact in centric relation than it is when they touch at the front end of the "long centric" area, light closure (which would be slightly protruded from centric closure) would direct the lower teeth against upper inclines instead of into stable contacts. If the patient requires a "long centric" and does not get its built-in freedom, the lower incisors may strike the lingual inclines of the upper incisors in a manner that has a tendency to wedge the upper teeth labially. It is probably this "wedging effect" that causes most of the instability of occlusions that have not been provided with a "long centric."

It might be argued that the wedging contacts would occur with such light pressure that they would not possibly cause any harm. Such reasoning would continue to point out that when firm muscular pressure is exerted, the condyles would then be pulled into centric relation, and at this point the pressure would be properly directed by correct centric stops.

To understand how such light pressure on such minute interferences can cause problems of comfort and stability, it is necessary to have an acute appreciation for the exquisite sensitivity of the proprioceptive mechanism. When teeth are in the way of any functional border position, the muscles moving the mandible have two choices: they can move the mandible in a pattern of closure and function that *avoids* the interference, or they can move the mandible in a pattern of erasure to get rid of the interference.

Careful observation will convince one of the consistent pattern of grinding or clenching that occurs when an interference restricts functional jaw movements. Patterns of wear or movement of teeth are too routinely found in relation to such interferences to ignore their potential as targets for bruxism, if not the actual trigger that activates much of the parafunction. It appears that the erasure mechanism may actually be part of the adaptive process that is activated to regain lost equilibrium in the system by grinding away or moving the offending interference. What is not generally appreciated is how the bruxism pattern can be activated by such delicate contact on tooth surfaces that interfere so minimally with functional jaw patterns.

Clinical experience has been consistent, however, in the observation of accelerated wear of anterior teeth when inclines strike before full closure, or when an anterior guidance is restricted in any way from functional movements that occur during upright posture. The patterns of wear will be noticed on the labial surfaces of the lower incisors, or on the lingual surfaces of the upper incisors, or both.

Often the patient's subconscious attempt to regain the freedom of a muscularly coordinated closure ends up as forced protrusion, with the lower jaw trying to push the upper teeth forward to move them out of the way. Because of this forward thrust against the upper teeth, it is not uncommon for "locked-in occlusions" to develop slides. If the centric holding contacts on posterior teeth have been locked in with steep inclines that also interfere in the protrusive range of long centric, pressure against upper distal inclines can have a tendency to move them forward. This brings the upper mesial inclines into interference, and the slide results.

Not all patients require "long centric." Their centric closure and their light closure when they are in a postural position are identical. If such patients are given a "long centric," they will not use it, but it will not hurt them either. In fact, there are no contraindications for providing the freedom that goes with "long centric." Problems occur when we fail to realize that *"long centric" starts with a perfectly harmonized centric relation* and that all we are doing is providing patients with the freedom to close slightly anterior to that point at the same vertical. They are not forced to use either position, but they are free to use both positions or any point in between.

PROVIDING "LONG CENTRIC" BY EQUILIBRATION

When interferences to centric relation are eliminated by equilibration, "long centric" is usually provided automatically unless the vertical dimension is closed.

If the vertical dimension of the acquired occlusion is maintained, the first step in equilibration consists simply in eliminating all interferences from that point back to centric relation. The result is a "long centric" area that goes from centric relation all the way to the point of the original "acquired centric" (Fig. 15-5). The equilibrated patient is then free to close either into centric relation or into his

original convenience position or anywhere in between.

Our clinical experience has clearly and consistently shown that when interferences to centric relation are eliminated, the acquired position of occlusion is immediately forgotten. There is no need to maintain a "long centric" *that includes the original acquired position* because, given the freedom to do so, the mandible will either close directly into centric relation or within a fraction of a millimeter forward of it, the amount depending on vagaries of anatomy and on how much pressure is exerted by the closing musculature.

There is no relationship between the length of a "slide" and the length of the "long centric." The length of the "slide" is a result of interferences of the teeth. The length of the needed "long centric" is dependent on the anatomy of the condyle-disk relationship and the varying patterns of muscle activity in different persons. Many patients with long slides require no "long centric" when the interferences are eliminated. However, when the equilibrated mouth ends up with a longer "long centric" than the patient needs, it is not usually an indication for restoration of the entire occlusion. It will cause no discomfort or harm, since the patient will use only as much of the "long centric" as is needed.

In some patients, the interferences to centric relation are so severe that their elimination requires extensive flattening out of the occlusal areas between the convenience contacts and centric relation. Although such gross contouring will not cause any actual discomfort,

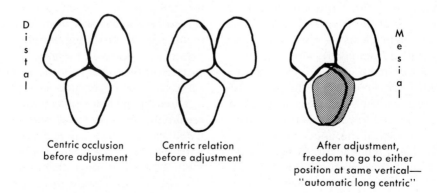

Fig. 15-5. Equilibration usually results in an "automatic long centric." This results from elimination of the inclines that interfere with closure into centric relation so that contact can be made at the most closed vertical *either* in centric relation or the original centric occlusion. The patient is free to use either position, or both.

some patients may complain that the flat surfaces make it difficult to chew meat or other fibrous foods. They may relate the feeling that their teeth are not "sharp enough." It is sometimes necessary to restore cuspal anatomy to such occlusions to give patients efficiency along with the comfort that goes with a harmonious gnathic system.

If there are no indications for restorative procedures other than a feeling of inefficiency, it would always be wise to give the patient a little time to see whether it is just a matter of adapting to the changed occlusion. The improvement in comfort is usually so great after proper equilibration that most patients will gladly accept the change in chewing efficiency that sometimes occurs when severe malocclusions are corrected. In many cases it would be the lesser of evils when compared with the otherwise unnecessary restoration of an entire occlusion.

It should be very clearly stated that reduced chewing efficiency should not result from normal equilibration procedures. The preceding discussion refers *only* to the unusual occlusal problems that cannot be corrected without extensive flattening out of the occlusal surfaces from the acquired position of maximum occlusal contact back to centric relation—in other words, the patient who ends up with the much too long "long centric." In almost all other cases, judicious and correct equilibration

should not "flatten out" an occlusion. The careful use of small stones on interfering inclines almost always improves efficiency without destroying the occlusal anatomy.

It should also be pointed out that orthodontic procedures should be considered as an alternative to equilibration procedures that would mutilate. In many instances, minor tooth movement through use of simple appliances will minimize the need for occlusal reshaping.

Although the establishment of "long centric" is usually an automatic part of equilibration, it is not always so. There is never a concern about this if both condyles are deviated to some degree of protrusive movement. If occlusal interferences cause a definite lateral shift of the mandible with no protrusion whatsoever of the rotating condyle, elimination of the interferences could produce a "locked-in bite."

To determine a patient's need for freedom of a "long centric," it is necessary to use two different colors of marking ribbon. First, the red ribbon is used to mark the light closure from the postural rest position. The patient should sit up in a postural position with no head rest and tap lightly on the ribbon (Fig. 15-6). The patient should be instructed to relax the jaw and lips and then tap lightly. Both anterior and posterior teeth should be checked for contacts in this manner.

After all contacts are marked in rest closure

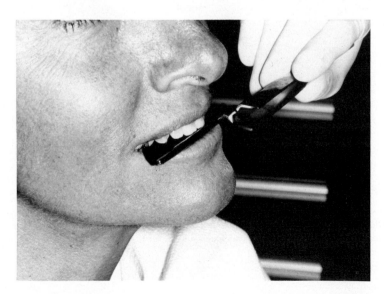

Fig. 15-6. In determining the length of the "long centric," the patient is seated upright, no headrest, lips relaxed. Red ribbon is used.

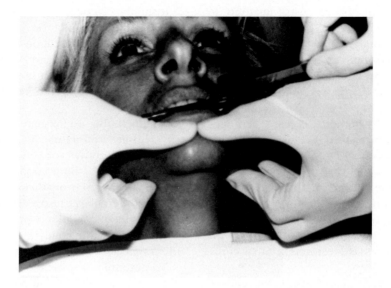

Fig. 15-7. With the patient in the supine position, the mandible is manipulated into the terminal axis. Centric relation contact is marked with a darker ribbon. If the red mark extends forward of the dark mark, the centric relation stop should be extended forward at the same vertical to include it.

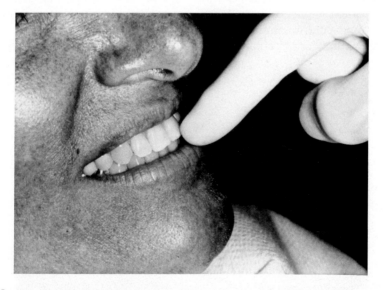

Fig. 15-8. Each tooth should be checked for movement when the patient taps the teeth together. The fingernail tip is very sensitive to any movement. If a tooth is jarred by functional tapping, it should be held in place and remarked for further refinement.

with the red ribbon, the patient should hold the mouth open to keep from losing the red marks. Then the patient is moved back so that the mandible may be manipulated correctly to record centric relation contacts (Fig. 15-7). By using a green or blue ribbon for centric relation, you may compare the centric contacts with the contacts made by allowing the patient to close from the rest position. Variations in marking may occur if red is used for light closure from rest and green is used for a manipulated centric marking. The following is a list of the various marking combinations along with the interpretation and treatment suggestions for each combination.

1. **When each red mark is covered by the green centric mark.** Exact coverage would indicate that terminal hinge closure and light closure from rest are identical. A "long centric" is not essential in such cases.

2. **When red marks extend forward from green centric marks.** Forward extension would show a need for "long centric." To provide the necessary amount, each centric stop should be extended forward at the same vertical for the length of the red mark. *One should not grind the green centric marks.* Equilibration for long centric is completed when there are no red marks on inclines. Allowing the patient to tap the teeth together should not cause movement of any tooth. This should be noted by careful digital examination of each tooth while the patient taps. Teeth that are jarred by the tapping (Fig. 15-8) should be remarked while being held in place and then adjusted accordingly by selective grinding. The final result should produce no perceptible jarring of any tooth on closing, either when manipulated into centric relation or when the patient closes from the relaxed postural rest position.

The red marks on the perfected occlusion will still extend forward from the green centric marks, but both red and green marks should be at the same vertical dimension of occlusion, as measured in the anterior part of the mouth. The vertical dimension of occlusion will open slightly in the posterior region as the protruding condyles move downward, but because of the minute distances involved, the differences in vertical between the front and the back of the average "long centric" is minimal.

3. **When red marks extend backward from green centric marks.** Backward extension can mean only one thing: the dentist has not manipulated correctly into centric closure. The green marks made by correct manipulation into centric closure will always be at the back border of any red mark. The red mark may be the same as the green mark, but it cannot be behind it.

4. **When green centric marks are missing from red marks.** If posterior teeth are marked by the red ribbon when the patient taps but some of them do not mark with the green ribbon when the mandible is manipulated into a centric closure, the equilibration for centric relation is incomplete. The equilibration *must* be perfected to permit free, unobstructed access into centric relation before the correct "long centric" can be determined. If red marks are not accompanied by green marks, it may be because teeth with some degree of mobility are being moved when the teeth are tapped together. Compression of mobile teeth permits more teeth to mark when they are squeezed together into the red ribbon than are permitted to touch with controlled manipulation for centric relation.

To check for such mobility, the dentist should manipulate into centric relation with different degrees of firmness, varying from a feather touch to a very firm contact. A different-color ribbon should be used for comparing the light contacts with the firm contacts. There should be no difference in the position of marks made by varying degrees of firmness when the mandible is manipulated into centric relation. This is accomplished by grinding interferences that are detected by marking with the lightest pressure so that the interfering tooth is not moved out of the way.

When the centric stops have been perfected to this degree, you are then ready to determine the "long centric." An occlusion that has been properly equilibrated in this manner will always show the green centric marks contiguously with the red marks made by allowing the patient to close from the postural rest position.

PROVIDING "LONG CENTRIC" WHEN THE OCCLUSION IS TO BE RESTORED

If all posterior teeth of either arch are to be restored, an excellent opportunity is presented to see the difference, if there is one, between a firm closure into centric relation and a light closure from the postural rest position.

By preparing all the upper or lower posterior teeth, you eliminate the possibility of any proprioceptive influence from them. Since the prepared teeth have been reduced occlusally and cannot contact the teeth in the opposing arch, they certainly cannot interfere with any pattern of closure. With all such chance of any posterior interference eliminated, it is then rather simple, when needed, to correct any inclines on the anterior teeth that cause a deviation from terminal hinge closure. By manipulating the mandible to make sure it does not deviate off its terminal axis, mark and reshape the interferences by selective grinding to provide centric relation stops on as many anterior teeth as possible. Properly adjusted centric stops on anterior teeth should be stable enough that not one of the teeth is jarred when the teeth are firmly tapped together in a terminal hinge closure.

When this is accomplished, the muscles that move the mandible are free to close it in any manner that best suits them. Since there are no interferences to terminal axis closure, the mandible is free to go there if the physiologic action of the muscles dictates. if the muscles close the mandible into any position other than centric relation, it is easily observed by checking with thin marking ribbon on the anterior teeth. Consequently, this is the ideal time to determine whether the restorative patient requires a "long centric" and, if so, how much.

After the anterior centric relation stops have been perfected, the patient should sit up in a normal postural position. The head rest should be removed, and then the patient should lightly tap his teeth together from a relaxed jaw position. Thin red ribbon should be interposed between the teeth, and the patient should repeat the light tapping. The red marks made from this procedure will indicate on the lingual surfaces of the upper anterior teeth the first points that the lower teeth contact when the mandible is closed lightly by the unrestricted, unaided, physiologic action of the muscles when the patient is in a postural position.

For comparison of such a closure with the terminal axis closure of centric relation, the mouth should be held open to preserve the red marks while the patient is placed back into a supine position for marking of centric relation with a darker colored ribbon. If green ribbon is used to mark centric relation contacts over the red marks, it is simple to see whether there is a difference between a manipulated terminal hinge closure and the unmanipulated light closure from a postural rest position.

If the patient requires the freedom of a "long centric," the red marks will extend forward from the green centric marks. If the red marks are on wedging inclines, the centric stops should be extended forward at the same vertical dimension for the length of the red marks.

When extending the centric stops to include closure from postural rest position, the dentist should be sure never to grind on the green centric marks. A knife-edged inverted-cone Carborundum stone is practical to use for accurate grinding (Fig. 15-9).

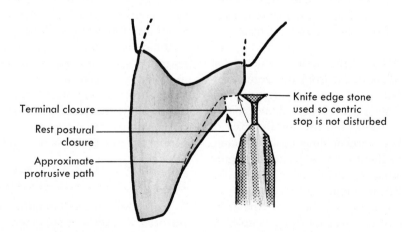

Terminal closure
Rest postural closure
Approximate protrusive path
Knife edge stone used so centric stop is not disturbed

Fig. 15-9. A knife-edge stone is ideal for extending the centric stops forward. It permits delicate extension of the stops without disturbing the preestablished centric relation stops.

It is very important to check each tooth digitally for any jarring from the light rest closure. It is easy for mobile teeth to be moved rather than marked by the ribbon. Checking each tooth for such movement while the patient taps is sometimes the only way such interferences are picked up. It is often necessary to hold mobile teeth in place with one finger while the patient taps in order to correctly mark them.

For those who are skeptical about the value of "long centric," the preceding procedures can be very enlightening. It is quite convincing to see teeth jarred when the patient sits up and taps that were not jarred by tapping when the patient was lying back. It is also quite enlightening to see other patients who tap directly and precisely into a terminal hinge axis closure, despite the fact that before the interferences to centric relation were removed their habitual closure was far from their centric closure.

When patients tell us that their teeth feel fine when they are lying down but that the teeth are in the way when they are sitting up, they are really giving us important information. They are telling us, in effect, that their centric relation is all right but they need the freedom of a "long centric." To provide them with less than both is to fall short of potential comfort and stability. We would like to provide our patients with occlusions that are comfortable when they are either sitting up or lying down, whether biting hard or lightly closing. This is not always possible to do with an occlusion that is restricted by tooth inclines to terminal hinge closure only.

If patients complain that their teeth fit fine when the dentists "push the jaw back" but hit only on the front teeth if they close it themselves, they are referring to the same type of restricted occlusion that often occurs when the dentists fail to provide a needed "long centric."

If restricting an occlusion only to centric relation is sometimes bad, restricting it only to an acquired habitual closure is worse. We have never seen a temporomandibular joint disorder that was directly caused by failure to provide a "long centric" if centric relation was correct. Failure to provide a needed "long centric" may lead to clenching and bruxism and a locked-in feeling of mild discomfort, but in itself it cannot cause a true joint pain-dysfunction syndrome.

On the other hand, failure to provide access to centric relation not only can cause severe problems of discomfort, clenching, and bruxism, but, as already pointed out, can also cause pain and dysfunction of the muscles that move the mandible.

Occlusal inclines restricting mandibular movement are potential stress producers. "Long centric" is permissive. It frees the mandible to close either into centric relation or slightly anterior to it. When the mandible is free to go where the muscles wish to move it, the result is predictable comfort with minimal stress to the entire gnathic system.

Because of the permissiveness of "long centric," there are really no disadvantages to providing it. Since we are talking about a freedom of rarely more than 0.5 mm, it does not create any problems for restoring the posterior occlusal form with good morphology. If the patient has it and does not need it, he does not have to use it. These are probably the reasons why Pankey has been telling us for years: "Any occlusion that is worthy of restoration, is worthy of 'long centric.'"

SUGGESTED READINGS

Ramfjord, S.P., and Ash, M.M.: Occlusion, ed. 3, Philadelphia, 1983, W.B. Saunders Co.

Schuyler, C.H.: Factors in occlusion related to restorative dentistry, J. Prosthet. Dent. **3**:772-782, 1953.

Schuyler, C.H.: Freedom in centric, Dent. Clin. North Am. **13**:681, 1972.

16

Anterior guidance

Next to centric relation, the anterior guidance is the most important determination that must be made when one is restoring an occlusion. The success or failure of many occlusal treatments hinges on the correctness of the anterior guidance. Yet the dentist who clearly determines specific guidelines and communicates precise information to the technician about the anterior guidance is a rarity. Dentists who are not utilizing methods for precisely establishing correct anterior guidance can make a quantum improvement in patient satisfaction with their restorative efforts by adhering to some very learnable concepts for determining, communicating, and verifying the accuracy of every anterior restoration.

The anterior guidance has similar importance in orthodontic treatment. Failure to properly establish the correct guidance is a major cause of posttreatment instability. Unfortunately, the occlusal problems that result from an inadequate anterior guidance are usually slow enough in causing damage that the orthodontist is not aware of the problems or the reason for the instability. Furthermore, a clear understanding of the functional rationale for a correct anterior guidance can simplify orthodontic treatment planning and often shorten the time required for treatment.

Besides being the most visible part of the smile, the relationship of the anterior teeth in function, is the principal determinant of posterior occlusal form. How precisely the anterior guidance is harmonized to individual patterns of function determines each patient's comfort; it is also, as we now know, critically important to the coordinated muscle function of the entire masticatory system. Normal function includes the lips and tongue in a variety of functional relationships, and the anterior teeth must fit into all those relationships with far greater preciseness than is possible without definitive methods of determination.

The contour and position of upper and lower anterior teeth is so critical that an error of less than a millimeter in incisal edge location can feel grotesque to some patients. It is a rare dentist who has not been stung by a patient's displeasure at what the dentist felt were beautiful anterior restorations. We have all heard the adage, "It is harder to fit the patient's mind than it is to fit the mouth," and we tend to explain away most patient dissatisfaction as more psychologic than real. There is no question that there are some patients with irrational expectations, but I have come to believe they are rare. We have learned that anterior relationships must be determined with extreme preciseness if we are to be predictably successful in restorations involving anterior teeth. Fortunately we do have definitive guidelines for determining every aspect of anterior teeth relationships, and so there is no reason to guess at a single determination of position, contour, or arch-to-arch correlation. Radical change in lip support, incisal edge position, and lingual

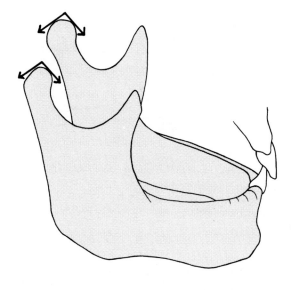

Fig. 16-1. Visualization of the mandible as a stable inverted tripod at centric relation. The posterior determinants (the condyles) have a stable uppermost stop in centric relation, and the anterior determinant (anterior guidance) also has an uppermost stable stop in centric relation. No posterior tooth should ever interfere with any one of the three legs of the tripod. The condyles should be free to move forward of the apex, but the anterior contact should never force either condyle down the distal path.

contours may affect more than a patient's natural appearance. Along with the discomfort and the look of artificiality, improperly restored anterior teeth may contribute to the destruction of the entire dentition.

One thing every dentist should know before attempting to restore anterior teeth is that besides being the key to esthetics, the anterior teeth are also the key factor in *protecting the posterior teeth.* So important is this job of anterior relationship that posterior teeth that are not protected from lateral or protrusive stresses by the discluding effect of the anterior teeth will, in time, almost certainly be stressed or worn detrimentally.

Despite how good the upper front teeth may look, their chance of staying healthy and keeping the back teeth healthy depends on their lingual contours, specifically the contact of the lower anterior teeth against the upper anterior teeth in centric, "long centric," straight protrusive, and lateral excursions. This dynamic relationship of the lower anterior teeth against the upper anterior teeth through all ranges of function is called the *anterior guidance.* As such, it literally sets the limits of movement of the front end of the mandible.

For the time being, to grasp the perspective of anterior guidance a little better, we will ignore the back teeth, since they should not interfere with either anterior guidance or condylar guidance anyway. We will imagine that all the back teeth have been shortened through

preparation so that they cannot touch in any position of the mandible. Now without any possibility of posterior tooth interference, we visualize the mandible closing in a terminal axis closure until the front teeth contact. If all the lower anterior teeth contact simultaneously against stable centric stops at the correct vertical dimension, the first requirement of good anterior relationship has been fulfilled. The mandible should be closed into a stable tripod relationship with the solid anterior contact as the front leg of the inverted tripod and the upwardly braced condyles serving as the other two legs (Fig. 16-1).

Since this mandible tripod is a lever that hinges at the condyles, it will be apparent that the power for closing this lever is in muscles that exert the closing force *between* the condyles and the front teeth. The anterior teeth are all forward of the closing muscle power; so to exert stress on the anterior teeth, the mechanical result of the closing muscles would be like trying to crack a walnut by placing it at the tips of the handles of a nutcracker and squeezing the handles back at the hinge (Fig. 16-2, *A*). Even though the mandible is shaped differently from the typical nutcrackers, it does not change the mechanical effect (Fig. 16-2, *B*). This is the unique position of resistance to stress that the anterior teeth enjoy by virtue of their relationship to the condylar fulcrum and the source of muscle power.

The condyle-disk assemblies, braced firmly

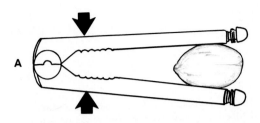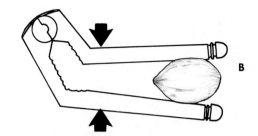

Fig. 16-2. This nutcracker drawing, **A**, illustrates the unique position of resistance to stress that the anterior teeth are in. Muscle power, *arrows*, is exerted back close to the hinge, and the force diminishes as the distance from the fulcrum increases. Visualizing the mandible as a nutcracker type of lever, **B**, and relating the anterior teeth to the illustrated nut show why the anterior teeth are in a position to protect the posterior teeth. Making the anterior "nut" as strong as possible by correctly contoured stops enhances the protective role of the anterior teeth.

against bone, form a very strong hinge that is completely capable of resisting the power of the closing muscles. The anterior teeth, when their position allows it, should be made to form a very stable stop for the front of the mandible and thereby limit its closing motion. If the closing motion of the mandible is stopped by the incisal edges of all six lower anterior teeth against stable holding contacts of the six upper anteriors, we have not only taken advantage of the *position* of the front teeth, we have also strengthened that position by *distributing* the stresses. Wear is also diminished to the maximum degree possible because of the distribution to more surfaces.

With correct contouring and distribution of centric stops, there is really no logical reason why the anterior teeth should not contact in centric relation. It should be obvious that there are in fact distinct advantages to such contact, especially if "long centric" concepts are understood.

Up to now, we have been discussing just one position of the mandible, the terminally braced condyles in the back and the corresponding anterior centric contacts that serve as the front leg of the tripod. What happens when the mandible moves out of its centric position?

We will continue to visualize the stable tripod relationship. Since the back two legs of our tripod represent the two condyle-disk assemblies that are braced against bone, they obviously cannot go any farther up the eminentiae. What happens when they slide forward down the curved pathways of the eminentiae? Well of course, if the condyles slide forward, the lower anterior teeth have to move forward

too. It is a popular fallacy, however, that whatever path the condyles follow must be duplicated in the lingual surfaces of the upper anterior teeth so the lower anterior teeth can follow the same path. This is wrong. *Condylar paths do not dictate anterior guidance,* and there is no need or even advantage to try to make the anterior guidance duplicate condylar guidance. Advocates of such a concept have failed to recognize that the condyles can rotate as they move along their protrusive pathways. This allows the front end of the mandible to follow a completely different path without interfering with the condylar path.

The path that the condyles travel dictates the outer limits to which the mandible can move. These outer limitations are referred to as the *envelope of motion.* The path that the front end of the mandible follows is dictated by *functional movements of muscle* as it relates the lower anterior teeth to the upper anterior teeth in the chewing cycle. The outer limits of these functional movements are referred to as the *envelope of function.* Such functional movements occur *within* the limits of condylar border movements and consequently should be treated as a separate entity (Fig. 16-3).

To better understand how the anterior guidance differs from the condylar guidance, we return to our visualization of the upside-down tripod. Since the condyles on the back two legs of the tripod are rounded (so that the mandible can rotate around them), it is easy to see how the lower incisors that form the front leg of the tripod can slide forward on a variety of paths without conflict to either the front path or the condyle path. The same condylar

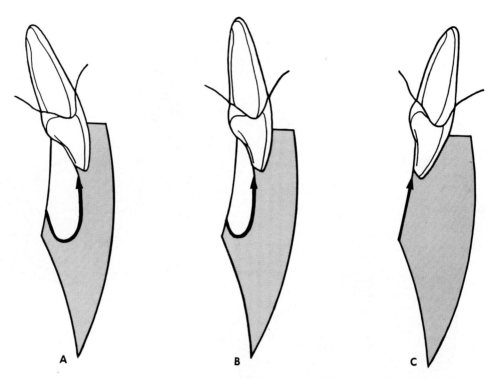

Fig. 16-3. Condylar border movements determine the outer limits of movement of the lower anterior teeth, but they do not dictate the lingual contours of the upper anterior teeth. Each of these three patients has the same outer limits of motion, but each has a different envelope of function. Even though the condylar guidance is the same, the anterior teeth would have to be contoured differently for each patient. Patient **A** has a fairly flat function and so would require an anterior guidance with more horizontal freedom. Patient **B** has a tighter lip with more of a tendency for uprighting the anterior teeth. The envelope of function is more vertical. Patient **C** has vertical chop-chop function with no horizontal movement. Since functional movements occur *within* the envelope of motion borders, merely recording the outer limits of motion would not supply enough needed information for optimally restoring anterior teeth. The envelope of function that controls the anterior relationship must be treated as a separate entity.

path that permits the lower anterior teeth to follow a horizontal path forward will just as easily permit them to follow a 10-degree, a 30-degree, or even a steeper path. It does not matter whether the anterior path is flat or curved, concave, convex, or parabolic, the rotating condyles sliding down the unchanged condylar path permit the lower anterior teeth to follow any number of path variations without interference (Fig. 16-4).

Slavicek[1] has shown from axiographic studies of over 3000 patients that the anterior guidance is *not* similar in contour to condylar guidance. In fact, the anterior guidance pathway is most often more similar to a mirror image of the condylar path. In healthy dentitions, the lower incisal edges usually follow a forward, fairly horizontal path as the condyles are traveling down the steepest part of the eminentiae. As the condyles start to move more horizontally on the flatter part of the eminen-

tiae, the anterior tooth contours become steeper (Fig. 16-5).

There does not appear to be any clinical evidence to support the early gnathologic dictum that the anterior guidance must be an analog of condylar guidance. Nor is there any functional reason to support the concept. Arbitrarily making the anterior guidance the same or nearly the same as the condylar guidance can cause some significant problems. It can result in restriction of the envelope of function if it causes the anterior guidance to be made too steep: It can cause interference with the lip-closure path, the neutral zone, and functional phonetic relationships if the condylar path dictates a too-horizontal anterior guidance because copying the condylar path may result in upper incisal edges that are too far forward, thus creating an interference with lip function and the neutral zone (Fig. 16-6).

If the condylar path does not dictate the an-

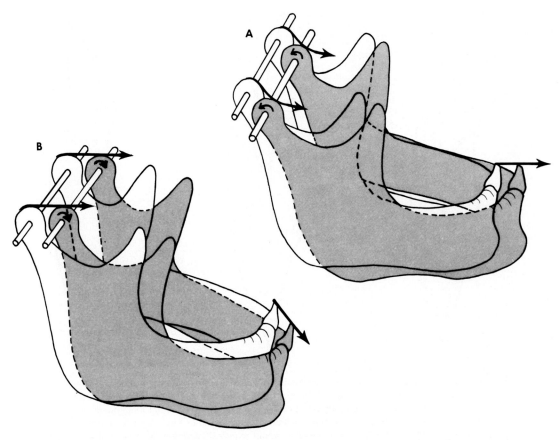

Fig. 16-4. It is not necessary or even desirable for the anterior guidance to duplicate condylar guidance. Because the condyles can rotate, the front of the mandible can travel a different path without producing any conflict for the condylar path. If the condyles follow a normal convex path, **A**, there is no reason why the anterior guidance cannot follow a flat path forward, a condition found in many healthy mouths. **B**, Although condyles do not follow a flat condylar path, there would be no mechanical reason why it could not function with a steeper anterior guidance because the condyles are free to rotate as they protrude.

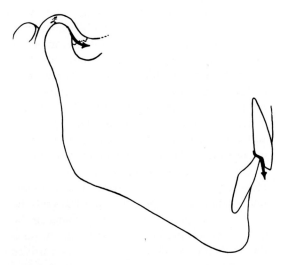

Fig. 16-5. The anterior guidance is not similar to the condylar guidance in nature. The condylar path is normally convex. The anterior guidance is normally concave.

terior guidance, it should be clear that the anterior guidance cannot be determined on an articulator regardless of how perfectly the condylar path is duplicated. It is a separate entity and must be determined in the mouth where the determinants of anterior tooth position can be observed in function. Unless each important guideline for specific contour and placement of anterior teeth is determined in the mouth and communicated precisely to the technician, the best any technician can do is to guess at where and how the anterior teeth should be contoured. That is almost always unsatisfactory, and guesswork is certainly unnecessary because there are very effective ways of determining every specific position and contour with great accuracy.

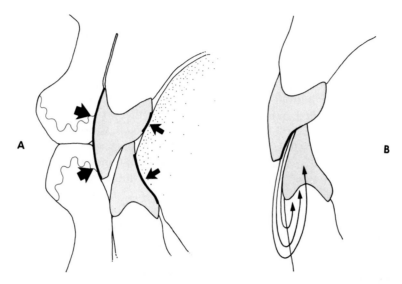

Fig. 16-6. A, The lips are the dominant controlling factor in determining the inclination of the anterior teeth. The inward pressure exerted by the lips when they seal for swallowing is a natural positioner for the anterior teeth. Forward pressure by the tongue opposes the inward lip pressure. The neutral zone between these two forces dictates the position of stability for the anterior teeth. It is unrelated to condylar guidance. Interference to the neutral zone and lip-closure path results if the anterior teeth are too far forward. **B,** The envelope of function is related to neutral zone positioning. Interference to functional harmony results if the anterior teeth are too far lingually. The envelope of function is also unrelated to condylar guidance.

The importance of condylar pathways should not be belittled. They are extremely important, and capturing the effect of condylar pathways by some method is one bit of information that cannot be ignored, but it is only part of the needed information, and it does not determine the correct anterior guidance.

Correctly recorded condylar pathways do not tell the technician how long the upper anterior teeth should be or how far out the labial contours should be for proper lip support and harmony with the upper and lower lip musculature.

Condylar pathways do not dictate the correct smile line. The precise incisal edge position varies greatly as the length of the lip and the degree of flaccidity or tightness of the lip vary. People with tight lips usually have anterior teeth that are positioned more vertically than those of people with flaccid lips, and even if the condylar guidance were the same in both types of patients, the anterior guidance would be different. It would almost always be steeper in the tight-lipped person.

There is another factor that cannot be determined from stone models on any articulator, and it is one of the most important determinants of anterior contours. That is the character of the periodontal support. The sick mouth should be treated differently from the healthy mouth, and when periodontal support has been reduced, it is often necessary to also reduce the lateral forces on the anterior teeth. We do this by opening out the lingual contours and reducing steep inclines. Lateral stresses on the anterior teeth must be reduced to a level that does not stress any tooth into noticeable movement during function. How do we know whether a tooth is being moved during function? We observe it visually and test it digitally as changes are made to the upper lingual inclines. When we reach an acceptable point of comfort with stability in all excursions, we stop.

It is both practical and logical to work out the details of anterior contours in the mouth. When done in an orderly sequence, we can determine precisely how much "long centric" is needed, we can test variations in incisal edge position for phonetic correctness, and we can be guided by the mobility patterns of teeth as they are subjected to varying degrees of lateral stress. The greater the hypermobility, the greater is the need for minimizing lateral stresses. The less the mobility, the less is the need for changing even steep anterior inclines.

By making any changes directly in the mouth, we give the patient the opportunity of approving the appearance and trying out the function, comfort, and phonetics before accepting the changed contours. Once the correctness of the incisal edge positions, labial contours, and lingual curvatures has been verified and accepted by the patient, the permanent restorations can be fabricated with confidence. All the information must be preserved in a usable manner, however, so that the finished anterior restorations duplicate the contours that have been tested in the mouth and confirmed as correct.

LATERAL ANTERIOR GUIDANCE

Our reason for not using the term "incisal guidance" is that the connoted limitation to the four incisors is often confusing. Incisal guidance is frequently described in terms of protrusive movements only. Actually, the *lateral* pathways that are established on the anterior teeth have a far greater influence on posterior occlusal form, and the cuspids play a major role in determining the lateral stress-bearing capabilities of all the anterior teeth.

The occlusal contours of all the posterior teeth are dictated by both condylar guidance and anterior guidance. No posterior tooth should interfere with either anterior guidance or condylar guidance. Either posterior teeth may be discluded from any lateral contact by the anterior teeth, or they must be in perfect, harmonious group function with them and the condyles. Either way, the anterior guidance, as a *determinant* of posterior occlusal form, must be perfected *before* occlusal contours can be finalized.

Whenever it is practical to eliminate posterior contact while working out the anterior guidance, it is helpful. This can be accomplished in mouths that require posterior occlusal restorations by completion of the preparation of the posterior teeth before the anterior guidance is worked out. If the posterior teeth do not require restorations, the anterior guidance must be worked out simultaneously with equilibration of the posterior teeth.

Since the anterior guidance is a protector of the posterior teeth, the goal is to make the anterior teeth as strong as possible so that they may carry out their protective function. Adjusting the anterior inclines when there is no support from posterior teeth enables us to fully evaluate the stress-resistance capabilities of the anterior teeth and to correct them accordingly.

The ultimate goal of a correct anterior guidance is that it should be comfortable, functional, and stable even without posterior contact. In other words, a good anterior guidance should be able to stand on its own without any help from posterior teeth.

The importance of anterior guidance is better understood as a result of the research of Williamson.[2] He demonstrated that disclusion of all posterior teeth in eccentric jaw position reduces muscle contraction in two of the three elevator muscles. This is an important finding because it enables us to reduce the load on both the temporomandibular joints and the posterior teeth in all excursive movements. But it has equal importance for the anterior teeth. When all posterior teeth are taken out of any excursive contact, the load applied to the anterior teeth is actually lessened even though they are the only teeth in contact.

As long as the anterior guidance remains intact, capable of discluding the posterior teeth in eccentric jaw positions, the protection of the posterior teeth is assured. For that reason it is critically important to make the anterior guidance as stable as possible. If the anterior teeth wear away, or move, or get loose, they may lose the capacity for separating the posterior teeth. The moment any posterior tooth comes into premature excursive contact, not only the anterior guidance loses its capability for shutting off elevator muscle contraction, but also the elevator muscles are hyperactivated by the posterior contact. This increases the load on the whole system, including the joints and the teeth and especially the anterior teeth themselves.

Because of our new understanding of muscle responses to posterior disclusion, we no longer attempt to bring posterior teeth into working-side group function to help weak anterior teeth. Even when anterior teeth are weakened by loss of supporting structure, it is preferable to have them carry the whole load during jaw excursions because by doing so we actually lessen the load on the anterior teeth because of the reduction in elevator muscle contraction to only one actively contracting muscle on each side (Fig. 16-7).

If the anterior teeth are too weak to func-

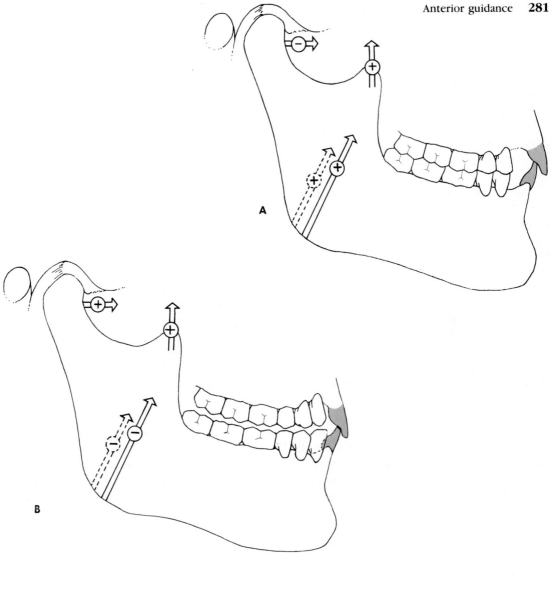

Fig. 16-7. A, Equal contact on anterior and posterior teeth in centric relation results in release of the inferior lateral pterygoid muscle (−) and active contraction of all elevator muscles (+). In this relationship, no excess horizontal stress is directed at the upper anterior teeth. **B,** When the mandible is protruded by the inferior lateral pterygoid muscle (+) and *all* contact is on the anterior teeth, elevator muscle activity is reduced to partial contraction of the temporalis. This effectively reduces the horizontal forces on the anterior teeth even though they are the only teeth in contact. **C,** If a posterior interference prevents the anterior guidance from discluding the posterior teeth in excursions, the effect is hyperactivity of all the elevator muscles plus the incoordination and hyperactivation of the lateral pterygoid muscles.

tion as discluders of the posterior teeth, it is usually better to stabilize them by splinting than it is to bring the posterior teeth into excursive function. Clinically, our long-term results appear to be consistently better whenever we have been able to fully utilize the disclusive capacity of the anterior teeth, even when they have been compromised by loss of bone support.

The beneficial effect on muscle contraction does not appear to be related to any special proprioceptive sensitivity of the anterior teeth. Rather it appears to be entirely related to disclusion of the posterior teeth. The moment total posterior disclusion occurs seems to be the signal for active contraction of all but one elevator muscle on each side to shut off. Williamson's research indicates that in straight protrusion the temporalis muscle is the only actively contracting muscle whereas in lateral movements the internal pterygoid replaces the temporalis contraction on the balancing side while the temporalis remains in contraction on the working side.

Making every anterior relationship conform to a stereotyped ideal is not always possible because tongue-thrust swallowing patterns or lip-biting habits may alter the relationship. In the absence of such habit patterns, which may or may not be detrimental, maximum comfort with stability can be predictably achieved if the following conditions are met for the anterior teeth.

1. Stable holding contacts for each anterior tooth.
2. Centric relation contacts occurring simultaneously with equal-intensity posterior tooth contacts.
3. Position and contour of anterior teeth in harmony with the envelope of function.
4. Immediate disclusion of all posterior teeth the moment the mandible leaves centric relation.
5. Position and contour of all anterior teeth in harmony with the neutral zone and the lip closure path.

Whenever possible to achieve, the above conditions should result in long-term stability of the anterior teeth because when all the conditions are met the teeth are in anatomic as well as functional harmony. When such harmony exists, there is no need for adaptive changes. In fact, the forces applied from various directions have a tendency to hold the teeth in place vertically as well as horizontally. As long as the anterior teeth remain in a stable position with no excessive wear occurring, they will continue to serve as the very important protector of the posterior teeth and the signal for reduction of muscle loading in all eccentric jaw positions.

Anterior teeth that are in anatomic and functional harmony can take advantage of a system that was designed to reduce the forces on them in three significant ways:

1. The position of the teeth in relation to the fulcrum and the muscular power source reduces the effect of muscle contraction loading.
2. The effect of proprioceptors around the anterior roots on programming the muscles to function within the limits imposed by the teeth. The more upright the anterior teeth, the more vertical is the envelope of function, thus reducing horizontal forces.
3. The reduction of muscle loading when only anterior teeth are in contact.

Like all other parts of the masticatory system, the anterior guidance serves as an integrated part of the system, and the anterior teeth are designed to last a lifetime if harmony in the total system is maintained. When there is a problem with anterior teeth, it is the diagnostician's job to find where the disharmony exists.

Close observation of the anterior teeth in the mouth is the best way to determine whether lateral movements are stressing them. Both visual and digital examination should be used to determine whether any teeth are being moved during lateral excursions. Noting the contact area between the cuspid and the lateral incisor during lateral excursions is often a good indicator of stress. Movement of the cuspid will frequently open the contact as the jaw is moved laterally.

Upper anterior teeth that are noticeably moved by any functional excursion should be corrected. Correction usually consists in reshaping the upper lingual contours. Centric stops should always be established before refinement of excursive inclines; so the lower incisal edges are rarely involved in the correction of any lateral excursion interferences. Changes in the lower anterior teeth should be limited to minimal adjustments that do not involve the centric stops on the incisal edges.

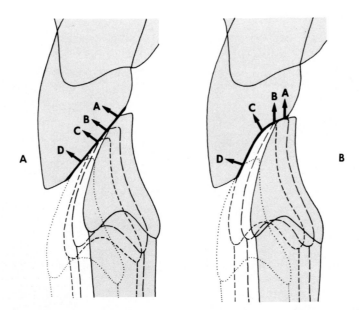

Fig. 16-8. A, The main vector of force is at a right angle to the surface contacted. As the lower cuspid moves in lateral excursion from position *a* to position *d*, the vector of force is maintained in a nearly horizontal direction. **B,** Changing the contour of the contacted surface changes the vectors of force. As the lower cuspid moves from position *a* (centric relation) to position *b*, the force vector is nearly parallel with the long axis. The only lateral stress exerted is the result of frictional drag across the horizontal surface. As the lower tooth moves from position *b* to position *c*, the force vector starts to change toward the horizontal, but at that point other anterior teeth can usually share the stress by joining into group function with the cuspid. From position *c* to position *d* the vector of force is nearly horizontal, but that surface should be slightly outside the functional border pathways, so that it may contact but not interfere. The downward path of the lower tooth follows the natural movement of the mandible as the orbiting condyle moves down and initiates the opening part of the lateral cycle.

Correction of upper lingual contours is patterned to accomplish two effects: redirection of forces and improved distribution of forces. Forces are redirected when the shape of the contacting surfaces is changed. The main vector of force is at a right angle to the surface contacted. Changing the surface changes the vector. The main vector of force against a steep incline is directed nearly horizontally (Fig. 16-8, *A*). Changing the steep incline to a flat incline would redirect the forces more nearly up the long axis (Fig. 16-8, *B*).

Improved distribution of forces is accomplished when more teeth are brought into simultaneous contact during excursions. This is often accomplished as a side benefit when force direction is improved because more anterior teeth are brought into lateral function as steep convex inclines are changed to concave.

In some mouths with good periodontal support, it may only be necessary to slightly improve the direction of forces to stabilize the teeth. Hypermobility patterns may be eliminated by even slight reductions in stress. If sta-

bility can be achieved with minimal changes, there is no reason for drastic recontouring.

In mouths with poor periodontal support, poor crown-root ratios, poorly shaped roots, or poor quality alveolar bone, drastic changes in contour may be necessary. To reduce stresses to the minimum, it is almost always necessary to both redirect and redistribute all lateral forces on the teeth.

Somewhere between the two extremes just given lie the majority of anterior guidance problems. The dentist who learns to understand mobility patterns and correlate them with improved vectors of force and better stress distribution will be able to achieve predictable success in treating anterior guidance problems without destroying the esthetics in the process.

All of this discussion boils down to this: correction of upper lingual contours is accomplished either by reduction of the steepness of any incline that, when contacted, causes the tooth to move, or by movement of the incline so that it does not interfere with functional jaw

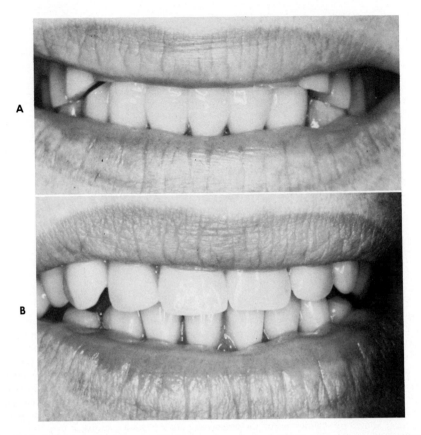

Fig. 16-9. It is not necessary to cut all the way through the teeth to reduce stress, **A.** A curved anterior guidance permits the stresses to be directed nearly up the long axis through the range of posterior function but permits better incising action in protrusive function. The esthetic "smile line," **B,** not only looks better, but also functions better.

movements. Steep inclines next to the centric stops are the most common source of stress. The need for corrective flattening from centric stops out is greatest close to the stops and then diminishes as the jaw moves laterally. This most often produces concave lingual inclines that are flattest near the centric stops but may then curve into quite steep inclines to permit effective incising.

It is almost never necessary to reduce the length of an esthetically correct tooth. It is not necessary to flatten the lateral or protrusive angles all the way through the teeth to reduce stress (Fig. 16-9). To do so in protrusion is esthetically disastrous, and the resultant reverse smile line "ages" the patient many years. If lateral stresses cannot be minimized enough with concave contouring of upper lingual inclines, it would be better to stabilize the anterior teeth by splinting than to ruin the appearance of a person's smile.

The determination of whether splinting is needed or not is dependent on whether or not an esthetically acceptable anterior guidance can be worked out that does not stress the anterior teeth to noticeable movement when firm excursions are made.

It may be quite surprising how practically the correct concave inclines can be worked out in the mouth. As the mandible moves laterally, the orbiting condyle moves downward and the natural tendency of the jaw is to open as it moves to the side. The resultant over and down movement of the lower anterior teeth produces the concavity in the upper lingual contours, which permits lateral function with minimal stress.

An anterior occlusal problem that will have to be solved quite often involves hypermobile cuspids in a cuspid-protected occlusion. The lingual incline of the cuspids is too steep to permit any other tooth inclines from sharing the lateral stresses. Very often the cuspid inclines are convex, which forces the cuspid laterally when the jaw moves to the side. If very little bone has been lost around the cuspids, it may be possible to eliminate the hypermobility with minimal changes to the cuspids. Changing the convexity to a straight steep incline with just a little concavity at and just lateral to the centric stops may solve the problem and be very compatible to a vertical envelope of function. This may sometimes be accomplished without even bringing other teeth into group function. Slight changes very often make major improvements in function and stability. Making such corrections in the mouth, where patterns of tooth mobility can be observed, enables you to keep changes to the minimum.

One might wonder what it could hurt to open the upper anterior lingual inclines out in all cases. If it is good for a sick mouth, why wouldn't it be just as good for healthy mouths? The answer, I think, should be obvious. It would be foolish to remove tooth structure (sometimes to the point of exposing dentin) unless it is necessary for the reduction of stresses that are contributing to accelerated deterioration. Although changing steep inclines to a more opened out chewing cycle may not actually cause harm, if it is not in harmony with the chop-chop shearing action that some patients are used to, they may complain that their modified teeth are "not sharp enough." For these reasons we change lateral inclines only as necessary to reduce stresses causing harm. Stresses that move teeth noticeably when excursions are made are harmful and should be corrected.

The cuspid with steep or convex lingual inclines that has lost a considerable amount of bony support will need to have the inclines opened out to allow an almost flat area from centric relation laterally to reduce horizontal stress and to permit other anterior teeth to come into group function with it. As more teeth are brought in to share the lateral stresses, the flat inclines can then curve into steeper ones to produce the concavity. At the same time, the mobility of the cuspid will diminish until even moving the mandible laterally with firm help from the operator will not cause noticeable movement of the teeth. (If this cannot be accomplished because of extreme hypermobility, it will be necessary to

consider either splinting or a removable retainer to be worn at night. Bringing more anterior teeth into group function not only distributes the stresses over more teeth, but it also distributes them to teeth that are progressively farther from the condylar fulcrum and in a better position to withstand the stresses. It is often possible to extend group function around to include both central teeth, and sometimes even the balancing side lateral incisor can contribute support.

Concave contours on upper anterior teeth feel very natural to the patient as they allow the tongue to fit against the teeth without irritation. The dentist must be careful not to leave sharp line angles at the junction of the centric stop and the lingual incline. The lingual edge of the stop should be rounded and smooth. Contours shoud always be compatible with maintaining healthy gingival tissues.

Although concave lingual contours usually work out quite naturally for patients with normal to deep overbite, they may be contraindicated for patients with minimal overbite. The near end-to-end anterior relationship will end up with an anterior guidance that is almost flat. Lateral guide pathways may have no curvatures at all. As long as the inclines permit firm excursions without noticeable movement of teeth, the centric stops are stable, and the esthetics and function are acceptable, all requirements for the anterior guidance have been fulfilled. The procedures for correcting or evaluating any anterior guidance are the same, regardless of the amount of overbite present, as long as arch relationships permit centric contact. Anterior relationships that do not permit centric contacts are discussed in separate chapters.

When anterior guidance inclines must follow straight paths, better esthetics usually results from having protrusive inclines that are steeper than lateral inclines. This gives the upper smile line a more natural curvature. Flat protrusive paths in combination with steeper lateral paths accentuate the cuspids and produce a harsh, unesthetic, reversed smile line.

STEPS IN HARMONIZING THE ANTERIOR GUIDANCE

The refinement and restoration of anterior guidance contours should not be attempted on a pure technique basis. It is essential to understand the reason for any change made. The effect on esthetics and phonetics should be considered in advance, and a clear insight should be developed regarding the variations of periodontal support, the mechanics of stress, and the role of the anterior teeth as protectors of the posterior teeth. Unless these factors are understood and tempered with clinical judgment, no technique will achieve dependable results. This is true for the procedures that follow. Nevertheless, it is a practical sequence to use when the anterior guidance needs modification. The same steps can be utilized to determine whether changes are needed. The procedures are practical whether the anterior teeth are to be restored or merely modified. If restoration is necessary, the correctness of any changes can be tested before they are accepted.

Preliminary steps

1. When indicated, lower anterior teeth should be reshaped or restored first.
2. If restorations are not needed on the posterior teeth, they must be equilibrated *before* the anterior guidance can be worked out. All interferences to centric relation must be eliminated on both anterior and posterior teeth to establish stable contacts at the most closed position. Eccentric interferences should then be eliminated on the posterior teeth. The goal is to move all excursive contact on to the anterior teeth if they are in a position to function in that capacity. Thus any posterior incline that causes separation of the anterior teeth should be reduced until anterior contact can be maintained through the complete excursion. As long as posterior interferences that prevent a full range of anterior guidance function are present, it will not be possible to determine or work out a correct anterior guidance.

Remember that full functional contact of the anterior teeth depends on their being able to contact in centric relation. If there is no anterior contact because of tongue or lip postures, or arch malrelationships, a normal anterior guidance may not be achievable. Various degrees of anterior open bite should be analyzed carefully before you make an attempt to achieve anterior contact (see Chapter 33).

If restoration of the posterior teeth is indicated, an opportunity for precise harmonizing of anterior guidance can be taken advantage of. By preparing the posterior teeth in one arch before completing the correction of the anterior inclines, you can eliminate the influence of posterior contacts completely. This is helpful because taking the posterior teeth out of contact eliminates their proprioceptive influence and makes it easier to record centric relation stops on the anterior teeth. It also makes it easier to observe mobility patterns during function when the anterior teeth are the only teeth in contact.

Any reduction of posterior support is helpful because the fewer posterior teeth that contact, the easier occlusal adjustments can be made and the simpler it is to observe hypermobility patterns on the teeth that remain in contact.

The four steps to harmony

STEP **1.** *Establish coordinated centric relation stops on all anterior teeth* (Fig. 16-10).

The dentist must manipulate the mandible and guide it into a terminal axis closure, marking with thin marking ribbon and adjusting until each lower incisor makes a definite mark. In most mouths, minimal adjustment is required to establish good centric stops. In others, major decisions may have to be made. Some of the common problems faced at this step are the following.

Deviation from first centric contact into a more closed position. All interferences should be eliminated so that the mandible may close all the way to maximum closure without any deviation. This is the most common problem and the easiest to solve.

No contact on some teeth after deviation is eliminated. This condition occurs in the patient who has solid centric stops, but not on all teeth. What do we do with the teeth that are not in contact? We have three choices:

1. *We can close the vertical* by grinding down the centric stops until all teeth contact. This may sound harsh, but a slight *closure* of vertical does no harm. In teeth with severe bone loss, it may have an advantage by improving the crown-root ratio. Even with firm teeth, slight closure to gain contact is usually better than having to restore teeth to contact.
2. *We can build up teeth to contact.* It is often necessary to make temporary resto-

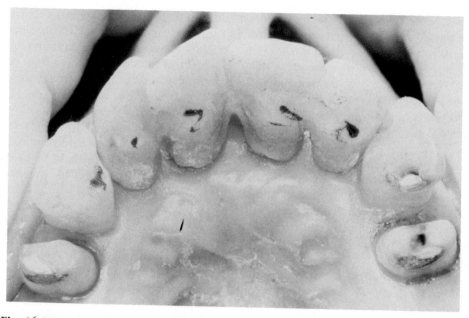

Fig. 16-10. Coordinated centric relation stops on the anterior teeth. Posterior teeth have been prepared. Temporary acrylic restorations were placed on the four incisors to bring them into centric contact that they did not have. The anterior guidance can then be harmonized on the acrylic surface.

rations to build out the lingual contours into contact. All the steps of working out the anterior guidance are then finalized on the temporary restorations before the contours are accepted as a guide for the permanent restorations.

3. *We can "do nothing."* Sometimes nothing is what we should do. Anterior teeth that are not in contact but that are stable because of a substitute contact such as lip or tongue position are sometimes better left as they are. We must just be certain that they are stable without tooth contact before electing to leave them that way. If noncontacting teeth need to be restored and if we can establish enough centric stops from other teeth to program the customized guide table, we do not have to worry about missing contacts. The restorations can be corrected on the articulator.

Missing anterior teeth. This problem is solved when a temporary anterior bridge is made from articulated casts and then all contours are finalized on the temporary bridge in the mouth. Correct esthetics can be established right along with correct lingual contours.

Arch-relationship problems that do not allow centric contact on all teeth. These problems are discussed in separate chapters. However, as a general rule, we must determine which teeth should contact in centric relation before proceeding to the next step. If lower anterior teeth need to be moved or reshaped, their position and contours must be correct before we proceed with finalizing the anterior guidance.

If orthodontic movement or gross reshaping of either upper or lower anterior teeth can improve the finished result, such changes should always be worked out in advance on articulated casts. Temporary acrylic restorations that reflect the changes can be placed after orthodontic movement has been completed. Refinements can be made in the mouth.

Habits that keep anterior teeth from contacting. Before any noncontacting tooth is brought into contact, we must make sure it is not being held out of contact by an unbreakable habit. Many habits of lip biting actually result from unconscious attempts to cushion the teeth from interfering contacts. Such habits usually disappear when the occlusion is corrected. Other habits such as chewing on a pipe stem can be broken if the patient wants to, but this should be determined before we restore the lost contact. If the habit remains, the restored teeth will simply be pushed further out of alignment. Equilibration procedures should be carried out to produce as much stability as possible before preparation. Any anterior teeth that could touch but do not should be evaluated carefully before they are brought into contact.

Contouring the centric stops. It is not necessary for the entire incisal edge of the lower incisors to contact in centric relation. This usually produces too much of a ledge in the upper teeth. If upper contours are rounded, contact with just the labial portion of the incisal edge is sufficient. The shape of the upper contacts should direct the forces as near up the long axis as possible, but contacts on slight inclines are not as stressful as they may seem because the labial vector of force is counteracted by inward pressure from the lips. Posterior support that is harmonized to the anterior stops will also minimize the potential stress.

When all centric stops have been refined, each tooth should be checked digitally to make sure it is not being moved by centric closure. Any teeth jarred by a manipulated closure should be remarked while slight pressure is applied to keep the tooth from moving.

STEP **2.** *Extend centric stops forward at the same vertical to include light closure from the postural rest position.*

Such extension occurs when we determine how much "long centric" the patient requires. It is also the step that enables us to have centric contact with the anterior teeth without fear of stressing them excessively toward the labial. "Long centric" is explained in detail in Chapter 15, and so there is no need for repetition here regarding its rationale.

After centric stops have been established by manipulation of the mandible into terminal axis closure, the patient should sit up in a postural position. The head rest is removed, and the patient is instructed to "tap lightly with the lips relaxed." Red ribbon is inserted between the teeth, and the tapping is repeated. The mouth should be held open while the patient is returned to the supine position and a manipulated centric closure into a darker marking ribbon made (green or blue works fine). If the red marks extend onto inclines forward of the centric marks, the centric stops should be ex-

tended at the same vertical so that the teeth can be closed either into centric relation or slightly forward of it without bumping into inclines. The amount of freedom from centric relation required rarely exceeds 0.5 mm. Regardless of the amount needed, we can determine it quite precisely by following this procedure.

Extension of the centric stops is accomplished nicely with a sharp inverted-cone Carborundum stone. Care should be taken not to touch the centric stops themselves. The results should be checked digitally to make sure that no teeth are jarred when the patient taps.

STEP **3.** *Establish group function in straight protrusion.*

Before protrusive pathways can be established, the precise location of each incisal edge must be determined. Since there are so many factors that determine the incisal edge position, this is discussed in separate detail in Chapters 17 and 18. For simplicity's sake now, let us assume that all the aspects of lip support, phonetics, and esthetics that dictate incisal edge position are correct. If so, all we need to do is selectively grind from the centric and "long centric" stops forward to the incisal edges. In most cases the four incisors fall right into group function as individual tooth interferences are reduced (Fig. 16-11). All reductions should be done on the upper teeth. Interferences are marked by sliding forward on marking ribbon from centric to end-to-end. If one tooth marks by itself, the marked area is hollow ground until the second tooth shares the load and on until all four incisors have continuous contact forward.

With patients who have a regular to deep overbite the protrusive pathways are almost always concave. However, as the amount of overbite lessens, the pathway becomes progressively straighter. Near end-to-end relationships produce nearly straight line protrusion. By maintaining incisal edge positions and being careful not to destroy centric or "long centric" contacts, we can work out the protrusive pathways with amazing simplicity for a variety of arch relationship problems. Patients with very large central and small lateral teeth may have to be content with protrusive group function on the central incisors only. If the central incisors are not strong enough to carry the load, it would be better to splint them to other teeth than it would be to give the lateral incisors a bizarre shape to bring them into func-

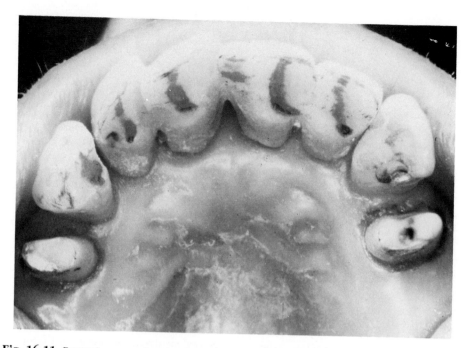

Fig. 16-11. Protrusive group function from centric relation to incisal edge. The incisal edge was established in temporary restorations first according to esthetic and phonetic requirements.

tion. Protrusive pathways should always be checked digitally. It is easy for an interfering, hypermobile tooth to move slightly and allow other teeth to mark evenly. If an individual tooth is displaced by protrusive movements, the tooth is simply held in place with the finger and remarked. It is adjusted by selective grinding until it is no longer moved.

If all incisors are stressed to movement, even with good group function, the incisal edge position should be reevaluated. It may be too far lingually. If it is necessary to shorten the upper incisors or move the incisal edges labially to flatten the protrusive guidance, the patient should test the changes under function before accepting them as final. If the hypermobility results from loss of bone support, splinting should be considered. At the completion of the protrusive movement, the incisal edges of the lower central incisors should meet the incisal edges of the upper centrals. If the lateral incisors can also meet edge to edge, so much the better, but it is not always possible without ruining the esthetics.

STEP 4. *Establish ideal anterior stress distribution in lateral excursions.*

It is wrong to think that *every* mouth should have anterior group function in lateral excur-

sions. It is just as big a fallacy as giving every mouth cuspid protection. Some dentitions function well and maintain excellent stability with only the cuspids carrying all lateral excursions, and there is no reason to change such an occlusion. However, if the cuspid is showing signs of hypermobility, accelerated wear, or loss of periodontal support, both stress and wear can be diminished when the cuspid is brought into group function with other anterior teeth. Although it is often advantageous to change a cuspid-protected occlusion to anterior group function, there appears to be no sound reason for changing anterior group function to cuspid protection.

Since we do not know for sure what the resistance level is in a deteriorating mouth, the safest approach is to minimize stresses as much as practical. Group function of the anterior teeth accomplishes this, and if the teeth in group function are also in harmony with the envelope of function and if their inclines have been adjusted according to the quality of periodontal support, the lateral anterior guidance can be said to be customized to produce minimal stress.

The procedure for customizing the lateral anterior guidance starts with closing the man-

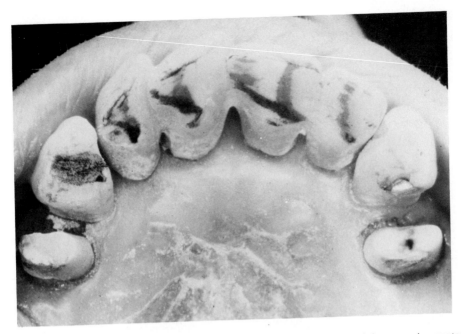

Fig. 16-12. Group function in lateral excursion. Notice how the direction of the excursive contact changes from the cuspid to a more forward path on the central incisors.

dible into centric contact. With firm help from the operator, the patient is asked to slide the jaw laterally and any movement of any teeth is noted. The excursion is repeated with marking ribbon interposed between the teeth and the marked lateral contacts selectively ground until there is continuous contact from centric to the incisal edge of the upper cuspid. In some mouths this will bring the lateral and central teeth into contact (Fig. 16-12), but it may not be sufficient to stop individual teeth from being moved by the stresses.

To reduce the lateral stress on any tooth or teeth, the contacting surfaces must be flattened from centric contact laterally. However, it is not necessary to extend the flat surface all the way through the teeth. The cuspid is the key tooth in lateral excursions, and as the jaw moves laterally on a fairly flat plane, teeth in front of the cuspid begin to share more of the load. This permits the lateral lingual inclines to be *gradually* steepened, forming a concave pathway. The downward excursion of the balancing condyle also contributes to a tendency for a natural opening movement as the jaw moves laterally to form a concave over-and-down pathway of the lower front teeth.

Just as in protrusive excursions, the ten-

dency toward concave inclines lessens as the amount of overbite decreases. However, it is not uncommon to have fairly straight lateral inclines that are compatible with concave protrusive inclines. For best esthetics, protrusive inclines are almost always steeper than lateral inclines.

In working out the lateral inclines we reach a point when the lower anterior teeth seem to function *smoothly* against the upper inclines. The patient may volunteer that the teeth feel good. Stressful movement of the teeth has been minimized or eliminated when the jaw moves laterally. There are no hangups. Esthetics is good, and there is fairly even symmetry to right and left inclines. Now the inescapable need for clinical judgment enters the picture. Do we accept what we have worked out or do we adjust further? If in doubt, the patient should try it for a few days and see whether he can find fault with any aspect of the anterior teeth. Any dentist who understands the importance of the anterior teeth to the success of the entire restorative case will be willing to make sure that all aspects of anterior guidance are correct before proceeding. Once the dentist and the patient have accepted the anterior relationship as correct, we are ready to capture that relationship so that it cannot be lost. We must duplicate it carefully. There are a number of ways of accomplishing this. Making a *customized anterior guide table* is a most effective yet simple method of transferring the guidance pathways to an instrument. It can be used with any instrument that has an anterior guide table.

CUSTOMIZED ANTERIOR GUIDE TABLE

The customized anterior guide table is only needed when anterior teeth are being restored. If anterior teeth are not being restored, the teeth themselves (on the casts) act to guide the front end of the articulator when the posterior teeth are being fabricated.

If both the anterior and the posterior teeth are to be completely fabricated on a fully adjustable articulator, the condylar guidances must all be set before the custom guide table is made. An articulator that is correctly programmed in this manner gives a reliable duplication of mandibular excursions because when both the front and the back guidances are correct, the casts can be made to duplicate mandibular border movements.

If the border movements of the posterior teeth are to be recorded *directly* through functionally generated path techniques, there is rarely a need to precisely duplicate condyle pathways on the instrument. The *result* of condylar pathways will be captured three dimensionally by the functionally generated path technique at the site of the teeth themselves, rather than by recording condyle movements and then interpolating tooth movement from the condyle paths. Either technique can be used effectively and with great accuracy.

If the posterior teeth are to be fabricated later on a semiadjustable articulator or if functionally generated path techniques are to be used later for fabrication of the posterior teeth, the customized anterior guide table can be fabricated with arbitrarily set condyle paths. A setting of 20 degrees horizontal and 15 degrees lateral will ensure posterior disclusion with even a flat anterior guidance. Unless there has been severe remodeling of the condyle and eminence to flatten the condylar path, the arbitrary settings will result in posterior disclusion because healthy joints will almost always be found to be steeper, thus posterior occlusions that relate to a correct anterior guidance will

automatically disclude in excursions if the condylar paths in the patient are steeper than those on the articulator.

If a preliminary test of the patient's protrusive function shows separation of the anterior teeth by the posterior teeth, that is a signal to note the condylar path as well as the occlusal plane. If a problem is found in either the occlusal plane or the condylar path so that anterior teeth are discluded in protrusion, it may be necessary to record the condylar path. Regardless of the method used (that is, checkbite, pantograph, or stereograph), casts must be mounted on the articulator with a facebow, and the condylar paths must be set *before* the customized anterior guide table is fabricated.

Condylar settings cannot be changed after the customized anterior guidance is completed.

Fabricating the customized anterior guide table

1. The anterior guidance must first be determined in the mouth. Determination should include the precise location of each upper and lower incisal edge, as well as all excursive pathways from centric relation to an edge-to-edge relationship in both protrusive and lateral jaw positions. Labial contours should also be finalized. If there is a question about whether the anterior relationships are acceptable, the patient should be allowed to try out the reshaped anteriors or the provisional restorations to see if any modifications are needed before impressions are made.

After the anterior relationship, including the anterior guidance is accepted by the patient, upper and lower impressions should be made.

2. Using indentations in the bite record, of posterior teeth only, a centric relation bite record is taken. If the posterior teeth have been prepared, the interocclusal record can be made at the exact correct vertical with the front teeth contacting. A facebow record should also be taken. If posterior teeth do not require restorations, the centric relation record should be made at a slightly opened vertical and then closed back to contact on the articulator. Equilibration should be completed before this step (Fig. 16-13).

3. After the centric relation bite record is taken, preparation of the anterior teeth can begin. If changes are necessary in incisal edge po-

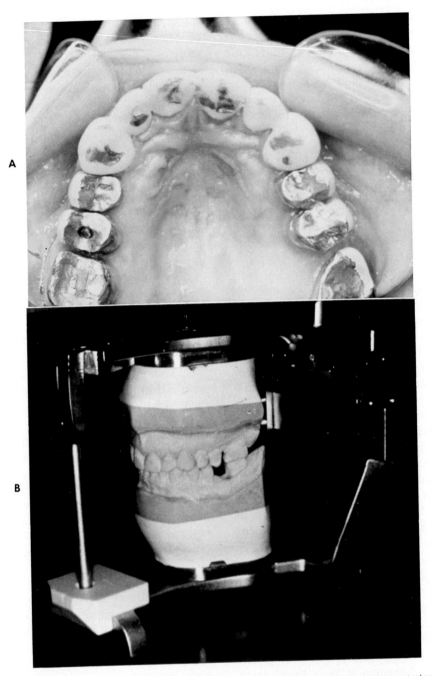

Fig. 16-13. A, Provisional restorations have been harmonized to the patient's correct anterior guidance. **B,** Casts of the corrected provisional restorations are mounted in centric relation.

sition or other modifications of contour are needed, it is better to prepare the teeth first so that changes can be made in provisional restorations. If provisional restorations are used to finalize anterior contours, the master impression of the prepared teeth can be made before the anterior provisional restorations are placed, and then an impression of the corrected provisionals can be made after their acceptability has been confirmed. It is from the cast of the anterior teeth or the cast of the corrected anterior provisional restorations in place that the anterior guide table will be fabricated.

To simplify the above:

a. If the anterior restorations are to copy the patient's teeth without changes, the impression for fabricating the custom anterior guide is made before the anterior teeth are prepared.

b. If changes in incisal edge position or tooth contour are desired, the changes should be made in provisional restorations. The custom anterior guide is fabricated from a cast of those corrected provision restorations in place.

c. Regardless of which method is used, a verified centric relation bite record is taken on the posterior teeth only, so that both the cast of the prepared anterior teeth and the cast of the correct anterior contours can be mounted interchangeably.

d. A facebow mounting is essential.

e. Either the centric bite record should be made at the correct vertical or the casts should be closed to the correct vertical before the customized guide table is fabricated.

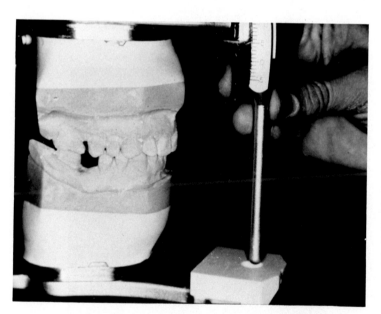

Fig. 16-14

4. With the casts of corrected anterior teeth in place on the articulator, a flat plastic guide table is placed, and the incisal guide pin is raised about 1 mm (Fig. 16-14). If the articulator in use does not have interchangeable plastic guide tables, the mechanical anterior guide table should be flattened to 0 degrees. A self-centering guide pin is essential.

5. Self-curing acrylic resin is mixed and placed on the guide table (Fig. 16-15). The plastic table is first dampened with monomer so that the acrylic will bond.

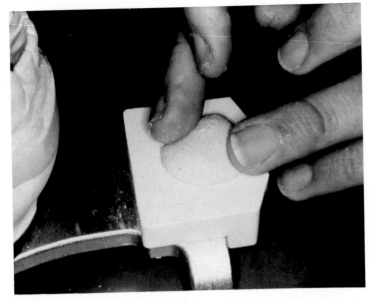

Fig. 16-15

The articulator is closed. When the anterior teeth are in centric contact, the guide pin should indent about 3 mm into the acrylic dough (Fig. 16-16).

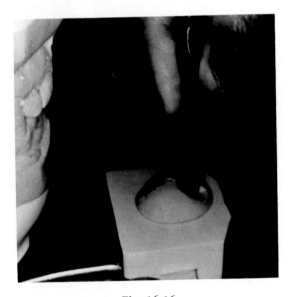

Fig. 16-16

6. The upper cast should then be moved back so that the anterior teeth slide over the lower incisal edges moving the guide pin through the acrylic dough along a similar path. The movement of the upper bow of the articulator should stop at the exact point at which the upper and lower labial surfaces are aligned and the incisal edges are in contact (Fig. 16-17).

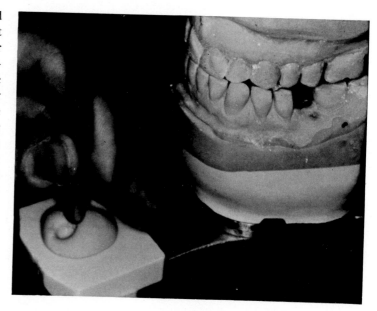

Fig. 16-17

7. The articulator should then be moved laterally in both directions, stopping exactly at the point of alignment of the labial surfaces of the upper and lower cuspids. This should result in a definite stop built into the custom guide table that relates to the labial-to-labial alignment of upper and lower teeth in protrusive and lateral excursions (Fig. 16-18).

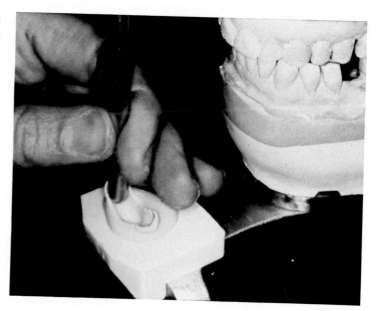

Fig. 16-18

8. The articulator is then moved into edge-to-edge relationships in all intermediate protrusive lateral excursions between the straight protrusive and the lateral border movements. This guides the pin to form similar pathways in the acrylic dough that represent the complete functional range for the anterior guidance. The acrylic is then allowed to harden (Fig. 16-19).

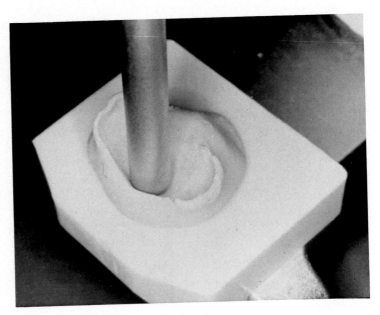

Fig. 16-19

A customized anterior guide table formed in this manner is in precise harmony with the guiding lingual inclines of the upper anterior teeth. As long as the condylar pathways are not changed, the anterior guide pin, sliding on the custom guidance inclines, will produce the same movements of the upper bow of the articulator whether the casts are on it or not. If the cast of the *prepared* teeth is mounted with the same centric relation record that was used to mount the cast of the correctly harmonized anterior teeth, its pathways will be identical.

One may be concerned that failure to precisely duplicate the patient's condylar paths on the articulator will create an error in the paths of movement of the anterior teeth on the casts. It is true that there could be minute discrepancies in the *direction* of the pathways around the vertical axes, but this will not produce an error on the lingual inclines of the upper anterior teeth. As long as the custom guide table is formed from guiding contact on all parts of the upper lingual surfaces, the guide table will dictate duplication of those surfaces. If the mandible needs to follow slightly different paths across those surfaces, it will be free to do so with preciseness and without interference.

When the customized guide table is completed, it is always wise to check it for accuracy. One can do this easily by observing if the pin maintains contact against the acrylic resin through complete excursions in all directions without losing contact of the lower teeth to the upper on the casts. Any loss of contact either between the teeth on the casts or between the pin and the acrylic indicates an erroneous anterior guide table. Such errors can be corrected by adjustment of the guide table by selective grinding on the acrylic resin where it separates the casts, or by adding acrylic resin where there is separation of the pin. Where there are gross errors, it may be easier to hollow out the guide table slightly and then repeat the excursive movements with a wash of freshly mixed acrylic resin in the relieved part of the guide table.

Fabrication of the customized guide table is not difficult, but it does require careful attention to make sure it is accurate when completed. Small errors in anterior guidance can ruin an otherwise successful restorative result. When done carefully, this procedure ensures accuracy of all excursive movements on the finished restorations.

Use of the customized anterior guide table is one of the most reliable and practical procedures we can use in restorative dentistry. It is only logical however if the anterior guidance that is being duplicated is correct in the mouth.

17

Restoring lower anterior teeth

The arrangement of the entire occlusal scheme starts with the lower anterior teeth. Just as the erupting lower incisors are guided into position by the tongue and lips before the upper anterior teeth erupt, so too must lower incisal edge position be determined before the position and contour of the upper anterior teeth can be finalized.

Determining the correct position for lower anterior teeth is one of the most important decisions we must make in planning restorative treatment. The position of the lower incisors is also recognized as the first priority in orthodontic diagnosis and treatment planning. Occlusal stability, esthetics, and space available in the mandibular arch all depend on correct positioning of the lower anterior segment. Many of the failures we see in orthodontics and restorative dentistry could have been avoided with even slight modifications in position or contour of the incisal edges of the lower anterior teeth.

There are five important goals in occlusal treatment that depend on correct position and contour of the lower incisal edges, as follows:

1. *Esthetics.* During speaking, the most visible part of the dentition is the incisal half of the lower anterior teeth (Fig. 17-1); also correct positioning of the upper anterior teeth depends on correct lower incisal edge placement.

2. *Phonetics.* The spacial relationships between the lower incisal edges and the opposing tooth surfaces are critical to the formation of various sound patterns. Their relationship to the tongue and lips also affects phonetic formations.

3. *The occlusal plane.* The lower incisal plane is the starting point in front for the occlusal plane. An incorrect incisal plane on the lower jaw may require compensations to be made in all other occlusal segments including the upper anterior teeth.

4. *The anterior guidance.* The lingual surfaces of the upper anterior teeth are determined by how the mandible, in function, moves the lower incisal edges. If the lower edges are incorrectly positioned or contoured, the position or contour of the upper anterior teeth must be compromised.

5. *Stability.* Long-term stability depends on harmony between the teeth and the structures that relate to them in function. If the teeth interfere with anatomic or functional harmony of those structures, the adaptive process will attempt to correct the imbalance. The result will be either loosening of teeth, excessive wear, or tooth migration.

Analysis of lower anterior teeth. The correctness of the lower anterior segment can

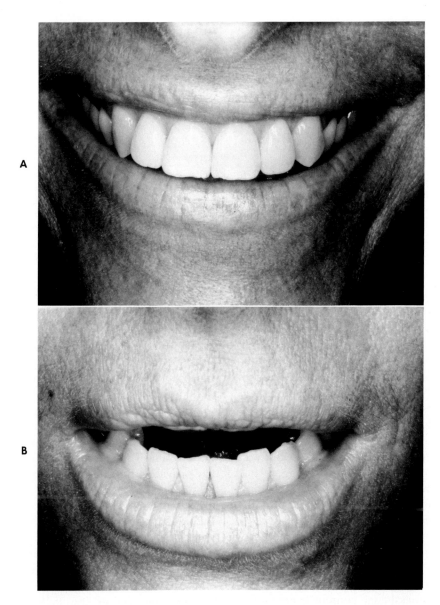

Fig. 17-1. A, When one is smiling, the lower anterior teeth are normally covered by the lower lip, which ideally relates to the incisal edges of the upper teeth (the smile line). **B,** Same patient, when speaking, shows the lower incisal edges prominently. The lower incisors are more in view than the upper anterior teeth during speech.

be analyzed from several different perspectives. If the teeth are stable, function comfortably, and are esthetically acceptable to the patient, there would rarely be a need to change them. If there are signs of instability, evidenced by excessive wear, hypermobility, or tooth migration, or if functional or esthetic problems are present, changes in tooth position or contour may be required. Likewise, if teeth are missing or improperly restored, so that positional landmarks have been lost, the correct relationship can be determined if a se-

quential approach is used in analysis. Some determinations must be made in a certain order. As an example, it is difficult to finalize incisal edge contours until after incisal edge position is determined. Incisal edge position cannot be refined until an acceptable incisal plane determines the height of each incisal edge.

Analysis to determine the best esthetics may seem unrelated to occlusion, but every contour has a purpose that is related to function. Thus it is almost always so, that the better the esthetics, the better the function will be, and

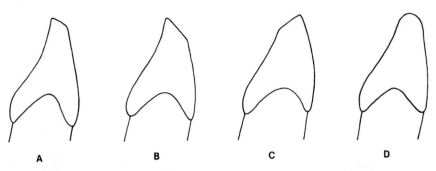

Fig. 17-2. Various contours of lower incisal edges from a lateral view. **A,** Correct lingual line angle is higher than labio-incisal line angle. **B,** Labio-incisal line angle is too low and angle of incisal edge is too high for stability as a holding stop. **C,** Lingual line angle is too low. Results in poor esthetics and problems with excursive function. **D,** Rounded edges. This is the worst esthetic contour and is not an acceptable holding contact.

vice versa. It is also important to the patient that occlusal therapy should not destroy the appearance of a natural smile. For that reason, esthetically correct contour should always be a goal along with the determination of what is functionally correct. Since the incisal edges are the most visible part of the lower teeth when speaking, I will start the analysis there.

Analyzing incisal edge outline. Except in very young patients, the incisal edges have lost any remnant of the mammelons and are flattened across the entire incisal edge. This produces definite line angles that clearly outline the incisal edge. When lower anterior teeth are being restored, a common mistake is to round the edges, instead of preserving the line angles. This not only creates a very artificial appearance but also affects the stability of the centric holding contacts with the upper teeth. Proper incisal edge contour is necessary for optimum occlusal stability. It can be analyzed from two perspectives: a lateral view and an incisal view.

From a lateral veiwpoint, the line angles should form a definite outline. The linguoincisal line angle should be slightly higher than the labioincisal line. This exposes the lingual outline of the incisal edge from a front view, which is important for a natural appearance. The angled incisal edge relates to the contour of the upper lingual surface it contacts. In a healthy dentition, upper lingual surfaces dictate an angled lower incisal edge with the lingual side being higher (Fig. 17-2, *A*).

If the upper lingual surfaces are restored improperly with too much convexity, the result is a lower incisal edge that wears to a steep angle (Fig. 17-2, *B*). This can eliminate the im-

portant labioincisal line angle, which provides stability to the centric stop. It is rarely stable and generally always leads to progressive wear of the labial line angle. It is also unesthetic. Correction of the problem requires altering the shape of the upper lingual surface as well as the lower incisal edges (Fig. 17-3).

If the lingual line angle is too low (Fig. 17-2, *C*), the natural view of normal incisal edges is distorted, and so it creates an unacceptable esthetic result. The sharp labioincisal line angle may provide a definite holding contact in centric relation but often fails to function properly in excursive movements.

Rounded incisal edges (Fig. 17-2, *D*) are neither esthetic nor stable. Many porcelain restorations are made with too much roundness because porcelain naturally rounds off when it is fired. It may be necessary for the technician to grind and polish the incisal portion to achieve the ideal contour. Line angles should be slightly polished to modify very sharp edges, but the appearance of line angles should not be lost (Fig. 17-4).

From an incisal viewpoint, since the incisal edge is clearly defined by line angles that form a line around the edge of a fairly flat surface, analyzing or correcting that shape can be easily accomplished. The definite line angles that outline the incisal edges are maintained even as the teeth are severely worn. As teeth wear, the shape of the incisal edges becomes thicker and rounder (Fig. 17-5). If you wish to make severely worn teeth appear younger and more attractive, you must remove enough labial and lingual tooth structure to make the incisal edges thinner and less convex. When severe wear has caused the incisal edges to become

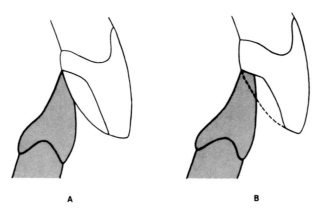

Fig. 17-3. Convex upper lingual contour results in steep angle of lower edge, **A.** Correction requires alteration of upper contour and reshaping of lower incisal edge to provide a stable stop, **B.**

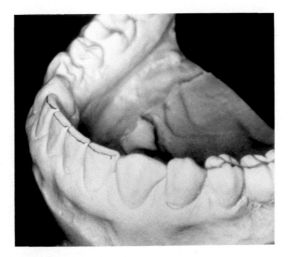

Fig. 17-4. Lower anterior restorations should be made with definite labioincisal line angle. Care must be taken to prevent edges from rounding off too much during firing of porcelain.

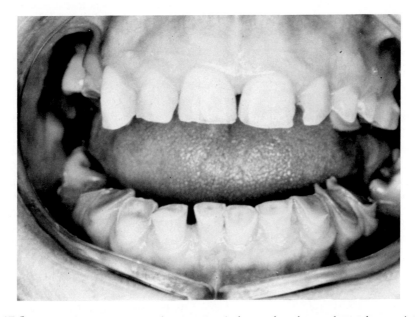

Fig. 17-5. Wear on lower incisors produces progressively rounder edges as the tooth wears into the thicker cingulum area.

too thick and too round, or too slanted, it will usually be necessary to alter the shape of the upper lingual contour so that the lower incisal edge can be reshaped to provide a more natural contour. The following illustrates the changes that occur as the teeth wear:

In a young person, notice that definite line angles outline the incisal edge. The lingual contour is slightly concave. The labial contour is quite flat.

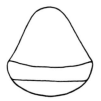

As wear occurs, the incisal edge moves down to the thicker part of the tooth. The lingual concavity changes to straight contour. The flat labial contour starts to develop a convex curve as wear progresses down onto the more convex part of the tooth on the labial surface.

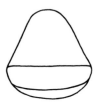

As more wear continues, both labial and lingual contours become more convex. The incisal edge becomes thicker and dentin color starts to show. At this stage the upper anterior teeth have also started to adapt to the changing shape of the lower incisal edges.

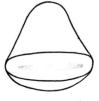

When wear progresses into the thicker part of the tooth, the incisal edge becomes more and more round. The dentin loses its enamel protection and starts to cup, permitting the wear to accelerate. Gross changes will be noticed on the opposing upper teeth, and there is a tendency for the anterior teeth to migrate into a more edge-to-edge relationship as they wear.

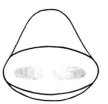

RELATING THE INCISAL PLANE

The lower incisal edges, when viewed together, form the incisal plane. The relationship of this plane is critical to esthetics because there is almost nothing that can detract from the appearance of the teeth as much as a slanted incisal plane. As is so often the case, the same factors that affect esthetics also affect function, and in regard to the incisal plane, this is particularly so, because the relationship of the plane, including its contour, is as important to phonetics as it is to esthetics.

In making *s* sounds, the flow of air must be constricted into a flat, wide band between the hard surfaces of the lower and upper teeth. Because the air must be constricted rather uniformly for the width of the incisal plane, the lower incisal edges must relate to the upper teeth with near contact at the jaw relationship that is used for the *s* sound. That position may vary from near contact against the upper lingual surfaces in some patients to near edge-to-edge contact in others. If the *s* sound is made at an overlap position, the lower incisal plane is more likely to have a convex bow to its contour so that it can fit the concavity of the upper lingual surfaces (Fig. 17-6). If the *s* sound is made at the edge-to-edge position, the lower incisal plane is more likely to be flatter (Fig. 17-7).

As a general rule, the more convex the incisal plane is on the upper teeth, the more

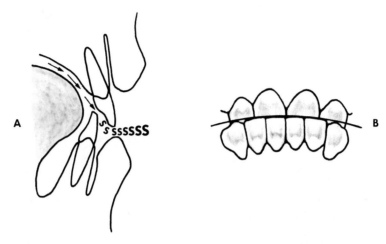

Fig. 17-6. Relation of anterior teeth during *s* sound when made at an overlapping position, **A**. Over-lapped relationship is used whenever there is a convex upper smile line because only a lower convex smile line will provide near contact on the full width of the incisors against the concave lingual contour, **B**.

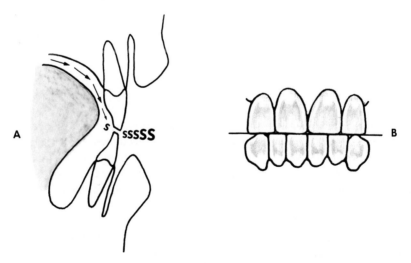

Fig. 17-7. The *s* sound is routinely made at the end-to-end relationship, **A**, by patients who have a flat incisal plane because the flat plane permits uniform proximity of the hard surfaces across the full width of the incisal edges, **B**. This wide flat band of air is necessary for producing a clear, crisp *s* sound.

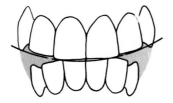

Fig. 17-8. Convex upper and lower incisal planes cannot make a clear *s* sound at the end-to-end position because air leaks out at the sides. A broad band of air is necessary for a clear *s* sound.

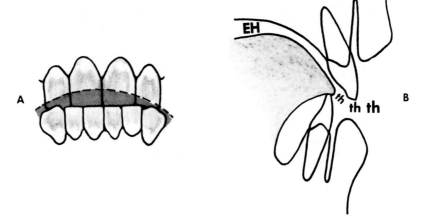

Fig. 17-9. If a convex lower incisal plane is flattened, it will no longer relate correctly to the concave upper lingual contour, **A**. This will create an open area in the center and destroys the relationship required for a clear *s* sound. To compensate, the patient must fill the space with the tongue, **B**, but this results in a lisp and produces a typical *eth* sound. This is a common mistake that is made because of an erroneous belief that all incisal edges must contact edge-to-edge during the protrusive position.

convex it will be on the lower teeth. The reason for that relationship is apparent if one understands the necessity of a wide, flat flow of air to make the sharp *s* sound. A convex upper incisal plane cannot fit end to end with a convex or flat plane on the lower teeth without leaking air out the sides (Fig. 17-8). Thus the *s* sound is necessarily made with the upper teeth overlapping the lower teeth so that the lower edges can evenly approximate the concavity of the lingual arch form.

If a patient with convex incisal planes is accustomed to making *s* sounds with an overlapped anterior relationship, altering the lower incisal plane can create a significant problem with speech. If a naturally convex lower incisal plane is mistakenly flattened, it will no longer fit the concave lingual arch form and the air will be funneled into an open area in the cen-

ter, rather than maintained as the flat band that is required for a crisp clear *s* sound (Fig. 17-9).

If the lower incisal plane is made concave to fit the convex upper plane in protrusive relation, the patient will be able to make a clear *s* sound by protruding the mandible to the edge-to-edge position. But such mandibular movements are not normal for patients who are used to speaking with less horizontal motion of the jaw, and they will routinely complain of tiredness or strain when they talk a lot. In addition, the natural harmony of the lower incisal edges is lost, and the esthetic result is often severely compromised.

It is a common but very erroneous belief that all upper and lower incisors must be in contact throughout the entire protrusive range and that all four incisors should meet edge to edge at the end of the protrusive path. If the

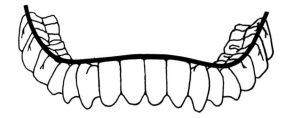

Fig. 17-10. An ideal incisal plane forms a continuous gentle curve with the posterior occlusal curve of Spee.

upper and lower anterior teeth are in harmony with the functional movements of the mandible, there is no tendency to overload them whether there be two teeth or four teeth in protrusive contact with the opposing arch. With very convex upper incisal planes it would be unusual to have more teeth in edge-to-edge contact than the central incisors in the maxillary arch and the four incisors in the lower arch. It is not unusual for the lower lateral incisors to also be discluded.

If the lower incisal plane does not closely approximate the contour of the upper arch during the *s* sound, another common problem of speech may also be caused. *Lisping* is the result of using the tongue to fill in the void so that the air can be squeezed into the flattened band that is necessary for making a crisp *s* sound. There is a characteristic difference however between the *eth* sound made with the soft tongue surface versus the clear *ess* sound that comes from approximation of hard tooth surfaces.

If the lower incisal plane relates to the upper arch form in a manner that produces a small roundish opening instead of the uniform space across the width of the incisors, the result is a whistle.

Remember that the organ of mastication is also a critical component of the organ of speech. The masticatory system was designed to be compatible with both functions. By using phonetics as a guide for functional relationships we will rarely find that it is inconsistent with either masticatory function or esthetics.

Analyzing height of the lower incisal edges

In ideal instances the lower incisal edges form a continuous gentle curve that is an extension of the posterior occlusal plane (Fig. 17-10). There should be no sudden variation in height between the incisal edges and the posterior cusp tips. As wear occurs, there is a tendency for the plane to become flatter, but

there should still be no sudden changes in height.

If the incisal plane is greatly higher than the posterior occlusal plane, that is an indication of elongation of the anterior segment, almost always the result of no stable holding contacts on the anterior teeth. When the lower incisors erupt, they do not erupt out of the alveolar bone. Rather the alveolar process itself elongates, moving the teeth vertically until a stable stop is met. That stop preferably is the opposing tooth, but it also may be the tongue or the lip. The absence of any stop allows the lower anteriors to erupt all the way to the palatal tissue, creating an incisal plane that is at a different level from the posterior plane of occlusion.

The critical element in determining the height of the lower incisal edges will in most instances be the relationship with the upper anterior teeth. It is often necessary to reshape or reposition the upper anterior teeth to get an acceptable position and contour of the lower incisors. This working out of both the upper and lower anterior teeth relationship is the first step in solving most of the complex problems of occlusal malrelationships. The goal is to establish stable holding contacts for the lower incisors at an esthetically acceptable height.

Relating lower incisal edges to the lips

Every patient does not look like the ideal norm in the textbook, so trying to adapt every patient's dentition to the average can result in some very unacceptable results. There is merit however in knowing what the norms are because they serve as basic guidelines toward which treatment can be directed.

There are three norms by which we can relate the height of the incisal edges to the lips. If we analyze a large number of attractive dentitions, we find a consistency in the amount of lower anterior tooth surface that is exposed during certain lip relationships, as listed in the following:

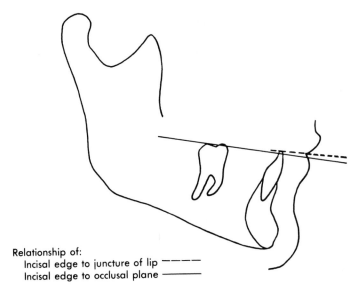

Relationship of:
   Incisal edge to juncture of lip – – – –
   Incisal edge to occlusal plane ————

Fig. 17-11

1. *Lips sealed.* The lower incisal edge is at the height of the juncture of the upper and lower lips when the teeth are together. On a lateral cephalometric radiograph this usually positions the incisal edge slightly above the functional occlusal plane (Fig. 17-11). If the lower incisal edges are much below that juncture, there is a tendency for the upper anterior teeth to be positioned too low, producing a gummy smile.

2. *Lips slightly parted, jaw at rest.* At this position, the upper lip completely covers the maxillary teeth while the lower lip droops down to expose approximately one half of the labial surface of the mandibular incisors (Fig. 17-12). The lower teeth are in the shadow of the lips and so are not prominently displayed when the jaw is at rest.

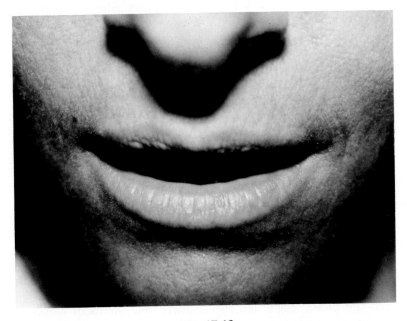

Fig. 17-12

3. *Relation to lips during speech.* During speech, the lower anterior teeth are in view and the upper teeth are generally covered. Exposure of the lower teeth varies with the different lip positions required for phonetics. Asking the patient to count from 1 to 20 is a simple exercise for observing the minimum to the maximum exposure while speaking occurs. During pronunciation of the number *four* there is almost no exposure, whereas pronunciation of the number *eight* may expose the entire labial surface of the lower anterior teeth and even show some gingival tissue (Fig. 17-13).

During smiling, the lower teeth are completely covered and the upper anterior teeth are exposed. Smiling during speech often exposes both upper and lower anterior teeth to varying degrees.

There are attractive smiles that do not fit the norms described above, and there are many situations wherein the length of the lips or other configurations simply do not permit a "normal" relationship. Common sense and clinical judgment must prevail. If the dentition is stable and function is acceptable, there is no need to alter the relationship unless the patient finds the esthetics unacceptable.

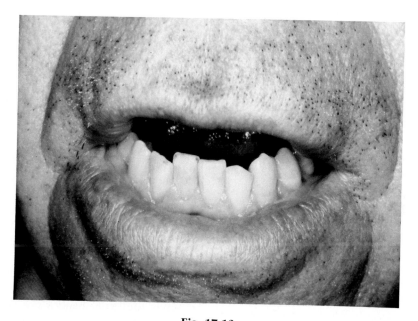

Fig. 17-13

Relating lower anterior teeth to the neutral zone

The outward pressure of the tongue and the inward pressure of the perioral musculature set the limits within which the teeth can be stable. This is the *neutral zone* between opposing forces. The contracted length of the buccinator muscles, which decusate into and become part of the orbicularis oris muscle, are, in effect, then tethered to the anterior bony base by the depressor muscles below and the elevator muscles above. Posen[1] in 1976 correlated the strength of the perioral musculature with the position of the incisors. Class II, Division 2 cases had the strongest perioral musculature, whereas bimaxillary protrusion cases had the weakest. He also observed that correction of arch form was often accompanied by more normal tonicity of the lips, thus reducing the tendency for incisor relapse. One needs to understand how the buccinator–orbicularis oris complex functions before assuming that orthodontic correction will predictably improve tonicity of the perioral musculature. Arbitrarily correcting the anterior segments to "ideal" angulations may in some patients result in failure to achieve acceptable stability. Observing the *effects* of the buccinator–orbicularis oris complex before treatment provides some clues as to which patients may be successfully treated and which ones require special attention.

Frederick[2] observed the varied effects of different perioral muscular complexes and concluded that changes in both soft and bony tissues were obviously the result of pressure resorption. Since the areas of resorption exactly matched specific bands of the buccinator muscle, it was clear that the length of the contracted buccinator muscle strictly limited the size of the arch, and if the arch was expanded beyond the acceptable length of the muscle, the pressure against the labial surfaces of the tissue overlying the roots resulted in thinning of both the bone and the soft tissues and sometimes jammed the roots against the lingual plate of bone. Clefting of the gingival margins is also a later consequence in some patients. The degree of soft-tissue damage and bony resorption varies as the severity of the abnormal pressure differs from the healthy norm.

Just as the contracted length of the elevator muscles determines the *vertical* size of the alveolar processes, the *horizontal* size of the alveolar processes is determined by the contracted lengh of the three bands of the buccinator muscle. The three bands of the buccinator muscle can vary in strength and length and may effect either arch or both. Often the effects are seen primarily on the lower arch, with the deformity being the greatest at the anterior segment.

In the lower anterior area, the effect of pressure varies according to where the lower band overlays the anterior segment.

The tissues that compose the zone of attached gingiva lie under the weaker middle band of the buccinator. That zone of bound-down gingiva extends down to the top of the stronger lower band of muscle that forms an indented line of resorbed bone covered from that line down by loose tissue that is not bound to the underlying bone. The more excessive the muscle pressure is from the contraction of the lower band, the thinner the tissue will be over the roots. If the lower band of the buccinator is of a shorter length than the bone base needs, the entire alveolar process may be moved lingually off its normal relationship to the basal bone.

Since the upper margin of the lower band of the buccinator determines where the zone of attached gingiva stops, examination of that area can be helpful in determination of both the position of the lower band and its strength of contraction. In the lower anterior area, the lower band can be classified as "high-middle-low." Frederick has described the effects of each position, as follows.

When the lower band is positioned high on the labial, the result is featheredging of the soft tissues and thinning of the labial bone. This is often associated with gingival recession and sometimes gingival clefts.

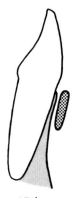

High

When the lower band is positioned at the middle, the bound-down portion of attached gingiva is normal, but it is greatly reduced in dimension. The line of demarcation where the loose tissue starts is higher than normal.

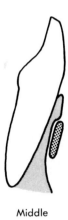

Middle

The low band is the condition seen most often. There is usually 3 to 4 mm of attached gingiva present and then the line of demarcation is usually very definite at the start of the un–bound down tissue.

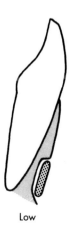

Low

The determination of height and pressure from the lower band of the buccinator muscle is mostly achieved by observation of the position and contour of the line of demarcation between bound down and loose tissues. But there is another condition that may also be seen in some patients when the line of demarcation is rather obscure and is located within a

flattened facet across the lower anterior area between the attached and detached tissue. This occurs when the fibers of the mentalis muscle extend up under the middle band of the buccinator where they are in turn pressed against the labial surfaces of the dentition. Pressure from the middle band is not of sufficient strength to cause detachment of the bound-down gingiva but is strong enough to cause some deleterious effects, and so it does not appear as normal, healthy attached gingiva.

The effect of the mentalis muscle on the lower anterior segment can be substantial, but its role is often misunderstood. The mentalis muscle is considered by some to be the most important cause of lower labial deformity, but the mentalis cannot of itself apply pressure against the bone from which it originates. Its purpose is to raise the skin over the chin, but its location under the buccinator band positions it just like a pressure bandage when the buccinator contracts. If the mentalis is hyperactive, its dimensions increase in thickness when contracted. This increased thickness under the contracting buccinator–orbicularis oris complex intensifies the pressure against the teeth and their supporting structure (Fig. 17-14).

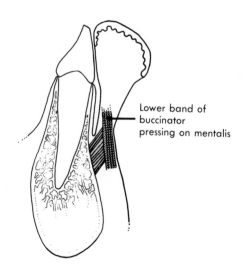

Lower band of buccinator pressing on mentalis

Fig. 17-14. A strong lower band of the buccinator muscle overlaps the mentalis muscle and compresses it against the root surfaces.

Detection of neutral zone problems for lower anterior teeth

If a neutral zone problem exists, it can be detected by the following:

1. Observing the condition of the alveolar process on the labial surface and noting its contour. If there are severe and sudden contour changes underlying the lower buccinator band or the bone over the roots is abnormally thin, suspect a very restrictive perioral musculature.

2. Observing the height and contour of the line of demarcation between the attached and unattached tissues on the labial surfaces. The top of the lower buccinator band starts at that line.

3. Observing the angulation of the anterior teeth (Fig. 17-15). From this, one can get a reasonable appraisal of the varying strengths of the different bands of the buccinator. Very vertical, or lingually inclined anterior teeth indicate a strong influence from the perioral musculature.

   The presence of root tips forced against the lingual plate with incisal edges forward indicates a strong lower band in a low position combined with active pressure from the tongue.

4. Observing facial contour in profile. A deep cleft over a button chin indicates a restriction of the neutral zone by a strong buccinator-mentalis combination. The lower lip is often folded up behind the upper anterior teeth, forcing the lower anterior teeth even more lingually. The upper teeth may be pushed forward into an excessive overjet position (Fig. 17-16).

5. Palpation of the dental alveolus. By use of thumb and finger palpation of the labial and lingual surfaces, the thickness of the bone can be noted at the level of the roots. A very thin dimension indicates a tight neutral zone from strong perioral musculature combined with equally strong tongue pressure. Movement of teeth or severe contour changes by restorations have a poor prognosis for stability if this neutral zone is violated.

6. Observing the relationship of the anterior teeth to the A-Po plane. If the position of the lower teeth is too far from the norm of plus 1 mm at the incisal edge or the angulation diverges too far from 22 degrees to the A-Po plane, suspect the possibility of a neutral zone problem. The direction of the divergence indicates whether the tongue or the perioral musculature is the dominant disruptive force.
   NOTE: Divergence from accepted cephalometric norms is not in itself indicative of instability. If stable holding contacts are present, a restrictive neutral zone can actually add to the stability regardless of the divergence. However if such teeth are to be moved or restored, caution is indicated.

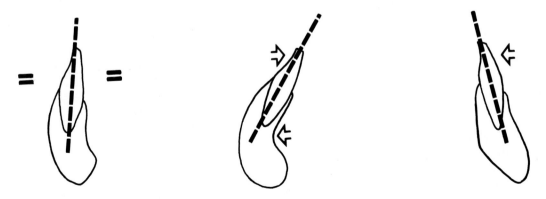

Fig. 17-15. Inclination of lower incisors is directly related to neutral zone pressures that result from the tongue and the perioral musculature. The strength and level of the bands of the buccinator muscle create varied inclinations in combination with variations of tongue pressures.

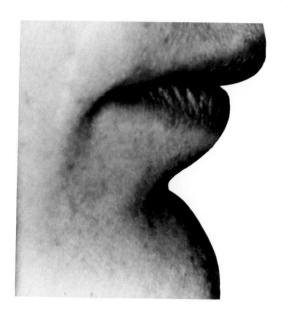

Fig. 17-16. Typical deep-cleft button chin results from strong lower band of buccinator. Protruded position of upper incisors results from lower lip being squeezed up behind them, forcing them forward.

Correction of neutral zone restriction

When the restriction of arch form is severe enough to prevent an acceptable alignment of the teeth to a stable relationship, or when the labial bone support is thinned to the point of danger to the attached gingiva, intervention is required.

A simple surgical procedure has been developed to reduce excessive perioral muscle pressure. After the pressure against the labial plate is reduced, the bone over the roots thickens and regains a more proportionate relationship to the dentition. The soft tissue also normalizes, and the zone of attached gingiva can be maintained. With the increased bone thickness and the decreased muscle pressure against it, lower incisors can then be moved anteriorly with greater assurance of long-term stability.

Surgical procedures

The procedure advocated by Frederick involves a surgical cut vertically through the lower band of the buccinator muscle just anterior to the mental foramen. This is followed at the same appointment by vestibuloplasty from the mesial of the second bicuspid around to the opposite side at the same position.

The combination of vestibuloplasty and sectioning of the muscle's lower band has the effect of reducing the muscular pressure on the arch and thus permits more expansion without relapse.

Relating lower incisor position with cephalometrics

The use of cephalometrics as a guide for positioning lower anterior teeth must be tempered with an understanding of the effect of the perioral musculature that determines the neutral zone.

Many orthodontists have observed that forward movement of lower anterior teeth too often ends with relapse back to their original position. The difficulty of treating lower anterior teeth without relapse has been the topic of many studies, and it has been generally accepted that lower incisors should preferably remain in their pretreatment position.

If proper tooth position is determined on an individual basis, lower incisors can be moved in many patients, and the result can be stable. The one place to which lower incisors cannot be moved is any position that is not harmonious with the neutral zone. There is no tooth alignment that can overcome the effect of imbalanced pressure from the musculature. Muscle always wins, but the effects of strong, arch-confining perioral musculature can be observed clinically and related to facial profile, and so those effects can be considered along with the cephalometric analysis. Tooth arrangements can often be improved within the confinement of the neutral zone, and remember, the neutral zone can often be changed if you alter the relationship of the upper teeth to

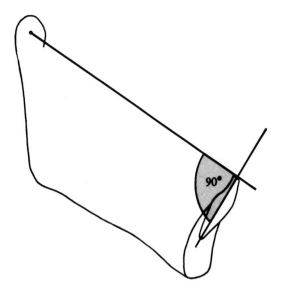

Fig. 17-17. "Norm" for inclination of lower incisors is 90 degrees to a line drawn from the incisal edge to the center of the condyle (the hinge axis angle).

the lower teeth, or through changes in arch form, or through surgery to release the confining pull of the buccinator muscle.

Unless there are contraindications directly related to neutral zone pressures, the lower incisors seem to remain stable if they are positioned at a 90-degree angulation to a line drawn from the hinge axis point to the incisal edge (Fig. 17-17). This is referred to as the *hinge axis angle.* Fuqua[3] found that cases treated to a value of near 90 degrees had a tendency to remain stable after the retention period of orthodontic treatment. This position aligns with the arc of closure and relates mechanically to the best alignment for resisting forces during penetration of food. If it is opposed by a correctly contoured contact on the upper anterior teeth, the prime vector of force at tooth contact will be favorable. At the risk of repetition, "normal" angulation values should not be the goal of treatment unless they are in harmony with the functional patterns of the soft tissues.

Ricketts[4] has advocated relating the lower incisors to the A-Po plane. This plane is a straight-line connection between the A point, which is the deepest point of the curvature of the maxilla between the anterior nasal spine and the alveolar process of the anterior teeth, and the Po point, or pogonion, which is the most anterior point on the midsagittal symphysis.

If the labial surface of the lower incisor is approximately 1 mm forward of the A-Po plane, its position is in harmony with the basal jaw relationship (Fig. 17-18). Incisor segments that appear to remain the most stable have an approximate angle of 22 degrees when related to the A-Po plane (Fig. 17-19).

In relation to cephalometric norms, using the A-Po plane is a logical choice for determining the position and inclination of the lower incisors because it relates them to both the mandible and the maxilla. The reliability of Ricketts' work regarding the relationship of the lower incisors to the A-Po plane has been confirmed, and it permits an easy and quick analysis of relative position of the lower anterior teeth.

Whether lower anterior teeth are being restored or repositioned, the incisal edge position and the axial inclination are both critical to the diagnosis and treatment planning of the entire dentition. In adults, these relationships are often disturbed by improper contour of restorations on the upper anterior teeth. When adults are being analyzed, all lingual restorations on upper anterior teeth should be evaluated as a possible causative factor for problems with lower anterior tooth position. It is not possible to correct lower anterior alignment to a point of stability if the lower incisal edges contact upper inclines that do not provide adequate holding contacts.

It is a fairly safe assumption that problems are minimal if the lower anterior teeth can be made to contact in centric relation at the correct vertical dimension. It is ideal if the contact is on the cingulum of the upper anterior teeth, but contact on any part of the upper lingual surface can usually be adapted to the requirements of good function when a stop is provided to prevent supraeruption. Even an end-to-end relationship can be made functional and stable with minor alteration. Shaping the lower incisal edge back slightly may be all that is required to provide a protrusive pathway against the upper anterior teeth.

Even a short horizontal path of the lower incisor teeth against the upper incisal edges is sufficient to disclude the posterior teeth in protrusion if the occlusal plane is correct. A flat lateral anterior guidance can disclude the balancing side because of the downward movement of the orbiting condyle, if cusp-fossae angles are coordinated.

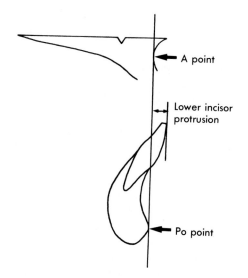

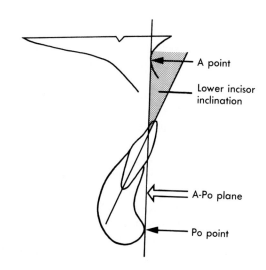

Fig. 17-18. Relation of lower incisor to A-Po line. Norm for lower incisor protrusion positions the lower incisal edge approximately 1 mm anterior to the A-Po line (±2.3 mm).

Fig. 17-19. Norm for lower incisor inclination is approximately 22 degrees from the A-Po line.

Sometimes a too steep anterior guidance can be flattened by shortening the lower anterior teeth and restoring the lingual surfaces of the upper teeth. The cingulum is brought down into contact with the shortened lower anterior teeth, making the angle flatter between centric contact and the upper incisal edge.

Any modifications of this nature should always be worked out on mounted models and the changes duplicated in the upper temporary restoration for refinement in the mouth and testing by the patient.

Crowded lower anterior teeth present a variety of problems that can be solved in a variety of ways. The first determination to make is whether the crowding is really a problem. It is not an occlusal problem if the teeth are stable and cleanable and can function without interference in the excursions. It may be an esthetic problem if the crowding is too noticeable. However, a slight irregularity of lower incisors is usually not the esthetic shortcoming that some patients may think. It is most often better to keep the slightly crowded condition than it would be to do unnecessary restorative procedures.

If crowded lower anterior teeth need to be restored for any reason, minor tooth movement can often be simplified when it is combined with the restorative procedures. If prep-

aration of the lower anteriors is going to be required anyway, the teeth can be narrowed, usually enough to allow the alignment to be perfected. If posterior teeth are to be restored also, those preparations can be completed and the orthodontic appliance for the front teeth can be incorporated into the temporary restorations on the posterior teeth. After the alignment is corrected, a temporary restoration can be used as an esthetic yet very effective retainer for a few weeks while the bone and periodontal fibers reorganize around the moved teeth.

Combining minor tooth movement with restorative preparation of lower anterior teeth makes possible a myriad of simplified and practical approaches to solving problems of irregularity or crowding. The key to solving such problems, however, is predetermination of where we want the teeth to be. We must work out the corrections on mounted models and then determine the most practical way of accomplishing it

A lower incisor that has supraerupted up above the incisal edge line of the other incisors should never be shortened back to correct alignment unless a centric stop is provided for it. If a centric stop cannot be provided, the tooth must be splinted to another tooth that does have a centric stop. Otherwise the shortened tooth will erupt right back up where it was.

Separated lower anterior teeth constitute another "problem" that should very often be left as is. Separation in itself is not an occlusal problem if the teeth are stable, maintainable, and esthetically acceptable. If the spaces must be closed for esthetics, closing the spaces should cause no problem of stability as long as the arch form is maintained. If the space to be closed is not too wide, composite bonding procedures may be effective.

If there is doubt about the esthetics, the waxed-up cast should be duplicated in stone, a heat-formed matrix should be made, and acrylic overlays reflecting the changes should be fabricated on the original cast. The plastic overlays can be tried on the patient's separated teeth in the mouth to see whether the wider teeth would look acceptable. To ensure accuracy, the dentist must be sure that the acrylic overlays are tapered all the way back to the tooth at the gingival margin. Overlapping the gingiva with the plastic overlays gives a very false picture of what the finished restorations would look like.

If the space between lower anterior teeth is too great to be widened acceptably, it may be necessary to move the teeth together orthodontically and add a fifth incisor. The extra incisor presents no esthetic problems and is hardly noticeable even with close observation.

Worn lower anterior teeth can present some difficult problems to solve if the wear has shortened the teeth to an extreme degree. The usual tendency is to assume that vertical dimension has been lost and the treatment is merely a matter of lengthening the teeth back to their original length to "restore the lost vertical." This is a dangerous assumption; such treatment is clearly contraindicated in most cases.

As teeth wear, they erupt, taking the alveolar process with them. When you see anterior teeth with excessive wear and posterior teeth with minimal wear, you observe how much higher the alveolar bone level is around the anterior teeth. Because the eruptive process keeps up with the wear, lengthening worn lower anterior teeth actually constitutes opening the bite, unless the contacting lingual surface of the upper anterior teeth is shortened commensurately. This is true if the worn teeth are in contact in centric relation.

Frequently the cause of anterior wear is a posterior interference that deviates the mandible forward into an acquired position that causes increased stress and wear on the front teeth. If the interference is eliminated, it often permits the patient to close on a more retruded arc to the same vertical dimension, with ample room provided horizontally between the upper and lower incisors. The lower anterior teeth can then be lengthened to regain centric contact and to restore the worn incisal edges.

If the lower anterior teeth are worn so short that they cannot adequately retain a restoration, it may be necessary to surgically remove some bony support from around the teeth to lengthen the clinical crown.

The problem of excessive wear on lower anterior teeth must usually be solved by restoration, and the restoration of choice is usually full coverage. If full coverage is indicated, it should be either porcelain jacket or porcelain veneer. Using acrylic resin on lower anterior teeth is absolutely contraindicated. The shape and position of the incisal edges are critical to the anterior guidance, and once precisely established, they should be maintained just as precisely. Acrylic incisal edges wear too rapidly. Worn acrylic veneers expose the underlying gold at the incisal edge, presenting a very unsightly appearance.

Onlaying worn incisal edges with gold fulfills the requirements of maintainability but certainly falls short on esthetics. It is true that some patients have no concern at all about the appearance of their teeth and for them this solution may be applicable. Normal patients do care about their appearance, however, and whether they express concern about the esthetic result, gold incisal edges are a crude departure from a normal appearance.

Not all worn lower anterior teeth need to be restored. Even if the wear has penetrated to the dentin, it may be possible to maintain the incisal edges without restoration. Lower incisors make contact at their labioincisal line angle. Even with worn edges, the contact will still be on enamel (Fig. 17-20). Correction of occlusal discrepancies to minimize wear and reduce bruxism is frequently all that is needed to slow the wear on the lower incisors to a manageable level. Depending on the age of the patient, the condition of the labio-incisal enamel, and other clinical factors, it is sometimes the most prudent treatment to leave worn incisal edges as they are.

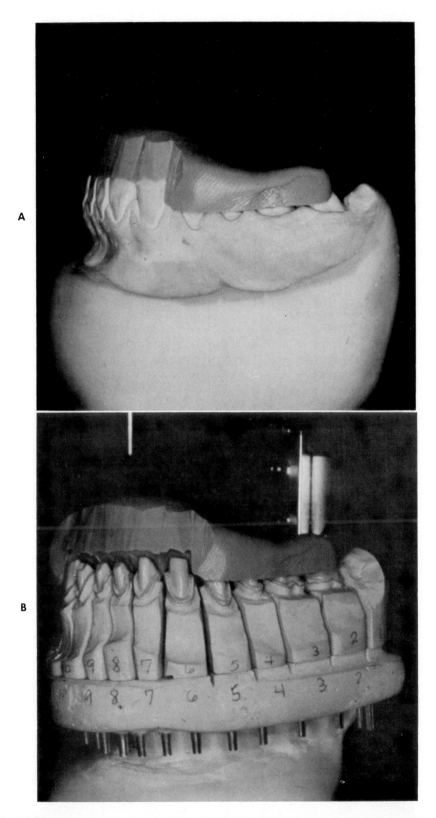

Fig. 17-20. An index, made from firm silicone putty is excellent for communicating incisal edge position. It should be adapted to the lower cast of corrected provisional restorations, **A** (or natural teeth before preparation, if no changes in contour are needed). The index is positioned on the master die model, **B.**   *Continued.*

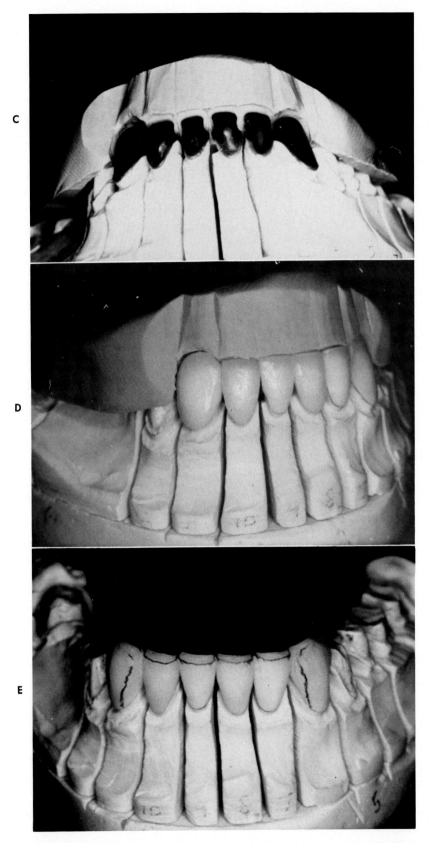

Fig. 17-20, cont'd. The index can be used as an aid in fabricating copings, **C**, so that there is room for a uniform thickness of porcelain, **D**, and it may be used for final contouring of the porcelain veneer, **E**.

If the dentin is cupped out but the enamel around it is intact, restoration of the cupped area with one of the hard filled resin materials is sometimes a logical choice of treatment. It is conservative, the esthetics is good, and it does not preclude the later use of full coverage if it becomes necessary.

Hypermobility of lower anterior teeth frequently results from occlusal stress. Occlusal correction often produces amazing results in eliminating hypermobility completely, but then so does periodontal treatment and even intensified mouth hygiene procedures. Any hypermobility should be treated as an unhealthy situation, and *all* necessary steps should be taken to correct it. If mobility patterns cannot be controlled by combined occlusal and periodontal therapy, splinting may be considered.

The decision of whether or not to splint lower anterior teeth, however, is based on different criteria of mobility from those of any other occlusal segment. Lower incisors can be maintained with a higher degree of mobility than other teeth. As long as gingival health is being maintained and the lower incisors are firm enough to function comfortably, my tendency is to avoid splinting. If restorative procedures are required on the lower incisors for other reasons and hypermobility patterns are present, it would be practical to go ahead and splint the restorations rather than having to destroy them at a later time if the need for splinting was determined.

If present restorative needs would be rendered obsolete by a later need for splinting lower incisor teeth, they should be included in the plan if they are hypermobile. Otherwise these teeth should be left unsplinted if they appear maintainable and are comfortable.

Lower incisors with extreme bone loss should not be splinted unless they offer support to other teeth. It is more practical to replace lower incisors with a fixed bridge than to splint them if the splinted teeth present problems of maintenance and offer no advantages to the treatment plan.

If splinting is required but full coverage is not needed, the method of choice is the non-parallel horizontal pin technique. It offers nut-and-bolt retention with minimal tooth preparation, and the enamel incisal edges are maintained intact. The main requirements for the technique are that there must be sufficient room for the pins between the pulp and the incisal edge and there must be sufficient thickness of the teeth to provide a layer of dentin between the labial and lingual enamel.

The use of embedded wire combined with bonded resin is also an acceptable method for conservatively strengthening weak lower anterior teeth.

The replacement of ***missing lower anterior teeth*** requires the same preplanning as other anterior problems. The teeth should be set up or waxed up tentatively on mounted models so that the incisal edges are in the best relationship for stable centric contact. Temporary restorations that reflect the planning should be made and checked in the mouth for esthetics, phonetics, and function. Corrections should be made in the temporary restorations and the permanent restorations should be fabricated accordingly.

Duplicating correct incisal edge position

After the position of incisal edges has been determined and verified in the mouth, that position must be precisely communicated to the laboratory technician. The method of communication is unacceptable unless the finished result can be verified regarding its accuracy.

The best method I have found for precisely communicating both the incisal edge position and contour is a firm silicone index made on a cast of the corrected lower incisors. If no changes are required in the teeth, the index can be made on a cast of the original teeth before they are prepared. If changes are necessary in incisal edge position, those changes should always be made in provisional restorations so that they can be tested in the mouth before they are copied in the finished restorations.

The use of the index (Fig. 17-20) is very practical for any type of restoration, including porcelain veneer restorations. Metal copings can be waxed in relation to the index to provide uniform thickness of porcelain, thus saving time for the waxup procedure and ensuring that there will be sufficient room for porcelain.

The index also can be used to locate the labioincisal line angle and is an excellent guide

LOWER ANTERIORS

FOR _____
DUE _____
DR. _____

INCISAL PLANE
- ☐ COPY CAST of TEMPS
- ☐ INCISAL PLANE aligned with bench top
- ☐ LABIAL EMBRASURES aligned with VERTICAL
- ☐ _____

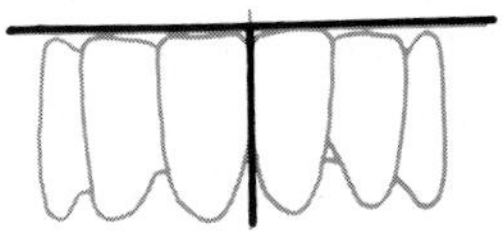

INCISAL EDGE POSITION
- ☐ FOLLOW E/O CAST
- ☐ COPY CAST of TEMPS
- ☐ COPY CAST of ORIGINAL
- ☐ INCISAL EDGES MEET DEFINITE STOP
- ☐ NO ANTERIOR CONTACT

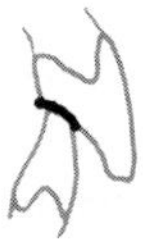

INCISAL EDGE CONTOUR
- ☐ OUTLINED BY LINE ANGLES 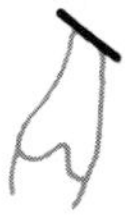
- ☐ INCISAL EDGE HIGHER ON LINGUAL
- ☐ INCISAL EDGE WIDER AT LINGUAL 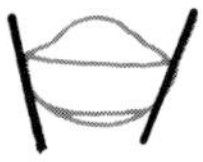
- ☐ DEFINITE LABIO-INCISAL LINE ANGLE 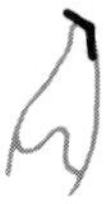
- ☐ LINGUAL STRAIGHT or SLIGHTLY CONCAVE

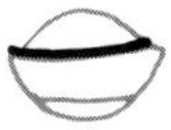

LABIAL EMBRASURES
☐
- ☐ FORMED BY CONVEX PROXIMAL SURFACES

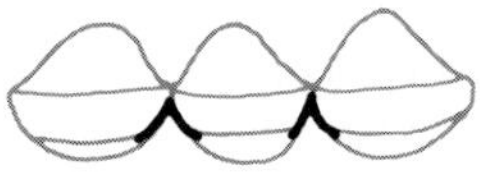

LINGUAL SILHOUETTE
☐
- ☐ FROM SLIGHT OFFSET OF INCISAL EDGES

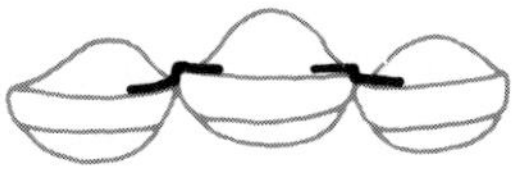

INCISAL EDGE SILHOUETTE
☐
- ☐ FROM SLIGHT ANGULATION OF FLAT EDGES
- ☐ PATIENT WANTS EVEN

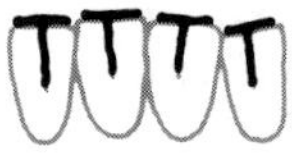

CUSPID
- ☐ MES-LAB LINE ANGLE POINTS FORWARD 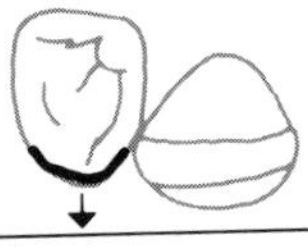
- ☐ SHOW LINGUAL OF CUSPID FROM LABIAL VIEW

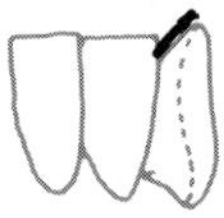

EMERGENCE CONTOUR
- ☐ RELATE TO SOFT-TISSUE MODEL
- ☐ NO METAL EXPOSED
- ☐ PORCELAIN MARGIN
- ☐ METAL EXPOSURE OK

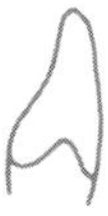

LABIAL CONTOUR
- ☐ RELATE LABIAL CONTOUR TO E/O
- ☐ TO CAST OF ORIGINAL
- ☐ TO CAST OF TEMPS
- ☐ NO BULGE AT MARGIN

- ☐ SPECIAL INSTRUCTIONS 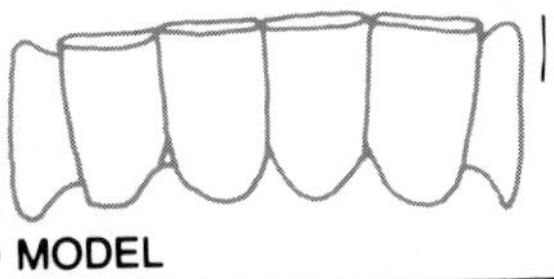
- ☐ SHADE INSTRUCTIONS

- ☐ CHECK CONTACTS ON SOLID MODEL

ESTHETIC CHECKLIST ©1984 PETER E. DAWSON, D.D.S.

Fig. 17-21. The *esthetic and restorative check list* is an excellent means for communicating all the important guidelines for the laboratory technician. The appropriate check boxes should be circled for each guideline. Every box that is circled must then be checked off by the technician indicating that instructions have been followed. The check list is then returned with the prosthesis, at which time each request is checked off by the doctor to verify that instructions have been followed. Special instructions can also be added.

for labial contour. It can be used for either in-dividual restorations or when splinting is to be done.

The use of the *Esthetic and Restorative Check List* (Fig. 17-21) has been an important advancement in our communication with the laboratory. It serves as a quality-control check for both the doctor and the technician to ensure that all information is provided to the laboratory and then to verify that all communications are adhered to.

If it is necessary to reshape the incisal edge of a natural tooth to improve its alignment, the ground surface will have a tendency to chip unless it is polished. Any rough tooth surface should be polished to a smooth sheen.

Whether the occlusal problem requires restorative procedures, orthodontics, maxillofacial surgery, or just simple equilibration, the position and contour of the lower incisal edges must be determined before completion of any other part of the occlusal scheme. All other occlusal considerations relate to lower incisal edge position. Whenever modifications are needed, the lower incisal edges should be finalized before you proceed to any permanent restorations. If the lower anterior teeth have been correctly analyzed and necessary alterations are complete, further changes in that segment should not be required regardless of the complexity of the remaining occlusal treatment.

18

Restoring upper anterior teeth

There is no part of the occlusal scheme that demands more understanding and skill than the upper anterior teeth. There is no part of the dentition that is more important to the patient because it is the part that is clearly visible with every smile. It is the part that is most important to phonetics, and it is the part that is most critical in regard to function. The stability of the entire dentition depends on a correct relationship of the upper anterior teeth, which, in function with the lower anterior teeth, dictates the anterior guidance. The principal role of the anterior guidance is to protect the posterior teeth, and it must do this job without destroying itself. To accomplish all these objectives requires meticulous care in determining the correct position and contour of each upper anterior tooth. Fortunately there is an understandable reason for every aspect of position and contour, and these reasons provide a practical basis for restoring upper anterior teeth.

For years our group has been observing and photographing beautiful smiles and then carefully analyzing what similarities exist in attractive smiles and what similarities are found in unattractive smiles. What we have learned is that there are definite interrelationships between functional requirements and the goals of natural esthetics. Through understanding these interrelationships, a set of guidelines has emerged by which we can analyze any smile and quickly determine whether it is in anatomic and functional harmony. If it lacks either, it will be apparent what must be done to correct the disharmony.

DETERMINING POSITION AND CONTOUR

The position and contour determinations for upper anterior teeth require more preciseness than is generally practiced. There are three essential determinations that must be made if anterior restorations are to be fabricated accurately. Each of those determinations must be made *in the mouth* before they can be communicated to the laboratory. None of those decisions can be accurately determined from any articulator because they are not dictated by condylar guidance, and so the technician must be given specific information in addition to the correctly articulated cast.

If upper anterior teeth are to be restored or altered, you must *determine in the mouth* the following:

1. Precise position of each incisal edge
2. Correct lingual contour of each tooth
3. Correct labial contour of each tooth

There are seven factors that work together to dictate the above determinations. Each dictating factor must be understood and must be used as a cross-check against the dictates of each of the other factors. If this is done, all guesswork is removed from the determination of position and contour of upper anterior teeth. Let's take each of those factors and see how it affects the determinations that must be made.

The seven factors that determine labial and lingual contour and relate them to the correct incisal edge position are as follows:

1. Mandible-to-maxilla relationship at centric relation
2. Lip support
3. Lip-closure path
4. Tooth-to-lip relationship during formation of *f* and *v* sounds
5. Envelope of function
6. Tooth-to-tooth relationships during the *s* sound
7. Neutral zone

These seven determining factors should be employed in proper sequence and should not be used until the following three basic preparatory steps are taken:

The first preparatory step is to make certain that the lower incisal edges are correct. If needed, any reshaping, repositioning, or restoring of lower anterior teeth should be completed. On some occasions when both upper and lower anterior teeth are to be restored, it will not be practical to complete the finished lower restorations until the upper anterior teeth are reshaped. If so, the lower incisal edge position and contour should at least be finalized in provisional restorations before you attempt to complete the permanent restorations on the upper teeth.

The second preparatory step requires that all occlusal interferences on posterior teeth be eliminated so that the condyles have free access to centric relation at the correct vertical dimension. Also, excursive interferences must be eliminated so that the posterior teeth do not interfere with anterior contact in protrusive or lateral excursions. If posterior teeth are to be restored, it is often helpful to prepare them on one arch to eliminate any possibility of posterior interferences while working out the anterior guidance. If they are not to be re-

stored, equilibration should be completed before anterior restorations are finalized.

A third determination should precede any contour decisions on anterior teeth: it must be determined that there are no habit patterns of tongue or lips to prevent anterior tooth contact. This is determined at the maximum intercuspation position. If there is no anterior tooth contact when the posterior teeth are intercuspated in the most closed position, the anterior teeth should be evaluated as an anterior open bite condition (see Chapter 33). If the anterior teeth are in contact in centric occlusion, it is correct to give them contact in centric relation. This is such an important determination that it should never be overlooked before treatment planning for anterior teeth.

With those three preliminary steps completed, you are ready to determine the contour and position of the upper anterior teeth. By using the seven factors that determine position and contour, you can ascertain every part of the contour of each tooth as seen from a lateral view. Let's assume you must restore upper incisors that are missing and have elected to make a six-tooth anterior bridge using the cuspids as abutments. There are no clues to tell us where the incisal edges should be or how the labial surfaces should be contoured. Let's assume also that the anterior guidance has been destroyed, and so you must make every determination of position and contour. This is the same type of situation you face when you must replace upper anterior restorations that have been improperly restored, or in any anterior restorations that require a change of incisal edge position.

In upper anterior restorative situations that require a change of incisal edge position or in which the incisal edge positions are unknown, utilize the seven factors to make all determinations in provisional restorations first before proceeding with the permanent restorations. It is necessary to use those factors in correct sequence and only after the preliminary steps have been completed.

SEQUENCE OF DETERMINATION
Step 1: Centric relation stops

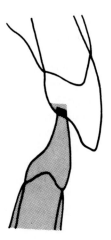

The position of the lower incisal edges in centric relation determine the start of contour for each upper anterior tooth. This is the starting point for function and must be determined first. It should be obvious why the lower incisal edge position and contour must be final-

ized before this step. If the lower incisal edges are in final form, all you must do to start the contour of the upper anterior teeth is to hinge the mandible closed on the centric relation axis, to the correct vertical dimension. The lower incisal edges at that position determine the reciprocal contours for each holding contact on the upper teeth.

This starting point for upper anterior contour is determined horizontally by the precise centric relation position of the condylar axis and vertically by the length of the elevator muscles during repetitive functional contraction (Fig. 18-1).

You can easily ascertain the vertical position by closing the jaw to the level of maximum intercuspation, after deviating occlusal interferences have been equilibrated.

Holding contacts at centric relation can be determined on correctly articulated casts. It is the one contour relationship for the anterior teeth that must be meticulously related to condylar position. If provisional restorations are fabricated on the articulator, the centric re-

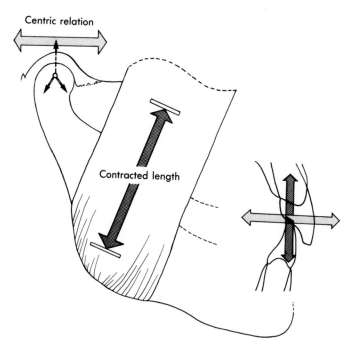

Fig. 18-1. Diagram showing how the lower incisal edge is positioned to determine the starting point for upper anterior contour. The horizontal position is determined by the position of the condyles at the apex of force (centric relation). The vertical dimension is determined by the repetitive contracted length of the elevator muscles.

lation contacts can be completed on the articulator. As a matter of practicality, though, provisional restorations that are so fabricated should always be carefully evaluated in the mouth and adjusted if necessary in centric relation before you proceed with further contour decisions. All contours, other than centric relation stops, should be refined from observation in the mouth.

Step 2: Lip support

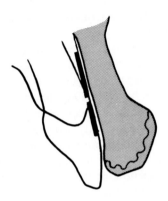

The labial contours of the upper anterior teeth must support the upper lip at rest. It should neither sink in nor bulge out to form a "monkey lip." It should drape naturally at rest and feel comfortable to the patient. For this to be accomplished in a predictable manner the labial surface of each tooth must be divided into two separate planes.

The upper half of the labial contour relates directly to the labial contour of the alveolus. Unless the alveolus is misshapen, the upper half of the labial tooth surface is nearly parallel and continuous in contour with the tissue over the root. If the incisors are missing, the labial contour of the alveolar ridge will serve as an excellent guide. If there has been extensive resorption of the ridge or the labial plate of bone has been lost, it is generally not too difficult to determine where the normal contour of the ridge should be. The provisional restorations should be contoured at this section until the lip is comfortably supported with no abrupt changes of contour.

A common mistake in contouring is to create a bulge at the gingival part of the labial surface. Bulges create potential problems for stability, especially if they result in extra inward pressure from a tight perioral musculature. The transition from the alveolus to the labial surface of the teeth should be just as smooth and continuous as the inner surface of the lip. There should be no bulges and no sudden changes in contour. A slight overall convexity is normal.

The upper half of the labial contour can usually be determined reasonably close from a cast of the upper arch if it includes a good reproduction of the entire alveolar ridge. The rest of the labial surface cannot be accurately determined outside the mouth because it relates to the functional activity of the lip. So the lower half of the labial surface involves a distinctly different determination.

Step 3: Lip-closure path

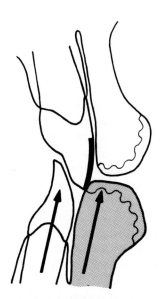

When the lips come together to seal so that a swallow can be made, the lower lip should be able to slide smoothly past the labio-incisal line angle of the upper incisors. The incisal third to one half of the labial surface should be contoured back to permit the lips to come together without interference from the teeth. It should be comfortable for the patient to hold the lip seal without any feeling of strain on the perioral musculature.

Failure to taper the labial surface back in this manner is one of the most common errors in restoring anterior teeth (Fig. 18-2). Often the slightest amount of reduction in bulk is all that is required to change patient displeasure to acceptance of anterior restorations.

The incisal half of the labial surface is particularly important because of its relationship to the lower band of the buccinator. The greatest pressure is applied at the incisal third; so if it is too bulky, there will be a tendency to move the upper teeth lingually and thereby move the upper lingual inclines into interference. Evidence of this is the complaint that the front teeth bump or hit first on closure. Reduction of the lingual surface relieves the problem, but it reoccurs and must be readjusted several times. If the labial surface is corrected, the problem often is resolved without the need for multiple adjustments on the lingual.

Determination of the correct labial contour is as critical to occlusal stability as many of the procedures we do on posterior teeth. It is also a prerequisite for determining the position of the incisal edges. In working with correct ante-

rior relationships, it is helpful to start with some extra length because it is easier and quicker to reduce the length than it is to add on. The added length does not interfere with the lip-closure path and may even help define it more easily. After the two planes of contour have been determined to provide comfortable lip support and lip-closure path, you are ready to proceed with locating the vertical height of each incisal edge. Determine this and refine it with great preciseness by relating it to the functional relationships of phonetics and the smile line.

LOCATING THE INCISAL EDGE POSITIONS. Location of the incisal edges is second in importance only to a correct centric relation. Centric relation determines where the starting position is for function; the upper incisal edges determine the end point of function. If you can precisely determine the correct starting point and end point that the lower incisal edges travel in comfortable function, you can fabricate upper anterior restorations that are in harmony with the mandibular envelope of function, as well as the neutral zone. The intermediate functional paths can be worked out very practically if you have correctly determined the two end points.

Incisal edge positions can be located with extreme preciseness by utilizing the functional relationships that are a necessity for correct speech. A basic understanding of how certain sounds are formed by the relationship of the upper anterior teeth to the lips should make it clear why the use of phonetics is such an accurate determinant of incisal edge position.

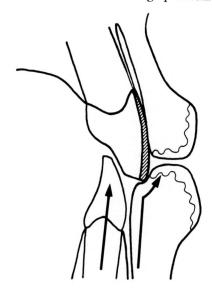

Fig. 18-2. Labioincisal edge too far forward. Interferes with the lip-closure path and the neutral zone.

Step 4: Tooth-to-lip relationships during formation of *f* and *v* sounds

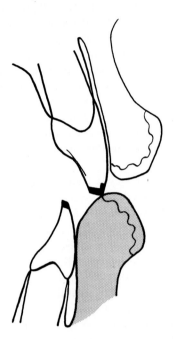

The muscle memory pattern involved with making the *f* or *v* sounds is amazingly consistent. Make an *f* sound and note the relationship of your upper incisal edges to the exact position along the vermilion border of your lower lip. Now repeat the *f* sound at different intervals and different volumes.

You will find that whether you repeat it at a slow or a fast repetitive rate or whether you say *f* softly or loudly, the relationship of upper incisal edges to the lower vermilion border of your lip does not change. There is a reason for this consistency. Correct formation of the *f* sound requires the flowing air to be constricted into a wide flat band where the *ehh* sound is closed down so that the flat band of rushing air is constricted between the hard surfaces of the upper incisal edges and the soft surface of the lower lip. As the two dissimilar surfaces approximate each other, the *ehh* sound becomes an *ehhff* sound.

There are two dimensions involved with the incisal edge to lip relationship. One is the correct alignment from a lateral viewpoint. The other is related to the frontal view of the incisal plane to lip relationship, which we refer to as the *smile line*. This is very important be-

cause the axial alignment of the teeth has a great effect on their apparent length. From a labial viewpoint, a vertically positioned anterior tooth becomes progressively shorter in appearance as its incisal edge is moved out (Fig. 18-3).

For that reason, we must position the labial surface and determine its contour before locating the smile line. After the smile line is used to determine the vertical position of the incisal edges, the horizontal position can then be refined with great preciseness by careful observation and patient input regarding the naturalness of the *f* sound.

USING THE SMILE LINE. The normal curve of the lower lip when smiling is one of the most important factors in determining the contour of the upper incisal plane. The upper incisal edges naturally follow the curve of the lower lip for a functional reason. When one is making *f* or *v* sounds, the air is constricted against the lip in a flattened band for the full width of the upper incisal plane. If the edges of the teeth do not fit the natural curve of the lip, the patient must strain the lip to constrict the air for proper phonetics. This is such a delicately coordinated balance that even slight changes can be very bothersome to the patient, even when no noticeable change in speech can be observed.

This is one of the most graphic examples of how closely related form is to function, and it explains how the observation of functional relationships can be used as very dependable guides for determining tooth position and contour (Fig. 18-4).

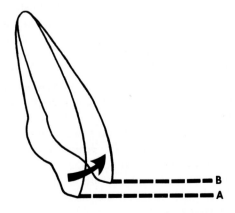

Fig. 18-3. As an upper incisor is inclined toward the labial, it appears to be shorter. Notice the difference in apparent length between position *A* and position *B*.

After the labial relationship has been determined in acrylic provisional restorations, the lip when smiling can be used as a template and the contour can simply be drawn on the surface of the acrylic provisionals. The incisal edges can then be trimmed back to that line.

After the temporaries are trimmed to the smile line, the incisal edge length and labiolingual position can be tested and precisely refined at the *f* and *v* position. Refinements in lip-closure path can now be finalized, and the overall labial contour can be observed for naturalness of the lip at rest or in function.

By following this procedure, the incisal edges can be located so precisely that they rarely require changes to be made after the initial determination. However, there are some patients who have such exquisite sensitivity to *any* change, they will need minor modifications made before they become totally comfortable. Many times, just a slight polishing off of a tooth surface makes a noticeable difference to the patient.

There are also patients who have such a strong opinion of how the teeth should look that the slightest alteration may be important to them. This is one of the advantages of working with provisional acrylic restorations to work out all the contour details before proceeding with the permanent restorations. The patient has the opportunity to test the feel and function of the provisional restorations, and changes can be made until the patient approves.

Sadly (but realistically) there are some patients who are not totally rational in their demands for anterior segment contour. There are limitations regarding length and position if we are to have stability or a functional anterior guidance. It is far better to work out those compromises in the provisional restorations where the shortcomings can be clearly explained to the patient who must assume responsibility for failure if the doctor's clinical recommendations are not accepted. It is my personal experience, however, that such patients are rare, and most will be cooperative if meticulous attention is given to refining the contours and subjecting them to the functional criteria outlined in this chapter.

The incisal edge of each tooth has a relationship to its own root that is an added guideline for better understanding of correct position, in addition to its relationship to the lip. If you were to equally bisect the long axis of an anterior tooth, the line would go through the root tip and the incisal edge (Fig. 18-5).

One of the most common mistakes we see in restorations is positioning the incisal edge too far to the labial. After the smile line is refined, be sure to recheck the lip-closure path to be certain the labioincisal line angle is contoured back enough to permit easy pass-by of the lower lip during lip closure.

After the incisal edges have been located and contoured, we are ready to work out the anterior guidance. We now have the beginning contact in centric relation and the end point of function when the anterior teeth meet in end-to-end alignment. We cannot finalize the anterior guidance until both of those determinations have been made.

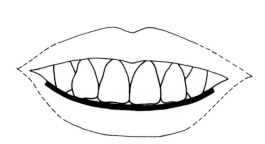

Fig. 18-4. The smile line. The incisal edges should contact the smiling lip line contour without strain.

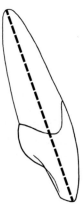

Fig. 18-5. The incisal edge is on a line that bisects the long axis of the tooth.

Step 5: Determining lingual contours for upper anterior teeth

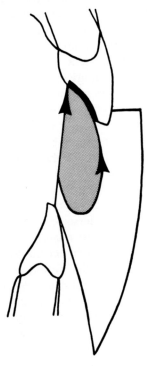

Fig. 18-6. The envelope of function is incorporated into the lingual contours *after* the incisal edges are determined.

The lingual contour from centric relation out to the incisal edges in all excursions constitutes the anterior guidance. The anterior guidance must be in harmony with the envelope of function or the anterior teeth will lack stability. Just being in noninterference is not enough. Tilting the axis of the upper teeth outward can eliminate interference to the envelope of function but would place the incisal edges in interference with the lip-closure path and the neutral zone. It also interferes with phonetic relationships, especially the *f* and *v* sounds.

The envelope of function. As discussed in Chapter 16, the functional movements of the lower incisal edges determine the envelope of function (Fig. 18-6). Any interference to these functional movements by restrictive inclines seems invariably to result in excessive wear on the lingual inclines of the upper anterior teeth, or the labial surfaces of the lower teeth.

Restriction of the patient's established envelope of function does not necessarily cause discomfort. As long as there are no interferences to centric relation contact of the anterior teeth, protrusive or lateral function restrictions are not always noticed by patients, but even when the patient is comfortable, there is the probability that interferences to functional patterns will create stress or wear on the interfering inclines. If the upper lingual surfaces are too far to the lingual, too steep, or not concave enough, excessive wear, hypermobility, or development of spaces between the teeth will almost certainly be the result.

To avoid the problems of a restricted envelope of function, the four steps outlined in Chapter 16 for harmonizing the anterior guidance should be followed every time upper anterior restorations are being fabricated. If the teeth being restored do not require any changes, they can be copied, but whenever any change is made to the anterior relationship, the guidance should be meticulously determined. This includes an analysis in proper sequence of the following:

1. Verification of centric relation holding contacts.
2. Evaluation of gentle closure while patient is in an upright posture to determine if any "long centric" is needed.
3. Development of smooth protrusive function between the centric–long centric stops and the predetermined incisal edges. This most often tends to develop a slightly concave contour of the upper lingual surfaces.
4. Determination of the lateral anterior guidance between the centric stops and the edge or tip of the cuspids. This determination includes a decision regarding the number of anterior teeth in contact during lateral excursions.

For details on making each of the above determinations, please review Chapter 16.

Step 6: Analyzing cingulum contour

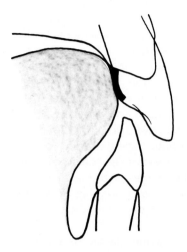

Fig. 18-7. The cingulum contour should conform with the natural position of the tongue during formation of *t* and *d* sounds.

The lingual contours are now completed through the functional range of occlusal contact. But there is still a contour to be refined that is often overlooked. It is the lingual contour between the centric relation stop and the gingival margin. Analyze its correctness using the phonetic relationships during *t* and *d* sounds. If the contour of the upper cingulum is too bulky, the tongue may bump into it when making *t* and *d* sounds. Sometimes there is left a sharp-line angle at the junction of the centric stop and the lingual contour toward the gingiva. This sharp-line angle can almost always be rounded off without the stability of the holding contacts being affected (Fig. 18-7).

If the lingual surface must be extended to provide a holding contact for the lower incisors, some slight interference to the *t-d* tongue position may be unavoidable. If so, it is an advantage to explain the problem to the patient in advance. Most patients will adapt to the change in time, if they understand the reason for it.

In patients with a strong tongue thrust, added bulk on the lingual may increase tongue pressure against the teeth, causing them to be moved labially.

Step 7: Verifying correct contour with *s* sounds

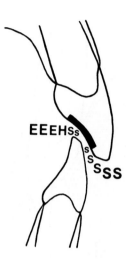

Because tooth-to-tooth relationships can vary during the *s* sound, it is not the best determinant of upper anterior contour. It does, however, serve as an excellent *verification* procedure. Since air can be restricted for the *s* sound between the lower incisal edges and *either* the lingual contour or the incisal edges of the upper teeth, an error on any part of the upper contour might affect the *s* sound. Too much space causes a lisp. Too little space causes the teeth to bump.

Step 8: Relating upper anterior teeth to the neutral zone

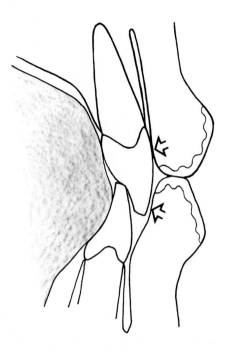

If the procedures just outlined are followed in sequence, they will result in upper anterior teeth being in their precisely correct neutral zone. The reason for this is basic. The tongue and the perioral musculature determine the neutral zone limitations by their functional activity. The same muscular components that establish the lip-closure path, and the various phonetic relationships, also form the functional matrix for the neutral zone. When the muscles contract in function, they set the boundaries for tooth position and contour. The steps outlined for determining the contour of the various tooth surfaces are related to those same muscles in function.

The same neutral zone that was shaped by the tongue versus the contracting perioral musculature is also the dominant factor in determining the envelope of function. Whether the mandible functions in a very restricted arc of closure or functions with much horizontal motion is directly related to proprioceptive input from periodontal receptors around teeth that were, during eruption, guided into position within the neutral zone. That tooth-directed envelope of function stays pretty much intact as long as no disruptive forces are introduced, such as occlusal interferences, improper orthodontics, or poorly contoured restorations. Any such disturbing factors that

cause the teeth to be in disharmony with the neutral zone may also affect the envelope of function. Habit patterns such as tobacco chewing or bruxing may also significantly alter the envelope of function by wearing the anterior guidance flatter. If posterior disclusion is not affected, a flatter guidance is well tolerated, but it has been my experience that once the anterior guidance is flattened it is difficult to restrict function back to a more vertical guidance without paying a price for it. It appears that the response to restricted function is almost always one of trying to regain the horizontal freedom by wearing away the restrictive inclines or by spreading the teeth or loosening them.

Despite some claims for successful restriction of flat anterior guidances to verticalized function, I do not see this occur without some degree of one or more of the signs of instability. Usually wear of the upper lingual surfaces is the most common sign. I have been very carefully monitoring patients for many years with anterior guidances that have been steepened. I find, almost without exception, a greater tendency to anterior wear problems when this is done. It does not, however, seem to adversely affect the patient's comfort, and even though there is a tendency toward hyperfunction against the steepened inclines, countermeasures can be taken to reduce the wear and stress problem. Splinting of the anterior teeth or the use of a retainer at night can keep them from spreading, and the same appliance can include occlusal coverage to reduce wear from parafunction during sleep.

There are some problems of anterior wear that cannot be resolved with acceptable esthetics unless the upper anterior teeth are lengthened. Since severe wear tends to result in a more end-to-end relationship of the anterior teeth, it is difficult to lengthen the upper teeth without either steepening the guidance or moving the labial surfaces forward. The lower incisal edges can sometimes be moved lingually by reduction of their thickness on the labial surface. This in turn makes it possible to develop a concave lingual guidance on the upper anterior teeth, thus reducing the need for severe steepness forward of the centric relation stops. It also makes it possible to lengthen the upper incisal edges without increasing the vertical dimension or intruding too much into the lip-closure path or the neutral zone. These procedures are illustrated in Chapter 30, since they relate to solving problems of wear. They are mentioned here because such problems are so often treated improperly.

When you are restoring anterior teeth, if the importance of the neutral zone or the envelope of function is not considered, the restorations will probably be unacceptable. It is far too common to see anterior restorations that not only are stressful, but are also terribly unesthetic because the factors that determine their position and contour have not been considered. When you are restoring severely worn anterior teeth, the process of determining the position of the incisal edges and the contour of the labial and lingual surfaces involves the same steps as described for restoring any anterior teeth if the incisal edge position is being changed. The only difference may be that you must sometimes compromise on some contour relationships with the neutral zone or lip-closure path or the envelope of function. When compromise is necessary, it will be apparent in advance, and so the patient can be prepared for the changes.

By making all changes in provisional restorations first, you allow the patient to be able to determine whether the modifications are acceptable before the final restorations are fabricated. With all the treatment options that are available to us today, there are very few problems of anterior relationships that cannot be restored to both good function and good esthetics if the patient is willing to do what is necessary.

Relating upper incisor position with cephalometrics

The A-Po plane is a simple-to-use reference plane that is practical for comparison of the position of upper incisors with the norm. Because the A-Po plane relates to both the upper and lower skeletal bases, relating tooth position and alignment with that plane can provide some valuable clues for determining approaches to treatment.

The principal value of cephalometrics in diagnosing adult occlusal problems is that it gives us a quick appraisal of which segments are malposed and which segments are in a normal relationship. In trying to correct a dentition to normal, you must know which segments are normal so that you can preserve those relationships and confine treatment as much as possible to those malposed segments that need correction. As an example, if the upper incisal edges are too far forward of the A-Po plane while the lower incisors are in a normal relationship, you would not try to correct the problem by moving the lower anterior teeth forward. You would first consider the effect of moving the malposed upper teeth back into a more normal relationship.

There are three principal evaluations that you can relate to the A-Po plane to give a quick analysis of anterior tooth position compared to the norm. They are as follows.

Upper incisor protrusion. The norm according to Ricketts and co-workers is 3.5 mm of protrusion forward of the A-Po plane with a clinical deviation of +1 to 2.3 mm.

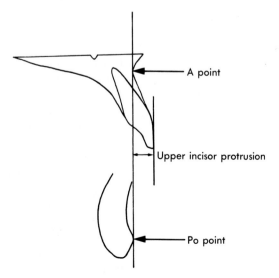

A point

Upper incisor protrusion

Po point

Norm 3.5 mm ± 2.3 mm

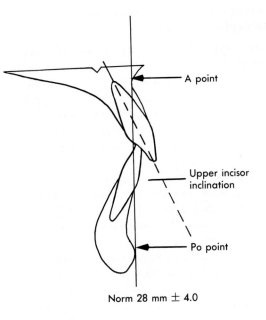

Norm 28 mm ± 4.0

Upper incisor inclination. The normal angulation of the upper incisor to the A-Po plane is 28 degrees with a clinical deviation of +1 to 4 degrees. When the inclination varies too much from the norm in either direction, the influence of the neutral zone must be evaluated carefully. Lip and tongue posture must be observed in function.

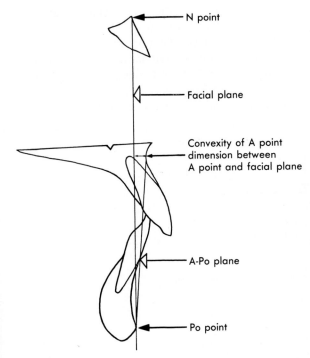

Convexity of A point. This analysis can show us the relationship of the skeletal base. The measurement between point A and the facial plane can either be positive (forward of the line) or negative (posterior to the line). The norm for adults is 0 mm, meaning that point A is on the facial-plane line. A high convexity indicates a Class II skeletal relationship. A negative measurement indicates a Class III skeletal relationship.

The cephalometric norms are useful guidelines for treating adult patients. They must be used, however, in combination with other observations. Tooth position and even the skeletal base relationships must be evaluated in relation to the perioral musculature. Habit patterns and lip posture must be analyzed to learn if their effect on tooth position is correctable. If one remembers that the teeth and to a large extent the alveolar processes go where the tongue and the perioral musculature move them it will be apparent that stability within a strong neutral zone does not always have to be consistent with cephalometric norms. As long as vertical stability is achieved with stable holding contacts, in combination with horizontal stability within the neutral zone confinement, the dentition can function and stay healthy.

Communicating upper anterior guidelines to the laboratory

If it is important to determine accurate position and contour for anterior teeth in the mouth, it should be equally important to communicate each determination to the technician in such a precise manner that there is no need for guesswork related to any tooth surface.

The main criteria that determines if a method of communication is acceptable relates to whether the accuracy of the finished restorations can be verified. A method of communication that cannot also be used to *verify* the accuracy of results is not an acceptable method of communication.

There are five practical methods of communicating tooth position and contour. Each method permits verification that each communicated guideline has been accurately followed. The five methods are as follows:

1. Use of alternate tooth preparations and an "every-other" cast
2. Use of a matrix
3. Use of an index as a guide for incisal edge position and labial contour
4. Use of full casts of corrected anterior teeth
5. Use of the custom anterior guide

Alternate-tooth preparation method. Surprisingly, the method that provides the most precise detail is also the simplest to use. In fact, it can noticeably cut the laboratory time required for shaping anterior restorations if the restorations do not require splinting by means of a multiple-unit casting. If restorations are to be individually made and then soldered together or if they are to be placed as single units, the alternate-tooth preparation method is the most accurate of all the methods for precisely copying all the details of the teeth to be restored.

Since this method duplicates what is in the mouth, the anterior teeth must have satisfactory shape and position before preparation. Corrections should be made, if needed, by reshaping or by use of provisional restorations so that correct position and contour is confirmed (Fig. 18-8).

If the posterior teeth are to be prepared in addition to the anterior teeth, it is helpful but not necessary to prepare them in one arch before the anterior preparations (Fig. 18-9). This eliminates any possibility of posterior interferences to the anterior guidance so that the guidance can be evaluated in detail and refined if necessary. Preparation of the posterior teeth also makes it possible for you to make a centric relation bite record at the exactly correct vertical by recording centric at the point of anterior tooth contact.

If the posterior teeth are not to be prepared, the occlusion should be equilibrated before preparation of the anterior teeth so that there will be no interferences to either centric relation or any excursion that prevents the anterior guidance from functioning correctly be-

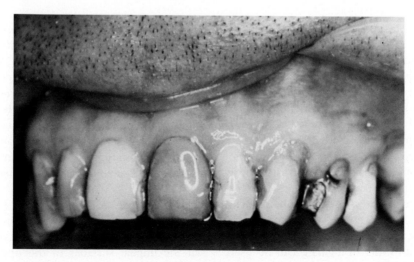

Fig. 18-8. Labial view before restoring. Notice that the shape of the teeth is good. The lip support is correct, and the incisal edge position should not be changed.

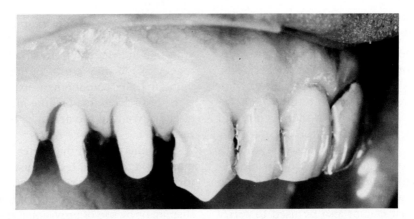

Fig. 18-9. All posterior teeth that need it are prepared in one arch so that there is no possibility of interference to functional movement. This also facilitates making the centric bite record at the correct vertical.

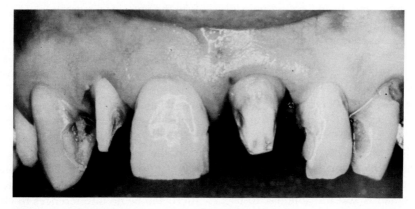

Fig. 18-10. Every other incisor is prepared. The teeth that are left should be the best shaped, since they are the ones that will be duplicated. The anterior guidance is corrected, if necessary, on the unprepared teeth, following the procedures outlined in Chapter 16.

fore being duplicated. After that the steps are as follows:

1. One central incisor and the lateral incisor on the opposite side should be prepared. The unprepared central incisor should be the one with the better shape or function, since it will serve as the guide tooth for contouring the other restoration (Fig. 18-10).

2. The steps for customizing the anterior guidance should be rechecked on the unprepared teeth to verify correctness.

3. A full-arch impression should be made. It is not necessary to capture the gingival margins with total accuracy on this impression, and so a smooth mix of alginate can be used. Wipe some of the mix into the gingival sulci before seating the tray.

4. A centric relation bite record should be made using the posterior teeth only. If the posterior teeth have been prepared, the interocclusal record can be made at the correct vertical dimension. If the posterior teeth have not been prepared, the bite record is made at a slightly opened vertical. The casts are closed to the correct vertical (usually anterior contact) after mounting procedures are completed. A facebow is always used for the mounting.

5. The custom anterior guide is fabricated from these mounted casts as outlined in Chapter 16. This will facilitate correct contouring of all the lingual surfaces of the upper anterior teeth. Fig. 18-11 shows the mounting of an alternate preparation cast on a Hanau articulator.

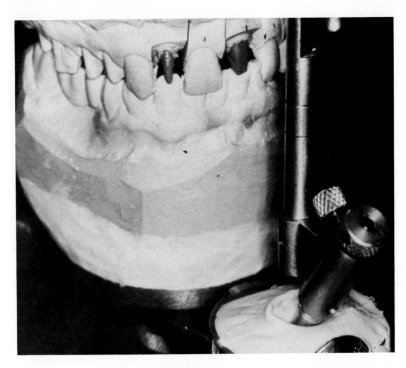

Fig. 18-11. The "every-other" cast is used to guide the incisal pin in making the customized anterior guide table (shown here on a Hanau articulator).

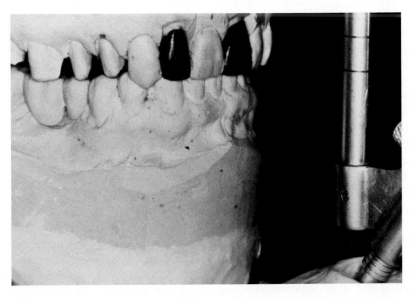

Fig. 18-12. Waxup or porcelain buildup of the dies is completed to match the incisal edge position and labial contours of the unprepared teeth. Lingual contours are determined by the customized guide table.

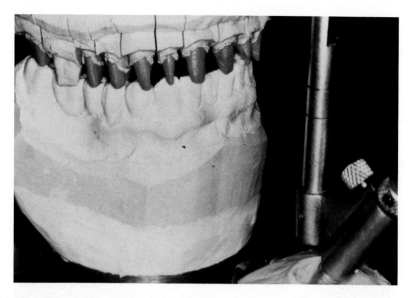

Fig. 18-13. The master die cast is mounted with the same centric bite record that was used for the every-other cast. Wax "throw-away patterns" that are shaped on the every-other cast can be transferred to this cast to be used as guides for either waxup or porcelain contouring of the remaining dies.

With the Hanau, use of the special guide pin is essential when you are making a custom anterior guide.

6. On the alternate preparation cast, which our group calls the "every-other cast," the prepared teeth should be painted with die spacer and then wax patterns are fabricated. The wax patterns are contoured to precisely duplicate the labial contours of the adjacent teeth (Fig. 18-12). Particular attention is paid to copying the correct incisal edge position. Even the texture of the labial surfaces can be duplicated in the wax pattern. The same accuracy is possible that would be expected if only one central or lateral tooth were being restored. Lingual contours are determined by the customized anterior guide table.

7. For the sake of continuity, I have described the laboratory procedures for the every-other cast before discussing the completion of the preparations. Actually the remaining anterior preparations are completed as soon as the first impression has been taken and the centric bite record has been made. In other words, all upper anterior preparations are completed at the same appointment, and the second impression is then made for the master die cast.

8. The master die cast will fit the same centric bite record that is used to articulate the every-other cast. It is mounted on its own ring

and is interchangeable with the first cast (Fig. 18-13).

The wax patterns that are fabricated on the every-other cast are referred to as "throw-away patterns" because they are never actually used for casting. They are used only as contour guides for waxing the dies on the master cast and also for guiding the ceramist in shaping the porcelain veneers. They can also be used as contour guide for fabrication of porcelain jackets or cast ceramic crowns.

After the throw-away patterns are fabricated, they are simply transferred to the master die model (Fig. 18-13) when needed. When the adjacent dies are waxed to conform to the throw-away patterns (Fig. 18-14), the patterns are returned to the every-other cast for later use by the ceramist. The waxup is then completed to conform to the patterns on the master die model.

If porcelain veneer restorations are to be made, the wax patterns are then cut back to provide a uniform thickness of porcelain, and the patterns are cast. The ceramist then uses the throw-away patterns as a guide for applying the porcelain on the copings. The throw-away patterns can be used as a guide for final finishing of the veneers so that incisal edge position and all other contours can be exactly matched.

The throw-away patterns are returned with

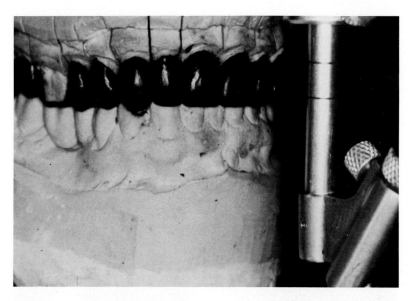

Fig. 18-14. All patterns are waxed, preferably to completion. They are then cut back a uniform amount to ensure correct thickness for the porcelain veneer. Combining the every-other cast method with the *index method* eliminates the need for complete contour waxups but provides an ideal guide for porcelain fabrication on correctly formed copings.

the finished restorations to the doctor. They can be used to verify that all contours are correct. It should be possible to place restorations done in this manner, without the need for any reshaping, since all restorations should exactly conform to precise dimensions that were predetermined in the mouth (Fig. 18-15).

There are many possible variations to the "every-other" method. On some occasions it will be advantageous to prepare two incisors on the same side in order to use the better teeth on the opposite side as guides (Fig. 18-16).

The throw-away pattern is used because it is easier and faster than using removable every-other dies that have had the gingival margins accurately exposed. Precise accuracy of the margins is not necessary for copying labial and lingual contours. Margins can be refined on the master die. However, the every-other cast can be made from impressions that capture the margins accurately so that the finished restoration can be directly related to the adjacent teeth with correct contour (Fig. 18-17). When the contoured restorations are then transferred to the master die cast, they, in turn, become the contour guide for the remaining restorations (Fig. 18-18).

If individual restorations are to be part of a splint or a fixed bridge, the restorations are soldered after the porcelain is applied. On

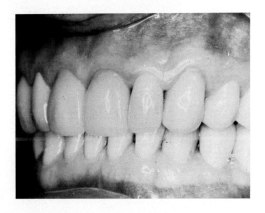

Fig. 18-15. The completed case. Lip support is unchanged, incisal edge position is correct and so there will be no chance of phonetic problems, the lingual contours are quite steep, but they are exactly correct for the near-vertical functional movements that were dictated by a very tight lip. The success of the anterior restorations was assured by the information that was supplied to the technician.

some occasions it will be advantageous to prepare one cuspid along with a central and a lateral incisor. If that cuspid is needed for making the customized guide table, it will be necessary to take an extra impression before you prepare it, so that the guidance inclines will be correctly recorded. However, if the lateral incisor shares all lateral excursive movements with the cuspid, the lateral incisor will provide

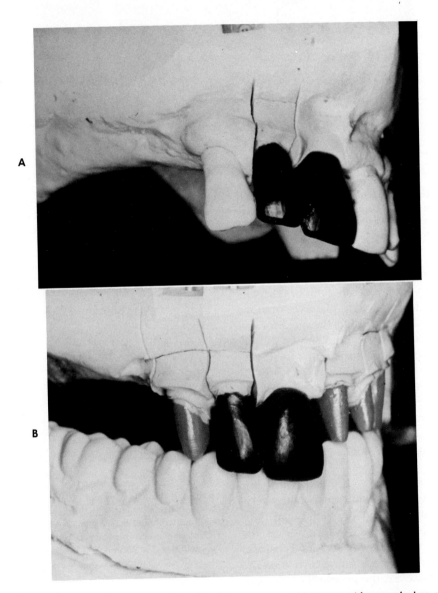

Fig. 18-16. A, Adjacent central and lateral incisors are prepared because neither one had an acceptable shape to use as a contour guide. **B,** Notice the shape of the patterns in comparison to the master dies. It is highly improbable that any technician would carve the pattern to this correct shape by chance.

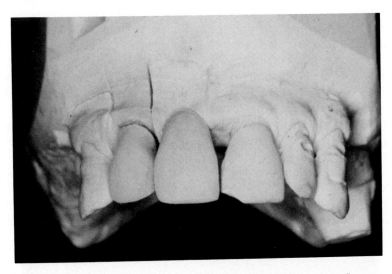

Fig. 18-17. Porcelain veneer application is accomplished on the same "every-other" or contour guide model. The shaping of the porcelain can be refined with extreme accuracy on this model.

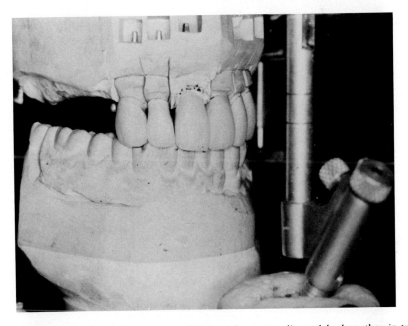

Fig. 18-18. The contoured restorations are placed on the master die model where they in turn become the contour guide for the remaining porcelain application. When splinting is required, the restorations are soldered after the porcelain is applied.

sufficient guidance inclines for making the guide table, and an extra model will not be necessary.

In mouths that have good contours on one side but all the anterior teeth on the other side are poorly shaped, you may elect to prepare adjacent teeth on the same side. It is important, though, to always have one correctly contoured central incisor as the main guide to incisal edge position.

When the two upper central incisors are the only anterior teeth that require full-coverage restorations, I would never think of preparing both teeth without first preparing one by itself and making a separate die model for establishing the correct contours. However, if the adjacent lateral incisors share the protrusive pathways with the central incisors, it is not neces-

sary to mount this model. Incisal edge position and labial contours can be duplicated on the unmounted model, and the pattern or jacket can then be transferred to the mounted master model (both centrals prepared) to finalize the lingual contours. A customized guide table is not needed if the unprepared teeth can serve as the guiding inclines.

When there is no contact between the upper and lower anterior teeth in centric relation but the relation is stable, the stability is often the result of delicately balanced lip or tongue habits. In some arch relationships the position of the lips or tongue in swallowing may be all that keeps unopposed teeth from shifting or supraerupting. It is extremely important to maintain the lingual contours of the upper anterior teeth so that new and possibly

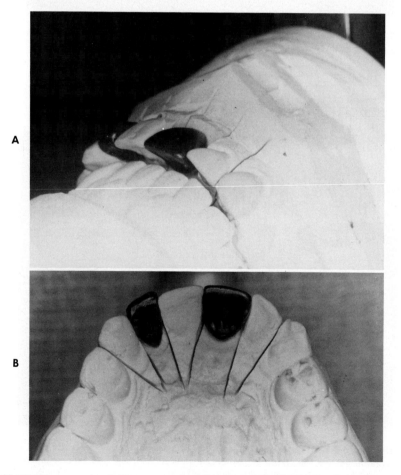

Fig. 18-19. When an unbreakable tongue or lip habit prevents stable anterior teeth from contacting in centric relation, the lingual contours should be duplicated if the teeth are restored. This can be accomplished when one prepares one central and the opposite side lateral incisor. The adjacent unprepared teeth are used as guides to lingual contouring as well as for labial contour and incisal edge position. The wax patterns or porcelain restorations are then transferred to become the guides for contouring on the master die model with the remaining teeth prepared.

destructive habit patterns are not initiated. The customized guide table does not work for such cases because there is no contact against the upper lingual surfaces. In this type of case the *lingual* contours should be duplicated on the "every-other-tooth" model in the same manner that labial contours are copied. It can be done with the same preciseness (Fig. 18-19).

When a central incisor is missing, only the opposite lateral incisor should be prepared. The shaped pontic should be used as the guide for contouring the other central incisor. If a lateral incisor is missing, the opposite-side central incisor should be prepared. The advantage of preparing every other tooth is that the width of the prepared teeth can be established very quickly when the die has properly shaped teeth on both sides of it.

If adjacent teeth are missing or the incisors do not have satisfactory shape. If one central incisor is intact, it is often all that is needed to set incisal edge position and labial contours, but when both central incisors are missing, it is almost always necessary to work out the contours in temporary restorations. The contours for the temporary restorations are worked out on articulated casts, but refinements are made in the mouth. Esthetics, phonetics, and comfort are checked before the final result is accepted for duplication in the permanent restorations.

The same procedure is followed when any gross changes are made in the shape of the anterior teeth. Since the corrected temporary restorations need to be worn by the patient until the permanent restorations are completed, it sometimes presents a problem to use the "every-other-tooth" method. To provide an "every-other-tooth" model would necessitate cutting the temporary restorations into sections, and if there are missing teeth, this would sometimes make the temporary restorations unusable. There are several ways of solving this problem, and the versatile operator will vary the methods to suit the individual needs in the most practical way. Some suggested approaches are as follows:

FIRST METHOD. The temporary restorations should be separated at the midline if each segment is stable. An impression is taken with both segments in to make the customized anterior guide table, and a second impression is taken with only one segment in for alignment of contours.

SECOND METHOD. The temporary restorations may be separated in "every-other-tooth" fashion for the model and then the segments joined back with self-curing acrylic resin.

THIRD METHOD. Sometimes it is easier just to fabricate two sets of temporary restorations, one to be segmented for the "every-other-tooth" model and one for the patient to wear during fabrication of the permanent restorations. This may seem like a lot of trouble, but there are times when absolute preciseness is so important that making an extra temporary restoration is a small price to pay.

FOURTH METHOD. A full-arch impression is taken of the finalized temporary restoration and the model poured. The model is mounted with a centric bite record and used to make the customized guide table. After the guide table is completed, a fine-toothed coping saw is used to carefully saw through the contacts and saw out one central and the opposite lateral by cutting through these teeth just short of the gingival margin. The contours of the adjacent teeth are carefully preserved. The precedure is the same as the one illustrated for maintaining the contours of a worn-out anterior bridge (Figs. 18-20 through 18-24). The model is lubricated and the sawed-out portions are replaced in wax to the correct labial contours and incisal edge positions. A double thickness of base plate wax is warmed and pressed firmly against the posterior teeth to form an index. The index fits the upper posterior teeth in the same manner as a bite record except that the wafer is extended forward to be joined with hot wax to the lingual of the two waxed-in teeth. The dies for the teeth that were sawed off and waxed up are removed, and the wax index is fitted to the posterior teeth. This will place the waxed-up central and lateral incisors in perfect relationship to the other dies. The other dies can then be waxed to the correct contour and incisal edge position. When they have been contoured, the indexed waxup of the cut-off central and lateral incisors can be discarded, and those dies can be replaced and waxed. Lingual contours are established from the customized guide table.

This technique has many possible modifications. The index can be made in the palate when necessary, and this same procedure can be used to relocate lost incisal edge positions from old study models made before periodontal surgery or improperly done anterior resto-

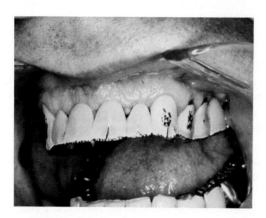

Fig. 18-20. This full upper restoration needs to be replaced because of the badly worn facings. The incisal edge position and lingual contours are correct. The labial contours need only slight modification to compensate for the worn acrylic material.

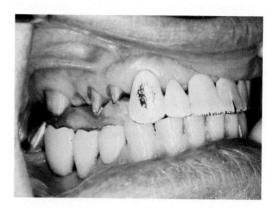

Fig. 18-21. The posterior segments are removed, and the correctness of the anterior guidance is verified or modified if needed. An impression and centric relation bite record are made.

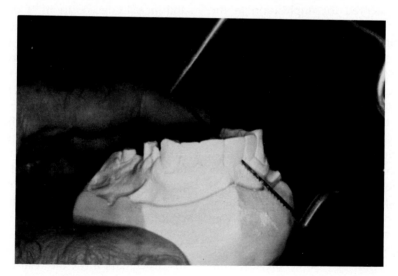

Fig. 18-22. The model made from the impression is used to fabricate a customized guide table, and then one central incisor is sawed out of the model.

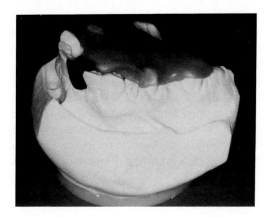

Fig. 18-23. The model is lubricated and the sawed-out pontic is waxed back to shape. It is joined to an index that fits the prepared posterior teeth on the model.

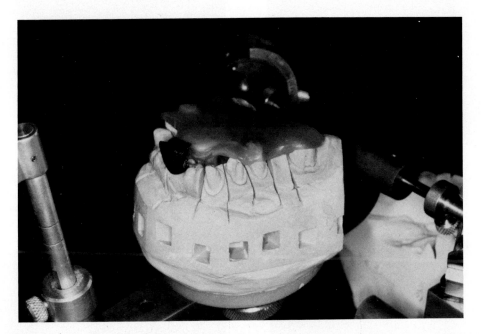

Fig. 18-24. The index is transferred to the master die model and the waxed-up pontic is used as the guide for labial contouring and precise duplication of the incisal edge position for the other anterior pontics. Lingual contours are dictated by the customized anterior guidance. Modifications of this procedure are almost unlimited for reproducing contours on either pontics or full crowns. If it is used as a guide for full-coverage contouring, a die must be removed when the index is in place. It is returned to the model when the adjacent teeth have been waxed and the index is removed.

rations. The possible variations are limited only by the operator's imagination. It is almost always possible to find some place on a model, even an old one, that can serve as a usable index if the need arises.

Using a matrix for contour duplication
(Figs. 18-25 to 18-34)

This method is for use when all incisors are missing. After the anterior temporary restorations have been refined to correct labial and lingual contour, a full-arch impression and a centric bite record are taken. This model will be used to customize the anterior guide table. Before mounting the model, make a matrix of temporary matrix material using an Omnivac or similar heat-vacuum device. If care is taken

to use melted wax that is not too hot, the wax can be flowed into the lightly lubricated matrix with care being taken not to distort it. The contours of the corrected four incisors can be duplicated in this manner with considerable ease. They can be positioned on the master die model by use of the fit of the posterior teeth into the matrix as an index. Once positioned, the matrix is removed. Lingual contours should be refined through use of the customized anterior guide table. When the four incisors have been correctly contoured, the cuspids can be shaped with relative ease by careful observation of the corrected model and copying of the contours. The matrix does not work as well on dies as it does for forming pontics.

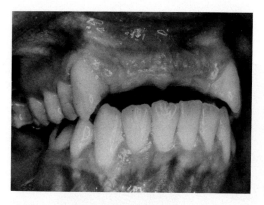

Fig. 18-25. Replacement of missing upper anterior teeth requires special care to make certain that the incisal edge position is correct.

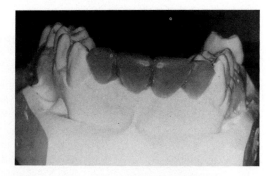

Fig. 18-26. All anterior contours should be finished on temporary restorations before the permanent restorations are completed. Overcontouring the waxup for making the matrix for the temporary restorations is helpful because it provides extra bulk with which to work.

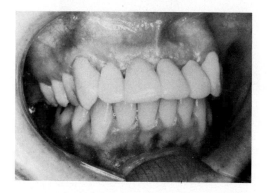

Fig. 18-27. After the cuspids are prepared, the temporary anterior bridge is fabricated from the prepared matrix and seated without cement.

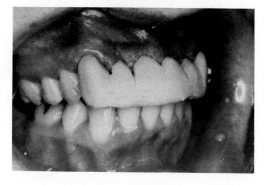

Fig. 18-28. The first analysis should be concerned with proper lip support. Incisal edge position cannot be determined until the inclination of the anterior teeth is determined. Making the temporary restorations bulky to start with enables the dentist to reduce the contours little by little until the lip support is acceptable.

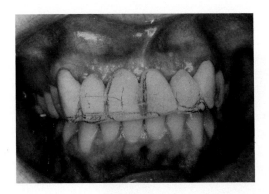

Fig. 18-29. When acceptable lip support and inclination have been achieved, the next step is to determine the length. It is always easier to start long and reduce the length. Drawing contours on the labial surface is helpful in the analysis of the smile line for esthetics. As the length is reduced and the incisal edge positions are being determined, they should be repeatedly checked phonetically for correctness. The upper incisal edges should just touch the lower vermilion border when *f* and *v* sounds are made.

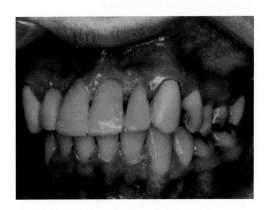

Fig. 18-30. When labial and incisal contours have been established, the patient should approve the appearance before the incisal edge position is accepted.

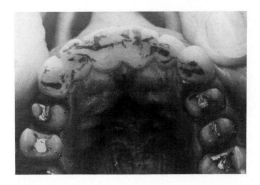

Fig. 18-31. After the incisal edge position has been finalized, the anterior guidance can be worked out. The completed lingual contours should again be tested phonetically, this time with *s* and *x* sounds to make certain there is sufficient horizontal freeway space. The posterior teeth can be prepared any time after the anterior centric relation stops have been established, since they will maintain the correct vertical dimension.

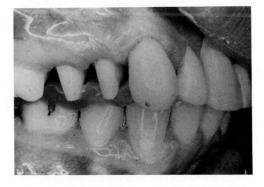

Fig. 18-32. A centric relation bite record is made at the correct vertical dimension (if posterior teeth were prepared). An impression is made with the anterior temporary restorations in place.

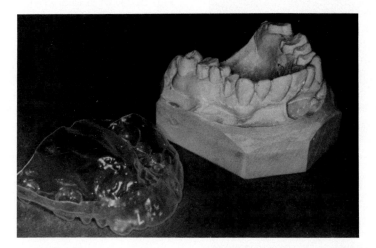

Fig. 18-33. One method of reproducing the anterior contours in wax is to make a matrix on the model of the corrected temporary restorations in place. The pontic areas of the matrix can then be filled with wax (not too hot).

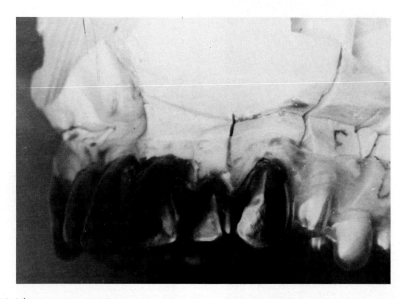

Fig. 18-34. The matrix is then placed on the master die model. Further refinement is still necessary, but the matrix can be used to get the general shape established rapidly. The customized guide table is used for refinement of lingual contours. A cut-out procedure as described in Figs. 18-21 through 18-24 can be used for refinement of porcelain veneer contours.

Using an index as a guide for incisal edge position and labial contour

The index method is by far the most popular method with our technicians because it is so simple to use whether restorations are individual or splinted. With the availability of firm silicone putty, an ideal material is obtainable for making an excellent index for almost any situation. The silicone material is easy to mix and can be trimmed easily. Yet it is firm enough to hold its shape (Fig. 18-35). It is accurate, and because it is slightly flexible, it can snap into undercuts for good stability on the master cast.

By including the lingual surfaces along with the incisal edges in the index, you need not use a waxup to full contour for veneer restorations. The full waxup method is often used to determine contour, and then each pattern is cut back to provide for a uniform thickness of porcelain. This time-consuming step can be eliminated with a properly made index because the index shows the relationship of the lingual and incisal surfaces so that the coping can be waxed to provide uniform thickness for porcelain (Fig. 18-36).

The index should always be trimmed in a straight line that is continuous with the labial surfaces of each tooth to be copied. This provides a good guideline for the fabrication of the cast coping and the porcelain veneer (Figs. 18-37 and 18-38).

The index method can be supplemented with an "every-other" cast for precise verification of labial contour and texture. Since a full cast of the corrected anterior teeth is always needed for making the index, it is also available for further contour analysis.

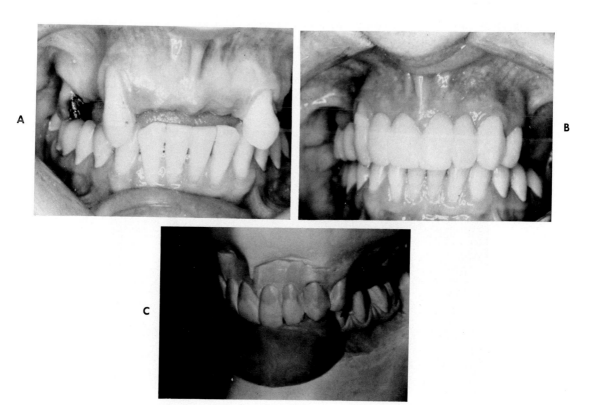

Fig. 18-35. A, Patient before preparation for upper fixed/removable prosthesis. **B,** Provisional restorations in place before final contours are worked out. **C,** Putty silicone index in place, adapted to cast of provisional restorations after refinement in the mouth.

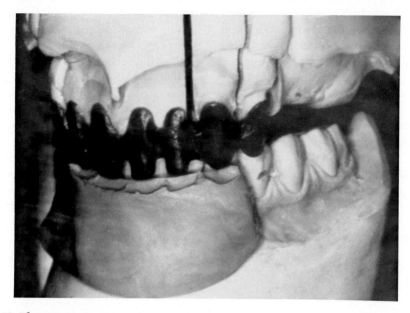

Fig. 18-36. Index in place for carving copings. Patterns can be carved to provide uniform thickness of porcelain without one having to first wax up to the full contour.

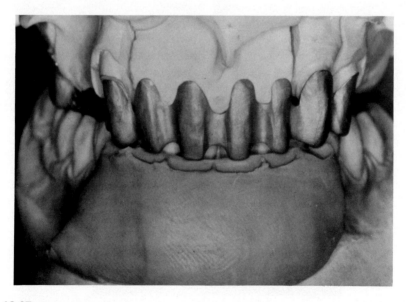

Fig. 18-37. Cast copings related to index. Verification should be made at this point to make certain there is ample room for porcelain.

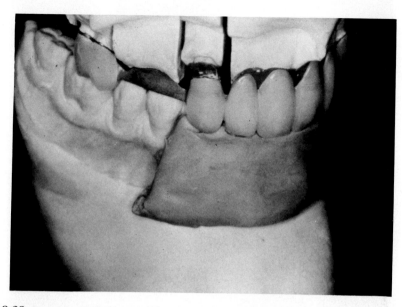

Fig. 18-38. Porcelain fabrication related to index. Labial contour should be continuous and on same plane as index. Bar between cuspid and molar is for stabilization of removable prosthesis (bar partial).

Use of full casts for communicating contours

A full cast of the corrected teeth is always beneficial for the technician. It serves as a quick reference for all contours regardless of what other methods may be used. To accurately communicate overjet, anterior guidance, or precise relationships to any contours, the cast must be mounted with an accurate centric relation bite record.

Shortcuts in using the full cast should be avoided. Outlining the incisal plane with a sharp pencil drawing on the lower anterior teeth is a very common procedure, but it is not so accurate as an index, and it does not communicate horizontal positioning of the incisal edges.

Using the custom guide table for incisal edge position

The reason for making the custom guide table is principally for communicating the upper lingual contours, but it also serves as an excellent method for showing where the incisal edges should be as well as giving a quick reference for labial contours.

When the custom guide table is being made (see Chapter 16), it is important to have definite stops for the guide pin that relate to the end-to-end position of the anterior teeth in straight protrusive relation. At this position, the labial surfaces should be aligned. Lateral excursions should be stopped at the tip-to-tip or labial alignment of the cuspids.

If the master cast is mounted interchangeably with the cast of the corrected anterior teeth, the technician can quickly determine incisal edge positions by moving the guide pin into the stop that corresponds with edge-to-edge position. The same can be done laterally (Fig. 18-39).

The custom guide serves as a quick verification method when the restorations are completed. By moving the pin to protrusive or lateral stops, you can verify the incisal edge position. If the pin is held off the guide table when the anterior teeth are end to end, that indicates that the restorations are too long. If the teeth are separated, it indicates they are too short. If the labial surfaces are not precisely aligned, it indicates improper contour of the restorations. It will be obvious whether the labial surface is too far forward or too far to the lingual.

CAUTION: Make certain that the master die cast is set at the same vertical as the cast that was used to make the custom guide.

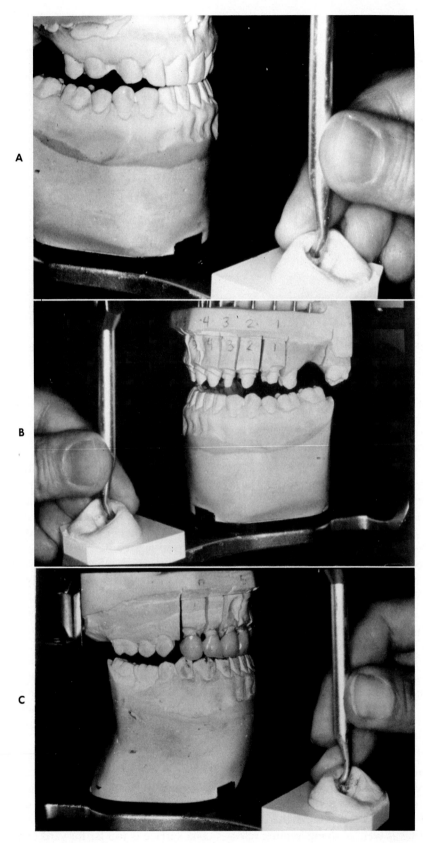

Fig. 18-39. Using the customized anterior guide table for incisal edge position and labial contour. **A,** Casts of corrected anterior teeth with labial surfaces aligned and edges in protrusive contact. Notice that the pin is at a definite stop on the guide table. **B,** Die model related to lower incisal edges when pin is at protrusive stop. Patterns should be aligned at this position. **C,** Finished restorations must be aligned edge to edge and labial surfaces in line when the incisal pin is at the protrusive stop.

UPPER ANTERIORS

FOR _____
DUE _____
DR. _____

INCISAL PLANE

☐ ALIGNED WITH BENCH TOP
☐ SAME AS MOUNTED CAST of TEMPS
☐ CENTRAL EMBRASURE VERTICAL

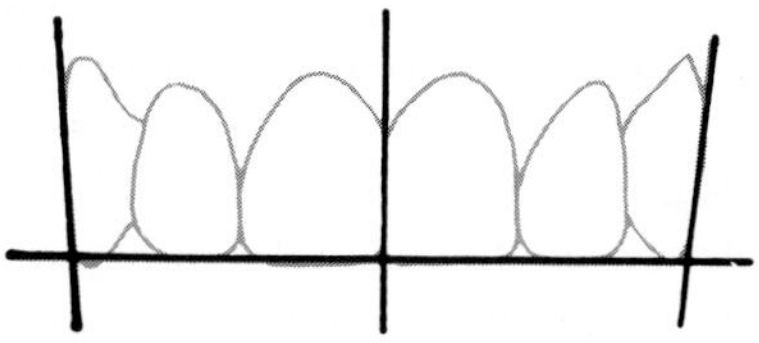

INCISAL EDGE POSITION

☐ FOLLOW E/O CAST
☐ COPY CAST of TEMPS
☐ COPY CAST of ORIGINAL

☐ NO CONTACT
☐ LABIALS ALIGNED IN PROTRUSIVE
　 EDGE-TO-EDGE with AG TABLE

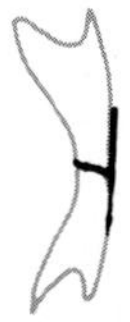

LABIAL EMBRASURES

☐ FORMED BY
　 CONVEX PROXIMALS

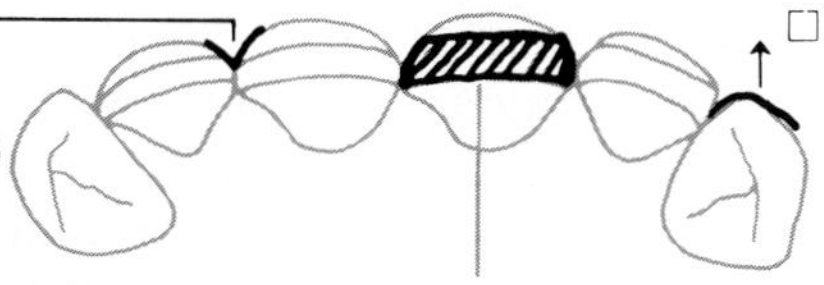

☐ CUSPID
　 MES-LAB
　 LINE ANGLE
　 FACES FORWARD

☐ INCISAL EDGES OUTLINED BY LINE ANGLES

☐ _____

EMERGENCE CONTOUR

☐ STRAIGHT or CONCAVE
☐ FOLLOW TISSUE MODEL
☐ NO BULGE AT MARGIN
☐ ALL SPACES CLOSED

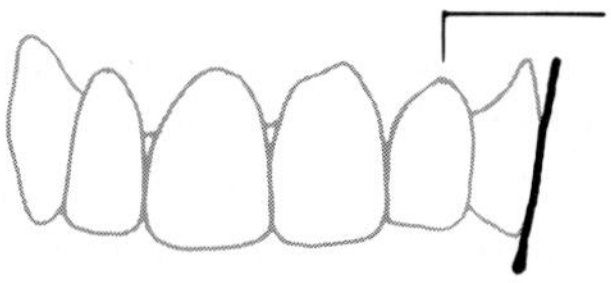

☐ TRIGONAL SHAPE
　 ON PONTICS
☐ GINGIVAL MARGIN
　 SAME AS TEMPS
☐ CUSPID PROFILE

LABIAL CONTOUR

☐ ALIGNED WITH
　 ALVEOLAR CONTOUR

☐ 2 PLANES FOR
　 LABIAL CONTOUR

☐ COPY TEMPS

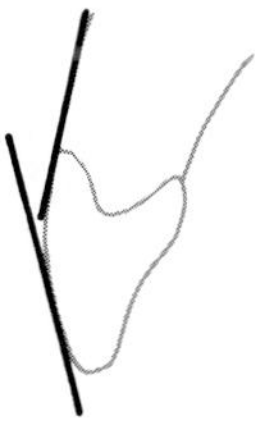

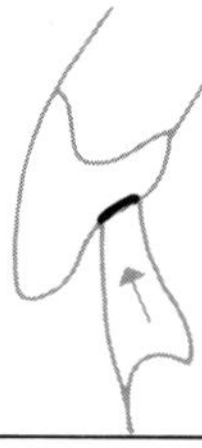

☐ DEFINITE STOP
　 FOR LOWER ANTERIORS

☐ NO CONTACT

☐ SPECIAL
　 INSTRUCTIONS

☐ SHADE
　 INSTRUCTIONS

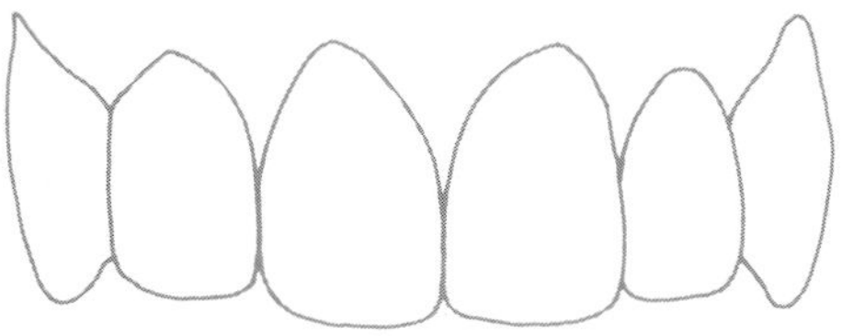

☐ CHECK CONTACTS ON SOLID MODEL

Fig. 18-40. Esthetic and restorative check list for upper anterior teeth. (Available from Center for Advanced Dental Study, Suite 1109, 111 Second Ave., N.E., St. Petersburg, FL 33701; see also p. 318.)

Relationships of anterior teeth to solving problems of occlusion

In the analysis of occlusal problems the importance of the anterior teeth is second only to centric relation. After the acceptability of the temporomandibular articulation is confirmed, the relationship between the upper and lower anterior teeth is always the first concern to be studied.

In every occlusal analysis, it must be remembered that the anterior guidance is a determinant of posterior occlusion and thus must itself be confirmed before posterior occlusal decisions can be made in complete detail.

Regardless of how complicated an occlusal problem may appear, it can generally be solved with minimal complications if you can establish stable holding contacts in centric relation on all the anterior teeth. That relationship is the critical starting point for occlusions, and until that starting point is correctly located, you are not ready to proceed with any further decisions about the occlusal relationship.

If tongue or lip habits prevent the anterior teeth from contacting in centric relation, that must be known and accounted for, but in the absence of unbreakable habit patterns that keep the upper and lower anterior teeth from contacting, the strategy of treatment planning gives first priority to finding the best way for providing stable holding contacts on each anterior tooth. The second priority is to determine the correct incisal edge position so that the full range of anterior guidance can be worked out in harmony with the envelope of function and the neutral zone.

Every aspect of treatment planning for occlusal stability relates in some manner to these determinations regarding the anterior teeth. In the chapters on problem solving, notice how consistently the resolution of various problems depends on first solving the problems of disharmony of the anterior teeth.

The procedures outlined for *determining* the contour and position of anterior teeth are the same procedures to use for any restorative patient if the position of the incisal edges is to be changed or is unknown.

The procedures used for *communicating* contour and position must be clear enough to eliminate any and all guesswork on the part of the technician. The esthetic and restorative check list (Fig. 18-40) serves that purpose quite well.

If the temporomandibular articulation is acceptable and the anterior guidance is correct, you are ready to proceed with completing the restorative needs on the posterior teeth.

19

Determining the type of posterior occlusal contours

There are three basic decisions to make regarding the design of posterior occlusal contours:

1. Selection of the type of centric relation contacts
2. Determination of the type and distribution of contact in lateral excursions
3. Determination of how to provide stability to the occlusal form

For each of the preceeding decisions, we have several options from which to choose. Because there are many different arch-to-arch relationships, we must sometimes vary from standardized tooth contours. *There is no one type of occlusal form that is optimum for all patients.* Nor is there only one type of occlusal form that is correct. There are several ways to satisfy all the requirements for stability without sacrificing function. So even if stereotyped occlusal contours may work well for most patients, the varied problems of stress associated with sick mouths can be solved better by flexibility of form that enables us to vary the direction and distribution of forces. Rather than designing occlusal surfaces on the basis of what they *look* like, we should instead approach each occlusal surface design to definitively accomplish specific effects.

For achieving functional efficiency with stability, the critical objectives of posterior occlusal contours are as follows:

1. Multiple equal-intensity contacts on each tooth in centric relation at the correct vertical
2. Occlusal forces directed parallel to the long axis of each tooth
3. Noninterference with any border path of the condyles or the anterior guidance

Posterior teeth should not interfere either with the centric relation position of the condyles or with any contact of the anterior teeth in protrusive or lateral excursions. This means that when the mandible moves forward, only the anterior teeth should be in contact. The anterior teeth should also disclude all the posterior teeth on the nonworking side. Posterior teeth on the working side *may* contact in group function with the anterior teeth but rarely do. In most healthy occlusions the only contact on posterior teeth is in centric relation. As soon as the mandible moves in any direction, all the posterior teeth are discluded, but that decision should be made on an individual basis.

In the design of occlusal contours, the first decision is where to locate each of the multiple contacts that meet the opposing teeth when the mandible is in centric relation. These decisions are determined when each holding contact is related to how it would direct the occlusal forces. Teeth can withstand tremendous force if the force is directed up or down

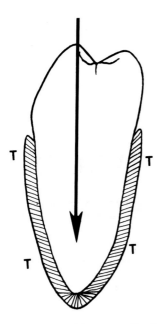

Fig. 19-1. When occlusal forces are directed axially, all the periodontal fibers (except at the apex) are in a state of tension, *T*. Thus forces are resisted equally by fibers around the root.

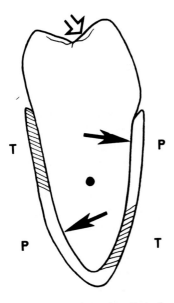

Fig. 19-2. Lateral forces have the effect of rotating the tooth around a pivotal point within the suspended root. This results in a combination of pressure areas and a reduction of tensive resistance by approximately half the periodontal fibers.

the long axis of each tooth because when force is directed parallel to the long axis it is uniformly resisted by all of the supporting periodontal ligaments except those at the apex (Fig. 19-1). If forces are misdirected laterally, the tooth loses the support of about half of the ligaments that are compressed and puts almost the entire load on the half under tension (Fig. 19-2). So the starting point in designing occlusal contours is to shape and locate the centric contacts so that the forces are directed as nearly parallel as possible to the long axis of both upper and lower teeth.

There are many ways to design occlusal contours if direction of forces in centric relation were the only consideration. A perfectly flat occlusal surface contacting another flat surface could be made to fulfill this first requirement, but it would not be a very good design for penetrating or grinding fibrous foods. Proper placement of a sharp cusp against a flat surface could penetrate foods easily and still direct the forces correctly, but a single sharp cusp against a flat surface might lack resistance to the lateral forces that come from the cheeks versus the tongue. The addition of more contacts seems to be an aid to the requirement of occlusal stability though it is unlikely that any kind of occlusal contour is capable of stabilizing posterior teeth if they are not in horizontal harmony with the neutral zone.

The posterior teeth must do more than penetrate food; they must also be capable of crushing and grinding it. To fulfill these roles, they must be able to work one surface against another in enough proximity to masticate efficiently. To accomplish this, the sharp cusps are broadened at the base and rounded at the tips. The flat surfaces are changed to fossae, and the walls of the fossae are curved and angled to relate to the lateral movements of the mandible as guided by the lower anterior teeth against the lingual surfaces of the upper anterior teeth. Blades are made to emanate from the lower buccal cusps to function in reasonable closeness to the upper inclines.

Our thinking has changed somewhat regarding how closely the lower cusps should function in relation to upper inclines. We once believed a near miss was essential for function, making it mandatory for all inclines to be precisely related to border paths of the mandible. This does not appear to be the case. Patients with fairly flat occlusal contours seem to function as well with a steep anterior guidance that prohibits proximation of cusps in excursive movements. The one essential factor that relates to whether patients are content with function seems to be the number of tooth contacts in centric relation. If a patient complains of inability to masticate properly, we invariably find a lack of tooth contacts in centric relation. This is tested by whether or not a Mylar strip is held tightly by the teeth at the closed position. If centric relation contacts can be reestablished, the patients complaints are almost always satisfied, regardless of how close or how far apart the cusp inclines approximate each other during excursions.

Nevertheless, since it is such a practical matter to restore occlusions so that their fossae walls do relate to the lateral function dictated by the anterior guidance, it is logical to give that benefit to most occlusions that must be restored. It is not practical however for occlusions with very steep anterior guidances because such an occlusal scheme would require fossae that are too deep to be self-cleaning.

In selecting which option to use regarding occlusal contour, we should first determine the desired effect. If the same effect can be accomplished in more than one way, the selection of which option to use would be logically made on the basis of which option can be achieved in the most practical way. We will keep our primary focus on the effect we must achieve and allow the operator to choose the method that is most practical to use on his or her own terms. I will start with defining the choices for centric relation contacts.

TYPES OF CENTRIC HOLDING CONTACTS

There are three basic ways by which centric relation contact is usually established on restorations:

1. Surface-to-surface contact
2. Tripod contact
3. Cusp tip-to-fossa contact

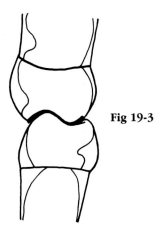

Fig 19-3

Surface-to-surface contact (Fig. 19-3). We refer to this as "mashed-potato occlusion." It is the form that results if the articulator is simply closed together when the wax on the dies is soft. There is never any valid reason for using this type of contact. It is stressful and it produces lateral interferences in anything other than near-vertical chop-chop function.

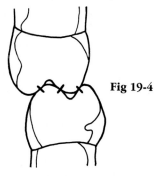

Fig 19-4

Tripod contact (Fig. 19-4). In tripod contact the tip of the cusp never touches the opposing tooth. Instead, contact is made on the sides of the cusps that are convexly shaped. Three points are selected from the sides of the cusps, and each point in turn is made to contact the side of the opposing fossa. Contacts of the stamp cusps must be made at the brim of the fossa wall so that all posterior teeth can disengage from any contact immediately upon leaving centric relation. Lateral and protrusive disclusion of posterior teeth is essential whenever tripod contact is used because convex lower cusps cannot follow normally concave border pathways against upper teeth, which are also convex. This is especially true when the contacts are on the *sides* of convex cusps. Consequently, if the lateral anterior guidance starts with a near-horizontal path and if rest closure function dictates the need for a "long centric," it would be necessary to use flatter occlusal surfaces and wider cusp tips with the contacts distributed more on the tips than on the sides of the cusps. Fossa contacts have to be more on ridges and fossa brims than on the walls of the fossa. Some advocates of tripodism do recommend this.

When the working-side condyle translates laterally on a horizontal plane and the lateral anterior guidance permits the front end of the mandible to also move laterally on a horizontal plane before curving down a concave pathway, there is no way to make tripod contact work if the contacts are on the sides of convex cusps. Allowing the cusps to move through grooves is not practical because contacts aligned on the sides of the cusps to facilitate travel through a straight lateral pathway groove would interfere with a slightly protrusive lateral pathway. There is no way to align the contacts around the sides of the cusps to permit the full range of lateral and protrusive pathways if the anterior guidance starts out with horizontal paths. This is important to understand because many periodontally involved mouths are best served by such concave anterior guidances.

If tripod contact is to be used with concave anterior guidances, the contacts must be confined to the tip of broad flat cusps. A tripodism of sorts can be achieved if you keep the tips of the cusps wider than the grooves and fossae that they rest against or pass over. This type of pseudotripodism can even be made to function in lateral excursions if the upper cusp inclines are matched to the concave border pathways of the mandible. If there is any horizontal movement of the mandible in lateral and protrusive excursions, convex surfaces simply cannot function against the *sides* of other convex surfaces without creating stressful interferences.

Tripod contact is difficult to accomplish, but it can be done as long as the anterior teeth are capable of discluding the posterior teeth in all excursions. For patients whose functional movements, anterior periodontal support, arch relation, and tooth position are best served by posterior disclusion, tripod contact can be very comfortable, functional, and beautiful to behold.

Tripod contact should *not* be used when lateral stress distribution is best served by including posterior teeth into group function to help out weak or missing anterior teeth or when the arch relationship does not permit the anterior guidance to do its job.

With tripod contact, any degree of shifting of any tooth produces an *incline interference.* Any wear on a centric contact leaves the remaining centric stops for that cusp to be on inclines. Since upper and lower arches are usually restored together, even a minute error in recording or transferring centric relation causes loss of tripodism on all teeth.

Tripod contact is extremely difficult or impossible to equilibrate without losing tripodism and ending up with contacts on inclines. However, this is mostly academic because usually enough counteracting inclines can be kept in contact to maintain reasonably good direction of force.

If tripod contact is so difficult to achieve and has so many limitations, why is it used? Probably the main reason for the popularity of tripodism is the impression that it is so stable if it is properly done. This certainly has been one of the main reasons for advocating its use. However, there is no scientific evidence to show that tripod contact is more stable than proper tip-to-fossa contact. Development of "slides" is common, even among the most meticulous operators.

It should be brought out that some of the real advocates of tripod contact are among the most meticulous operators in our profession. The precise attention that they give to every detail is probably far more responsible for their success than the tripod contact. A precisely recorded centric relation will make the majority of patients very happy even if little else is accomplished, and eccentric disclusion of posterior teeth is always better than posterior interference in excursions. Combined with the clinical observation that most patients can also function quite well with excursive disclusion of the posterior teeth, one can readily see why there are many patients who are very happy with their tripod-contact occlusions.

Nevertheless, I believe that there are no actual *indications* for tripod contact. Although it can be used successfully in a large number of patients, it has definite limitations in many others. It offers no advantages over proper cusp tip-to-fossa contact, and since it is more difficult to achieve, is hard to adjust, and is limited in its use, we would probably do well to thoughtfully evaluate its practicality.

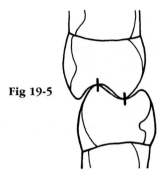

Fig 19-5

Cusp tip-to-fossa contact (Fig. 19-5). If cusp tips are properly located in the most advantageous fossae, this type of occlusion offers excellent function and stability with the flexibility to choose any degree of distribution of lateral forces that is warranted. It is the easiest occlusion to equilibrate. Resistance to wear is excellent, since the centric stops are on the cusp tips, whereas in working excursions, contact is on the sides of the cusp tips as they travel along the inclines of the opposing teeth. If disclusion of any tooth is desired in any eccentric excursion, it is accomplished easily by adjustment of the fossa inclines without disturbing the centric holding contacts.

With cusp tip-to-fossa contact, it is not necessary to restore upper and lower teeth together. In fact, there is no advantage whatsoever to preparing both arches together. Location of cusp tips can be determined with extreme accuracy against unprepared teeth, and cusp height and fossa contours can be established one arch at a time with complete assurance that the contours will be correct.

Location of cusp tip-to-fossa contacts is decided according to the best interest of each tooth on the basis of direction of forces as near parallel to the long axis of each tooth as possible and stability without interference to eccentric movements.

Cusp tip-to-fossa contact is not a by-product of any specific technique. It serves the goal of

function rather than form. It can be accomplished with the aid of gnathologic instrumentation, functional path procedures, or a myriad of other instrumentation techniques. The one essential for accomplishing it correctly is an understanding of what we are after. Properly done, it can be beautiful as well as functional and stable.

VARIATIONS OF POSTERIOR CONTACT IN LATERAL EXCURSIONS

As the mandible moves laterally, the lower posterior teeth leave their centric contact with the upper teeth and travel sideways down a path dictated by the condyles in the back and by the lateral anterior guidance in the front. Each lower posterior tooth is limited to these border pathways, meaning that they cannot follow a path from centric relation that is any flatter or more concave than the condyles and the lateral anterior guidance permit.

As the lower posterior teeth follow this lateral border pathway, there are several options regarding their contact with the upper tooth inclines. They may maintain contact with upper teeth, or the cusp inclines may be contoured so that there is no contact at all between any of the back teeth in any jaw position except centric relation. There may be variations in numbers of teeth in lateral contact or in the length of the incline contacts. The reason for bringing any teeth into lateral function is to distribute stress and wear over more teeth. Whether the distribution is beneficial depends on how well it is accomplished and whether it is needed.

To make meaningful judgments about the distribution of lateral stress, we must first distinguish the difference between the rotating condyle and the orbiting condyle. Each side has physical characteristics that are important to understand before an occlusal scheme can be planned with any degree of dependability. In discussing lateral excursions I divide the movements accordingly into working-side occlusion and nonfunctioning-side occlusion (also referred to as the balancing side).

Working-side occlusion refers to the contact relationship of lower teeth to upper teeth on the side of the rotating condyle. The side toward which the mandible moves is the working side. The condyle on the working side can be braced against bone or ligament throughout the working excursion, and so it is possible and quite practical to accurately record and restore the posterior teeth to precise working-side border movement contacts.

Nonfunctioning-side occlusion is the side of the orbiting condyle. When the condyle leaves its braced position and slides forward down the slippery incline of the eminentia, it is no longer solidly fixed against the unyielding bone and ligament. Rather, it can move up a little, since the mandible bends slightly under firm muscle pressure. Consequently, tooth contact during nonfunctioning-side excursions should not be allowed. Because of the flexibility of the mandible, it would not be possible to harmonize occlusal contours to all the variations resulting from the differences in muscle force from light to heavy. Hence we have the rule: *whenever lower teeth move toward the tongue, they should not contact.*

The job of discluding the nonfunctioning side is always the responsibility of the working side. *How* the working side discludes the nonfunctioning side is an important decision that must be made for each individual patient. While the teeth on the working side are discluding the teeth on the nonfunctioning side, they must also function as cutters, holders, and grinders.

The dentist must decide how all this is done by selecting one of the following choices for working-side occlusion:

1. Group function
2. Partial group function
3. Posterior disclusion

None of these choices is optimum for all cases. Selecting the one that offers the most advantages for each different patient is just good treatment planning.

Group function refers to the distribution of lateral forces to a group of teeth rather than protecting those teeth from contact in function by assigning all the forces to one particular tooth.

To paraphrase a law of physics—the more teeth that carry the load, the less load any one tooth must carry. We must decide which teeth are capable of carrying how much load and assign the load accordingly. As an example, we would not use a loose cuspid with little bone support to protect strong posterior teeth from contacting in a working excursion. Instead, we would allow the posterior teeth to *share* the load by bringing them into group function with the cuspid and the other front teeth on that side.

Group function of the working side is indicated whenever the arch relationship does not allow the anterior guidance to do its job of discluding the nonfunctioning side. The anterior guidance cannot do its job in the following situations:

1. Class II occlusions with extreme overjet
2. Class III occlusions when all lower anterior teeth are outside of the upper anterior teeth
3. Some end-to-end bites
4. Anterior open bite cases

When you are using posterior group function, the following rule applies: *contacting inclines must be perfectly harmonized to border movements of the condyles and the anterior guidance.* Convex-to-convex contacts cannot be used to accomplish this.

Partial group function refers to allowing some of the posterior teeth to share the load in excursions whereas others contact only in centric relation. As an example, a second molar may be very firm vertically but be hypermobile buccolingually. Such a tooth should touch only in centric relation and be discluded immediately by the other teeth in excursions. A very strong first premolar may work with a moderately strong cuspid and incisors to disclude a weak second premolar and molars.

Because of arch relationships, a first and second molar may be the only source of disclusion for balancing-side contact. Group function had better be *perfectly* harmonized to border movements in such a case, but it can be done successfully. Anterior teeth with postorthodontic root resorption or congenitally poor crown-root ratios should sometimes be harmonized to group function with the working side.

Whether any tooth should share the lateral stresses should be decided on the basis of each tooth's resistance to lateral stress. There is no good reason why such a decision cannot be made on a tooth-by-tooth basis. If a tooth is weak laterally, it should contact in centric relation only. If a tooth is firm and clinical judgment says that it would be beneficial to the other teeth to let that tooth share the lateral stress and wear, that is what should be done.

Some dentists object to ever having posterior teeth contact in lateral excursions. Strenuous objection to group function usually comes from having had problems with it. Because of the resultant problems, objectors may think that group function is actually harmful. I want to make it clear that problems with group function result from improper harmony of the contacting inclines. Attempts at group function with convex inclines, as an example, are invitations to hypermobility. Some patients do change their pattern of function to conform to the restrictive inclines of convex cusps, but it is unpredictable at best. For group function to be effective in reducing stress, the cusp inclines must be in perfect harmony with the lateral border movements of the jaw. Posterior cusp inclines that are not contoured to match the mandibular border movements are discluded if the inclines are opened out too much, or they interfere if any part of the incline is steeper than the corresponding part of the lateral jaw movement. Incline interferences on posterior teeth get progressively more stressful as they get closer to the condyle fulcrum, so that a slight interference on a second molar would probably be more stressful than a more noticeable interference on a cuspid. If this rule of stress distribution is understood, it is quite practical to distribute lateral stress over some or all of the posterior teeth. It can be done effectively by restorative means and by occlusal adjustments of the natural teeth.

Posterior disclusion refers to no contact on any posterior teeth in any position but centric relation. It can be accomplished easily with cusp tip-to-fossa morphology. It *must* be accomplished with tripod or surface-to-surface morphology to prevent lateral interferences in any case with centric contact on inclines that are steeper than the lateral border movements of the mandible. It occurs automatically if tripod contacts are distributed on the tips of broad flat cusps or the lateral guidance angle is steeper than the contacting posterior surfaces, or both conditions.

In healthy mouths or in mouths with normally strong anterior teeth, it is an excellent occlusion, since normal anterior teeth are quite capable of carrying the whole excursive load, particularly if they are in harmony with functional border movements.

Posterior disclusion in all jaw positions except centric relation is the most desirable occlusion whenever it can be achieved by an acceptable anterior guidance. Even some weakened anterior teeth may actually be stressed less by separation of the posterior teeth from contact in excursions. The reason

for this phenomenon is the effect that posterior disclusion has on the contractive force of the elevator muscles. The moment complete posterior disclusion occurs in protrusive, the masseter muscle stops contracting, the internal pterygoid muscle stops contracting, and the temporalis muscle contraction is reduced. In lateral excursions, internal pterygoid contraction controls the balancing side.

There are two methods of accomplishing posterior disclusion:

1. The anterior guidance is harmonized to functional border movements *first* and then the lateral inclines of the posterior teeth are opened up so that they are discluded by a correct anterior guidance.
2. The posterior teeth are built first and then discluded by restriction of the anterior guidance. This method is backward. Anterior guidance is a proper *determinant* of posterior occlusal form and thus should be done first. When posterior occlusal form determines the anterior guidance, the correctness of the anterior guidance is a product of chance.

Posterior disclusion can be achieved by two different types of anterior guidance: anterior group function and cuspid protected occlusion. Neither is applicable for all cases.

Anterior group function is the most practical method for discluding the posterior teeth when arch relationships and tooth alignment permit it. Anterior group function is beneficial in three ways:

1. It distributes wear over more teeth.
2. It distributes the stresses to more teeth.
3. It distributes stress to teeth that are progressively farther from the condyle fulcrum.

Any one of these considerations would be reason enough to recommend anterior group function, but in addition to its effect on stress and wear, anterior group function is extremely comfortable and efficient. It improves the efficiency of incising movements by providing lateral as well as protrusive shearing contacts.

Despite its advantages, anterior group function is not applicable in all cases. Some arch relationships do not permit the incisors to contact in lateral excursions. Concave anterior guidances permit group function, whereas convex lateral guidances make it difficult to accomplish. When it is impractical to distribute the lateral guidance stresses over several teeth, disclusion of the posterior teeth can be accomplished by use of the cuspids in one form or another of cuspid-protected occlusion.

Cuspid-protected occlusion refers to disclusion by the cuspids of all other teeth in lateral excursions. It usually serves as the cornerstone of what is called *mutually protected occlusion*. Mutually protected occlusion has been defined in several ways, but the usual connotation refers to an occlusal arrangement in which the posterior teeth contact in centric relation only, the incisors are the only teeth contacting in protrusion, and the cuspids are the only teeth contacting in lateral excursion. It is an ideal relationship for some patients, is tolerated by some, and is detrimental to others. Clinical judgment should be developed so that cuspid-protected occlusion is used only when it offers advantages over other occlusal arrangements.

In cuspid-protected occlusion, all lateral stresses must be resisted solely by the cuspid. Therefore the predominant prerequisite for its use is the capability of the cuspid to withstand the entire lateral stress load without any help from other teeth.

It may seem unlikely that any one tooth could have enough stability to carry such a load over a long period of time without becoming subjected to excessive wear or hypermobility. The fact is that the lateral stresses are minimal if the lingual contours are in harmony with the functional border movements. In other words, lateral stress becomes insignificant if the mandible functions normally within the lingual inclines of the upper cuspids.

It is impossible to exert excessive stresses against the cuspids in centric relation because the posterior teeth also resist the stresses in that position, if the occlusion is correct.

In natural cuspid-protected occlusions, the pattern of function is rather vertical, and so the mandible does not use lateral movements that would subject the cuspids to stress in that direction either.

The cuspids actually assume the role more as a guidance that actuates vertical function rather than as a resistor to lateral stress. Any attempt at lateral movement is felt by the pressoreceptors around the cuspids. *Within limits,* these exquisitely sensitive nerve endings protect the cuspids against too much lateral stress by redirecting the muscles to more vertical function. As long as the pressoreceptors can keep the muscles programmed to a vertical envelope of function, there is insufficient lateral stress generated to harm the cuspids.

Some clinicians have reported that the cuspids have the distinction of being protected by a greater number of pressoreceptor nerve endings than is found around any other tooth. This alleged density of proprioceptors is supposed to impart a unique capacity to the cuspid to redirect any functional pattern that would be destructive. If, for example, a horizontal chewing cycle would exert too much lateral stress against the cuspids, their special proprioceptive protectors would simply change the chewing cycle to a vertical, chop-chop function rather than let harm come to the cuspids or their supporting structures.

It is easy to see why such a concept would be popular. If the cuspids really did have the capacity to change functional movements from horizontal to vertical, it would eliminate much need for concern with occlusal morphology. Good centric contacts would be all that would be necessary for posterior teeth, since mandibular movements could be restricted by changing the cuspids to permit vertical opening and closing only. Some advocates of cuspid-protected occlusion actually subscribe to such a theory, but further research has failed to substantiate the report that there are more proprioceptors around the cuspids than there are around other teeth. Furthermore, clinical results over a period of time have shown that the cuspid, just like other teeth, is also subject to the usual problems of excessive lateral stress if it interferes with normal functional movements. Although the cuspids do have the benefit of normal proprioceptive protection, there does not appear to be any valid support for the cuspid-protection theory on the basis of special proprioceptive capacity to radically alter habitual patterns of function.

However, there are other valid reasons why cuspid-protected occlusion works well for many patients. The cuspids have extremely good crown-root ratios, and their long fluted roots are in some of the densest bone of the alveolar process. Furthermore, their position in the arch, far from the fulcrum, makes it more difficult to stress them. In short, they are very strong teeth. If their upper lingual inclines are in harmony with the envelope of function, they are usually quite capable of withstanding lateral stresses without help from other teeth.

Many patients have natural cuspid protection, and if the cuspids are firm and the occlusion is comfortable, I believe it should be maintained, even if the teeth must be restored.

The natural cuspid-protected mouth is easily distinguished by convex or very steep lingual inclines on the upper cuspids. The patient usually cannot move the jaw laterally, even when asked to do so. The chewing cycle is a vertical chop-chop. The patient has never functioned laterally and has no need for more than minimal lateral pressure on the closing stroke. If posterior tooth form were brought into group function with such steep inclines, even the slightest shifting of a posterior tooth could subject it to extreme lateral stress because it would be in interference to the powerful closing stroke. The vector of force against a steep incline interference is nearly horizontal and the stress is further amplified as it gets closer to the condyle. In near-vertical envelopes of function it is usually better to let the posterior teeth be discluded by the cuspids if the cuspid protection is natural and if the cuspids are firm. If the mouth requires extensive restorative treatment and minimal changes to the cuspids would affect anterior group function without noticeably altering the chewing cycle, it would be logical to make that change for the advantages that could be gained. However, changing from cuspid protection to anterior group function is contraindicated if it would require a major change in the envelope of function or extensive reduction of sound lingual enamel.

For simplicity, cuspid protection can be divided into two categories:

1. Posterior disclusion by cuspid inclines that are *in harmony with functional border movements*
2. Posterior disclusion by cuspid inclines that *restrict mandibular movements* within habitual functional border movements

Whether a patient functions normally in vertical chop-chop motions or wide horizontal strokes, it will still be possible to harmonize cuspid inclines. If the harmonized cuspid inclines are the discluding factor for all posterior teeth in lateral excursion, it may be considered a form of cuspid-protected occlusion. Because of their arch form or tooth arrangement, many patients will be served best by this type of occlusion.

Restrictive cuspid protection is usually used as an attempt to avoid stressful posterior contact in lateral excursion by forcing the patient into a changed pattern of function. It may result in a reduction of hypermobility of posterior teeth that have been under stress, but then so will proper posterior occlusal form. Restrictive cuspid protection falls far short of the immediate comfort that patients feel with a harmonious anterior guidance. They must get used to the restrictive guidance. Although some patients will change their functional patterns when the cuspids get sore enough to force them into a chop-chop bite, it is an unnecessary irritation to mouth comfort, and the long-term maintainability of such occlusal relationships is very unpredictable. If the cuspids are stressed into lateral movement, they are no longer able to protect the posterior inclines.

It should be reemphasized that from the standpoint of comfort many patients can tolerate a change to the more vertical function of a steeper cuspid rise. The problem is not so much one of comfort as it is of long-term stability. It is far better, whenever practical, to get posterior disclusion from an anterior guidance that is in harmony with the patient's envelope of function.

SELECTING OCCLUSAL FORM FOR STABILITY

Assuming that cusp-fossae relationships are correctly placed for ideal *direction* of stress, we still must make decisions regarding the number of contacting cusps that are needed for maximum stability under differing conditions. We generally have four basic types to choose from in normal arch relationships:

TYPE **1.** *Lower buccal cusps contact upper fossae. There are no other centric contacts* (Fig. 19-6). *Working-side excursive function is limited to the lingual inclines of upper buccal cusps.*

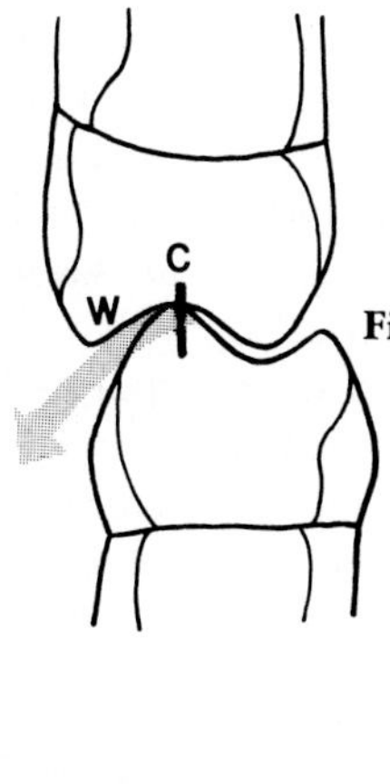

Fig. 19-6

If desired, continuous contact can be maintained in working excursions on the lingual incline of the upper buccal cusps, or if disclusion of posterior teeth is desired, it can be easily accomplished by modification of the upper inclines. Disclusion of balancing inclines can be easily accomplished.

This type of occlusal relationship can be very comfortable and can be made to function in a completely satisfactory manner. It is the easiest contour to fabricate when one is restoring posterior teeth because cusp-fossae angles on the lower are not critical. If functionally generated path procedures are used, the upper working inclines are formed automatically and the upper lingual cusps are wiped away if lower cusp-fossae angles are too steep.

The only apparent disadvantage to this type of occlusal relationship is its lack of dependable buccolingual stability. Pressure from the tongue can tilt the teeth toward the buccal with very little resistance. Because it lacks the stability that upper lingual cusp contact would give it, more follow-up occlusal adjustment is usually required than is necessary with more stable occlusal contours.

In periodontal prostheses utilizing around-the-arch splinting, buccolingual stabilization is ensured by the splinting itself. It is not necessary to stabilize the teeth with upper lingual cusp centric holding contacts. Lower buccal cusp contact is sufficient to satisfy all the needs of the splinted patient. Working excursion contact is an elective that can be used when needed for disclusion of the nonfunctioning side. From the standpoint of either function or comfort, patients seem to be just as happy with only contact of the lower buccal cusp as they are with more elaborate occlusal schemes. Since it is the easiest occlusal form to accomplish and the easiest to adjust, it is an acceptable choice of occlusal form whenever buccolingual stability has been assured by splinting.

TYPE 2. *Centric contact on the tips of lower buccal cusps and upper lingual cusps* (Fig. 19-7). *Working-side excursive function is limited to the lingual inclines of the upper buccal cusps. There is no excursive function on any lower incline.*

The addition of the upper lingual cusps as centric holding contacts contributes greatly to the stability of the posterior teeth. Lateral stress toward the buccal is resisted by the contact of the upper lingual cusps against the lower fossae. Stress toward the lingual is re-

sisted by the lower buccal cusps against the upper fossae. Furthermore, the vector of force against the cusp tip-to-fossae contacts is directed toward the long axis when the teeth are stressed laterally, because lateral movement takes place by rotation of the tooth around a point within the root.

Lateral excursion contact is limited to the lingual incline of upper buccal cusps, the same as in type 1. This presents no problem of lateral stress as long as the upper inclines are in perfect harmony with lateral border movements. The return to multiple cusp-holding contacts in each centric closure has sufficient stabilizing effect for maintenance of the occlusion within practical limits. Working incline contact can be discluded when desired by modification of upper inclines.

If the upper lingual cusp is to be used as a holding contact in centric, the inclines of the lower fossae must not be steeper than the lateral anterior guidance. If the upper lingual cusp is to be discluded in all lateral movements, the lower fossae inclines must be flatter than the lateral anterior guidance.

Because lower fossae inclines need only be flatter than lateral anterior guidance inclines, the fabrication of lower occlusal contours is simplified. The lower inclines do not need to be precisely identical to border pathways, since they are to be out of contact in excursions.

Contact in working excursions can be accomplished by use of functionally generated path techniques or any other procedure that accurately records lateral border movements.

From every clinical standpoint, the performance of this type of occlusal contour is acceptable. It is comfortable and functional, and because it fulfills all the requirements of good occlusal form and can be accomplished with clinical practicality, it is the type of occlusion for which we strive in unsplinted restorative cases when posterior group function is needed.

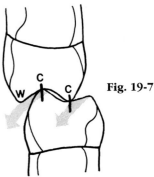

Fig. 19-7

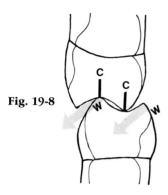

Fig. 19-8

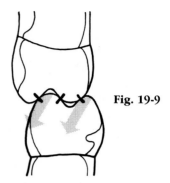

Fig. 19-9

TYPE 3. *Centric contact on tips of lower buccal cusps and upper lingual cusps. Working excursion contact is limited to the lingual incline of upper buccal cusps and buccal incline of lower lingual cusps* (Fig. 19-8).

This type of occlusal contour is identical to type 2 except that the buccal incline of the lower lingual cusp becomes a functioning incline.

There is no clinically discernible advantage in making the upper lingual cusps contact in lateral function. There is no recognizable difference in patient comfort or function, and if there is a difference between either long-term stability or wear, I have been unable to detect it in clinical comparison between types 2 and 3.

The major difference between this type of occlusal form and type 2 is the difficulty of accomplishing it. To bring the upper lingual cusps into working excursion contact, the buccal inclines of the lower lingual cusps must be precisely contoured to the exact lateral border movement of *both* the condyle and the anterior guidance. If the incline is made too flat, it will disclude. If it is made too steep, it will interfere.

Certainly there are methods available to us to record these border movements accurately and to refine the lower inclines to duplicate them, but unless the additional time, effort, and instrumentation produce an improvement in the result, it is time wasted.

Although complexity of fabrication seems to be the only disadvantage of type 3 occlusal form, it is reason enough not to advocate it because the result has no clinical advantage over type 2 occlusal form, which can be fabricated with less complicated and less time-consuming procedures without any reduction in the quality.

TYPE 4. *Tripod contact.*

There are two types of tripod contact: contact on the sides of cusps and the walls of fossae and contacts on the brims of fossae and on top of wide cusp tips.

Contact on the sides of cusps and the walls of fossae (Fig. 19-9). Contact on the sides of the cusps does not permit any lateral or protrusive movement on a horizontal plane; so if the anterior guidance has been flattened even for a short distance from the centric stops to permit a lateral side shift of the mandible, this type of occlusal form will be contraindicated. It is also contraindicated for any patient who requires a "long centric."

It may be used in vertical or near-vertical functional cycles with either cuspid-protected occlusion or anterior-protected occlusion.

In the cases permitting its use, its performance is clinically indistinguishable from type 2 or type 3 occlusions. Like type 3, its disadvantage comes from the difficulty in fabricating it. Tripod contact is the most difficult of all occlusal forms to fabricate.

Centric contact on the brims of fossae and the top of wide cusp tips with no contact in eccentric excursions (Fig. 19-10). This type of tripod contact can be made to function with any type of anterior guidance because it per-

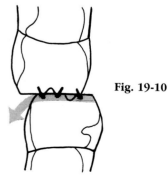

Fig. 19-10

mits horizontal lateral movement without interference. It is automatically discluded by any anterior guidance effect other than flat plane; so it cannot be used when posterior group function is indicated.

Since it is essentiallly a flat occlusal contour and cusp tips do not fit into fossae, it is only necessary to make sure the fossa width is narrower than the width of the cusp tip. Consequently it is not extremely difficult to fabricate. Elaborate fossa and groove contouring can be accomplished as long as the multiple centric contacts are not disturbed. Even though the contacts may stay the same, it is possible to develop very sophisticated contours within the framework of this type of occlusion.

When posterior disclusion is indicated, this type of occlusal form may be used with the same clinical success as type 2 occlusal form that has been modified to disclude. It is purely a matter of dentist preference. Patients will not be able to distinguish between the two forms.

SUMMARY

There are several types of occlusal form that can be used to restore posterior teeth. Whatever contour is selected should be chosen because it:

1. Directs the forces as near parallel as possible to the long axis of each tooth
2. Distributes the lateral stress to maximum advantage in varying situations of periodontal support
3. Provides maximum stability
4. Provides maximum wearability
5. Provides optimum function for gripping, grinding, and crushing

Practicality of fabrication is a factor that should be considered when the type of occlusal form is being selected. If additional time, effort, and expense are required to produce the same clinical result that could be accomplished with greater ease to the patient, the dentist, and the technician, technique orientation has in all probability taken the place of goal orientation.

20

Methods for determining the plane of occlusion

Establishment of a proper plane of occlusion is one of the most misunderstood aspects of restorative dentistry. A review of the purpose of the curve of Spee and the curve of Wilson may be in order before we proceed with posterior restorative procedures. Chapter 7 describes the physiologic rationale for the tooth inclinations that form the curves, but in the simplest of terms an occlusal plane is acceptable if it permits the anterior guidance to do its job. That is a basic goal in any posterior occlusal treatment.

A correct plane of occlusion allows protrusion without posterior interference. It allows noninterfering lateral excursions without loss of function on the working side.

When the mandible is protruded, the anterior guidance and the downward movement of the condyles should disclude all posterior teeth. If the curve of Spee is too concave or too high posteriorly, one or more posterior teeth may interfere in protrusive movement (Fig. 20-1). Likewise an improper curve can cause interferences on the nonfunctioning side because of the protrusive movement of the condyle on that side, or because of an exaggerated curve of Wilson.

There are other considerations that should not be disregarded, but they are secondary in importance to the primary requirement of protrusive and balancing-side disclusion of the posterior teeth. These two requirements can be accomplished with an amazingly wide degree of flexibility as far as the occlusal plane is concerned. This flexibility makes it possible in many patients to satisfy esthetic requirements without having to drastically alter an entire occlusion. Teeth should never be restored unnecessarily simply to conform with an arbitrary predetermined occlusal plane.

It is possible for an occlusal plane to be flat and still fulfill the basic requirements, but if optimum efficiency in function is the goal, the occlusal plane will usually have curvatures to it. Better esthetics is, in most cases, also dependent on the natural curvatures of the occlusal plane, the perfectly flat plane often being the epitome of artificiality. A flat occlusal plane can even be harmful, since it can create stressful crown-root ratios when the curvature of the supporting alveolar bone is not matched to a reasonable degree with the curvature of the occlusal plane.

A severely concave plane of occlusion on the lower arch may function acceptably if it is combined with a steep enough anterior guidance to disclude the posterior teeth in excursions. Appearance is not generally impaired with this combination as long as the level of the occlusal plane is fairly even on both sides.

The occlusal plane problem that is most detrimental to esthetics is the slanted plane,

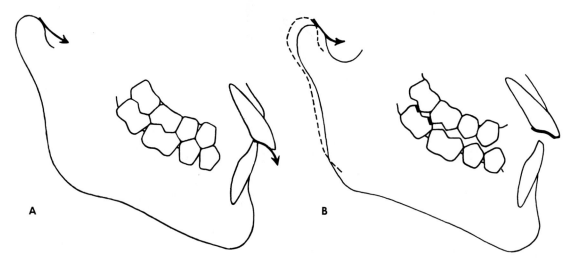

Fig. 20-1. A, Occlusal intercuspation at centric relation jaw position. **B**, Protrusive: posterior teeth separate the anterior teeth. This is indicative of an occlusal plane problem.

which is high on one side and low on the other. In fact, there is probably no single factor of occlusion that is more noticeably unattractive than a slanted plane of occlusion. Leveling of the occlusal plane always starts with the anterior teeth for the following two reasons.

Esthetics. The location of incisal edge position relates to the smile line and determines the incisal plane, which is the anterior starting point for the occlusal plane on each side. For best esthetics, it is an absolute requirement that the incisal plane be parallel with the interpupillary line.

Function. Since the functional acceptability of any occlusal plane is primarily related to letting the anterior guidance do its job, the anterior segments must be organized before we can know how effective the anterior guidance can be in discluding the posterior teeth. The importance of the occlusal plane increases as the steepness of the anterior guidance decreases. The flatter the anterior guidance, the less capable it is of discluding a severely curved occlusal plane.

Examination for occlusal plane problems

An occlusal examination is not complete unless it includes an analysis of the occlusal plane. Simply ask the patient to protrude the mandible. If the anterior teeth are separated by the posterior teeth, there is a problem with the occlusal plane (Fig. 20-2). The problem may be the result of a single misaligned tooth, or it

may be caused by improper curvature or alignment of the entire occlusal plane.

Because the condylar path is so important to protrusive disclusion of the posterior teeth, condylar paths should be recorded at least by a protrusive interocclusal record when an occlusal plane problem exists. The steeper the condylar path is in protrusive, the better able it is to help the anterior guidance disclude the posterior teeth.

When protrusive separation of the anterior teeth is accompanied by severe wear of the upper lingual cusps, there is a probability that bony changes have resulted in flattening of the condyles and the eminence. The resultant flatter condylar path is less capable of helping the anterior guidance and can create critical problems of working out an acceptable occlusal plane. In such cases, the condylar path should be accurately recorded so that its effect on the posterior occlusion can be analyzed along with the anterior guidance. Facebow-mounted diagnostic casts are essential for this analysis.

Correcting occlusal plane problems

There are two basic approaches to solving occlusal plane problems. One involves *leveling or flattening the occlusal plane* so that it can be discluded by the existing anterior guidance, which remains unchanged (Fig. 20-3). The second approach involves *steepening the anterior guidance* so that it can disclude the existing occlusal plane, which remains unchanged (Fig.

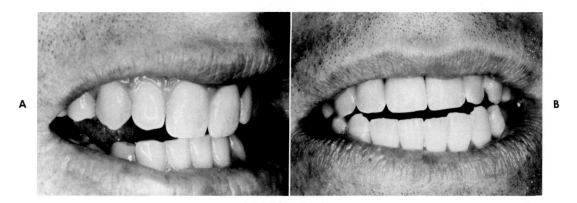

Fig. 20-2. Clinical test for acceptability of the occlusal plane. **A,** Acceptable occlusal plane. Anterior teeth disclude posteriors in protrusive. **B,** Unacceptable occlusal plane. Anterior teeth are separated in protrusive.

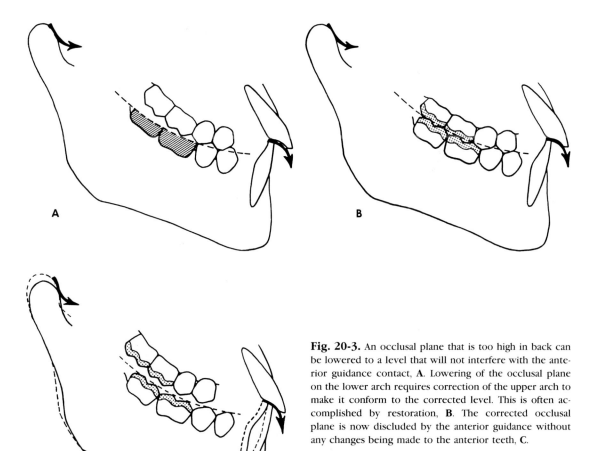

Fig. 20-3. An occlusal plane that is too high in back can be lowered to a level that will not interfere with the anterior guidance contact, **A.** Lowering of the occlusal plane on the lower arch requires correction of the upper arch to make it conform to the corrected level. This is often accomplished by restoration, **B.** The corrected occlusal plane is now discluded by the anterior guidance without any changes being made to the anterior teeth, **C.**

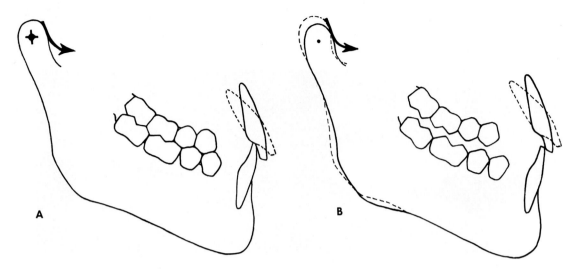

Fig. 20-4. Disclusion of the posterior teeth in protrusive may also be accomplished by steepening the anterior guidance, **A**. If the steeper guidance can be achieved without interfering with neutral zone or function jaw movements, it may be the best choice of treatment, **B**.

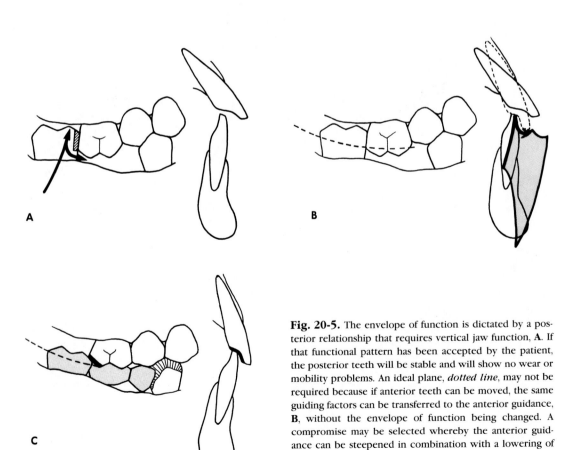

Fig. 20-5. The envelope of function is dictated by a posterior relationship that requires vertical jaw function, **A**. If that functional pattern has been accepted by the patient, the posterior teeth will be stable and will show no wear or mobility problems. An ideal plane, *dotted line*, may not be required because if anterior teeth can be moved, the same guiding factors can be transferred to the anterior guidance, **B**, without the envelope of function being changed. A compromise may be selected whereby the anterior guidance can be steepened in combination with a lowering of the occlusal plane in back and reduction of posterior protrusive interferences, **C**.

20-4). There is obviously a compromise alternative that combines both a steepening of the anterior guidance with alteration of the occlusal plane. Several considerations need to be understood before there is a decision on which approach to take on any given patient.

Whether the anterior guidance should be steepened depends on four factors:

1. Envelope of function
2. Arch-to-arch relationships
3. Esthetic factors
4. Periodontal support

The envelope of function is the principal determinant of the anterior guidance; so any steepening of the anterior guidance can result in restriction of the established pattern of function. However, when occlusal-plane problems separate the anterior teeth in protrusive, it is often possible to eliminate the posterior interferences by selective grinding so that anterior contact can be maintained from centric relation forward to the incisal edge-to-edge position. This is most often possible to accomplish without any major changes in the anterior guidance.

In some instances, however, changes to the posterior occlusion may be extensive enough to require posterior restorations in order to preserve the existing anterior guidance. This is an easier decision to make if extensive restoration of the posterior segments is needed anyway for other reasons. In mouths that have no other need for posterior restorations, orthodontic treatment should be considered to correct the occlusal plane rather than alter a potentially favorable anterior relationship.

Steepening the anterior guidance does not always restrict the envelope of function. *Posterior* tooth alignment can prevent the mandible from horizontal function and thus be the limiting factor that dictates verticalized function even though the anterior teeth are not in contact. In such cases, steepening the anterior guidance may simply transfer the guiding inclines from the posterior teeth to the anterior teeth without altering the envelope of function (Fig. 20-5).

When this procedure is done, even slight modification of the occlusal plane can result in disclusion of the posterior teeth in excursions.

The envelope of function should be evaluated in every case before extensive changes in the occlusal plane are recommended. Even though the occlusal plane prevents the anterior guidance from discluding posterior teeth in protrusion, a problem may not exist if the jaw has no protrusive movement as part of its functional envelope. Some patients with locked-in occlusions do not use protrusive movements. If they function solely in a chop-chop verticalized pattern, there is no need to disclude the posterior teeth in jaw relationships that are never used. Analyzing the teeth for signs of instability should make it evident if there is no horizontal component of function. There is rarely a functional occlusal plane problem in vertically restricted function if all the teeth are stable. If there is a need for esthetic improvement in such patients, the anterior guidance can generally be altered all the way to verticalized function with no ill effects, and the occlusal plane can be altered to improve the appearance with almost no concern that it will interfere with the anterior teeth.

Certain arch-to-arch relationships may make restorative alteration of the anterior guidance contraindicated. If the anterior teeth are in a stable relationship with strong tongue or lip pressures related to an anterior open bite or a severe overjet, it may create instability if the teeth are moved or restored to contact. The occlusal plane becomes a critical factor in some of those patients because posterior disclusion must be achieved off the flatter surfaces of the farthest forward teeth that can contact in centric relation. In such conditions, it is particularly important that the occlusal plane is low enough in the back to be discluded by the relatively flat anterior guidance.

In the resolution of arch-malrelationship problems the occlusal plane is always a factor to be considered. The less the anterior guidance is able to disclude the posterior teeth, the more critical is the occlusal plane.

Esthetics is often a key factor in determining what to do with a slanted or uneven occlusal plane. Very uneven planes can often be made to function acceptably, but the result is unacceptable esthetically. When teeth on one side have been unopposed, it is sometimes very difficult to level both sides because of the severe elongation on the unopposed side. Unless esthetics is of no concern whatever, every effort should be made to evenly align the occlusal plane, including endodontic procedures if needed. Fig. 20-6 illustrates a compromise

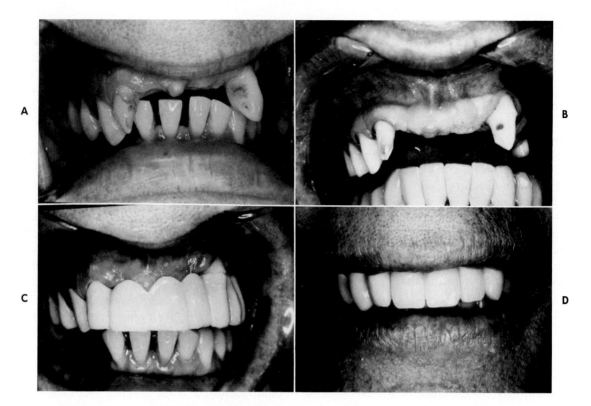

Fig. 20-6. Severe occlusal plane problem resulting from long-term lack of opposing teeth on the right side, **A**. Teeth are prepared as short as possible to avoid pulp exposure (at patient's request), **B**. **C**, U-shaped provisional restorations used to work out a correct occlusal plane. **D**, Compromised occlusal plane. Notice how much improvement could have been made if the pulps had been removed and the teeth shortened more on the patient's right side.

that could have been dramatically improved by further shortening of the teeth on the upper right side. Even though endodontics would have been required, the difference in appearance would have been worth it. Changes in the anterior segments must be related to the posterior segments or even the appearance of correctly aligned anterior teeth will suffer.

Periodontal support around the anterior teeth is critical if the anterior guidance is steepened to disclude the posterior teeth. It is tempting to solve an occlusal plane problem by steepening the anterior guidance, especially if it takes the place of correcting the occlusal plane by restoring anterior teeth that need to be restored. One must remember that if steepening the anterior guidance restricts habitual patterns of function, there will be a tendency for increased horizontal stress on the anterior teeth. If the supporting structures are already compromised, this may be a poor decision. It will be safer to keep the anterior guidance nonrestrictive and make the changes on the occlusal plane.

If there is no choice, and the steeper anterior guidance must be used, the teeth should be stabililized to prevent them from being forced out of alignment. Stabilization can be achieved by splinting, or by use of a retainer at night when restorations are not needed.

Irregular occlusal plane caused by lost but unreplaced posterior teeth. When a posterior tooth is lost and the patient is allowed to go without a replacement, it is almost inevitable that undesirable changes will take place in the plane of occlusion. Teeth behind the void have a tendency to lean into the space while unopposed teeth in the opposite arch supraerupt until they meet opposition. The result is a collapsed arch that prohibits protrusive or lateral excursions because of interference from the tilted or elongated teeth. The effect is the same as a curve of Spee that is too high posteriorly. The protruding mandible directs the stresses onto the teeth least able to resist it. In addition, these eccentric interferences hyperactivate the elevator muscles and thus intensify the stress. Tilted lower posterior teeth, riding against opposing elongated teeth cause the anterior teeth to disclude, thus preventing the anterior guidance from doing its job.

Correction of such an interfering occlusal plane is usually essential if supporting structure problems are to be prevented in all but the most fastidiously cared for mouth.

When an upper molar has supraerupted into a vacant space between two lower posterior teeth, the upper tooth should be shortened to permit protrusion of the mandible without posterior contact (Fig. 20-7). In some cases this should be done even if it requires devitalization of the elongated tooth. The same is true if a lower posterior tooth has elongated into a space above.

If the *terminal* tooth on the *upper* has erupted down *distal to the most posterior lower tooth,* it does not present a problem, even though it fails to conform to the picture of an "ideal" occlusal plane (Fig. 20-8). Devitalizing such a tooth just to make the occlusal plane conform would be wrong, since the upper tooth is behind the lower teeth and it does not restrict the mandible from moving forward under the guidance of the anterior teeth. Such a tooth should be prevented from excessive elongation into soft tissue by splinting or by extension of a lower tooth into contact, but it need not be reduced in length any more than the position of its pulp permits.

It should be pointed out that when the basic requirements of an occlusal plane are considered rather than an inflexible demand for a preconceived contour, it is rarely necessary to devitalize any tooth to provide an acceptable occlusal plane.

Curve of Spee too low posteriorly. Making the distal end of the occlusal plane too low presents no major problems, since it cannot interfere with the basic requirements of protrusive and balancing-side disclusion. If it is grossly overdone, however, it can create a poor esthetic result, can cause excessive stress on upper teeth by requiring an unfavorable crown-root ratio, and could conceivably reduce function in some mouths by causing too much separation of the posterior teeth in protrusion.

Curve of Spee too high or low in front. If the lower premolars are higher than the cuspids, they can interfere with the anterior pro-

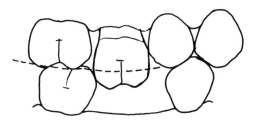

Fig. 20-7. A common occlusal plane problem. Any posterior tooth that interferes with the protrusive path of the mandible should be reduced to correct the plane of occlusion.

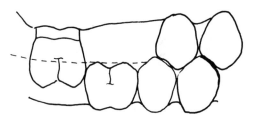

Fig. 20-8. Quiz yourself on this occlusal plane problem. Is it necessary for the upper molar to be reduced to an "ideal" occlusal plane when an upper fixed bridge is fabricated? When the mandible is protruded, it moves forward—*away* from the supraerupted upper molar. It is not necessary to reduce an upper tooth that is *distal* to all lower teeth to prevent an occlusal plane interference. It can be brought into better alignment to improve its crown-root ratio, but there would be no need to reduce the tooth to the point of requiring endodontics simply to satisfy an arbitrary occlusal plane requirement.

trusive guidance by bumping into the upper cuspids. If the lower premolars are considerably lower than the anterior teeth, the result is very poor esthetically. There is rarely a reason for such a relationship because it requires very simple clinical judgment to extend the incisal level of the lower anteriors into an esthetically acceptable occlusal plane. The upper teeth may, however, require some changes to accomplish an ideal plane.

CURVE OF WILSON

Because the curve of Wilson is always depicted on the lower arch, we may fail to understand that its real importance is related more to accommodating the *upper* lingual cusps into the lower occlusal scheme. Because of the normal outward tilt of upper posterior teeth, their lingual cusps are lower than their buccal cusps. Let us see how this affects the occlusal contours of lower posterior teeth

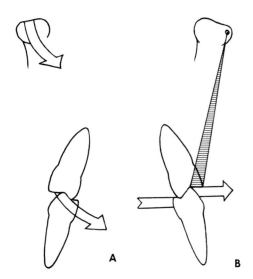

Fig. 20-9. Depiction of how the lower arch travels in lateral excursion. **A** represents balancing side. **B** represents working side. Opposite movement would reverse the pattern. Notice how this results in buccal cusps that are higher than lingual cusps on the lower arch. The result is a curve of Wilson.

Fig. 20-10. Curve of Wilson results from the relationship of the teeth to the normal pathways of the mandible in function.

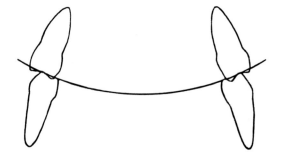

when the mandible is moved laterally. To emphasize the influence of condylar pathways, we will imagine that the lateral anterior guide angle is 0 degrees. In other words, the anterior guidance is flat.

When the mandible moves toward the working side with such a flat anterior guidance, the rotating condyle permits the posterior teeth on that side to move almost horizontally toward the cheek. The lower lingual cusp must be lowered to prevent it from interfering with the upper lingual cusp (Fig. 20-9, *B*).

On the balancing side, the orbiting condyle moves *downward* as it moves forward and permits lateral movement without interference to the upper lingual cusps (Fig. 20-9, *A*). The result in the lower arch is buccal cusps that are higher than lingual cusps and consequently a concave curve of Wilson (Fig. 20-10).

There are two ways of effectively changing the curve of Wilson. The first way is to change the lateral anterior guidance angle. The steeper

the lateral anterior guidance angle, the higher the lower lingual cusps may be on the same side. Raising the lower lingual cusps has the effect of flattening the curve of Wilson, and with a steep lateral guidance from the cuspids, there may be a flat curve of Wilson and still fairly steep cusp-fossae angles if the steep cuspid inclines direct the teeth on the working side down as they move laterally.

It rarely serves any purpose, however, to have high lingual cusps on the lower arch, since the lower lingual cusps are ordinarily not functioning cusps. At least they need not contact in any functional movement. One may wonder why we even worry about the height of these lower lingual cusps if they serve neither as a holding contact nor as a functioning incline, but they do act as useful *grippers* of coarse or fibrous foods and consequently they serve a useful purpose even though they need never be in actual contact (in normal arch relationships). Furthermore, the lingual cusps should also be lower than the buccal cusps to make it simpler for the tongue to get the food on the occlusal surface. If we understand the reasons for the curve of Wilson, it will become apparent that we have a fair amount of latitude in establishing an acceptable curve of Wilson.

The second way we may change the curve of Wilson is by changing the length of the upper lingual cusps. By shortening the upper lingual cusps and flattening the cusp-fossae angles, we can actually make a flat curve of Wilson. Such an occlusion can still function without interference and without losing the upper lingual cusps as centric holding contacts. All that would be lost is the maximum gripping effect that goes with closely approximating cusps in excursions. In some mouths the difference would not even be noticeable, but in others it could give the patient a feeling of lost efficiency. Since the establishment of an acceptable curve of Wilson can be accomplished so practically, there does not seem to be a good reason for denying any patient whatever increased function a proper occlusal plane can provide.

If the curve of Wilson is made too steep, it may eliminate the use of upper lingual cusps as holding contacts, since they would interfere with lateral movements of the mandible. Therefore it becomes a matter of practicality to establish a curve that serves the functional requirements within fairly broad limits of effectiveness, while avoiding overly steep inclines that could cause interference.

ESTABLISHING THE PLANE OF OCCLUSION

There are three practical methods for establishing an acceptable plane of occlusion. In selecting the method for a particular patient, remember that the purpose of the procedure is to cause the posterior teeth to be discluded by the anterior guidance. If there is an esthetic problem, there will be an added purpose of correcting the plane to a contour and height that is pleasant in appearance. If there is no esthetic problem, any method that satisfies the requirements of function and results in a stable occlusion is acceptable. There is no need to complicate it beyond these requirements.

The three most commonly used methods for establishing an acceptable occlusal plane are as follows:

1. Analysis on natural teeth through selective grinding
2. Analysis of facebow-mounted casts with properly set condylar paths
3. Use of Pankey-Mann-Schuyler method (PMS) of occlusal plane analysis

Analysis through selective grinding. If it is possible to eliminate excursive interferences without losing centric relation contacts, the plane of occlusion is acceptable as it is. Other than for appearance, there is no need to change an occlusal plane that permits the anterior guidance to disclude the posterior teeth in excursions unless centric stops are lost in the process.

Analysis through selective grinding does not eliminate the need for mounted diagnostic casts. In fact it should only be considered after mounted casts have been studied and a decision made to equilibrate the occlusion. If extensive posterior restorations are needed for purposes other than just correcting the occlusal plane, there is no harm in proceeding with equilibration. Teeth that will require later restorations regardless of the outcome of the equilibration can be reshaped until they are discluded by the anterior guidance in excursions. If the result is functional for the patient and the occlusal plane is esthetically acceptable, there is no reason to change it.

It is a good procedure to follow this process as part of the preliminary preparation of any extensive restorative plan.

If severe changes are required in the occlusal plane, it is often possible to avoid the need for endodontics by selective adjustment of the opposing arch. If it appears that sensitivity may be a problem after adjustment, the operator should be prepared to proceed with preparation for provisional restorations.

The patient should always be informed in advance about the need for eventual restoration of any teeth that are involved in the occlusal correction.

Analysis through use of instrumentation. Any articulator that can duplicate condylar border paths can be used to analyze or establish a correct occlusal plane, as long as an acceptable anterior guidance can also be programmed into the instrument. Selective grinding or preliminary waxup, or both, can be done on the casts to show the outer limits of occlusal plane contour and position. The preliminary correction and waxup can also be used for the fabrication of provisional restorations.

The need for fully adjustable instrumentation for analyzing occlusal plane problems is no longer so critical as once believed. Since there is rarely a need for posterior group function on the working side, and there is never a need for excursive contact on posterior teeth in protrusion or on the nonfunctioning side, disclusion can be effected by any articulator setting that is flatter than the actual condylar path in the patient. Condylar path settings can be accomplished with protrusive and lateral interocclusal records made at the edge-to-edge position of the incisors. Any protrusive curvature of the condylar path will be convex, and so it will provide a built-in added disclusive factor that works as a safety factor in the patient. There are no functional disadvantages to the added disclusion factor in excursions, and the method does not result in excessive changes in the occlusal plane.

The above approach can be depended on with confidence for any patient that has normal temporomandibular joints. However, as the disk has been lost and the condyle and eminentiae have been flattened, the condylar path becomes more critical to the disclusion of the posterior teeth. In combination with the usually worn flat anterior guidance, an occlusal plane problem may require precise duplication of the condylar path so that one can work out an acceptable occlusal plane that can be discluded by the anterior guidance.

Pankey-Mann-Schuyler (PMS) analysis of mounted models. If models are properly mounted with an accurate facebow record on either a fully adjustable or a semiadjustable instrument, an acceptable plane of occlusion can be determined with extreme simplicity. It should be made very clear that the PMS technique should *not* be used to determine *whether* a tooth should be restored. It is simply a technique for determining the occlusal plane when all or most of the posterior teeth have already been diagnosed as needing restoration. If a sound tooth can function adequately without interference, it should not be restored simply to make it conform to an arbitrary occlusal plane. Preliminary equilibration or analysis on the articulator should verify the need before a sound tooth is prepared for a restoration.

When it has been determined that restoration of all or most of the posterior teeth is necessary, the PMS technique provides an excellent and practical method for determining an occlusal plane that will fulfill all the requirements of a correct occlusion. The simplest method of implementing this part of the technique is through the use of the Broadrick Occlusal Plane Analyzer.

Broadrick Occlusal Plane Analyzer

For mouths requiring restoration of all or most of the posterior teeth, proper use of the occlusal plane analyzer will accomplish the following:

1. Preliminary determination of an acceptable plane of occlusion on the study models as an aid in treatment planning
2. Preliminary determination of the amount of reduction that will be required when each tooth is prepared
3. Extremely simple transfer to the mouth of predetermined preparation height for each tooth
4. In the laboratory waxup, simple determination of the height of each cusp tip. Through such a determination, the curve of Spee and the curve of Wilson are automatically established according to the predetermined plan of the dentist.
5. Predetermination of both the cusp height of the finished restoration and also the height of each prepared tooth. Thus room for a sufficient thickness of metal or metal and porcelain can be assured in advance. The technician never need be restricted in his occlusal carving because of insufficient tooth reduction.
6. A properly predetermined plane of occlusion on the lower arch, which enables the dentist to select virtually any type of acceptable occlusal contour scheme (posterior disclusion, group function, and so on) with complete assurance that the established plane of occlusion will permit it.

Using the Broadrick Occlusal Plane Analyzer. The so-called *flag* instrument can be adapted to almost any type of articulator that will accept a facebow mounting of the upper model. The lower model must be mounted with a centric bite record. By using a scribing caliper, a *survey center* is located on the plastic sheet attached to the flag. From that survey

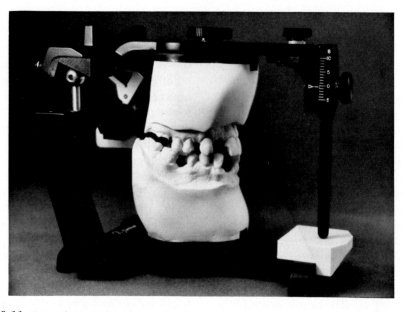

Fig. 20-11. Casts of a patient with an occlusal plane problem, mounted on a Combi articulator. The Broadrick flag attaches to the upper bow.

center, an acceptable plane of occlusion can be drawn on the lower model. The technique was adapted for restorative dentistry by Pankey from original anthropologic research by Monson. The "Monson curve" was originally applied to complete denture fabrication, but the practicality of the concept makes it especially useful for patients needing restoration if it has been predetermined that all or most of the posterior teeth need to be restored.

The technique consists in the following steps.

1. After the upper model has been oriented to the articulator by a carefully taken facebow registration, the mounting is completed and the lower model is then related to the upper by means of a centric bite record (Fig. 20-11). When the lower model has been mounted with stone, the upper model should be removed and set aside for later use.

2. The "flag" is secured to the upper bow of the articulator and the plastic sheet is snapped onto one side.

3. The pencil lead is inserted into one end of the caliper, and it is set at a radius of 4 inches from needle point to lead point. The width of the "flag" is 4 inches, and so it can be used as a convenient guide (Fig. 20-12). The selection of a 4-inch radius may seem to be a very arbitrary setting. The radius could be varied a little either way, but the change has so

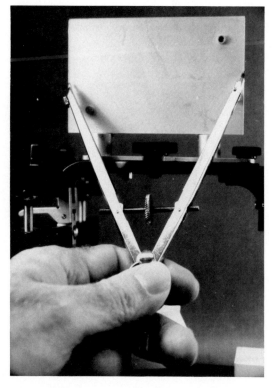

Fig. 20-12. The calipers are set at a 4-inch radius, the width of the flag.

little effect on the occlusal plane that there is nothing to be gained by it except in unusual cases where there is an extreme curve to the occlusal plane occurring naturally in an extremely small arch. Such cases are rare, and their uniqueness will be readily apparent to anyone who understands the basic requirements of an acceptable occlusal plane.

4. The point on the lower cuspid from which an esthetically pleasing occlusal plane would emanate is located. This will vary slightly according to the shape of the lower cuspid, but it is a matter of simple judgment. It will fall somewhere between the tip of the cuspid and the distoincisal line angle. Generally speaking, the flatter the cusp tip, the closer the point will be to the line angle. The more pointed the cuspid, the closer the survey point will be to the cusp tip. The needle point of the caliper is placed against the selected point on the cuspid and an arc scribed on the flag (Fig. 20-13). This arc will be referred to as the *anterior survey line*. The survey center that will be used to determine the occlusal plane will be located somewhere on this line.

5. Without varying the radius of the calipers, the point is held against the condyle ball of the articulator so that it aims near the center of the ball and another arc that will intersect the anterior survey line is scribed (Fig. 20-

14). We refer to this as the *condylar survey line*. The *survey center* for scribing the occlusal plane on the lower model is usually at the point where the lines intersect, but the point may be moved up to 1 cm from the intersect if necessary to favor either the upper or lower posterior tooth, as long as it remains on the anterior survey line. To determine the acceptability of the intersect as a survey center, the calipers are turned around, the point put at the intersect, and the height of the pencil mark, which would be made on the last lower tooth, checked. If too much reduction would be required to make the lower molar fit into such an occlusal plane, the survey center is moved forward on the anterior survey line *up to* 1 cm. The occlusal plane may be lowered in the back when the survey center is moved backward *up to* 1 cm.

If it appears necessary to move the survey center more than 1 cm forward or backward to establish an acceptable plane, the facebow mounting is incorrect. The models should be remounted with a new facebow record, and the procedure is repeated.

6. When an acceptable height has been established for the most distal lower tooth, a line is scribed on the model from that tooth forward to the cuspid. This line will represent the height of the buccal cusp tips (Fig. 20-15).

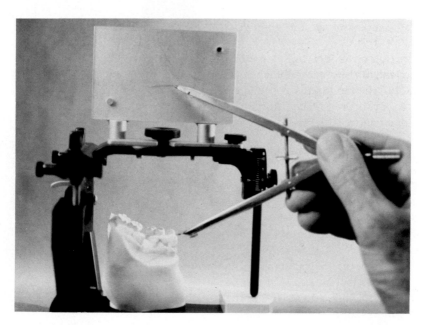

Fig. 20-13. Making the anterior survey line. The tip of the caliper point contacts the point selected on the cuspid.

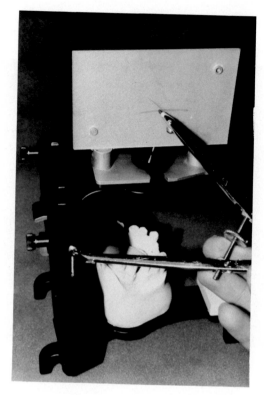

Fig. 20-14. Determining the posterior survey line. Without changing the caliper radius, position the point on the condyle ball as near the center as possible when the lead point is in contact with the flag. The arc formed is called the "condylar survey line."

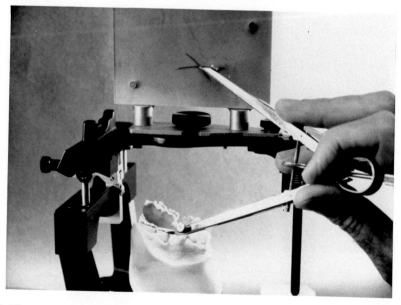

Fig. 20-15. The point is placed at the intersect, and using the pencil lead as an analyzing instrument, determine whether an acceptable plane of occlusion would result from using the intersect as a survey point. If the survey line on the back tooth is too low, it may be raised by moving the caliper point forward of the intersect. As long as the point stays within 1 cm of the intersect and is on the anterior survey line, the occlusal plane will be acceptable (if the facebow recording is correct).

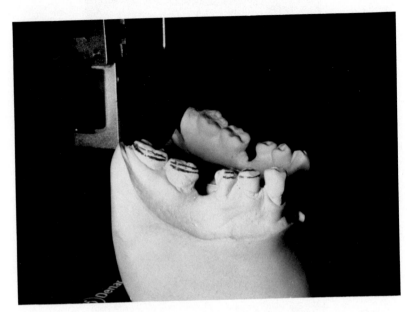

Fig. 20-16. Determine the preparation line by opening the calipers about 1.5 mm. This can vary according to the thickness of restorative material desired.

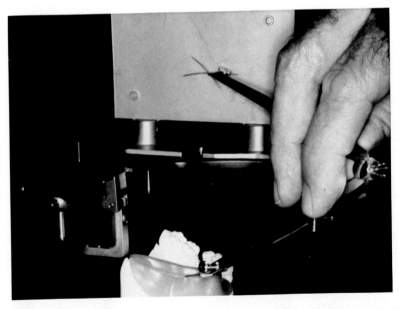

Fig. 20-17. A double layer of base plate wax is softened and adapted to the buccal contours on the cast. The preparation line is scribed on the wax.

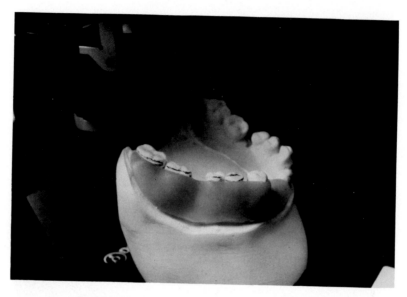

Fig. 20-18. The wax is trimmed to the preparation line.

7. To determine the *preparation line*, the calipers are opened an amount equal to the desired occlusal thickness of the proposed restoration (usually about 1½ mm), and a second line is scribed. This will represent the height of the buccal cusps after the teeth have been prepared (Fig. 20-16).

8. Some softened base plate wax is adapted to the buccal surfaces of the model and the preparation line scribed on the wax (Fig. 20-17). The wax is cut carefully back to this line (Fig. 20-18) and also trimmed along the mucobuccal fold line so that the wax can be fitted accurately in the mouth against the teeth. Extrahard base plate wax is used so that it will not distort when it is chilled and placed in the mouth. This is called the *occlusal plane cutting guide.*

9. When the lower posterior teeth are to be prepared, the cutting guide is placed snugly against the buccal surfaces of the dried teeth and a pencil line is drawn on the teeth according to the guide (Fig. 20-19).

10. The wax is removed and an inverted cone diamond is used to cut into the teeth along the line (Fig. 20-20). The entire occlusal surface of each tooth is reduced down to the preparation line. The preparation should be about 1½ mm lower on the lingual than it is on the buccal to accommodate for the curve

of Wilson. It is possible to make a lingual cutting guide to determine the lingual preparation line precisely, but it is more practical to just visualize the curve of Wilson and prepare the teeth sufficiently lower on the lingual than on the buccal.

11. The occlusal plane cutting guide represents only the preparation height for the buccal cusps. The lingual cusp preparation is 1½ mm lower. After reduction for correct cusp height has been completed, it is still necessary to reduce the central groove area to permit correct cusp-fossae contouring of the restorations. One must note the steepness of the lateral anterior guide angle to get a general idea of the steepness of the cusp-fossa angle. The steeper the lateral anterior guidance, the deeper one should hollow-grind the central groove part of the teeth.

12. After occlusal reduction has been accomplished, the preparation is completed according to the predetermined treatment plan.

If the teeth are being prepared for onlays and we wish to minimize any display of gold, it is practical to make the occlusal plane cutting guide to represent the height of the *finished* cusp tips. First, the teeth that need it are reduced to the predetermined finish height and then clinical judgment is used to reduce further from that level, with the esthetic require-

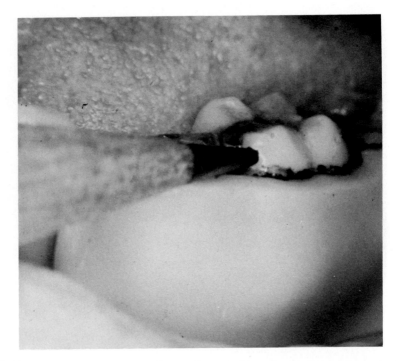

Fig. 20-19. A wax preparation guide in the mouth. It is held snugly against the dried teeth while the preparation line is drawn on the teeth.

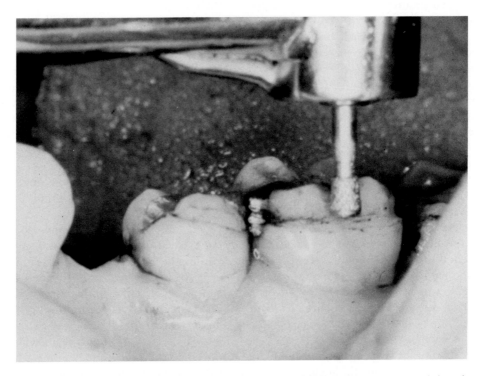

Fig. 20-20. An inverted-cone diamond stone can be used to etch the preparation line, and then the occlusal reduction is completed. The lingual side of the teeth is reduced more to allow for a curve of Wilson. A lingual guide is not necessary. The central groove area of each tooth should be hollow-ground to allow for occlusal contouring.

ments being kept in mind. The amount reduced at any given point will be the amount of thickness of the gold at that point.

When the occlusal plane is predetermined before the preparation of the teeth, it should never be necessary to grind through a restoration to adjust it. There should always be sufficient room to permit a correct waxup of each restoration, and there should be no need to make anything other than the most minor occlusal adjustment on the finished restoration.

The same procedure that is used for determining the plane of occlusion can also be used most effectively to establish the correct oc-

clusal plane on the wax patterns. By using a special wax cutting blade in the calipers, the overwaxed patterns can be cut back to the correct height. The angle of the blade automatically produces an acceptable curve of Wilson, making the lingual cusps lower than the buccal cusps.

Once the occlusal plane has been established on the wax patterns, the location of the cusp tips, the carving of buccal and lingual anatomy, and the contouring of fossae, ridges, and grooves can be accomplished easily and accurately. A complete procedure for waxing lower posterior teeth is detailed in Chapter 21.

21

Restoring lower posterior teeth

There are three important determinations that must be made for successful posterior occlusions. Each of these determinations involves the lower posterior teeth. These determinations in order of priority are as follows:

1. Plane of occlusion
2. Location of each lower buccal cusp tip
3. Position and contour of each lower fossa

The reason these three decisions are so important is that once these decisions are made all other aspects of posterior occlusion are relative to them.

Restoration of posterior teeth should not be considered until the condyles can be positioned with acceptable comfort in centric relation. Restoration of posterior teeth should not be attempted for the purpose of making uncomfortable condyles comfortable. Condyles should be comfortable *before* restorations are completed.

Restoration of posterior teeth should not be completed until the anterior guidance is correct. The fossa contours are directly related to the anterior guidance and cannot be determined accurately until after the anterior guidance pathways have been finalized.

It is not necessary to restore upper and lower posterior teeth together to ensure correct occlusal contours. Even when upper occlusal surfaces are to be changed, every aspect of lower occlusal form can be correctly determined and accurately restored before the upper posterior teeth are prepared.

There are advantages to completing the lower posterior segment before the upper teeth are prepared. It is easier on both the dentist and the patient. The lower posterior preparations can be made, and impressions, bite records, and temporization can be accomplished in a reasonably comfortable time period. There is no need for extremely long, tiring appointments, repeated removal of temporary restorations, and extra anesthetics. The cumulative errors of cementation are reduced to the effect of cement thickness on a single arch. Laboratory procedures are more easily carried out, and the coronal reference points left intact on the upper segment can be used to indicate the degree of buccolingual tilting of each tooth.

Every aspect of occlusal form has a purpose and every contour can be determined by measurable and recordable factors. As an example the lower cusp-fossae inclines are determined by the anterior guidance and the condylar guidance. If the lower lingual cusp is to have functional contact in working excursions, its buccal incline must be the same as the lateral anterior guidance, with some modifications to maintain simultaneous conformity to condylar paths. If the lower lingual cusp is to be discluded in working excursions, its buccal incline must be flatter than the lateral anterior guidance. These facts of occlusal morphology will hold true whether the upper and lower teeth are waxed up together or separately. The inclines will not change simply because the technique changes. If the controlling determinants can be recorded, the results of the determinants can be captured.

As already discussed, lingual cusp excursive contact unnecessarily complicates the fabrication of occlusal surfaces without any improvement in function or stability. So from a practical standpoint, lower cusp-fossae angles should be flatter than the lateral anterior guidance. This is one simplification that can be utilized without any concern that quality is being compromised.

Posterior teeth in the lower arch can be accurately restored with cusp tip-to-fossa contact if the following determinations can be made:

1. Correct height and placement of buccal cusps
2. Correct height and placement of lingual cusps
3. Correct placement of fossae
4. Correct inclines for fossae walls

None of the above ascertainments is complicated if the objectives and determinants of each occlusal segment are understood. Following a logical sequence simplifies each determination and provides a reference point from which the next decision can be made regarding occlusal configurations.

The starting point for determining lower occlusal contours should be the buccal cusps.

PLACEMENT OF LOWER BUCCAL CUSPS

Placement of lower buccal cusps is determined on the basis of providing the optimum effect for buccolingual stability, mesiodistal stability, and noninterfering excursions.

Buccal cusp placement for buccolingual stability

The correct location of each lower buccal cusp should be one of the first determinations made when the original treatment plan is outlined. Preparation for restorations should not be made until the lower teeth are in their most acceptable relationship to the upper teeth. When necessary, arch expansion is usually a simple orthodontic procedure that can be accomplished in a matter of weeks. Lower teeth that are not in acceptable buccolingual rela-

tionship with their related upper teeth should have their alignment corrected before restorative procedures are initiated, rather than be restored with "warped" contours that misdirect stresses off the long axis. The need for orthodontic correction can be determined from correctly mounted study casts. It is frequently necessary to equilibrate the casts to make a final determination regarding the acceptability of interarch relationships. To make such a determination, casts *must* be mounted with a facebow recording and an interocclusal bite record at the correct centric relation.

The buccolingual position of lower buccal cusps is determined in the following manner on mounted casts.

1. Upper central groove position is analyzed. On each upper occlusal surface, a line is drawn from mesial to distal in the central groove. The ideal contact point for each lower buccal cusp tip should usually be located somewhere on this line. However, the correctness of the central groove should be analyzed on each tooth. In some tilted teeth, it is advantageous to move the central groove to gain better direction of forces through the long axis. As an example, an upper second molar, which is tilted toward the buccal, can have the stresses directed to better advantage if the central groove is moved toward the lingual. When the upper teeth have not been prepared, the tilt of each tooth can be more easily determined and points of contact can be more accurately selected. If moving the central groove will enable the stresses to be directed more nearly through the long axis of any upper tooth, the improved central groove position should be so noted on the upper cast by drawing a new line.

2. Optimum contact for stress direction on lower posterior teeth should be determined. While we disregard the upper central groove position, the buccal cusp position that would most nearly direct stresses down through the long axis of each lower posterior tooth is determined. This may be done at the study model stage, or in cases with acceptable arch alignment, it may be done after the lower posterior teeth have been prepared. At this point we are concerned only with buccolingual relationships.

A mark is made on each lower tooth to indicate the position of the buccal cusp that would be optimum for buccolingual stability and di-

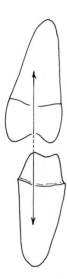

Fig. 21-1. When determining the buccolingual placement of the lower buccal cusp, the resultant direction of force should be favorable to *both* upper and lower teeth. The main force vector should be as parallel as possible to the long axis of both.

rection of force. In selecting this point we are disregarding the upper teeth and are determining only what is best for the lower teeth. Next, we will evaluate the relationship of the selected lower cusp position against the ideal upper central groove position.

3. The alignment of the optimum lower buccal cusp position against optimum upper central groove position is evaluated. This is easily done if we close the articulator and observe how the lower marks line up with the upper marks. If the marks do not line up precisely, the positions of both the upper central groove and the lower buccal cusp tip are equally changed. The new cusp-tip positions are reevaluated to make certain that they are compatible with acceptable stress direction through the long axis of each lower tooth. The upper groove position is similarly evaluated.

If the altered buccal cusp-tip position does not provide acceptable stress directioning for *both* upper and lower posterior teeth, the arch relationship is unacceptable and the treatment plan should be designed to correct the problem. Orthodontic movement is usually the best way to correct malrelated arches, but it is not always possible or practical. There are many subtle factors to be considered before arch expansion or contraction is initiated, and a competent orthodontist should be consulted.

When it is practical, arch expansion or contraction can usually be done rather easily and seldom takes very long to accomplish.

There are some arch relationship problems that are better off being left as they are. The chapters on solving crossbite problems and end-to-end bite relationships (Chapters 34 and 36) should be studied carefully. "Warping" posterior occlusal contours to "correct" such conditions is very often more damaging than corrective.

The basic rule to follow regarding the buccolingual position of the lower buccal cusp is: *The lower buccal cusp must be positioned so that its contact directs the stresses through the long axis of both upper and lower teeth* (Fig. 21-1).

When the buccolingual line of the lower buccal cusp tips has been determined, the next determination to make is the mesiodistal position of each cusp tip on that line.

Mesiodistal placement of lower buccal cusps

Two considerations should determine the mesiodistal position of lower buccal cusps: mesiodistal stability and noninterfering excursions.

Attaining mesiodistal stability. The best mesiodistal stability is attained by placement of the lower buccal cusps in upper fossae. Placement in the fossae directs the stresses properly through the long axis, eliminates any possibility of plunger cusp food impaction at contact, and is stable. There is no tendency for cusp tips to migrate out of properly contoured fossae (Fig. 21-2).

There will be times when it is not practical to place the lower buccal cusp in an upper fossa, and it will be necessary for it to contact on the marginal ridges of two upper teeth. Plunger cusp food impaction can be avoided by proper design. The upper marginal ridges should be contoured with sluiceways from the adjacent fossae that permit the crushed bolus to slide away from the contact. The contact itself should be wide enough to protect the interdental papilla. Whenever possible, another lower buccal cusp of the same tooth should be brought into centric contact, or the upper lingual cusp should be used as an additional centric stop to eliminate plunger activity. Of course, the main cause of plunger cusp impac-

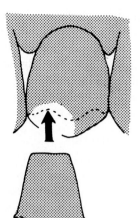

Fig. 21-2. For mesiodistal stability, the cusp tip has a tendency to stay centered in a correctly designed fossa far better than against an incline or even a flat suface contact.

MES

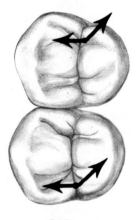

Fig. 21-3. When the lower buccal cusp tip placement is being located, the path of egress from the upper fossa should be evaluated. If the cusp tip is placed in the mesial fossa, *above*, it moves into space on its excursion toward the lingual. If it is placed in a distal fossa, *below*, it may meet interference with a lingual cusp.

DIS

tion is the wedging open effect of incline contacts. Incline contacts in centric relation should be avoided.

Although acceptable tooth–to–two teeth contact can be accomplished, it is usually rather simple to warp the lower buccal cusp mesially or distally the 1 or 2 mm required to place the cusp tip into an upper fossa. Whenever it can be done with practicality, this is what I try to do.

Locating the lower buccal cusps for noninterfering excursions

Determining which fossa the lower buccal cusp should contact depends on where the cusp travels when it leaves centric relation. The mesiodistal placement of each lower buccal cusp is determined when one locates it in the fossa that permits excursions from centric relation without interference (Fig. 21-3). This may sound complicated, but learning the border pathways of each lower tooth can be a rather simple exercise.

By first selecting appropriate fossae on the upper mounted model, one can quickly determine the paths of the lower cusps from each fossa, since they will travel at right angles to the rotating condyle. By visualization of a straight line from the rotating condyle to the selected contact point in the fossa, it is a simple matter to determine the general path of the lower cusp as it travels in either a working or balancing excursion (Fig. 21-4). Protrusive pathways are easy to determine since all cusps move straight forward in that excursion.

When each upper fossa position is selected, the articulator should be closed to see whether the upper fossa location would also be acceptable as a buccal cusp position for the lower tooth. The selected contact points should direct the forces through the long axes of both upper and lower teeth.

If stress direction is acceptable to both teeth, the paths of movement from the selected fossa should be evaluated. If the lower buccal cusp can move out of the fossa in protrusive working and balancing excursions without colliding with another cusp, its position is acceptable. By evaluating each lower buccal cusp placement in this manner, we are taking an essential step to assure in advance the correct contouring of the upper posterior teeth after the lower teeth are completed.

Placement of the lower cusp tip directly between the upper buccal and lingual cusps not only is unstable, but it also necessitates the destruction of upper occlusal anatomy to permit excursions. Placement of a lower premolar cusp tip in the distal fossa of the upper may provide a free path from centric relation out to a working excursion toward the buccal, but the upper lingual cusp could be in the way of balancing excursions toward the lingual.

It is usually best to place the lower buccal cusps of bicuspids in a mesial fossa when possible. This allows egress from centric relation through all excursions with the least chance of destroying tooth anatomy in the process.

Molar cusp tips should be placed so that they will not collide with upper cusps. They may be placed in the mesial fossa, the same as bicuspids, or in the distal fossa with nonfunctional egress through the transverse groove. Molar cusp-tip placement is also permissible in the upper central fossa, since it can pass to the mesial of the upper mesiolingual cusp in its nonfunctioning excursion and it can pass between the buccal cusps in working excursion.

Because the nonfunctioning-side condyle must move down the eminentia for a lateral excursion to take place to the opposite side, the buccal inclines of upper lingual cusps on the nonfunctioning side can usually be steeper than the anterior guidance. However, since we

never want those inclines to contact in any jaw position, it provides a safety factor to have the buccal inclines of upper lingual cusps slightly more concave than the anterior guidance. If the anterior guidance is very steep, there is rarely a problem, since jaw movements are restricted to near-vertical function.

Contouring cusp tips

For cusp tip-to-fossa contact, the tip of each lower buccal cusp should be small enough to fit into a normally contoured fossa. If the anterior guidance permits a lateral side shift, the cusp tip should be able to contact the base of the fossa without touching the fossa walls in centric relation. If the anterior guidance is steeper than the fossa walls and no lateral side shift is permitted, the side of the cusp may contact the fossa walls.

When the tip of the cusp serves as the centric contact, it should be wide enough to provide optimum wear resistance. A sharp, pointed cusp tip would have too little surface contact to resist accelerated wear. A broad flat cusp tip could require the upper fossa to be opened out too much to permit good occlusal contour. It is difficult to be specific about the size of a cusp tip that would be suitable for all fossae because contours vary as border pathways vary, but in general the tip of the cusp should have a fairly flat area about 1 mm or so wide. This is wide enough to withstand wear when the tip contacts in centric relation and small enough to permit good fossa contours in the upper. In lateral excursions, if group function is desired, the side of the cusp contacts the wall of the fossa rather than the tip (Fig. 21-5). The centric contact on the tip itself is subject to very little wear if the occlusal contours are correct.

If a cusp tip is to be placed in a fossa, the tip must not be wide mesiodistally. This is a common fault, and it should be remembered that each cusp must follow border pathways from its point of centric contact. If a cusp is too wide, the path that must be cleared for its excursive movements will destroy the anatomy of the opposing tooth.

Wide cusp tips require more force for bolus penetration, and therefore they put more stress on the supporting structures. Narrow cusps require less force, and so they produce less stress (Fig. 21-6).

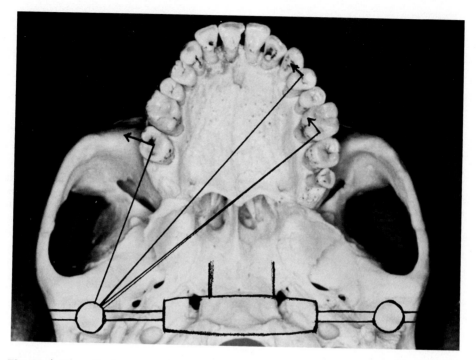

Fig. 21-4. The path of any lower cusp can quickly be determined either in the mouth or on an articulator when one visualizes the path as being at right angles to an imaginary line from the rotating condyle to the cusp in question. Paths depicted on the opposite side from the rotating condyle represent balancing excursions, whereas the path on the same side represents a working excursion.

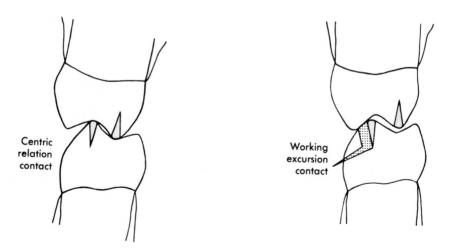

Centric
relation
contact

Working
excursion
contact

Fig. 21-5. In centric relation only the cusp tips contact. In lateral excursions, if contact is desired, the side of the cusp functions against the upper incline. The centric stop at the cusp tip is discluded. This minimizes wear on the centric holding contacts.

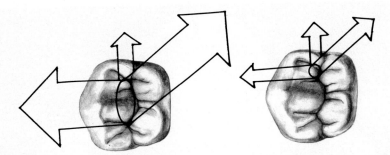

Fig. 21-6. Wide cusp tips produce neither better function nor better stability. A properly contoured small cusp tip fits into the base of a saucer-shaped fossa that helps to stabilize it because the cusp does not have a tendency to migrate down the inclines of the fossa. The smaller cusp can pass through opened-out grooves and does not destroy the occlusal anatomy. A cutter blade extends distally from the small lower cusp tip, but it does not touch in centric relation. It barely misses lateral contact with the grooved fossa walls of the upper tooth.

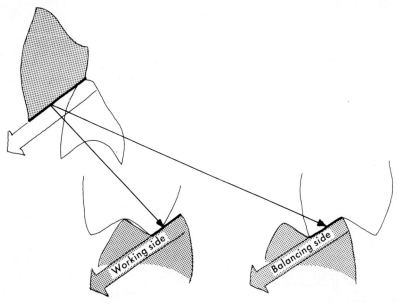

Fig. 21-7. The inner incline of the upper cuspid dictates the incline limitations of the lower posterior inclines facing it. The lower working side incline cannot be steeper than the lateral anterior guidance incline of the cuspid. From a practical standpoint, it should be made flatter, since it is not necessary for the lower incline to contact in function. The balancing incline should never be allowed to contact, so it too should be flatter than the lateral guidance of the cuspid. This incline also usually gets some downward movement from the orbiting condyle, but for simplicity this can just be considered as insurance. If the cuspid is steeper than the lower balancing incline that faces it, the balancing incline will be discluded (if occlusal plane is correct).

Placement of lower lingual cusps

In normal tooth-to-tooth relationships, the tip of the lower lingual cusp never comes into contact with the upper tooth. Even though the buccal incline of the lower lingual cusp can be made to contact in working excursions, there is no apparent advantage in doing so (type 3 occlusal form). For reasons of practicality we treat the lower lingual cusp as a nonfunctioning cusp as far as contact is concerned. This does not mean, however, that it should be ignored. It should still act as a gripper and a grinder by passing close enough to the upper lingual cusps to aid in tearing, crushing, and shearing the food that is caught between the opposing surfaces.

The lower lingual cusp has another job to do, since it is primarily responsible for keeping the tongue from getting pinched between the posterior teeth. The position and contour of the cusp tip should reflect this responsibility without causing irritation to the tongue. The cusp tip should be rounded and smooth on its lingual aspect. The position of the tip should have enough lingual overjet to hold the tongue out of the way, but it should always be located over the root, within the long axis.

The distance between the lower buccal and lingual cusp tips is the same as the distance between upper cusp tips; so once the lower buccal cusp tip has been located, this measurement can be applied to position the lingual cusp. The measurement between buccal cusp tip and lingual cusp tip should not be much greater than half the total buccolingual width of the tooth at its widest part.

The height of the lower lingual cusp is determined when one follows the concepts outlined in Chapter 22. The lingual cusp height can vary in relation to buccal cusp height because of variations in the lateral anterior guidance, but such variations are not necessary from a practical standpoint. Generally the lower lingual cusp height should be about a millimeter shorter than the buccal cusp. Cusp height can be lowered further in the first premolar. If upper and lower posterior teeth are to be restored, simply following the occlusal plane dictated by the PMS concept will be acceptable for both the curve of Spee and the curve of Wilson. Any one of the accepted types of occlusal form can be fabricated on such an occlusal plane.

Contouring the lower fossae

As the mandible moves right or left from centric relation, its front end should be guided down the lingual incline of the upper cuspid. When it serves as the lateral anterior guidance, the lingual incline of each upper cuspid dictates the fossa contour of each lower incline that faces it (Fig. 21-7).

The lateral guidance incline of each upper cuspid dictates the fossa contours of the buccal inclines of each lower lingual cusp on the same side and the lingual inclines of each lower buccal cusp on the opposite side. When the cuspid is not in position to function individually or in group function as the lateral anterior guidance, the lingual incline of the most anterior upper tooth that can assume the role becomes the dictator of the lower fossae inclines facing it. As the lower posterior teeth follow the mandible down its lateral path, any fixed upper lingual cusp seated into the lower fossa becomes an interference if the lower incline is steeper than the upper guiding incline it faces.

Since this is such an important aspect of occlusal form, we will look at lower lateral fossae contours in still another way. When the mandible moves right or left, the tooth with the steepest fossae incline carries all the stress. This is modified slightly on the balancing side by the downward movement of the orbiting condyle, but for now we do not need to consider that as anything but a safety factor to help disclude the balancing side. With that in mind, the following is a good rule to follow: from the contact point of each upper lingual cusp, the lower fossa inclines should be no steeper than the lateral guidance inclines they face. Any incline that is steeper discludes the lateral guidance and adds to its own lateral stress. If the lower cusp-fossa angle is steeper than the lateral anterior guidance, the upper lingual cusps will be locked into the lower fossae and the back teeth will clash stressfully when lateral excursions are made.

If functionally generated path procedures are carried out with lower posterior teeth that have such restricted fossae contours, the functional wax would be wiped away and the result would be no upper lingual cusp contact in centric relation.

To accommodate upper lingual cusps as centric holding contacts without interference to excursions, the cusp-fossa angle of the lower posteriors *must be the same as or flatter than the lateral anterior guidance angle.* If the anterior guidance has been freed laterally to permit a side shift of the mandible, the lower fossae *must* be opened up accordingly or interference will result. A concave anterior guidance requires concave fossae contours.

The simplest and most practical approach is to open up the lower fossae by providing more than enough freedom for a lateral side shift and making the cusp-fossa angle flatter than the lateral anterior guidance angle. This takes away nothing that is needed while facilitating an extremely stable centric holding pattern. A simplified method for accomplishing this is through the use of the fossa contour guide described later in this chapter.

Contouring ridges and grooves

Ridges and grooves give beauty and naturalness to the occlusal scheme. It is the action of ridges and grooves against their opponent counterparts that grasps the food and then crushes, tears, and shreds it as the lower teeth follow their cyclic paths of function against upper inclines. With proper occlusal relationships, it is not necessary for the lower teeth to actually contact the upper teeth in function. The bolus is nearly disintegrated by the time the first tooth contact is made, and so the arrangement of ridges and grooves is to permit the cusps to pass close enough to each other to mangle the food between the grooved surfaces without actual need for tooth contact.

Fairly accurate determination of ridge and groove direction is all that is needed. Extreme preciseness is not required because in tip-to-fossa contact only the base of the lower fossa contacts the upper lingual cusp. The walls of the fossae never contact, and grooves can be opened out just as fossae are opened out to avoid contact. The only part of any lower posterior tooth that ever needs to contact in any eccentric position is the buccal cusp, and it can be limited to centric contact only whenever group function is not required.

We must not make the mistake of designing grooves that are slotted so that a cusp can pass precisely through the slot on a given border path. As an example, the walls of such a groove may allow passageway of a cusp in a lateral working excursion, but the groove would not

accommodate the cusp in a protrusive lateral path. If we try to provide a groove to accommodate the upper lingual cusp for each path the lower tooth can follow, we would have contiguous grooves starting with a straight working excursion, all the way around through all the protrusive lateral paths, until we came to the border pathway of the balancing excursion. Thus we would end up with no groove at all. We would have an opened-out fossa that permitted centric contact of the upper lingual cusp in the bottom of the fossa concavity, and the walls of the fossa would not clash with the cusp no matter how the lower jaw was moved.

Since this is the effect we are after anyway, it seems practical to simply work out the fossae contours first and then functionalize and beautify the anatomy by placing the appropriate grooves at the working, protrusive, and balancing excursion. *There can be no entanglement of cusps in grooves that have been made into inclines that are already out of reach.* Other grooves may be added as desired to improve esthetics or to provide more ridges for better masticatory function.

The practicality of actual pathways through grooves increases as the difference increases between the lateral and the protrusive anterior guidance angles. A patient with a flat lateral guidance and a steep protrusive guidance could have very definite working excursion grooves that permit passage of prominent cusps because the steep anterior guidance separates the posterior teeth rapidly in protrusive excursions, eliminating the need for opened-out pathways except in the flatter lateral excursions. Whether there is any advantage of groove over generally opened-out fossae would be difficult to assess. There does not appear to be any noticeable clinical difference as far as we can tell.

The direction of any ridge or groove is determined by the path of the lower tooth as it moves with the mandible. Lateral excursion grooves are at right angles to a line drawn from the rotating condyle. The lateral shifting of the mandible may alter the groove direction slightly, but by the time the lateral shift occurs the posterior teeth have already been separated by the anterior guidance so that it has no consequence if a correct centric relation is the starting point.

WAXING TECHNIQUE FOR LOWER POSTERIOR TEETH

The following technique is a simplified procedure for waxing lower posterior teeth when all posterior teeth are to be restored. The simplicity of the procedures may be surprising, but one must not get the impression that we will be making any compromise on quality. The technique can achieve optimum stability, function, and beauty. Lower posterior teeth waxed in this manner can have natural, beautiful contours with all cusp tips precisely located for optimum stability and directioning of forces. All fossae will be in harmony with the lateral anterior guidance, and so any fossa may accept an upper lingual cusp as a holding contact. The plane of occlusion will be acceptable for allowing the anterior guidance to do its job.

The waxing technique can be used whenever cusp tip-to-fossa contact is used. It works equally as well on gnathologic instruments as it does on semiadjustable articulators. When lower cusp location and fossae contours have been correctly established on an acceptable occlusal plane, the upper occlusal surfaces may be accurately restored using several different methods including stereographic or pantographic techniques. Functionally generated path procedures, however, can be used against such lower occlusal contours with extreme accuracy in the full range of border movements without the loss of the upper lingual cusp as a centric contact. The correctly placed and contoured cusps of the lower teeth used against functionally generated path wax determine not only upper fossa contours but ridge and groove directions as well.

A major advantage of the procedures that follow is that they offer a unique method of communication between the dentist and the technician. Virtually every requirement of good occlusal form can be specified in a manner that is simple to understand and easy to fulfill. The specifics that the dentist gives to the technician actually make the technique procedures simpler and less time consuming. The finished result can be easily checked for accuracy by either the technician or the dentist, and even corrections to fossa inclines can be easily made in the finished restorations with extreme accuracy by the dentist.

The major part of the technique can be carried out on the lower model while it is off the articulator. There is no need for working against an upper model once the cusp tips have been located, and there is no need for the articulator once the occlusal plane has been finalized. The procedures can be modified in several ways, but the important steps of cusp-tip location, occlusal-plane analysis, and fossae contouring must be achieved. The simpler each of these steps can be accomplished, the better, so long as accuracy is not sacrificed by the simplification.

After the lower posterior teeth have been prepared, the anterior guidance should be checked for correctness. Impressions should then be made for the upper opposing model and the lower die models. They should be properly mounted with a facebow and centric bite record.

PROCEDURE FOR LOCATING THE BUCCAL AND LINGUAL CUSP TIPS

1. A line is drawing along the central groove of the upper posterior teeth (Fig. 21-8). The articulator is closed to see whether buccolingual stability of either the upper or lower teeth would be improved by movement of the contact more to the buccal or more to the lingual. This can usually be visualized quite easily. If some of the upper teeth are badly broken down or missing, it is often helpful to reshape the upper teeth by carving the stone model or reshaping the teeth with wax before finalizing the best cup tip placement.

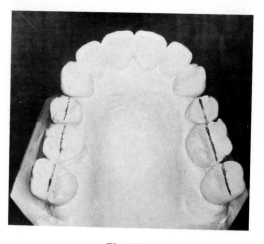

Fig. 21-8

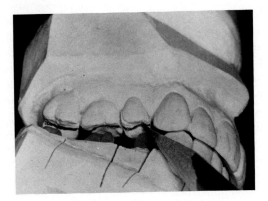

Fig. 21-9

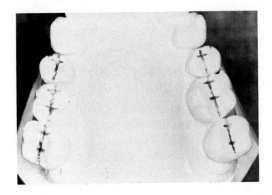

Fig. 21-10

2. Now, noting the mesiodistal relationship of each lower tooth to its opposing upper, we select the most advantageous placement of each lower buccal cusp. We should try to select fossae for cusp tip placement whenever possible. Each spot should be marked (Fig. 21-9). Buccal cusp tip placement will be where each line intersects (Fig. 21-10). We should check the selection of cusp tip placement by noting the direction of excursions from each point. Is it compatible with good tooth anatomy? Will cusp tips bypass each other without interference when the lower teeth move from centric relation out through excursive movements? If this can be improved, it should be marked accordingly.

3. Using a No. 6 round bur, a hole is drilled at each cusp tip location to the depth of the bur head (Fig. 21-11).

4. Dark-colored 14-gage wax sprues should be cut into 3 mm lengths and inserted into each drilled hole. The articulator should be closed to be sure the sprue wax does not interfere with opposing lower dies. It may be necessary to either shorten or lengthen sprue wax cores. This is easily determined by checking the space between the die and the opposing tooth before cutting and placing the wax core (Fig. 21-12).

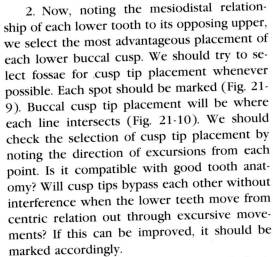

Fig. 21-11

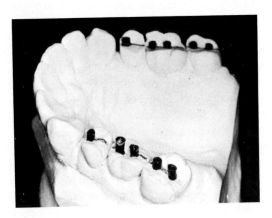

Fig. 21-12

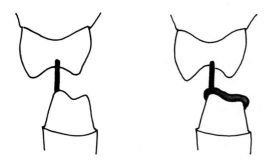

Fig. 21-13

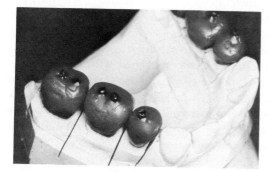

Fig. 21-14

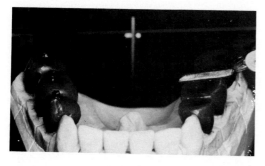

Fig. 21-15

5. With the articulator closed, red inlay wax is flowed around the occlusal part of the die to engage the dark sprue wax (Fig. 21-13). The sprue wax core should not be melted into the red wax. It is better to flow the red wax only on the occlusal part of the die to serve as an index because the sprue sometimes sticks in the upper hole when the articulator is opened. It can be easily removed and placed back on the die for continuation of the waxup.

6. The articulator is opened and more wax flowed around the dies until the crowns are overbuilt (Fig. 21-14). Interproximal contacts between teeth should be as close to correct as practical in this early waxup stage.

7. The flag instrument (Broadrick Occlusal Plane Analyzer) should be used to determine the heights of the buccal and lingual cusps through the establishment of the curve of Wilson (buccolingual curve) and the curve of Spee (mesiodistal curve) (Fig. 21-15). (Refer to Chapter 20 for details.) The correct occlusal plane must be determined before preparation of the teeth to ensure sufficient occlusal thicknesss for all the lower posterior restorations.

When the overbuilt wax patterns are reduced to the proper line and plane of occlusion, the precise position of each lower buccal cusp tip will show up in the dark wax (Fig. 21-16). *After the plane of occlusion is established, that dark cusp tip is never touched.* Its height and position mark the predetermined location ideal for stress direction and stability for both upper and lower teeth.

When this step is completed, there is no further need for keeping the lower model on the articulator. All the steps that follow can be accurately carried out with the lower model off the instrument. This adds greatly to the simplicity and reduces the time required for the waxup.

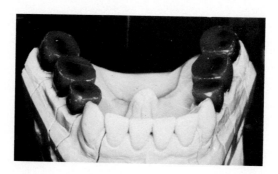

Fig. 21-16

8. Buccal anatomy is carved easily now. Using the cusp tip as one reference and the gingival margin as the other, the buccal contours can be carved quickly (Fig. 21-17). The crest of contour should be established at about the junction of the gingival and middle third. In waxing of full crowns, the contour of the gingival third should start with a concavity before becoming convex at the junction of the middle third. From the crest of contour to the cusp tip, the convexity should flatten somewhat to keep the cusp tip from being too broad. In contouring for tip-to-fossa contact, only the cusp tip is to touch in centric relation. Broad, bulbous cusp tips require wider flatter upper fossae and make it more difficult to achieve good occlusal form on the upper teeth.

9. Lingual cusp tips are located. The distance between the buccal and lingual cusps of the lower teeth is generally the same as that of the upper posterior teeth. It is a practical procedure to simply measure the upper teeth and transfer to the lower. A double-pointed caliper can be used to measure the upper tip-to-tip distance. One point of the caliper is then placed in the center of the buccal cusp tip and the location of the lingual cusp is marked with a slight depression being made in the wax with the other caliper point (Fig. 21-18).

10. Lingual contours can now be carved with the lingual cusp tip location being used as one reference and the gingival margin as the other. The crest of contour should be within the middle third.

At this point we must determine the type of occlusal relationship we wish to produce. Once we have located all the buccal and lingual cusps, we have a frame of reference that simplifies the carving of the result of the occlusal contours. There is no substitute for a knowledge of occlusal anatomy. We must still rely on our understanding of individual tooth form, marginal ridge contours, and general ridge and groove direction, but all of these carvings are accomplished with much greater ease and speed when cusp tips have been precisely located first. Location of the various fossae is a rather routine procedure, but how the walls of these fossae are carved will determine whether the upper lingual cusps can be used as centric holding contacts.

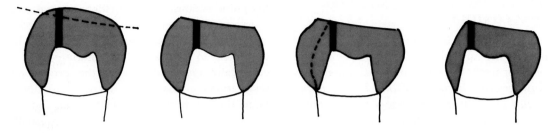

Fig. 21-17

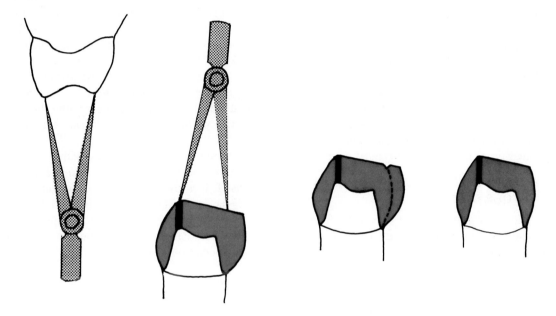

Fig. 21-18

DETERMINING AND CARVING LOWER FOSSA CONTOURS

The following technique was designed to *simplify* the carving of occlusal fossae of lower posterior teeth. It has one purpose: *to ensure a noninterfering accommodation for the upper lingual cusps.* It will provide a fossa contour that is compatible with the lateral anterior guidance regardless of the contour of the anterior guidance. It can be easily modified to provide extra freedom for Bennett shift. Lower posterior occlusions that are carved in this manner will not wipe away upper lingual cusps when functionally generated path procedures are used for the upper teeth.

The procedure involves making a *fossa contour guide* that can be used in any stage of waxup or even porcelain application. It can be fabricated by auxiliaries in the office in just a few minutes' time. The guide should accompany the articulated die model to the technician and should be returned with the finished restorations for use by the dentist in his or her evaluation of the finalized occlusal contours.

PROCEDURE FOR MAKING THE FOSSA CONTOUR GUIDE

The fossa guide is used only if both upper and lower posterior teeth are to be restored. The anterior guidance must be correct before the guide is fabricated or before occlusal contours can be determined for lower posterior restorations. The anterior guidance may be corrected in provisional restorations, and a centrically mounted cast of the provisional restorations in place may be used to determine the allowable fossa-wall angulation for the posterior restorations. The guide is usually made when the casts are mounted, but it is not used until the posterior waxup is done or the porcelain is being applied and contoured. Procedures for making a fossa guide are as follows:

1. The regular incisal guide pin is removed and replaced with the special fossa-contour pin. The blade of the pin is indented into a mound of wax on a flat plastic guide table (Fig. 21-19).

2. The upper bow is moved into left and right excursions, allowing the contours of the lateral anterior guidance to determine the path that the guide pin cuts into the wax (Fig. 21-20).

3. When the lateral guidance pathways have been cut sharply into the wax, the special pin is raised. It is then used to hold a handle for the fossa guide. Make the handle by cutting off the tip of a plastic protector for a disposable needle. The large end fits snugly onto the raised special pin (Fig. 21-21).

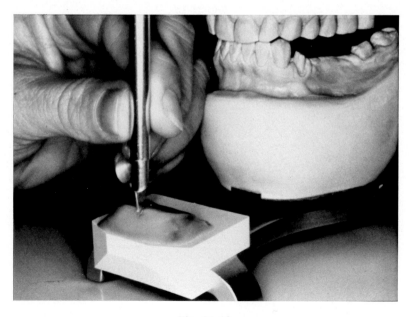

Fig. 21-19

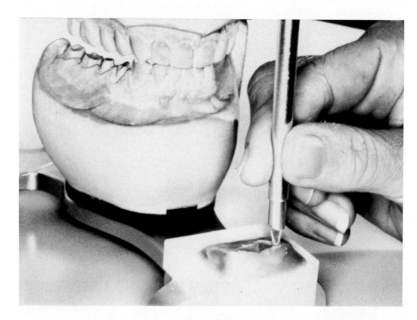

Fig. 21-20

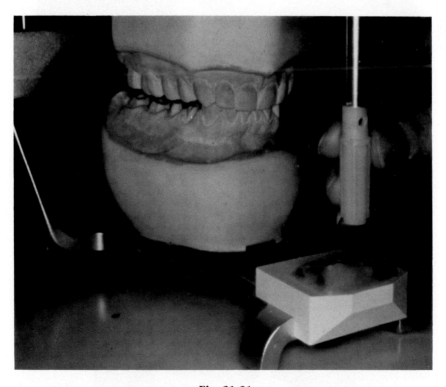

Fig. 21-21

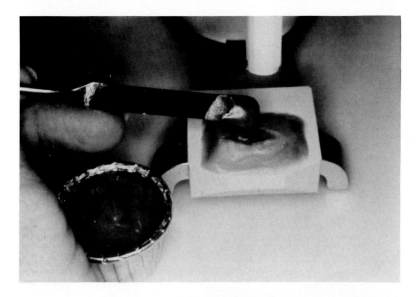

Fig. 21-22

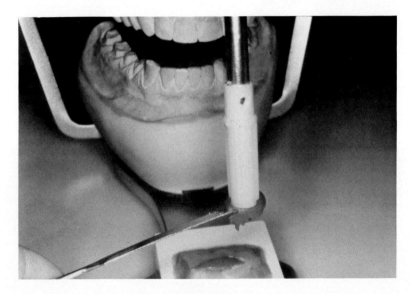

Fig. 21-23

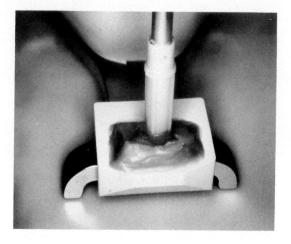

Fig. 21-24

4. A creamy mix of self-curing acrylic resin is flowed into the indentation in the wax (Fig. 21-22). Resin is wiped into the hollow end of the handle (Fig. 21-23), and the pin is lowered so that the two portions flow together (Fig. 21-24). The resin is allowed to set hard. The guide can then be removed. There is no further need for the wax on the guide table, and so it can be cleaned off after the guide is removed.

5. Because of the design of the special wax-cutter pin, the lateral anterior guidance angle will be evident as a sharp line running along the bottom edge of the acrylic guide. The edge is marked with a pencil (Fig. 21-25) and any excess acrylic resin may be ground off *in front of the line.* One may actually hollow-grind the front surface down to the line to make a scoop-shaped guide (Fig. 21-26), which is excellent for shaving out wax from the fossae.

6. To ensure posterior disclusion, the fossa walls must be flatter than the lateral anterior guidance, and so the fossa guide angle is flattened on the sides and the tip is rounded to a more opened-out fossa (Fig. 21-27).

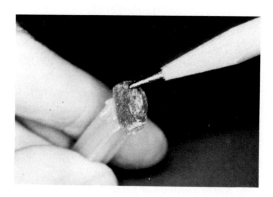

Fig. 21-25

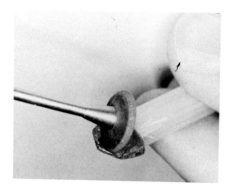

Fig. 21-26

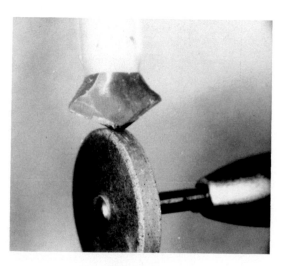

Fig. 21-27

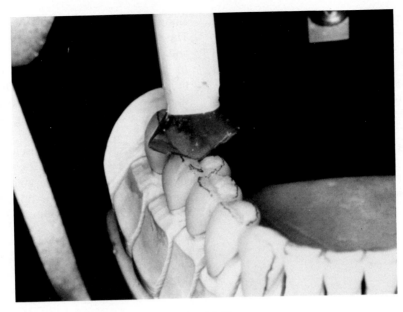

Fig. 21-28

7. The fossa guide can be used to contour the wax patterns or as a guide for shaping occlusal surfaces in porcelain (Fig. 21-28). The tip of the guide should be able to touch the base of the fossa without interference from the walls of the fossa. The shape of the special wax-cutter pin will provide for enough thickness of the back of the fossa guide, so that it will be strong enough to be used either as a guide to check the carving of the fossae or as a convenient instrument that can itself be used as a tool to scoop out fossae contours in the wax or the buildup-stage porcelain. If a rubber band is attached through a hole drilled in the handle, the guide can be attached to the articulator for convenience.

There are just three basic rules for using the fossae contour guide.

1. *Always hold the handle perpendicularly* (Fig. 21-29). The cusp-fossae angles were related to the handle when it was straight up and down on the articulator. Tilting the handle would produce an error in the fossae contours.

2. *Never destroy a predetermined cusp tip.* The depth of the fossae will be limited automatically if this rule is followed (Fig. 21-30).

3. *Locate fossae in proper relation to cusp tips.* A basic knowledge of anatomy is necessary for all techniques. Proper fossae location ensures saucer-like fossae contours and permits good occlusal form.

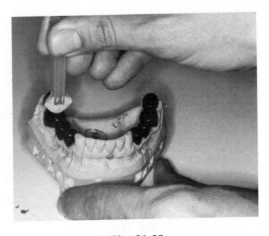

Fig. 21-29

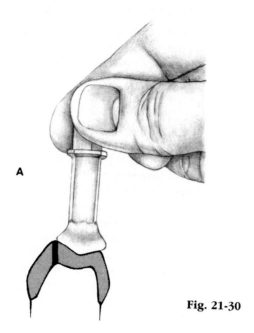

A

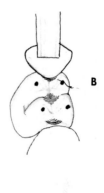

B

Fig. 21-30

The front of the guide always faces front, and in that position it is correct for either the right or the left side. When the handle is held perpendicular, it exactly reproduces the lateral anterior guidance. Flattening the bottom of the guide will provide extra room for lateral disclusion. Even though the side shift is usually built into the anterior guidance (and consequently duplicated in the fossae-contour guide), it is necessary to give a little extra lateral freedom to ensure posterior disclusion.

Modifications in using the fossae contour guide

As long as the base of the fossa is wide enough and the fossa inclines are not steeper than the lateral guidance inclines, supplemental grooves can be placed into the fossa walls and between cusps without fear of creating interferences to the upper lingual cusp. The fossae contour guide may be used before supplemental grooves are placed or it can be used to refine fossae wall inclinations after all the occlusal carvings have been completed. Carving the patterns with fairly deep grooves and slightly convex inclines will usually require an opening out of the fossae, but the result is an unusually natural looking occlusal contour, since it simulates normal wear. It is also the way most technicians will prefer because it does not require any change in their carving procedures. It merely adds the simple step of

using the fossae contour guide as a scoop to shave away any convexities in the wax that would interfere with the lateral guidance.

The fossae contour guide can be used in combination with dropped wax techniques and gnathologic mountings. It is especially useful when the dentist does not wish to prepare both upper and lower teeth together. The wax can be built up on the lower teeth to conform to a correct occlusal plane and cusp tip location and then the guide can be used to modify the fossae contours when necessary. The result will be compatible with the upper gnathologic waxup, which will be done later.

Finished castings and porcelain occlusals can be checked by the dentist and modified by selective grinding. The fossae contour guide is an easy tool to use. A quick analysis of each fossa can be made when the restorations are received from the laboratory. Fossa walls that are not in harmony with the guide can be opened out by grinding. This is a practical approach because corrections almost always involve taking material away. If inclines are flatter than the guide, the fossa can be deepened to steepen them, provided that there is enough thickness. Fossa walls that are too flat do not constitute an interference, however, and on the lower teeth none of the inclines contacts in function anyway.

If there is any consistency in occlusal contouring errors, it is carving convex or too steep fossa walls. The familiar "Parker House roll" occlusion does not provide room in the lower fossae for the upper lingual cusps. The fossae contour guide enables the dentist or the technician to correct this problem.

Carving the marginal ridges

When all cusp tips have been properly located and the fossae correctly placed and contoured, the marginal ridges seem to fall right into place. The most common error noted in marginal ridge contouring is failure to evenly line up the marginal ridges of contacting teeth. Uneven height of adjacent marginal ridges invites food entrapment and often becomes an interference.

The ridges should be contoured to reflect food away from the contact, which means directing it into the fossae. Sluiceways should provide an escape route for the bolus out of the fossae toward the lingual as the stamp cusps crush the food against the fossae walls.

At the risk of being repetitious, I should reemphasize that no technique will work without a basic understanding of occlusal contours. The procedures described merely provide reference points and guidelines to organize our occlusal form. Remember too that the fossa contour guide is used only when both upper and lower posterior teeth are being restored.

PORCELAIN OCCLUSAL VENEERS

When lower posterior teeth are to have veneered porcelain occlusal surfaces, the same procedures described previously can be used to advantage. Porcelain veneers are much stronger if the veneer thickness is kept fairly uniform. Waxing the teeth to contour first and then cutting the patterns back about 1 to 1.5 mm wherever porcelain is to be applied results in the strongest possible porcelain application. It also provides for the best esthetics because there will be no need for thin spots in the porcelain where the opaquer shows through.

To make certain that the porcelain cusp tips are in the correct position, a simple procedure that utilizes an easily made stone matrix can be followed. A creamy mix of stone can be jiggled over the waxed-up occlusal surfaces and extended around the arch onto the anterior teeth (which have been lubricated). The stone is allowed to set and then the matrix is removed. The wax patterns can then be cut back to receive the porcelain. The patterns are cast and prepared for porcelain application. With a marking pencil, a mark that represents the exact tip of each buccal cusp is put in each indentation (Fig. 21-31). The matrix is trimmed back on a model trimmer to the center of each cusp tip mark (Fig. 21-32). The matrix will fit back on the model, indexed to the front teeth,

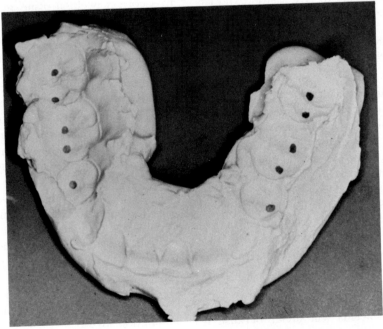

Fig. 21-31. To convert waxed-up occlusal contours to porcelain, a stone matrix of the occlusal is made of the completed waxup. The patterns are then cut back to provide a uniform thickness of porcelain and the patterns are cast. A mark is made in the matrix at the location of each buccal cusp tip.

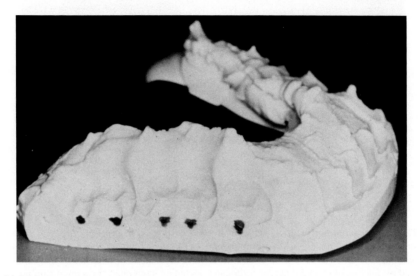

Fig. 21-32. The matrix is trimmed on a model trimmer back to the center of each cusp tip location. It will serve as an index to buccal cusp tip location.

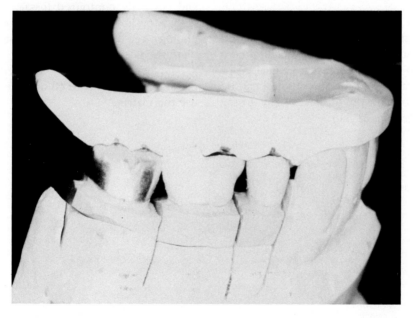

Fig. 21-33. The index is seated back on the model with the castings in place. The index acts merely as a guide to which each lower buccal cusp tip is related. The buccal porcelain is built to the cusp tip location. Once the buccal cusp tip is contoured in the right position, it serves as a point of reference for the ceramist. Occlusal contours can then be carved by the ceramist. The fossae contour guide can be used during application of the porcelain or as a guide in carving the occlusal surfaces after baking.

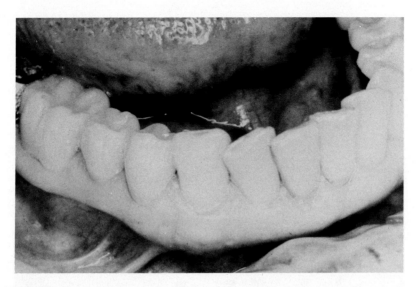

Fig. 21-34. Completed porcelain veneer crowns. Each cusp tip is in precisely the right position for optimum stability and function. Fossae contours have been opened out to permit centric contact with the upper lingual cusps without any interference in lateral excursion. Upper posterior teeth can now be fabricated by any one of several different techniques, including functionally generated path techniques.

and will serve as a series of reference points so that the ceramist can build the porcelain buccal cusp tips to the correct position (Fig. 21-33).

The matrix is used to locate only the *buccal* cusp tips for the ceramist, but once the buccal cusps are located, the rest of the occlusal contours fall into place more easily. Lingual cusps are easily located, and fossae contours can be carved or ground with the aid of the fossae contour guide (Fig. 21-34).

The two parts of each lower tooth that have functional occlusal contacts are assured with the correct location of the buccal cusp tips and correctly contoured fossae. The ceramist with a basic understanding of occlusal morphology can add the esthetic finery to complete the occlusal form.

The fossa guide can also be used directly on the porcelain if the technician elects not to use the matrix.

22

Restoring upper posterior teeth

The upper posterior teeth should be the last segment to be restored. It is the fixed posterior segment, and its cusps, inclines, grooves, and ridges are placed and contoured to accommodate the many border movements of the lower posterior teeth. If the upper contours are determined by the pathways of the lower posterior teeth, both the form and the paths of the lower teeth should be finalized before the upper teeth are restored.

Since the anterior guidance is the major determinant of the pathways that the lower teeth follow, it should logically be finalized before the attempt is made at harmonizing posterior inclines. When the lower cusp-fossae inclines are then designed to be discluded by the correct anterior guidance and the lower cusp tips are precisely located on an acceptable occlusal plane, upper contours can be refined to any desired degree.

Although it is possible to fabricate upper and lower posterior restorations together, upper posterior restorations should never be fabricated against lower posterior teeth that require correction of their occlusal plane, cusp tip placement, or fossa contours. If it is absolutely necessary to restore upper posterior teeth first, the lower teeth should be corrected as close to optimum as possible with selective grinding or temporary restorations. It seems

most inconsistent to build errors into restorations that are supposed to last for many years.

PREPARING UPPER POSTERIOR TEETH FOR OCCLUSAL RESTORATION

Many restorations are destroyed after they have been cemented in place because of corrective grinding to eliminate excursive interferences. It should never be necessary to grind through any restoration that has been placed on a properly prepared tooth.

When upper posterior teeth are being prepared, they should be checked *in all excursions* to make certain that there is room for a sufficient thickness of metal or metal and porcelain. Too often, preparations are checked in centric relation only, and it is impossible to provide sufficient thickness of the restoration when the tooth moves from its centric position.

If the anterior guidance has not been finalized and the lower posterior teeth are not also in their final form, it is not possible to determine the amount of clearance that is actually available for the upper prepared teeth. As an example, if upper fossae inclines are reduced to have clearance in lateral excursions that are guided by an incorrectly steep anterior guidance, flattening the anterior guidance will then bring the prepared posterior inclines into contact, leaving no room for the restorative material.

Following an orderly sequence of restoration, making certain each segment is correct before proceeding to the next, and checking the clearance in all excursions will guarantee that upper preparations will provide adequate room for the proper restoration of the occlusal surface.

MOST IMPORTANT CENTRIC RECORD

Of all the interocclusal records that are made during occlusal reconstruction, the most important one of all is the one for articulating the upper posterior die model. It is the final centric record, and the importance of having it accurate cannot be overemphasized.

Whenever possible, this final centric record should be taken at the correct vertical dimension. Allowing the anterior teeth to contact not only simplifies the record making, but also permits the condyles to seat all the way up into the superior terminal axis position when the record is being made. Taking the centric record at the correct vertical dimension eliminates any error that would have been associated with a missed axis of closure and provides the operator with a means of verifying the accuracy of the centrically articulated casts.

The next time we are tempted to rush through this important step, we must remember: it takes far longer to grind away all the carefully placed anatomy on the fnished restorations than it takes to record the centric position accurately in the first place.

RECORDING THE BORDER MOVEMENTS

All the upper occlusal inclines are related to the border pathways that the lower posterior teeth follow. In most patients, we do not want any contact against any incline during any excursive movement of the lower arch. We want immediate disclusion of all posterior teeth the moment the mandible moves out of centric relation in any direction. The effect of this disclusion is just recently understood, and the principle reason for advocating it is the reduction in elevator muscle activity at the moment of disclusion by the anterior guidance. The disclusion is easily accomplished if the anterior guidance is reasonably steep, or the condylar paths are healthy and sufficiently disclusive in their angulations. But if the anterior guidance

is fairly flat or nonfunctional or adaptive changes have flattened the condylar paths, the precise recording of border pathways becomes more important and more critical.

With normal condylar paths, we can effect posterior disclusion merely by setting the articulator paths flatter than the patient's in protrusive movements. Setting the progressive side shift at a greater angle than the patient's will cause disclusion of the balancing inclines. If the lower posterior occlusal surfaces have been contoured with fossae walls that are flatter than the anterior guidance, the upper posterior teeth can be constructed on an articulator, programmed with *arbitrarily* flatter condylar paths and greater progressive side shift. Disclusion in all excursions will be accomplished rather simply on semiadjustable instruments set in this manner.

If however, it is desirable to have excursive contact on certain inclines, or a near miss of precise dimensions, it will be necessary to record the border pathways with preciseness. Upper contours can be planned for group function or a measured miss only if we know exactly the path each lower cusp will be traveling.

For this type of preciseness, both the anterior and the posterior determinants of occlusion must be considered, and so the effect of the border movements of the condyles must be recorded at least to the extent that they can function within the envelope permitted by the anterior guidance. There are several methods of recording the border movements that will provide acceptable accuracy for completing the upper occlusal surfaces. Some of the various instruments that can be used are described in Chapter 12. The important thing to remember about capturing border movements is that it is actually the border movements of the lower teeth that determine upper occlusal contours. Whether condylar and anterior guidance determinants are captured directly to then reproduce tooth movements on an instrument or the tooth movements are captured directly at their site makes no difference, as long as the final upper tooth inclines are in harmony with the functional pathways that the *lower teeth* follow.

One of the most accurate methods of capturing border movements is the functionally generated path technique. Since it lends itself so well to the methods already described for restoring the lower posterior teeth, it is the method that I prefer for transferring lower tooth movements into three-dimensional upper occlusal contours.

SUPPLEMENTAL ANATOMY ON THE UPPER OCCLUSAL SURFACES

The dentist must decide whether the upper occlusal inclines are to be in group function, partial group function, or total disclusion in excursive movements. Whichever decision is made, it is accomplished by contouring and angulation of the inclines themselves. Supplemental grooves cut into inclines add to the natural appearance and increase the gripping and shredding ability of the tooth surfaces. If the incline *surfaces* are noninterfering, it will be impossible to create an interference by putting a groove in such a surface. For this reason it is a logical approach to first develop the incline surfaces according to the type of function desired and then carve into that surface the supplemental anatomy. The grooves are carved smaller than the cusp tips. The tips will just pass over the grooves with no effect on the actual contact through the excursive movement.

LENGTH OF GROUP FUNCTION CONTACT IN WORKING EXCURSION

If we elect to provide group function on the working side, we should be aware that all teeth do not stay in excursive contact for the same length of stroke. As the mandible starts its move to the working side, all the posterior teeth may contact in harmony with the anterior guidance and the condyle. As the mandible moves further to the side, the first teeth to disengage from contact are the most posterior molars. The disengagement is progressive, starting with the back molar, which has the shortest contact stroke, forward to the cuspid, which has the longest contact (Fig. 22-1).

The molar contact is maintained for only a fraction of the incline surface, whereas the cuspid contact is often maintained all the way to the incisal tip. The reason for giving the cuspid such a long contact ride and a progressive shorter contact as we go distally is based on factors of geometry and stress. As the working condyle rotates, the path traveled around the center of rotation lengthens as the distance

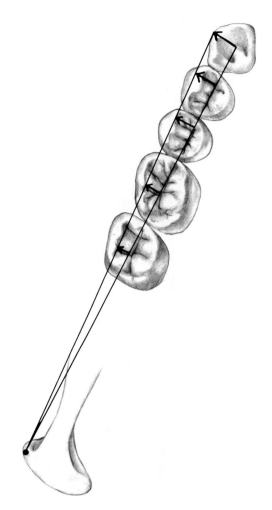

Fig. 22-1. The length of the contact stroke should be progressively shorter from the anterior teeth back. The molar contact is maintained for only a fraction of its incline surface, whereas contact against the upper cuspid incline is maintained all the way to incisal edge.

from the condyle increases. While the cuspid is traveling the full length of its incline from centric to its incisal edge, the second molar is traveling about half that far. When the cuspid reaches its incisal edge, the molar still has some incline left on which it could ride out. However, if the molar continued its contact after the cuspid was disengaged, the stress would be no longer shared by the protective anterior guidance. It would instead be loaded entirely onto the outer incline of the molar and would create considerable lateral torque in the extremely stressful position near the condylar fulcrum (Fig. 22-2).

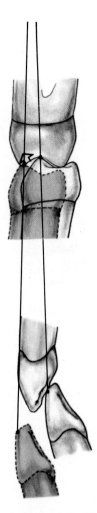

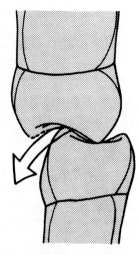

Fig. 22-3. Upper occlusal inclines should be contoured to disclude in a manner that allows the anterior teeth to maintain contact the longest. The second molar should contact in a working-side excursion for no more than half its incline length.

Fig. 22-2. If molar contact is maintained for the entire incline, the protection from the anterior guidance is lost. The stress exerted against the molar is severe because of its torqueing effect near the condylar fulcrum.

Because of these reasons, the lingual incline of the upper buccal cusps should be contoured to prevent posterior contact from occurring after the lower cuspid reaches the incisal edge of the upper cuspid (Fig. 22-3). More definitively, the anterior guidance contact should be maintained during all posterior contact in working excursions.

BALANCING EXCURSIONS

The term "balancing excursion" is a remnant of full denture terminology. It originally referred to actual balancing contact to stabilize the dentures on the side of the downward-moving, orbiting condyle. It is a part of the three-point contact concept, which for denture stability is a good concept. Many dentists have tried to apply the same concept of bilaterally balanced occlusion to the natural dentition but have abandoned the idea because of the disastrous clinical results. Hypermobility and periodontal breakdown seem to be the rule rather than the exception, since the posterior teeth succumb to the effects of the so-called balance.

As already discussed in Chapter 19, bilaterally balanced occlusion does not work because there is no way to harmonize the "balancing" inclines of the teeth to all of the variations of muscle force against the unbraced orbiting condyle. "Balancing" inclines must be relieved on all restorations regardless of the method used to record the border movements. The relief can be accomplished rather simply by slight hollow grinding of the buccal inclines of the upper lingual cusps between the centric contacts in the fossae and on the tips of the lingual cusps.

When the upper restorations are placed in the mouth and the centric contacts have been verified as correct, balancing inclines should be checked with marking ribbon while the mandible is manipulated into firmly guided excursions. The dentist must not rely on the patient to make lateral border movements unassisted. Patient tendency will be to go into a protruded lateral instead of the full border movement. Since balancing incline interferences are so stressful, extra care should be

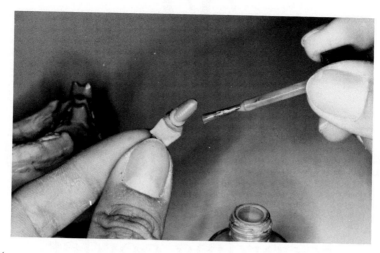

Fig. 22-4. The occlusion on restorations is often ruined by errors of cementation. Unless some form of relief is used to provide room for cement, even the most meticulously made crowns will be "high" after cementation. A practical way to relieve full crowns is by painting the dies with a sufficiently thick spacer before waxup. The die spacer provides room for cement and protects the dies at the same time.

taken to make sure such inclines are never allowed to contact.

When applied to natural teeth, the term "balancing side" is obviously not a correct connotation. Stuart and Thomas refer to the orbiting condyle side as the "idling side." The term that seems to be most commonly used now is "nonfunctioning side." It is certainly a better term, since it correctly indicates a lack of contact.

Regardless of the method used for restoring upper posterior teeth, it will almost always be necessary to spot-grind slight occlusal discrepancies that result from cementation. Such occlusal corrections should not require more than a few minutes and should not cause mutilation of any occlusal anatomy.

If the occlusion must be grossly adjusted on the finished restorations, one or more of the following errors has probably been committed:

Improper recording of centric relation. The bite record should fulfill all four criteria for acceptability outlined in Chapter 4. Careless recording of the bite records is one of the major sources of error and wasted time.

Errors in mounting. A perfect bite record can be ruined by anything less than extreme care in the laboratory. I believe that this step is so important that in my office it is carried out in the office and checked carefully before the case is turned over to the technician.

Improper fit of finished restorations. Castings that do not fit are responsible for a large share of occlusal problems. Casting techniques should be continually checked for accu-

racy using steel dies.* A second die model may also be reserved for careful and gentle seating of the castings by the dentist to check the fit. Precise casting accuracy requires continuous and meticulous attention to many laboratory details. Accuracy in this department cannot be left to chance.

Errors in cementation. Cementation does affect the position of the crown on the tooth. The best we can do is minimize the change. The type of cement, the way it is mixed, the fit of the crown, the taper of the preparation, and many other factors affect the accuracy of this step. The astute restorative dentist is always on the alert for information that can minimize cementation error. Failure to relieve the inner surfaces of crowns is a major cause of cementation errors. Painting the dies with a sufficiently thick layer of die spacer is the most practical method of supplying enough room for cement thickness (Fig. 22-4). It also protects the dies against chipping.

It has been my impression that improper mixing of oxyphosphate cements is an all too common error. Mixing too fast or too thick is a sure invitation for raised restorations. There is no substitute for meticulous attention to every detail when you are restoring an occlusion. However, the restoration of the upper posterior teeth is the sequence that can either complement or destroy all the prior restorative efforts. It is worthy of all the care and skill that might be expended on its perfection.

*Steel dies available from Sherwood Research, 9160 Brookville Road, Silver Spring, MD 20910.

23

Functionally generated path techniques for recording border movements intraorally

Despite its simplicity, the functionally generated path technique (FGP) can be an extremely sophisticated method of capturing in a usable way the precise border pathways that the lower posterior teeth follow. The technique has the distinct advantage of being able to record all dimensions of such border movements at the correct vertical as they are directly influenced by both condylar guidances and anterior guidance. The procedure can produce accuracy with fairly simple instrumentation, and it can be used in combination with almost any laboratory method for waxing upper posterior restorations. It can be used either in the actual fabrication of the restorations or as a three-dimensional checkbite technique after the restorations are completed.

FGP procedures are often misunderstood to be a technique that merely reproduces an existing occlusion. The common term "chew-in" is often placed on a par with the "mush bite," and the entire technique is written off as an inferior method that produces a "worn-out occlusion." Like any other technique for recording border pathways, the value of functional

path procedures is directly proportionate to the operator's understanding of what he is trying to accomplish and why. When properly used, FGP procedures are unsurpassed in accuracy and they require no compromise whatever in the finishing of occlusal contours.

If the following facts are understood, the value of FGP as a logical method of achieving precisely accurate occlusal contours will be obvious.

1. Border pathways of the lower posterior teeth are dictated by two different determinants:
   a. The anatomic limits of movement of the condyle-disk assemblies (posterior determinant)
   b. The anterior guidance (anterior determinant)
2. Functionally generated path procedures, properly used on upper posterior teeth, record directly all possible border pathways *of the lower posterior teeth,* as they are influenced by both the anterior and posterior determinants.
3. The shape of the occlusal surfaces of the

410

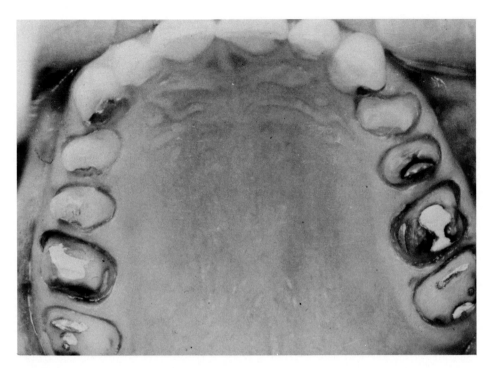

Fig. 23-1. Upper posterior teeth are prepared. The anterior guidance has been corrected if necessary, and the lower posterior cusp placement and fossae contours are correct. Patient is now ready for functionally generated path procedures. An impression is made of the prepared upper arch, and a model is poured while the patient waits.

lower posterior teeth has a profound influence on the type of occlusion that is dictated by moving said shapes along the border pathways through the functional wax.

In a nutshell, as each lower posterior tooth moves through the functional wax on the upper prepared teeth (according to the limiting effect of the condylar border movements and the anterior guidance), any wax *that is in the way* is wiped off. If the lower occlusal contours are in harmony with the combined effect of the anterior guidance and condylar border movements, nothing that is needed will be wiped away, including the wax representing the upper lingual cusps.

Obviously, any dentist who does not wish to reproduce an incorrect existing occlusion would not use FGP procedures until he has made certain that both the anterior guidance and the lower occlusal contours are correct. However, if either the anterior guidance or the lower occlusal contours are incorrect, there is *no technique* that can produce correct upper posterior teeth.

Since the most advantageous use of FGP procedures is for restoring all the upper posterior teeth, a technique for bilateral occlusal reconstruction is described first.

TECHNIQUE STEPS FOR BILATERALLY RECORDING THE FGP

After the anterior guidance has been harmonized according to the patient's functional, esthetic, and periodontal support requirements and *after* the lower posterior occlusal contours (fossae contours in particular) have been harmonized to the anterior guidance, the technique for recording the FGP is as follows:

Making the base for the FGP

1. Upper posterior teeth are prepared (Fig. 23-1).

2. An impression is made of the upper prepared arch and, while the patient waits, is poured immediately in hard stone. The impression material used for this step should have a soft consistency so that it will not distort the soft tissues. A smooth, creamy mix of alginate is acceptable.

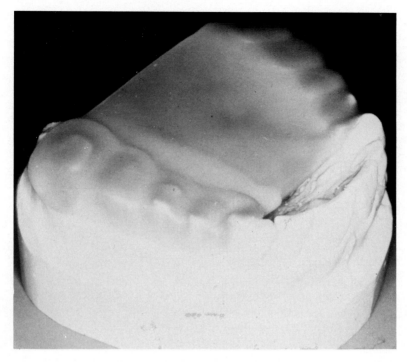

Fig. 23-2. Three layers of *extra-hard* base plate wax are softened and adapted to the model. The wax should be pressed thin over the occlusal surfaces and must be wrapped down around the prepared teeth so that the base will be completely stable in the mouth. The wax should extend straight across the arch. It should not be adapted to the palate.

3. When the model has set, *extra-hard* base plate wax is used to make a base for the functional wax. The wax used for this step should be brittle hard so that the base will not bend without breaking. Soft waxes that can bend during use create errors. Delar wax (extra hard) is a good wax for this step. The wax is softened over a flame and folded into three layers. While it is still soft, it is adapted around each tooth on the cast. It is pressed down very firmly over each tooth so that it will be thin enough to see through on the occlusal portion. Then the wax is adapted down around each tooth to completely cover all prepared teeth down to the gingival margins (Fig. 23-2). The wax wafer should *not* be adapted to the palate. It should go straight across. It should cover only the posterior teeth but should be extended right up to the unprepared cuspids.

4. The chilled base is removed from the model and inserted into the mouth. Soft-tissue impingement should not be a problem because the base was adapted to a model that had been made from soft impression material that is non-distorting to the soft tissues. This base *must be perfectly stable* in the mouth. The base is seated firmly and watched carefully for any spring back. If there is *any movement* whatever of the base, the wax is trimmed back on the underside wherever it touches soft tissue.

5. When it is certain that the base is stable, the patient should close his mouth. *There should be no tooth contact on the base.* Articulating ribbon will mark any contacts, which in turn can be reduced in the mouth with a discoid carver. Tooth contact on the hard base wax can move opposing teeth, cause the base to move, or prevent complete closure during the recording of border pathways. Contact in all excursions as well as centric relation closure should be checked. There must be no interferences that will restrict the anterior guidance from functioning in its normal manner.

Careless fabrication of the base is responsible for most FGP failures, and it is an unnecessary error to try to make accurate recordings on a poorly made base. The functional path recording can be no more precise than the stability of the base permits. If for any reason the base is not firm, stable, and retentive in the mouth, the procedure should be modified to satisfy these requirements. When there are fairly extensive edentulous areas (as an example), it may be necessary to cast the base of metal. Regardless of what is required, the base must fit the teeth and be absolutely stable.

The base should not be fabricated in the mouth. It is too easy to move a tooth or distort soft tissue. One actually saves time while improving accuracy by taking an impression and making the base on a model. Having a model at chairside when recording a functional path enables the dentist to go back to the model at any time to check for distortion of the base.

Use of acrylic and other hard materials for fabricating the base. Any material that can maintain accuracy through all the procedures is acceptable as a base. It must not be flimsy, and it must be stable and retentive. Furthermore, the base must fit the master die model as accurately as it fits the mouth, and it should not damage the dies when it is seated on and taken off the master model. I have not found acrylic bases to be consistently acceptable because of the distortion of the acrylic resin during or after setting and the damaging effect of the acrylic resin on the dies. Nevertheless, we have the flexibility to use any material or devise any technique for making the base as long as it fulfills the requirements of accuracy.

Cross-arch stabilization of the base. A common cause of error in FGP techniques is hypermobility of the teeth. If the teeth move during the functional movements, the inclines that are cut into the functional wax will be incorrect. Cross-arch stabilization can be affected by the base. Making the base on a model assures us that the prepared teeth will be stabilized in their correct position during all the functional procedures.

Cast bases. When there are missing teeth, bases can be cast in scrap gold or other metals. When the waxup is made, it should be kept very thin on the occlusal surface so that it will not contact the opposing teeth in either centric relation or any excursion. The functional wax table needs only to be wide enough to represent the upper occlusal surface with a little extra to hold the wax. Tables that are too wide interfere with the cheeks.

Beads can be added to hold the functional wax. The buccal and lingual edges of the cast table can be turned back to grip the wax (Fig. 23-3) or holes can be drilled in the cast table. Copings for the teeth should extend down

around the preparations far enough to assure stability. They do not have to cover the entire preparation, as a rule. A bar should connect the tables that will hold the wax. This is for cross-arch stabilization. It should not contact the soft tissue.

Recording the border movements

If a wax base is used, it should be tried in the mouth for fit and stability (Fig. 23-4).

After all posterior contact is cleared, the following procedure is performed:

1. The base is returned to the model and softened functional wax added for recording the FGP (Fig. 23-5). The functional wax is heated with a flame to make sure it is quite soft and sticky enough to securely adhere to the base. It may be sealed to the base with a hot spatula, but the base should not be softened too much or it will become distorted. A common problem is using too much functional wax. We want only enough to be impressed by about one third or less of each lower tooth. If too much wax is used, the excess bulk is too easily moved by the cheeks and tongue during the FGP recording and the path is useless. As stated before, the wax absolutely must not move during recording.

The functional pathways may be recorded in any material as long as that material records accurately and maintains that accuracy throughout all the laboratory procedures. There is an inherent problem with using any wax or material that can harden during the generation of the pathways. Inlay wax or sticky waxes work well while they are in their softened stage, but if they start to harden before all the border pathways have been recorded, an undetected error can occur. I prefer a functional wax that stays workable for as long as it is needed. Bosworth's Synthetic Tacky Wax is an ideal functional wax because of its good working qualities and ideal plasticity at mouth temperatures. It should be softened with a flame before being inserted into the mouth, and it will then maintain workable softness until it is chilled.

When the base with the Tacky Wax on it is placed back in the mouth, it must be completely seated. A little of the patient's saliva may be picked up on the tip of the finger and applied to the functional wax as a lubricant to prevent it from sticking to the lower teeth.

2. Using the same manipulative technique

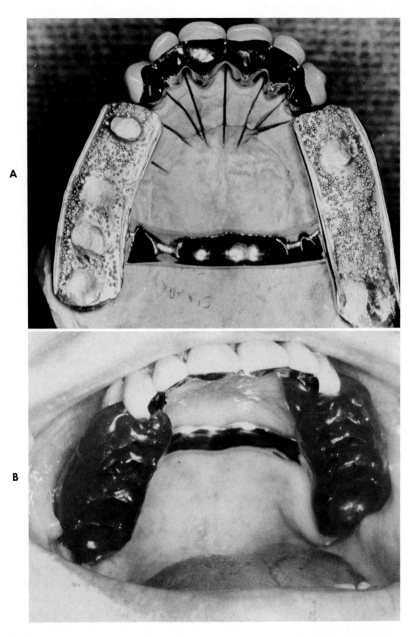

Fig. 23-3. A, A cast base is made if there are not enough teeth to adequately stabilize a wax base. It can be cast out of scrap metal. Beads and rolled edges are used to hold the functional wax in place. A cross arch stabilizing bar should be sturdy and should not touch soft tissue. (There is no need to polish the bar.) **B,** When a full arch splint is to be fabricated, the anterior restorations are completed, tried in, and checked for correctness. The cast base is seated and the functionally generated path is completed. The anterior restorations are returned to the master die model along with the cast base and the functional core for completion of the upper posterior restorations. The posterior restorations can then be soldered to the anterior splint if full arch splinting is desired.

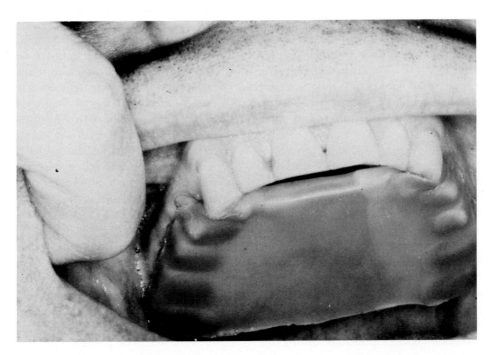

Fig. 23-4. If most posterior teeth are present and a wax base is to be used, it should be tried in and checked for stability. If the base springs back when seated, it is not acceptable. The extra-hard wax base should be checked at this point to make certain that no opposing teeth contact it. Only the anterior teeth should be in contact in any excursion. A discoid carver can be used to shave off interferences to the wax.

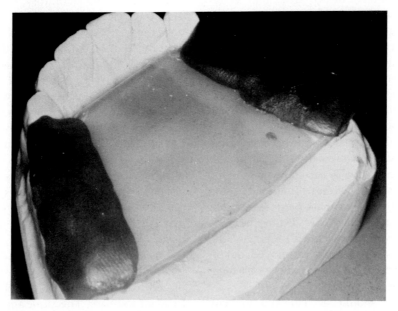

Fig. 23-5. After the base has been tried in and accepted, it is returned to the model for the addition of the functional wax. This softer wax must be luted securely to the base. One must not use too much functional wax; enough to impress one third of the lower tooth is sufficient.

that was used for recording centric relation, a closure is manipulated into the wax until the anterior teeth contact. The patient should be told in advance to hold that position and then slide forward until the anterior teeth are end to end. The patient should never open before going into an excursion, since this has a tendency to pull the base loose. After each opening the base should be checked to make sure it has not been dislodged.

3. The patient should close back into centric relation and the mandible is guided into lateral excursions. The dentist *must guide the mandible through all excursions* to ensure capturing of all border movements. If the excursive movements are left entirely to the patient, they will usually move in a protruded lateral direction and the mandible will not move the lower posterior teeth as far into the lateral path as it is really capable of doing in forceful movements. If the condyles are not forced to their outermost border positions during the generation of the path in the wax, tooth interferences to the extreme border positions will result in the restorations. These are the same interferences that usually go undetected by many dentists who do not use correct manipulative techniques in equilibration. They are potent triggers for bruxism and are the frequent cause of posterior tooth hypermobility.

The lateral shift of the condyles may be restricted in some degree by variations in the lateral anterior guidance, and it is the *combined* effect of anterior guidance and condylar guidance that dictates the border pathways of the posterior teeth. With proper manipulative technique, the exact outer pathways of the posterior teeth are captured three dimensionally in the functional wax (Fig. 23-6).

4. When all excursive movements have been recorded by manipulation of the mandible, the patient should be allowed to slide around however he wishes. This is the step that records the movements *between* straight lateral and straight protrusive. If there are any interferences to *any* movement of the jaw, the functional wax will simply be moved out of the way to record the outer limits of all functional movements.

5. The FGP should be checked for any movement during excursions and to make sure all pathways have been recorded in sufficient functional wax. If the dentist gently holds one cheek out of the way and the assistant holds

the other cheek, it is easy to observe the wax during jaw movements to see whether any distortion or movement of the wax base occurs. If everything appears to be in order, the wax is chilled with ice water to make it quite firm. The assistant should release the cheek while she mixes a creamy mix of Healey's Fast Setting Gray Rock or Whip Mix Bite Stone. When the stone is mixed, she should help hold the cheeks out again while the patient quickly goes through one last set of excursions. The cheeks should be held out while a creamy mix of stone is jiggled into all the depressions of the functional wax (Fig. 23-7).

The stone sets very fast and must be worked quickly once the mix is made. Vibrating the stone on the tip of the index finger while jiggling the mix ahead of the fingertip works quite well. Wiping the stone into the wax often traps air bubbles. The stone should be vibrated into the depressions in the same way an impression would be poured. Painting the wax with a detergent solution helps the stone flow smoothly with less trapping of air. *The fast-setting stone must cover at least one unprepared tooth in front and, if present, at least one distal to the prepared ones.* The stone index over the unprepared tooth on each side will serve as a definite vertical stop and a positive key to the master dies when the functional model is being used in the laboratory.

The cheeks should be held out of the way until the stone has set (about 2 to 3 minutes); then the FGP is removed from the mouth. The stone will stiffen the entire base and protect the functional wax. It also will make it easier to seat the FGP on the model without distorting the functional wax (Fig. 23-8). It is an unnecessary gamble to remove the FGP without first applying the stone in the mouth. I believe it is a major cause of error.

Application of the stone mix in the mouth has another important advantage. It enables the dentist to check for any distortion that may have occurred during the intraoral procedures.

Checking for distortion. When the FGP is removed from the mouth, it should be placed back on the same model that was used to adapt the base. The stone that covered over the unprepared tooth or teeth on each side should fit the same teeth on the model without any distortion whatsoever, that is, no space should be in evidence between the functional

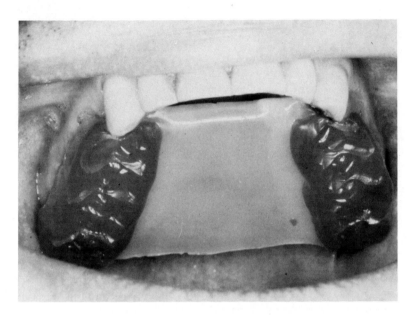

Fig. 23-6. A completed functional path recording. Notice how the pathways of each lower posterior tooth are recorded three dimensionally while the lower anterior teeth slide against the correct upper lingual inclines. The condyles control the movements of the back end of the mandible, and so the functionally generated path recording captures the movements of the posterior teeth as dictated by both anterior and posterior determinants.

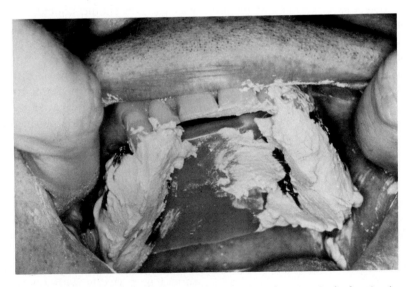

Fig. 23-7. A creamy mix of fast-setting stone is jiggled into the indentations in the functional wax. The stone must be extended to cover at least one unprepared "key" tooth (usually the cuspid).

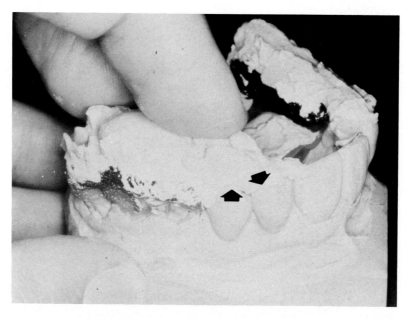

Fig. 23-8. A functionally generated path recording is tried on the model. The functional core stone *must* be adapted precisely to the key teeth in front or the functional record is unacceptable. There should be no space showing between the functional core and the model, *arrows.*

stone and the model stone. Even a slight crack between the model and the FGP stone should not be accepted, since it is an indication that the base has been distorted.

The distal end of the base should also be checked to see that it is in contact with the model. Both sides should be observed critically. If the FGP stone, now called the *stone core,* fits perfectly against the unprepared teeth in front and the wax base fits the model or unprepared teeth perfectly in the back, we may assume that there has been no distortion of the base. If there is any rock to the base on the model, it is usually easier and safer to start over and take a new FGP rather than to try to make a warped base fit. If proper procedures and materials are used, this will be a rare occurrence. Distortion of the base is usually the result of using wax that is too soft. The wax for the base must be brittle hard. A wax base should not be used when there are many missing teeth unless it can be thick enough to ensure strength.

Laboratory procedures

The upper master die model should be mounted with a facebow and should be articulated against the lower opposing model with a

centric bite record. The opposing anatomic model is not essential when FGP is used, but it serves as a doublecheck on the accuracy of the functional model.

In centric relation closure, the completed wax patterns should contact without interference against both the mounted functional model and the anatomic model. Any interference or lack of centric contact on either model indicates an error in either the FGP or the mounting of the anatomic model.

Many technicians prefer to wax the patterns against the anatomic model in the same manner they are used to, and then they refine the inclines against the functional model. This is a logical procedure. However, the skilled technician can soon "read" the functional model as effectively as the anatomic model.

Mounting the FGP

1. The opposing anatomic model is removed from the articulator and the FGP base placed on the mounted master die model. It should fit perfectly with no rock. The functional stone core should fit against the cuspids (or an unprepared tooth in front) without any crack showing. If a slight discrepancy is evident, it is almost always from some soft-tissue interference on the master model. The FGP is

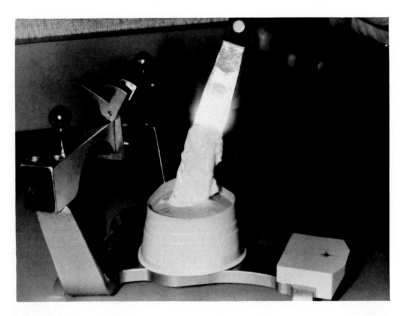

Fig. 23-9. One can make a built-up base in advance by cutting the bottom out of a plastic cup and inverting it over a mounting ring on the articulator. The cup is filled with stone or plaster and allowed to set completely before joining the function core to it.

removed, and the wax on the underside trimmed wherever it contacts the model. Trimming the dies before placement of the FGP often eliminates most of these problems, and such discrepancies are usually minor if the base is made and checked in the manner suggested. As long as the FGP base fits the first model perfectly, any discrepancies on the master die model can almost always be resolved by removal of soft-tissue contact on either the model or the underside of the base. There should be no loss of accuracy by such adjustments unless the base is warped in the process.

If the FGP base cannot be adapted to both models accurately, it is probable that one of the models is inaccurate.

2. Stone is built up from the lower articulator ring until it almost touches the stone core. An inverted plastic cup with the bottom cut out makes a good form for pouring the lower stone platform (Fig. 23-9). It is convenient to have several such platforms poured up for different heights. We can reuse them over and over by grinding the used stone core off on a model trimmer. This large mass of stone should set completely to take care of setting distortion before it is joined to the stone core (Fig. 23-10).

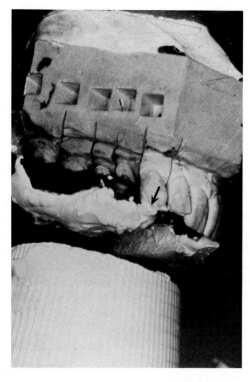

Fig. 23-10. The functionally generated path base with the stone attached is seated on the master die model. The stone core is checked for fit against the key tooth in front, *arrow.* The functional core is then joined to the base with a mix of stone.

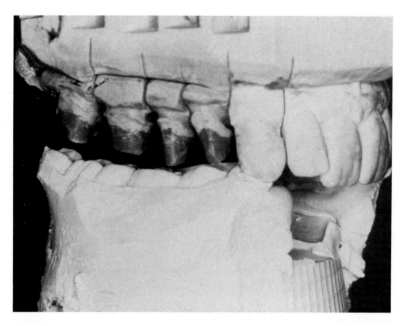

Fig. 23-11. The master die model related to the functional core. When the functional core is being used, *the articulator must be locked in centric relation.* The functional core is a three-dimensional record of border pathways, and so the articulator serves merely as a device to maintain the relationship of the dies to the recorded paths of movement of the lower teeth.

The stone core and the platform should be dampened and the two neatly joined together with another mix (Fig. 23-11). The guide pin should be set the same as it is for the anatomic model.

To check the accuracy of the FGP mounting, the upper die model is removed from the wax base and then the wax trimmed back to expose the occlusal edge of each upper tooth indentation. The upper model is then closed back into the FGP base to see whether there is any space between the dies and the base wax. If the die model does not seat perfectly into the FGP, the functional path recordings will be inaccurately related to the teeth. We can usually correct this error by knocking off the lower ring and redoing the mounting after making certain the die model is completely seated. On such a remount, the articulator is inverted and a new stone mix is used to join the platform to the lower ring.

There are several ways to check the accuracy of the FGP recording, and these accuracy checks are made at each step of the procedure from the intraoral steps through the completion of the mounting. None of the checks is complicated or time consuming, but each is important. The functional pathways that are recorded must be related perfectly to the dies,

or the entire procedure will be an exercise in futility. Every time we have had the opportunity of observing a dentist who was having poor results with FGP, the reason has been readily apparent: careless technique and failure to verify the accuracy of one step before proceeding to the next step. The simplicity of the FGP procedures should not be an invitation to sloppiness.

Using the functional model

The articulator is always locked in the position that allows absolutely no lateral movement when the functional model is in use. The articulator simply serves as a device to position the functional core in its proper relationship to the dies. Since the pathways of the lower teeth are recorded three dimensionally in the solid stone core, moving the articulator laterally produces an error. It must be kept locked in centric relation position.

The technician has the following three options for using the functional model:

1. Wax the restorations directly against the functional model (Fig. 23-12)
2. Wax against the anatomic model, and then refine the occlusal inclines and check for interferences against the functional model (stone core)

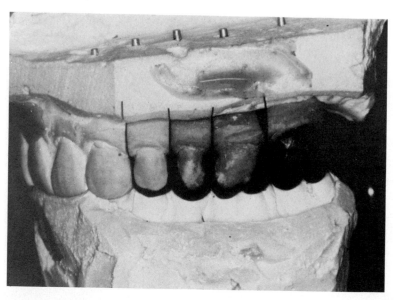

Fig. 23-12. One method of using the functional core is to wax directly against it. Inclines that should not contact are relieved. Inclines that are to be in functional contact are not relieved.

3. Complete the castings against the anatomic model, and then adjust the metal or porcelain occlusal surfaces against the functional model

Some dentists reserve the FGP model to do their own occlusal refinement when the restorations are returned from the laboratory. This is not the ideal method of using FGP, but it can serve as an alternative to accepting occlusal contours that have interfering inclines when the level of communication between the dentist and the technician falls a little short. It is a good learning experience for the dentist to adjust occlusal contours in this manner, since it provides a graphic illustration of the interferences that are so often built into the usual occlusal restorations. When the dentist develops a better understanding of correct occlusal contours, it is surprising how much more effectively he can communicate with his technician.

Since the most common mistake in occlusal contouring is carving inclines that are too steep, it will almost always be necessary to grind away interfering surfaces. Additionally and happily, the sum of all expansion and contraction of the materials used, from the hydrocolloid impression to the gold casting, seems to be slightly more on the expansion side. So adjusting the "finished" restoration against the FGP model has more application than might be suspected.

Making adjustments against the functional model. When the restorations are in place on the upper die model, it should be possible to close the articulator so that there is no crack between the "key" teeth and the functional stone core. All restorations should be in contact with the functional core. If there is any separation between these "key" teeth and the stone index (Fig. 23-13), it is an indication of an occlusal interference. Interferences can be marked with thin articulating ribbon and adjusted by selective grinding until the "key" teeth contact the index (Fig. 23-14).

We can observe infraocclusion by checking to see whether the die can be moved up and down when the restoration is in place and the key teeth are in contact against the index.

Group function is attained by adjustment of the lingual inclines of the upper buccal cusps to contact against the functional core (Fig. 23-15). *Disclusion* is attained when the inclines are taken out of contact with the functional core and only the selected centric stops are left in contact. The amount of space between the inclines and the functional model will represent the exact amount of clearance between the lower cusps and the upper inclines during excursions (Fig. 23-16).

Balancing inclines. All excursions made during the recording of the FGP represent actual contact. This includes balancing excur-

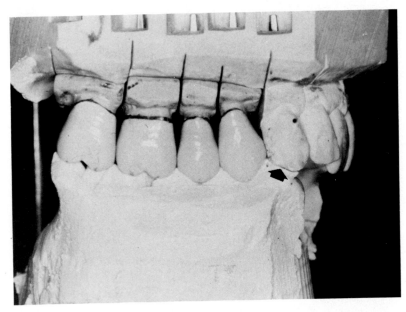

Fig. 23-13. Checking the finished restorations against the functional core. The slight separation between the core and the key index tooth indicates that an interference is present. The interference may be to any functional excursion. A marking ribbon may be used to find the interfering incline. It can then be adjusted by spot grinding.

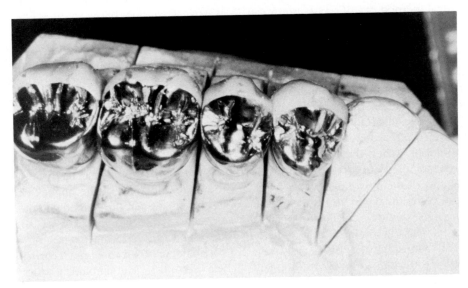

Fig. 23-14. Occlusal anatomy that has been fabricated and adjusted against a functional core. If the occlusal contours of the lower posterior teeth are correct, the upper occlusal anatomy can be made functional and stable without destroying occlusal contours.

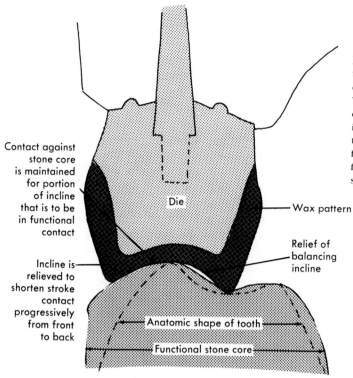

Contact against
stone core
is maintained
for portion
of incline
that is to be
in functional
contact

Die

Incline is
relieved to
shorten stroke
contact
progressively
from front
to back

Wax pattern

Relief of
balancing
incline

Anatomic shape of tooth
Functional stone core

Fig. 23-15. The relationship of the functional stone core to the upper occlusal inclines. Balancing inclines should be relieved. Working inclines remain in contact with the core if the tooth is to be in function in working excursions. The length of the stroke contact should be shortened progressively from front to back when the pattern is relieved from the buccal edge toward the centric stop.

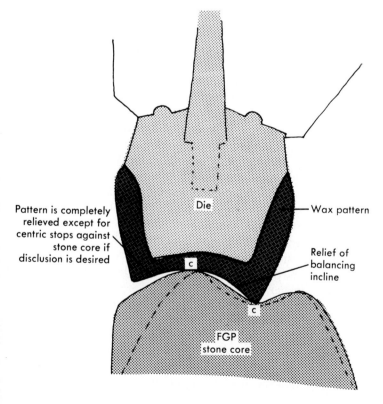

Pattern is completely
relieved except for
centric stops against
stone core if
disclusion is desired

Die

Wax pattern

Relief of
balancing
incline

FGP
stone core

Fig. 23-16. For posterior disclusion the pattern should be completely relieved so that only the centric stops contact the functional core.

sions. Since balancing-side contact is undesirable, *balancing-side disclusion must be effected by reduction of balancing inclines on the restorations so that they do not contact the functional stone at any point.* Heavy articulating paper may be used to mark these inclines to make sure there is ample clearance. A knowledgeable technician will establish this relationship in his wax carvings.

Wax patterns can be adjusted against the functional stone by use of white shoe polish on the functional model. It will mark interferences on the wax quite well. Talcum powder should not be used to mark interferences, since it becomes incorporated into the wax and causes a porous surface to the casting. With light-colored inlay waxes dark marking ribbon works well, and red marking ribbon can be seen against some blue or green waxes.

FGP CHECKBITE TECHNIQUE

The FGP technique can be used as outlined to check out castings that are already completed, after the castings have been tried in, checked for accuracy of fit, and then removed. To make sure the castings fit the mouth the same as they fit the model, they may be tried in and a stone matrix made along the occlusal surfaces. Fast-setting stone is ideal for the matrix because of its rapid setting time. The castings are then removed from the mouth and returned to the die model.

The stone matrix is trimmed back to the tip of the buccal cusps and placed on the castings. The matrix should fit the castings on the model as perfectly as it fit them in the mouth. Castings that have been checked in this manner and pass the test can be adjusted against an FGP model with complete assurance of accuracy. The whole procedure is simple enough that it can be accomplished easily while the patient waits.

No matter how perfect the occlusal contouring scheme may be, all accuracy is lost if the castings do not fit the teeth. Constant checking for casting accuracy is essential to ensure correct occlusal results without gross grinding of the finished restorations.

FGP FOR QUADRANT DENTISTRY

The real value of functional path procedures is more practically realized when it is used bilaterally because of the stabilizing effect on the teeth and the FGP base when it is attached to both sides of the arch. Nevertheless, functional paths can be recorded unilaterally if great care is exercised to assure the stability of the base and if hypermobility of the teeth in the quadrant is not a problem.

Because of the difficulty in stabilizing a unilateral base for FGP, I do not believe it should be used if both quadrants are to be restored. It would be far better to restore both together than to do one side at a time. Most often, unilateral quadrant restoration is done because of some uncertainty on the dentist's part to do both sides together. Sometimes it is believed that one side at a time is easier on the patient. Actually, it is usually less traumatic on the patient to have one master impression, one FGP, and (with good organization) half the appointments to complete both sides of the arch.

It is true that the appointment times will be longer for preparation and placement, but, within reason, patients usually prefer longer appointments if it means a reduction in the number of appointments. If the patient is not able to withstand the preparation of more than one quadrant at a time, the two quadrants can be prepared at separate appointments, temporary restorations can be constructed, and the FGP procedures can be carried out at a separate appointment so that the advantages of a bilaterally stabilized base can be realized. Organization and preplanning can make such appointments go very smoothly with minimal stress to the patient.

When only one quadrant is to be restored or when it is impractical to do both quadrants together, a single quadrant may be prepared and FGP procedures may be used to advantage *if the base can be stabilized.* In a unilateral quadrant it is often necessary to make a cast base in order to get enough stabilization. If the clinical crowns are long enough, it may be possible to use extra-hard wax as a base without fear of dislodgment, but the dentist should take extra precautions to make sure there is no movement of the base or of the teeth during generation of the path.

Care should be taken to be certain that only just enough functional wax is used, and it should be quite soft so that the drag on the wax is minimized when the lower teeth move through it. If there is any rock to the base or movement of the teeth, the FGP will be inaccurate. As long as that fact is understood, the method of making a stable base can be left to the unlimited imagination of the dentist. Whatever is used in the mouth for a base must be removable without distortion, and it must precisely fit the master dies without harm to them. All other procedures for completing the FGP are the same as already outlined.

After the path has been generated in the functional wax, a simple method for controlling the fast-setting stone application is to jiggle some into the FGP depressions and then carry some more into the mouth on a wooden tongue blade. The blade is vibrated to join the two portions and then held steady until the stone sets. The base, stone, and tongue blade are removed in one piece with little fear of distortion. The tongue blade is then removed, the excess stone is trimmed with a sharp scalpel, and the base is fitted on the upper dies. The functional stone is joined to the stone platform on the articulator with a creamy mix of fast-setting stone.

When preparing a single quadrant, special care should be taken to make sure the opposite side is perfectly equilibrated so that there are no deviating interferences to influence the functional paths. After preparation of one side, it is good to recheck the occlusion on the other side and to verify the correctness of the anterior guidance before proceeding with the FGP.

FGP FOR A SINGLE TOOTH

One of the most common uses for functional path procedures is the restoration of a single tooth. It is a helpful teaching exercise because it is easy for the student to relate the border movements recorded in the wax to the adjacent tooth inclines. As a practical clinical approach, however, FGP for a single tooth has minimal value. Using FGP for restoration of a single tooth involves unnecessary extra procedures that require longer chair time, and in many instances it produces unwanted results.

If there are occlusal interferences present, the FGP will perpetuate them in the restoration. Instead of condylar guidance serving as the posterior determinant, the offending incline interference becomes the determinant of the functional path and the new restoration will be restored into group function malocclusion. In such cases of "tooth-guided occlu-

sions," FGP accomplishes nothing that could not be acheived if one simply rubbed two hand-held models together with soft wax on the die. If tooth inclines limit the movement, the FGP can be done directly on the models. There is no clinically important difference between rubbing stone surfaces together and rubbing enamel surfaces together. In posterior tooth-guided occlusions, the direction of the pathways is insignificant because the models can be rubbed only in the paths that other tooth inclines permit. Regardless of the technique used, however, the entire occlusion should be in harmony before any restorations are made.

If the occlusion has been perfected in the mouth into precise group function, working inclines on the models will be in harmony with condylar and anterior guidance. Again, single-tooth FGP has no advantage over hand-held full arch models. If the occlusal pattern is determined by rubbing of the models together, the correct inclines will be patterned directly in the wax on the die. Correct disclusion of balancing inclines will even be duplicated in the restoration because the hand-held models permit the balancing inclines of adjacent teeth to contact and thereby duplicate the disclusive contour in the wax pattern or the restoration (Fig. 23-17).

Disclusion of balancing inclines is not achieved with FGP, however, even though the inclines in the mouth do disclude. Balancing inclines must be additionally reduced on the restoration whenever FGP is used.

The biggest shortcoming of single-tooth FGP occurs in mouths with posterior disclusion. Even if all other posterior inclines are discluded in working and balancing excursions, restoring against a functional model will put the restored inclines in full lateral contact. Such an occlusal requirement would rarely be desired for a single posterior tooth. If FGP is used in posterior disclusion cases, the restoration should be relieved on the working and balancing inclines. if full-arch hand-held models are used instead of FGP, the disclusion of both working and balancing inclines will be perfected right on the models, a decided advantage.

There is another potential disadvantage for single-tooth FGP. If adjacent teeth have any hypermobility, they can move during generation

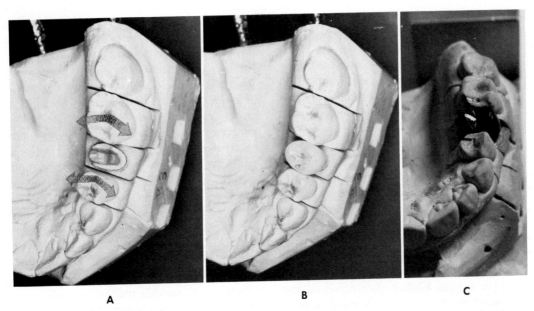

A   B   C

Fig. 23-17. A, Hand-held models permit the occlusal contours of adjacent teeth to be reproduced with maximum simplicity. The lower model is guided by the inclines on each side of the die. If balancing inclines have been relieved on the adjacent teeth, they will be relieved on the pattern. If the working inclines are in function, they will be in function on the pattern. If the working inclines are discluded, the disclusion will be effected on the pattern. As long as the teeth on each side of the prepared tooth are in centric relation contact, there is no possibility of losing centric contact on the pattern. **B,** The restoration in place. Notice the similarity of the inclines on the model with those on the porcelain occlusal surface. **C,** Notice the difference in the steepness of the balancing incline on the pattern made from a functional core compared with the adjacent inclines that have been equilibrated for disclusion. With functionally generated path techniques *all* inclines are in function unless specifically relieved. If this pattern were made by rubbing the models together, the adjacent corrected inclines would have been duplicated in the pattern and no further relief would have been necessary.

Fig. 23-18. The models articulated on a Johnson-Oglesby Spring Articulator. No bite record is needed, only an opposing model. The spring permits the models to be rubbed against each other in all directions so that each incline can come into contact. The *inclines of the adjacent teeth* must be in contact to be duplicated on the pattern. This method is only applicable for individual restorations, when the inclines of the adjacent teeth are to be repeated on the restoration. After the surface of the inclines is formed, grooves and ridges can be carved into the surface employing the same carving procedures used when a functional core is used.

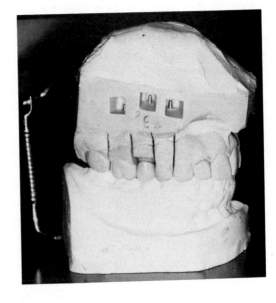

of the path and the path will be flatter in the wax than it is on the adjacent teeth. The restorative result is to disclude the restored tooth by letting the mobile teeth carry the load in excursions. However, if the tooth being restored is moved laterally during the generation of the path, its restored inclines will be steeper and it will have to continue moving laterally in excursions to bring its inclines into harmony with the adjacent teeth. This is a very common occurrence with single-tooth FGP. The drag of the functional wax can move an unstablized tooth back and forth with the lateral jaw movements. If FGP is used, the tooth being restored must be stabilized during generation of the path.

If full arch models are used, the position of the teeth stays the same as when the impression was made. If the other occlusal inclines are correct in the mouth, they will be correct on the models. Rubbing such models together with wax on the die will produce the same inclines in the wax that exist on the adjacent teeth, so that the wax pattern will also be correct. It should not require any further adjustments to provide either balancing or working disclusion.

If the anterior guidance is much steeper than the unprepared posterior inclines that are to be duplicated, it may be impossible for the posterior inclines to contact in excursions. This would prevent them from serving as the guiding influence for the hand-held models. Posterior inclines on each side of the die must be permitted to contact in order to have their working and balancing inclines duplicated in the soft wax on the die. If necesary, steep anterior teeth can be flattened on the model to permit full excursive contact of the posterior inclines. In this way the posterior inclines can serve as the guiding influence in contouring the occlusal surface of the wax pattern.

When the preceding model-rubbing procedure is used, the models must be free to move in all possible directions to assure no interferences in the wax pattern. Mounting the models on an articulator with limited incorrect excursions would permit interferences. The articulator would have to be fully adjusted to assure correct inclines and then the balancing inclines would still require additional relief.

The Johnson-Oglesby Spring Articulator (Fig 23-18) is a practical device for holding full arch models together while still permitting a full range of movement, including contact of the balancing inclines on the model. It may offend lovers of complexity, but it is the simplest way we know to achieve accuracy in a single restoration. The three essentials for a good result are as follows:

1. Occlusal correction before restoration
2. Full arch models
3. Reduction on the model of steep anterior inclines that prevent full excursive contact against the posterior inclines being copied

Some dentists seems to have an aversion to taking a full arch impression. They try to do restorative dentistry with quadrant impressions and absurdly inadequate little "crown and bridge articulators." Making a full arch impression requires no more time than a quadrant impression, but it saves time when the restoration is placed because occlusal adjustment is minimized. No centric bite record is required for mounting the full arch models. They are articulated without a bite, which is an acceptable method because they will be moved against each other in all possible contact positions.

There will be unusual occasions when it is not practical to take a full arch impression. Severe gaggers, patients with limited opening ability, and anatomic problems that make a full impression difficult are all resolvable by using FGP procedures. There are also some occasions when it may be advantageous to bring one or more posterior teeth into group function with the anterior guidance, even though other posterior teeth are discluded in lateral excursions. In such a case FGP would be a practical approach; the hand-held models would be contraindicated.

When we can relate the path that we wish to capture to the paths that are functionally generated in different circumstances, FGP will be a useful procedure for single teeth in certain situations.

Clinical procedure for single-tooth FGP

1. The occlusal reduction for the preparation is completed.

2. Before any proximal reduction is done, the tooth is stabilized with softened stick compound and the same compound is formed into

a broader occlusal table to receive the functional wax (Fig. 23-19).

3. The surface of the compound is roughened so that the functional wax will not slide off. Painting the occlusal surface of the tooth and the compound with copalite and then immediately sticking some cotton fibers to it helps to grip the functional wax.

4. Using a flame, the functional wax is softened (Bosworth's Synthetic Tacky Wax is a favorite) and stuck to the prepared occlusal table (Fig. 23-20). The occlusal portion is lubricated with saliva.

5. The patient should close into centric relation and move through all possible excursions. The wax should be checked to make sure it is firmly anchored to the base and that the base itself is absolutely stable. Any excess functional wax should be removed, and the patient should close and move his jaw in all directions with the teeth together. The wax is chilled with ice water.

6. A creamy mix of Healey's Fast Setting Gray Rock or Whipmix Bite Stone is made and vibrated into the FGP indentations. The stone is extended onto at least one tooth on each side of the prepared tooth (Fig. 23-21). There should be sufficient thickness to the stone so that it can be removed without breakage after

it hardens. The adjacent teeth are covered only enough to form a good matrix. A wooden tongue blade works well to carry additional stone to the teeth and makes removal easy.

NOTE: FGP can be done on a terminal tooth if the base and the wax can be made stable. On a terminal tooth, the fast-setting stone should be extended over at least three teeth in front of the prepared tooth.

7. The hardened stone is removed and set aside. The compound and the wax are removed and discarded, and the preparation is completed. An impression of the prepared tooth is made, including all teeth that will be covered with the stone functional core. An opposing model is not necessary.

Laboratory procedure

1. The impression with removable dies for the prepared tooth and each adjacent tooth is poured.

2. The functional core is positioned against the die model. The unprepared teeth on the die model should fit perfectly into the stone index. If there is any crack between the die model and the index, the relationship of the functional path will be incorrect.

3. Any instrument that can repeatedly reposition the functional model against the die

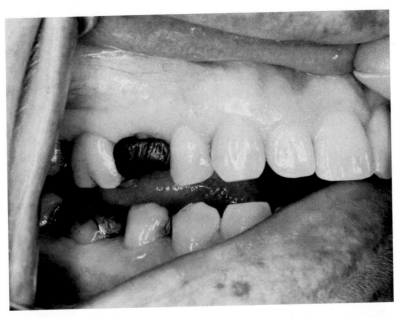

Fig. 23-19. Functionally generated path procedure for a single tooth. After preparation, red stick compound is formed over the occlusal surface and locked into adjacent contours to stabilize the teeth. The compound is flattened and roughened to receive the functional wax.

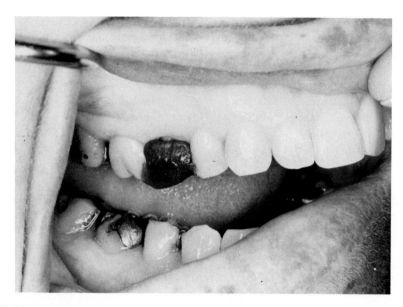

Fig. 23-20. The functional wax is stuck to the compound base, and the mandible is moved through the full range of border movements.

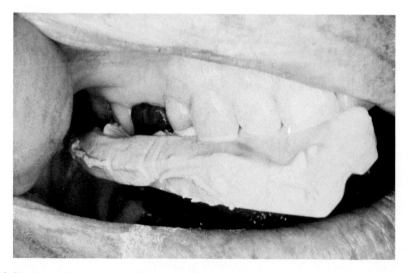

Fig. 23-21. Fast-setting stone is jiggled into the wax and at least one tooth on each side of the preparation is covered. More stone is held in place to provide sufficient thickness for strength. The additional stone can be carried to the mouth on a tongue blade or a special functional tray.

model with accuracy is acceptable for mounting the two models. They can be mounted in the joined position on a simple hinge articulator because the only requirement of the instrument is to permit the models to be separated and then returned to the same closed position. The arc of opening and closing has no importance, and of course no lateral movement is permitted. All pathways are represented on the functional model itself when it is closed. Instruments that have been especially designed for relating the functional model to the die model include the folowing:

a. The *verticulator* (Fig. 23-22), is a device that permits only an up or down movement. It is precision-made with a sturdy metal stop that permits the functional model to be struck forcefully against the die model without danger of model breakage. This facilitates very accurate marking of interferences on the restorations with silk marking ribbon. The verticulator is spring loaded so that with each closure it springs open to give access to the die or pattern.

b. The *twin-stage occluder* (Fig. 23-23) is a simple hinge articulator that will articulate both a functional core and an anatomic model interchangeably against the same die model.

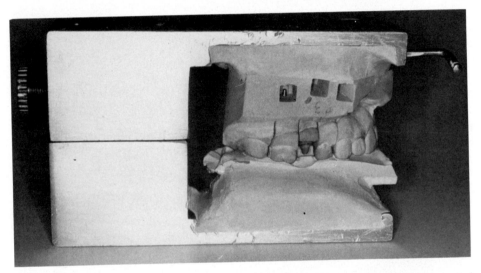

Fig. 23-22. The upper die model positioned into the functional core index. The models are mounted on a verticulator (Jelenko).

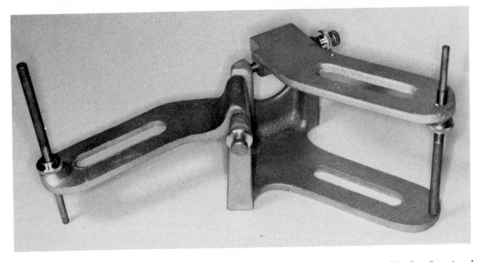

Fig. 23-23. The twin stage occluder (Hanau) is a device that permits mounting of both a functional model and an anatomic model against the die model. It serves the same purpose as the verticulator.

4. When using FGP for a single tooth, one generally waxes the pattern directly against the functional core. It is adjusted so that the stone index on each side fits together with no crack between the functional core and the die model. The pattern should contact the functional model but should not interfere with its closure. If the restoration is to be in group function, the lingual inclines of the upper buccal cusps should be in continuous contact with the functional model. If the inclines are to be discluded, they must be reduced so that there is no contact, but centric relation contacts must not be lost. In all cases, the balancing inclines should be relieved from any contact with the functional core.

White liquid shoe polish applied to the functional core is a good marking medium for locating interferences on the wax pattern (Figs. 23-24 and 23-25). Thin marking ribbon may be used when the casting is in place.

If group function of the restored working inclines is desired, the contact of the waxed incline against the functional core can be checked with the white shoe polish. The entire incline surface would be marked by the white polish when the models are closed (Fig. 23-26).

Anatomy is incorporated into the pattern by carving in grooves and sluiceways and making certain that blades remain but do not interfere. Working excursion contact is maintained by preserving enough of the white-coated incline to ensure good group function (Fig. 23-27).

FGP FOR LOWER TEETH

Functional path procedures are not generally used on lower teeth. If either the working or balancing inclines of the opposing upper teeth are too steep, the important lower buccal cusp will be wiped away in the functional wax. The restoration made from such an FGP would not contact in centric relation.

For FGP to work on the lower teeth, the upper inclines would have to be perfected first. This can be done by equilibration before the lower tooth is prepared. If the lower tooth is not in contact, it can be built up with compound or a well-made temporary restoration and the occlusion refined before the functional record is taken. This is referred to as *cusp-fossae analysis*. Except in unique situations, it would not be a practical use of time. It is a more logical approach to shape the upper tooth grossly into alignment with its adjacent

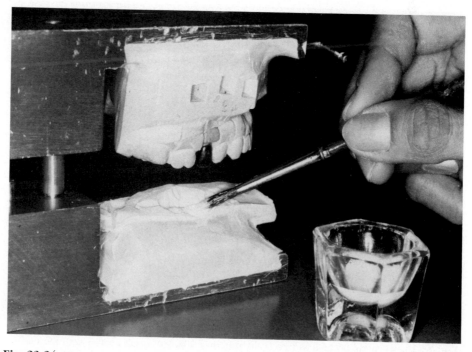

Fig. 23-24. The wax pattern is fabricated directly against the functional core. To check the occlusal contact, white shoe polish is painted on the core and the models are closed together. The white polish marks any contacting surface of the pattern.

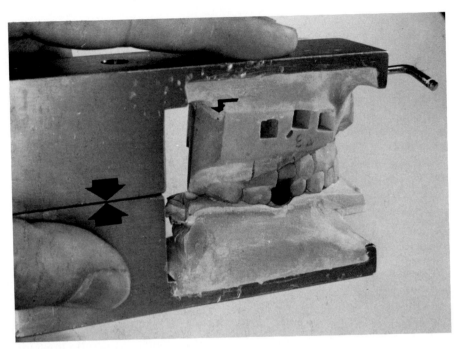

Fig. 23-25. Check the pattern for interferences by adjusting the occlusal surface until the two metal stops come into direct contact, *arrows.* The two halves of the verticulator are spring loaded, so that they spring apart after closing pressure is released.

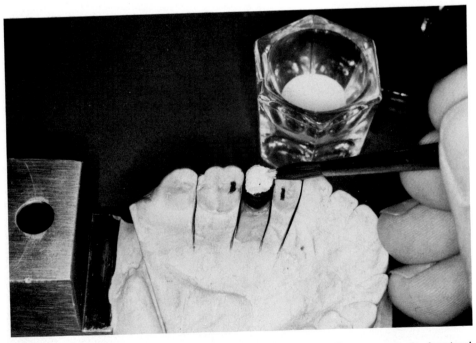

Fig. 23-26. When the occlusal surface of the pattern is adjusted to full contact with the functional core, selected parts of the surface must be relieved. An excellent method of controlling the contouring is to paint the entire surface with white shoe polish and then carve away whatever part of the occlusal surface that is not to be in centric or functional contact.

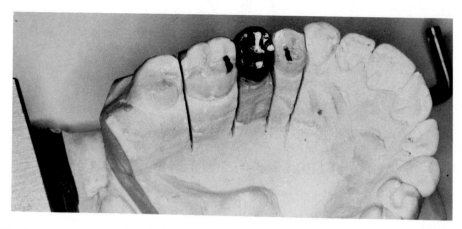

Fig. 23-27. The wax pattern is being carved to preserve centric relation stops and working excursion function. The white shoe polish is untouched wherever contact is desired. Black marks on adjacent balancing inclines serve as a guide to carving the balancing inclines on the pattern.

teeth when such shaping is needed and then to restore the lower tooth into good centric relation contact. Equilibration of the upper tooth can be done just as effectively against the finished restoration as it could be done against its compound facsimile.

Cusp-fossae analysis can be accomplished very effectively on the stone models. By sighting down the occlusal surfaces, we can align the inclines on the upper teeth opposite the lower preparation with reliable accuracy and adjust them on the model before fabrication of the lower pattern. The pattern can be given good centric stops and then the occlusion can be adjusted in the mouth when the restoration is placed. It is safer to adjust the occlusion against the finished restoration than to take the chance of wiping away the lower buccal cusp in FGP wax against upper inclines that may be in interference.

It is important to tell the patient *in advance* that the upper tooth will have to be adjusted when the lower restoration is placed. He should be told again when the lower tooth is being prepared and again just before the restoration is placed in the mouth for the first time. Unless it is explained in advance, the patient almost always believes that the dentist is grinding his good tooth to make the restoration fit. If he is warned ahead of time that it will be necessary to achieve a better occlusal alignment, he will not object.

FGP can be used on lower teeth, but only if the upper occlusal contours have been perfected first. This is true for a single tooth or for multiple teeth. For multiple teeth, there is the added problem of stabilizing the lower base against tongue and cheek action. It usually must be a cast base. In lower teeth the dentist is not interested in having any inclines in function, only functioning contacts on the buccal cusp tips and centric contact in the base of fossae. This can be accomplished in more practical ways than using FGP.

USING FGP FOR CROSSBITES

Posterior crossbites can be restored by use of FGP if lower cusp-tip placement and cusp-fossae contours have been perfected in advance. It is a practical approach when used on the upper teeth, particularly on bilateral restorations. If lower fossae contours are opened out as explained in Chapter 21, there will be no danger of losing the upper buccal cusps. The lower lingual cusp will serve as the functioning cusp, and it will create lingual inclines for the upper buccal cusp that are just as functional as if they were made by the lower buccal cusps. We have the option of keeping them in group function or discluding them. In all cases, the balancing inclines must be additionally reduced when FGP is used.

SUGGESTED READINGS

King, R.C.: Stabilizing functional chew in wax records, J. Prosthet. Dent. **26:**601-603, 1971.

Mann, A.W., and Pankey, L.D.: Oral rehabilitation utilizing the Pankey-Mann instrument and functional bite technique, Dent. Clin. North Am., p. 215, March 1959.

Pankey, L.D.: Seminar manual, Pankey Institute for Advanced Dental Education, Miami, Florida, 1973.

24

Occlusal equilibration

The term "occlusal equilibration" refers to the correction of stressful occlusal contacts through selective grinding. It involves the selective reshaping of tooth surfaces that interfere with normal jaw function.

From the time dentists first started to adjust occlusions in the mouth, there have been adversaries who have challenged the concept of equilibration. The general opposition to the procedure stems from a belief that it is impossible to adjust accurately enough *in the mouth.* Another reported disadvantage of selective grinding is that the entire adjustment must be accomplished by *removal* of tooth structure. Since it would appear that some occlusions could benefit from *adding on* tooth structure, the whole concept of intraoral selective grinding is rejected. An understanding of the principles and rationale of occlusal equilibration will permit refutation of either of these concerns.

Dentists who have learned to correctly manipulate the mandible into terminal hinge position without resistance from their patients find the mouth an extremely comfortable place to work. With good lighting and good assistance to keep the teeth and mouth dry, accuracy in occlusal adjustment can be realized to an amazing degree. Adjusting in the mouth provides the added advantage of being able to see or feel tooth movement under stressful contact. It permits a full range of adjustment to include all functional pathways. Variations of jaw

positions in various postural positions can be evaluated and adjusted. The actual effect of occlusal adjustment on the muscles can be observed, and occlusal comfort can be evaluated by the patients themselves.

It is true that intraoral selective grinding is limited to removal of tooth structure, but that does not eliminate the possibility of restoring tooth contours where indicated. It is not an "either-or" concept. It is merely a *part* of the overall plan to harmonize occlusal stresses. It is the phase of treatment that eliminates only that part of the tooth structure *that is in the way* of harmonious jaw function. Dentists who believe they must completely restore every patient with an occlusal problem are guilty of the worst type of technique-oriented tunnel vision. Combining occlusal equilibration with restorative dentistry very often minimizes the restorative needs. Equilibration procedures frequently eliminate the need for restorative dentistry altogether.

Probably the greatest distrust in occlusal equilibration procedures has resulted from observing the results of *improper* attempts at selective grinding. Doing a poor job of equilibration is far worse than leaving the malocclusion. Improper equilibration actually produces new interferences with which the patient must learn to cope. Proprioception of the new interferences can create an occlusal awareness and can trigger extreme discomfort of the teeth, the temporomandibular joints, and the masticatory muscles. Proper equilibration procedures do not cause these problems.

Proper equilibration procedures can never harm a patient. If equilibration procedures lead to an "occlusal awareness" or if they force a patient to function where the jaw is not comfortable, the equilibration has been done improperly or, at best, has just not been completed.

Proper equilibration never restricts. It *frees* the mandible to move wherever and however it wishes to move, consciously or unconsciously. It makes it possible for the muscles to move the mandible to any functional border position without deviation. It eliminates tooth-to-tooth interferences that trigger the "erasure" mechanism of bruxism.

Proper equilibration is stable. There is more to equilibration than just eliminating interferences. Resulting tooth contacts must properly distribute and direct forces for stable maintainability. It may take some time to achieve stability for teeth that have been depressed or moved by occlusal trauma. One of the biggest advantages of occlusal equilibration over immediate restorative correction is that adjustments can keep pace with the movement of teeth as they return to normal equilibrium as depressive stresses are reduced. Restoration should usually wait until maximum stability has been achieved.

EQUILIBRATION PROCEDURES

Equilibration procedures can be divided into four parts:

1. Reduction of all contacting tooth surfaces that interfere with the *terminal hinge axis closure* (centric relation)
2. Selective reduction of tooth structure that interferes with *lateral excursions.* This will vary as the influence of the anterior guidance varies to accommodate to individual chewing cycles. It will also vary, as necessary, to minimize lateral stresses on weak teeth.
3. Elimination of all posterior tooth structure that interferes with *protrusive excursions.* This must be varied in arch-to-arch relationships in which the anterior teeth are not in a position to disclude the posterior teeth in protrusion.
4. Harmonization of the *anterior guidance.* It is most often necessary to do this in conjunction with the correction of lat-

eral and protrusive interferences, but this is discussed as a separate entity for clarity in Chapter 16.

There are basic rules to follow for each of these procedures. Taking each procedure separately is a good way to understand the overall goals of equilibration.

Counseling patients before equilibration

Many dentists create problems for their patients and themselves because they do not adequately explain the reason for equilibration and the possible aftereffects. Worst of all, they may fail to adequately study the occlusal relationships in advance and thus mislead the patient into believing the adjustment requires less tooth reduction than is necessary. It is far better to prepare your patient for more grinding than is needed than to surprise him or her with unexpected reduction of tooth structure.

Proper communication regarding the need for equilibration should be an educational process. It should point out the specific problem as well as the reason for selecting a reshaping procedure over other methods of treatment. Patient understanding and receptivity to the process is usually resolved by the following:

1. *Proper diagnosis* in itself generally prepares the patient. Explain what you are doing as you align the condyle-disk assemblies and test for proper centric relation. Explain why the joints should be comfortable in the seated position and why the teeth should meet properly in harmony with that comfortable relationship.
2. *Point out loose teeth* and relate them to premature contacts or lateral excursion interferences. In the absence of pathosis or injury, loose teeth will always be related to occlusal interferences.
3. *Relate wear problems* to occlusal disharmony with the comfortable joint position. Explain that most excessive wear is an adaptive response that occurs when the teeth interfere with normal jaw movements.
4. *Study the occlusal relationship* on properly mounted diagnostic casts. Demonstrate the conflict between the teeth and the condyles on the articulator. Show how the joints must be displaced when the teeth intercuspate. Explain what

must be done to create harmony and distribute forces equally.

5. *Demonstrate on the mounted casts* the amount of tooth reshaping that will be required. If you believe there is a possibility that restorations will be required after equilibration, explain it to the patient.

6. *Tell the patient to expect further adjustments.* There is no sure way to predict the stability of an occlusion after the first equilibration. In my experience, an average of three appointments is required to achieve an acceptable stability. However some teeth continue to rebound from a stressed position, requiring more adjustments. Any need for adaptive remodeling of articular tissues could also result in a need for multiple equilibration appointments before stabilizing. The patient should be aware of this possibility before occlusal treatment is started. I prepare my patients to expect multiple adjustments as a possibility.

A cardinal rule that should not be violated is: *Never start an equilibration unless both you and the patient are committed to complete it.*

Locating the occlusal interferences

Improper manipulation of the mandible is responsible for most failures in equilibration. You cannot *force* the mandible into centric relation. Forcing will usually activate stretch-reflex contraction of the lateral pterygoid muscles, causing them to hold the condyles forward of centric relation. Too much pressure on the chin after neuromuscular release can force the condyles down and back from centric relation. For the equilibration to be successful, the condyle-disk assemblies must be free to seat in their most superior positions without any forced displacement when the teeth intercuspate. The centric relation position for each condyle must be confirmed before tooth contacts are marked. Failure to seat the condyles correctly results in imprecise marking of occlusal interferences, and so firm pressure should be used to test the position, but the pressure is not applied until after the condyles have been *gently* manipulated to the suspected centric relation seat. Loading pressure should be directed to seat the condyles against the eminence while firm upward pressure is also being applied. Distalization of the condyles must be avoided.

Centric relation must be located at the *open* position before any tooth contact occurs. When it is possible to freely arc the mandible without muscle interference, *then* apply firm pressure bilaterally. Test for centric relation. Both condyles should be completely comfortable, even when loaded with firm pressure. If there is any sign of tension or tenderness in either joint, equilibration procedures are contraindicated. Unless the posterior teeth need extensive occlusal restoration, bite planes should be used to optimize joint position before equilibration is started.

If centric relation can be verified at the open position, hold the mandible on its terminal axis and close on that arc by increments of a millimeter or two at a time. Do not jiggle. As the jaw closes and tooth contacts get closer, some resistance may be felt. Just delay for a moment and then start to close again. The patient may help the closure but loaded pressure toward the condyles should not be reduced. Continue a slow opening-closing movement until the first tooth contact occurs. That will be the first interference.

Have the patient feel the first contact. Hold that position for a second and then squeeze. This will determine the direction and degree of the "slide" from centric relation. The resultant slide must be completely eliminated to allow the mandible to close all the way to maximum intercuspation without any displacement by either condyle from its uppermost axis position.

To mark the interferences, the assistant should insert the marking ribbon on a Miller ribbon holder while the dentist manipulates the jaw with both hands.

Eliminating interferences to centric relation

For simplicity, centric relation interferences can be differentiated into two types:

1. Interferences to the *arc* of closure
2. Interferences to the *line* of closure

Interference to the arc of closure. As the condyles rotate on their terminal hinge axis, each lower tooth follow an arc of closure. It should be possible for each lower cusp tip and each incisal edge to follow this arc of closure all the way to the *most closed occlusal position* without any deviation off this arc

(Fig. 24-1, *A*). Any tooth structure that interferes with this closing arc has the effect of displacing the mandible (Fig. 24-1, *B*) forward of the interference to reach the most closed occlusal position. Most deviations from the arc of closure require the condyle to move forward. Primary interferences that deviate the condyle forward produce what is commonly called an *anterior slide.*

The basic grinding rule to correct an anterior slide is always MUDL: grind the mesial inclines of upper teeth or the distal inclines of lower teeth.

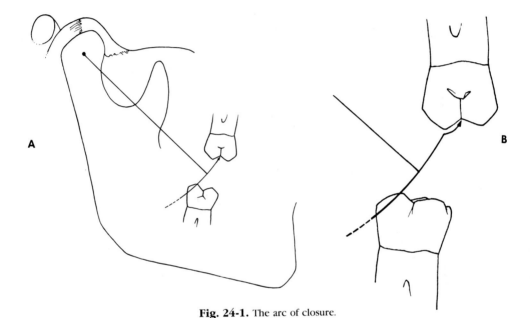

Fig. 24-1. The arc of closure.

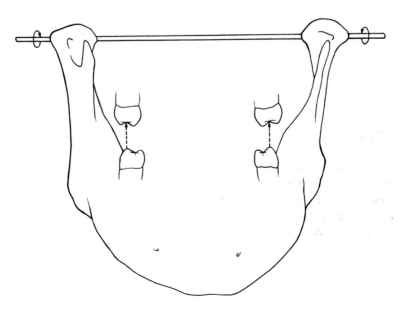

Fig. 24-2. The line of closure.

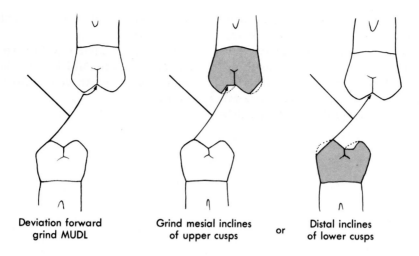

Note freedom to close *either* in centric relation or centric occlusion at the most closed vertical.

Interference to the line of closure. Line of closure interferences refer to those primary interferences that cause the mandible to deviate to the left or the right from the first point of contact to the most closed position (Fig. 24-2).

The basic grinding rules are as follows:

1. If the interfering incline causes the mandible to deviate off the line of closure *toward the cheek,* grind the buccal incline of the upper or the lingual incline of the lower, or both inclines. The selection of which incline to reduce depends on which adjustment will most nearly place the cusp tip in line with the center of its fossa contact or that will direct the force most favorably to the long axis of both upper and lower teeth.

2. If the interfering incline causes the mandible to deviate off the line of closure *toward the tongue,* the grinding rule is: grind the lingual incline of the upper or the buccal incline of the lower, or both inclines.

Both rules regarding deviations from the *line of closure* can apply to any cusp, and they

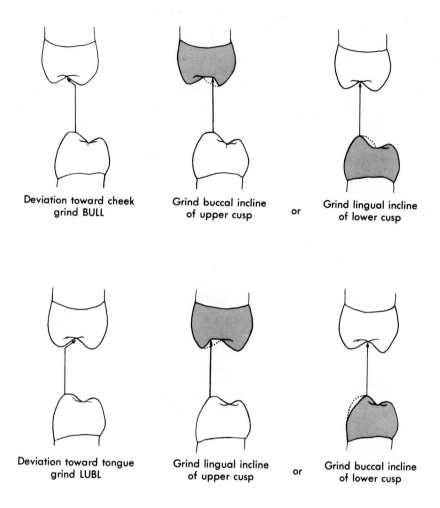

Deviation toward cheek
grind BULL

Grind buccal incline
of upper cusp

or

Grind lingual incline
of lower cusp

Deviation toward tongue
grind LUBL

Grind lingual incline
of upper cusp

or

Grind buccal incline
of lower cusp

are valid even if teeth are in a crossbite relationship. Remember that the grinding rules refer to *inclines,* not cusps.

Many interferences produce deviations off both the arc of closure and the line of closure at the same time. Upper teeth are always adjusted on the inclines that face the same direction as the slide. Lower teeth are adjusted by grinding of inclines that face the opposite direction from the path of the slide.

The vertical dimension of occlusion after equilibration at centric relation should remain the same as it is in the acquired centric occlusion before adjustment. If interferences that deviate the mandible forward are eliminated, a "long centric" will be provided automatically unless the vertical dimension is closed. The flat area of "long centric" will usually be longer than is needed, but the extra length will not generally create any problem.

Tilted teeth or wide cusp tips can be adjusted to improve stability as well as to eliminate interferences. If the mark on the upper tooth is buccal to the central fossa, the lower tooth is ground to move the cusp tip lingually *if* the shaping can be accomplished without shortening the cusp tip out of centric contact. Grinding on the upper teeth only may mutilate upper cusps unnecessarily (Fig. 24-3).

If the mark on the upper tooth is lingual to its central fossa and stability could be improved, if the lower cusp tip is moved toward the buccal, the lower cusp is reshaped by grinding its lingual inclines to move the contact buccally. This should not be done if it would require shortening of the cusp out of centric contact (Fig. 24-4). To grind the upper tooth only may mutilate the lingual cusp unnecessarily without improving the direction of forces as much as if the lower is adjusted.

Fig. 24-3

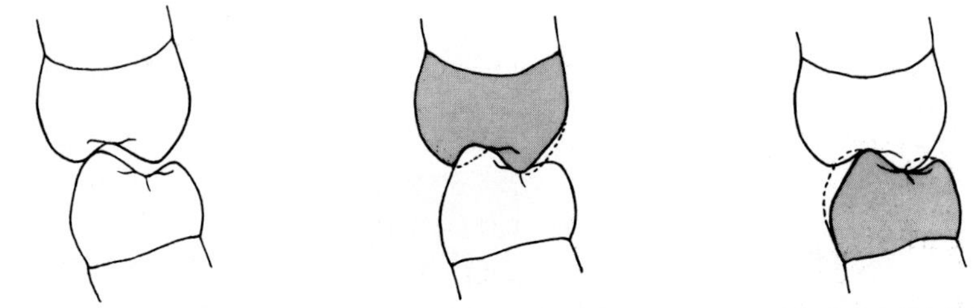

Moving cusp tip by selective grinding

Grinding upper fossa does not improve cusp tip position and mutilates upper

Grinding buccal of lower positions tip in center

Fig. 24-4

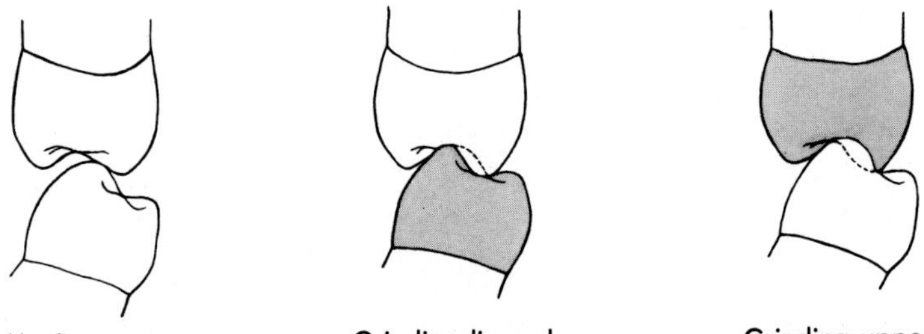

Moving cusp tip by selective grinding

Grinding lingual of lower positions tip in center

Grinding upper fossa does not improve cusp tip position and mutilates upper

Influence of skeletal contours. Facial contours that vary the shape of the mandible have a profound influence on the direction of the arc of closure. Because of shape variations, some centric slides that appear to be very long and very devious may be equilibrated with minimal tooth reduction even though a first impression may lead one to believe that equilibration would require mutilation of the teeth.

Other interferences are *frequently* missed completely because the deviation from the more vertical closure along steep inclines cannot even be noticed without exceptionally careful manipulation of the mandible so that it can be held with firmness on the centric relation axis while the interfering inclines are being marked.

If the incline that interferes nearly parallels the centric relation arc of closure, a slide from centric may be difficult to observe. Such interferences also occur in combination with enough tooth mobility to simply move the tooth rather than displace the mandible. Even such minute, hard-to-find interferences can however activate muscle incoordination. It has been a common experience for us to find such interferences in patients who have been unsuccessfully treated with occlusal therapy. The teeth should be dried thoroughly with air, and a fresh marking ribbon should be used to locate the interfering inclines. Firmly tapping the teeth together with sharp taps will produce better marks on steep inclines.

Adjusting centric interferences first. It is wise to give first priority to the elimination of all interferences to centric relation closure. There are three reasons for this:

1. By adjusting centric interferences first, you have the option of improving cusp-tip position. Most cusp tips are wide enough to permit narrowing toward a more favorable central groove relationship. Better placed, narrower cusp tips require less mutilation of opposing fossae walls when lateral excursions are adjusted.

2. When cusp-tip position is given first priority, occlusal grinding is more evenly distributed to both arches. Cusp-tip position is usually improved by narrowing the cusps on one arch. Excursive interferences are then corrected by grinding of the fossae walls of the opposite arch. After gross adjustments are made in this sequence, fine contouring can be selectively achieved on either arch.

3. If cusp-tip contours and position are improved first in centric relation, eccentric interferences can be eliminated with speed and simplicity. If all eccentric contacts on posterior teeth are to be eliminated, any incline that marks in any excursion can be reduced. Centric stops must be preserved, but all other contacts can be shaped so that they are discluded by the anterior guidance.

If lateral excursions are adjusted first, the option of precise cusp-tip placement is often lost or compromised and the grinding is usually done mostly on upper fossae walls. Although this is an effective way to eliminate interferences, it does not always produce optimum stability. If the posterior teeth are to be restored after equilibration, the sequence is not so important, however, because cusp-tip position can be improved in the restorations.

Lateral excursion interferences

The path that is followed by the lower posterior teeth as they leave centric relation and travel laterally is dictated by two determinants:

1. The border movements of the condyles, which act as the posterior determinant.
2. The anterior guidance, which acts as the anterior determinant.

When lateral excursions are being equilibrated, the mandible *must be guided* with firm upward pressure to ensure that all interferences are recorded and eliminated through the uppermost ranges of motion that can occur at true border paths for both the condyles and the anterior guidance.

If the patient is allowed to mark lateral interferences by unguided excursions, there will be a tendency to slide anterolaterally to the lateral border path. Guiding the mandible with firm pressure during excursions will routinely pick up posterior interferences that are missed with unguided movements. Lateral interferences that can be found only by firm manipulation from a verified centric relation are commonly the interferences that trigger muscle incoordination and excessive muscle loading during clenching or bruxing activity. The elimination of even minute interferences just lateral to centric holding contacts puts an end to many otherwise unsolvable occluso-muscle disorders.

Method of manipulation for lateral excursions. The reason for special manipulation is to ensure that we are moving the mandible all the way out to its border limit. The patient may not *use* the full range of freedom, but any posterior interference that prevents the mandible from reaching a functional border position is a potential trigger for bruxism and is a source of traumotogenic stress on the interfering tooth.

The procedure is easily accomplished once the method has been learned:

1. After all interferences to a terminal axis closure have been eliminated, the mandible should be manipulated into centric relation.
2. The teeth should be closed on the terminal axis arc until they contact. The patient should be asked to hold this position for a moment.
3. *On the working side,* the thumb is released and all four fingers used to exert upward pressure on the working condyle. The fingers must be placed on bone, not into the neck tissue.
4. *On the balancing side,* the same thumb-finger relationship that was used for centric manipulation should be maintained, except that *pressure should be exerted toward the working condyle.*
5. While maintaining pressure with both hands, the dentist should ask the patient to slide the jaw to the left or right (Fig. 24-5).
6. The assistant should insert the marking ribbon in the *dry* mouth to record any interferences. It makes no difference whether this record is from centric to outer border position or from outer border position into centric relation.
7. The manipulation is the same whether marking interferences on the working side or the balancing side.

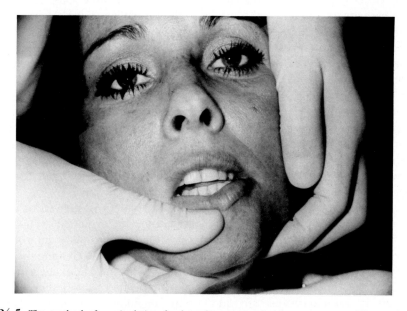

Fig. 24-5. The method of manipulation for lateral excursion border movements. The working-side condyle is held up on its terminal axis while firm guiding pressure is exerted to keep the orbiting condyle as far up and in as possible while the patient moves the jaw. Without firm guidance, the mandible is more likely to be moved on a protrusive lateral path. Manipulation is often the difference between correcting or not correcting the effects from a bruxism habit.

Eliminating lateral interferences. Lateral interferences can be divided into interferences of the *working side* and interferences of the *balancing side.* Both are adjusted together, but for simplicity I am discussing them separately. Since balancing side interferences are usually adjusted first and are the least complicated, let us start there.

BALANCING-SIDE INTERFERENCES. These interferences can be adjusted quickly and easily because the goal here is to eliminate all contact on inclines as soon as the lower teeth move out of centric relation and start toward the tongue.

The grinding rule for balancing incline interferences is BULL: grind the buccal inclines of the upper or the lingual inclines of the lower. The rule does not specify cusps. It refers to inclines and is applicable to all situations including crossbite

As balancing inclines are relieved, working-side inclines may start to interfere. As the working inclines are corrected, previously reduced balancing inclines may come back into interference and require further reduction. When adjusting lateral excursions, you will need to work with both balancing and working inclines together.

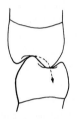

Path from centric
toward tongue

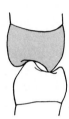

Grind buccal incline
of upper

or

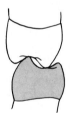

Lingual incline
of lower

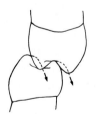

Crossbite with
balancing interferences

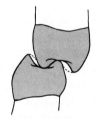

Grind both the buccal
incline of the upper and
the lingual incline of the
lower

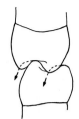

Working-side pathway

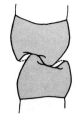

Grind lingual incline of
upper and buccal incline of
lower

WORKING-SIDE INTERFERENCES. Before adjustment of the excursions on the working side, it is necessary to determine the type of occlusion that will best suit the particular patient.

Group function. The working-side inclines are adjusted to precisely harmonize with both condylar movements and the anterior guidance. In group function, the lower posterior cusp tips *and* the lower working-side incisal edges maintain continuous contact from centric relation out toward the cheek. As the mandible swings laterally, the *length* of the stroke contact is progressive from the molar forward. This means the second molar disengages first, the cuspid last.

Posterior disclusion. In most patients, the posterior teeth should contact only in centric relation. The anterior guidance should immediately disclude all posterior tooth contact the moment the mandible moves from centric relation. The disclusion effect may come from the cuspids alone (cuspid-protected occlusion), or the anterior teeth may work in group function as the discluder.

Posterior disclusion is the occlusion of choice in most patients because of its effect on the elevator muscles. At the moment of posterior disclusion, most of the elevator muscle contraction is shut off, reducing the load on both the anterior teeth and the joints. It is necessary to have acceptable anterior guidance for this effect to take place, and so overjet patients will be more likely to benefit from a group-function occlusion in working-side excursions.

The rule for equilibrating working-side contacts is LUBL: starting at the centric stop, grind all marks on the lingual inclines of the upper teeth or the buccal inclines of lower teeth, or both sets of inclines. Since cusp tips are used for centric holding contacts, which have already been perfected, all adjusting is done on the walls of the fossae or the sides of the cusps.

Protrusive interferences

Only the front teeth should touch in protrusive excursions. All posterior contact should be eliminated in protrusion as soon as the posterior teeth move forward of their centric holding contacts.

The rule for eliminating protrusive interferences is DUML: grind the distal inclines of the upper or, in some instances, the mesial incline of the lower teeth.

In grinding away protrusive interferences, centric stops should be marked with a different colored ribbon so that they will not be inadvertently ground. The jaw should be positioned in centric relation, and the patient is asked to "slide forward and back, forward and back." The patient should do the sliding, but the dentist should maintain a firm hold on the mandible to make sure the condyles are staying up against the eminentiae during the movement.

One must look carefully for protrusive interferences because they are often missed. With careful observation they are frequently found as a little hangup on a slightly raised marginal ridge. The dentist must also note the linguo-occlusal line angle toward the distal of

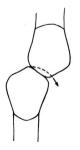

Protrusive pathway

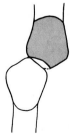

Grind distal of
upper most often

each upper tooth and also observe the fosse walls in the protrusive pathway. All posterior contact in protrusive interference must be relieved.

Posterior disclusion in protrusion is accomplished by both the anterior guidance and the downward movement of the protruding condyles. With steep anterior guidances, correction for protrusive interferences is usually minimal. Flat anterior guidances rely more on the condyles for disclusion, and the corrections required for protrusive interferences are usually more extensive.

Protrusive interferences are often corrected by some degree of "hollow grinding" of the offending inclines. The concave incline contours are easily discluded by the convex path of the condyles.

A frequent mistake in adjusting occlusions is to assume that the lower buccal cusp tips follow the upper central grooves in protrusion. This would occur only if both sides of the arch were parallel to each other (producing a perfectly square-jawed individual). Most arches taper from back to front so that when the mandible is protruded, the lower teeth *follow a straight path forward*, which results in the lower posterior teeth moving diagonally across the upper teeth (Fig. 24-6). Interferences to this pathway can be easily missed by misinterpretation of the marks as working excursions. Such interferences should be eliminated by concave grinding of the upper distal inclines or the lower mesial inclines. Such inclines are often polished very smooth by wear, and they do not mark easily unless the teeth are dry and the marking ribbon is fresh.

When the arch relationship does not permit the anterior teeth to disclude the posterior teeth, the farthest forward tooth on each side should serve as the discluder of the rest of the posterior teeth in protrusion.

Equilibrating hypermobile teeth

All teeth should be checked digitally for any hypermobility when occlusal adjustment is performed. Loose teeth that interfere can easily move to permit even marking with stable teeth. The mark on a loose tooth may even be less noticeable than marks on stable teeth. If the firm teeth are ground, the loose tooth is stressed all the more. Each tooth should be checked with the tip of the fingernail contact-

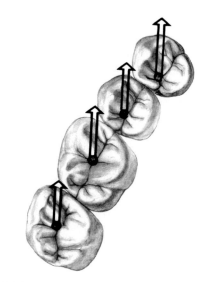

Fig. 24-6. Because of the shape of most arches, the protrusive path of the lower cusps is diagonally across upper occlusal surfaces. The distal inclines of upper cusps should be carefully observed for protrusive interferences. There should be no contact on posterior teeth in protrusive movements.

ing the facial surface while the patient closes and goes through all excursions. If there is any noticeable movement in any tooth contact position, the tooth should be held in place with the finger while it is marked.

Occlusions should be checked with both firm and light contact. The use of red ribbon for firm closure and black ribbon for light closure will show whether teeth are moving to permit equal contact at a forced closure. The red and black marks should be in the same locations.

If more marks are made on heavy closure than are recorded with light closure, the occlusion is adjusted further by grinding of the marks made with light contact until they are the same as those at firm contact.

Equilibration on patients with emotional problems

Patients with emotional problems may or may not be candidates for equilibration. There are many patients whose stress-related disorders can be profoundly improved by elimination of painful occluso-muscle incoordination. It has been my experience on numerous occasions that emotional symptoms disappeared when the occluso-muscle symptoms were relieved. The patient who is refused help for a diagnosable problem just because he or she is depressed is often caused greater stress. It may take extra time and extra compassion to help such patients, but good results can be achieved if the diagnosis is accurate and the patient is realistic about the symptoms that relate to occlusal imbalance.

If a patient has unrealistic expectations regarding the effect of treatment, no irreversible procedures should be started. All adjustments to the occlusion should be made on reversible occlusal splints. Only if all symptoms are resolved by the occlusal splints and the patient has a full understanding of the need for occlusal correction of the teeth, should direct occlusal equilibration be attempted.

Patients with irrational symptoms cannot be helped by occlusal equilibration, and it should never be attempted on such patients. Unless there is a definite, clearly defined diagnosis that explains the patients symptoms and those symptoms can be predictably resolvable by definitive treatment, occlusal equilibration is contraindicated.

Regardless of how obvious a causative factor may be or how predictable the occlusal treatment may be, equilibration should not be initiated on any patient with either irrational symptoms or irrational expectations.

If there is a definite problem of which the patient is aware and it can be resolved by correction of the occlusion, proper equilibration will not cause an occlusal awareness, even in an emotional patient as long as the patient is rational.

Occlusal splints are generally the method of choice for resolution of occluso-muscle disorders for patients with possible emotional side effects to treatment. In carefully selected patients who need complete posterior occlusal restoration, direct equilibration may be proper. It prevents the need for wearing an appliance, and the occlusal surfaces are going to be restored anyway.

If there is any question about the position or condition of the temporomandibular joints, a diagnostic occlusal splint should be used to verify a favorable response to occlusal correction before direct adjustments are started.

Prophylactic equilibration

There is no need to equilibrate any patient who is completely comfortable and who has no prospects for accelerated wear or periodontal breakdown, no hypermobile teeth, no excessive recession, pulpal sensitivity, wear facets, or bruxism habits, and no temporomandibular joint–related symptoms such as popping or cracking in the joint area, tenderness or pain, or headaches. If such patients have no requirements for restorative treatment, there would be no indication for occlusal correction. If equilibrating patients with none of these problems is what is meant by prophylactic equilibration, there would be no reason to endorse the concept.

Unfortunately, finding a patient with occlusal interferences and none of the preceding symptoms is more difficult than most dentists realize. Patients with occlusal disharmony who have "no problems" have in most cases not been examined carefully. There is no reason to postpone treatment until problems are bad enough to become obvious to the patient. Modern dentistry is capable of intercepting and correcting causative factors *before* the problem requires extensive treatment.

Occlusal stress is a causative factor that accelerates deterioration of oral health. Its correction is usually simple for the well-trained dentist. Correction makes the patient more comfortable and makes the teeth and the supporting tissues more maintainable.

Since proper equilibration cannot harm a patient and has the potential for being so beneficial, what are the objections to correcting occlusion before damage is apparent?

Dentists who have never seen the results of *properly* executed occlusal correction have no way to evaluate it and hence have little appreciation for its merits. Similarly, dentists who are not accustomed to thoroughness in examining their patients do not see the need for occlusal corrections because they are not aware that their patients have unhealthy mouths with problems that were caused by stress.

Dentists who think in terms of optimum oral health will embrace concepts of comprehensive, preventive dentistry. Correction of occlusal trauma is one of the preventive measures that noticeably improves the comfort and maintainable health of the teeth and surrounding tissues. If "prophylactic equilibration" refers to correcting problems of stress before the damage is serious, I recommend it. Waiting until *after* the damage has been wrought hardly seems like a worthwhile alternative. Careful examination is the key to determining whether or not there is a problem that requires correction.

CAUTION: One should never attempt to equilibrate any patient unless the problems of occlusal stress are first pointed out in the patient's own mouth. The patient should agree that there is a problem and should understnd *in advance* what will be involved in the treatment.

Dentists who are not totally confident of their expertise in equilibrating should not attempt any form of "prophylactic equilibration." The most unhappy patients I see are those who believed they had no problems until the dentist "just started grinding away my good teeth." Improper or incomplete equilibration can cause an occlusal awareness and sometimes even acute temporomandibular disorders. Such problems are amplified if the patients were reasonably comfortable before the attempted "equilibration."

Equilibrating the orthodontic patient

Every orthodontist should learn the principles and techniques of occlusal equilibration. No one can be in a better position to equilibrate orthodontic patients than the orthodontist himself. His understanding of directional growth factors may eliminate the need for reduction of inclines that will tend to move with growth into more favorable positions.

The orthodontist's appraisal of "rebound" movement of teeth after band removal gives him a better sense of timing as to *when* to equilibrate and *how much* to relieve certain inclines. The orthodontist is able to make slight corrections in individual tooth position when the alternative would mean grinding through enamel.

We are told by orthodontists who refine their finished cases with equilibration that they tend to constantly improve their orthodontic technique to minimize the need for selective grinding. The careful occlusal analysis that goes with equilibration has made them far more aware of factors of stability, and their results require less retention.

Equilibration should not be used to take the place of correct tooth positioning. Orthodontists who believe it is impossible to position teeth accurately enough to avoid extensive grinding should be aware that many orthodontists *are* finding it possible and practical to re-

late the teeth so well that minimal posttreatment spot grinding is all that is required.

Occlusal adjustment during treatment. It is permissible to change the shape of cusps, fossae, or inclines during treatment if such changes will benefit stability after the tooth is moved. Nonfunctioning inclines particularly can be reshaped at any time during treatment. Visualizing the final position of any tooth in question can help to determine what changes in shape would be beneficial.

Occlusal adjustment during retention. When the bands are removed and a removable retainer is inserted, gross occlusal correction should be initiated. If the occlusion can be corrected in the position of retention, stabilization of the teeth in that position will be enhanced.

If slight movement of any tooth would be beneficial to the occlusal relationship, additional finger springs can be added to the retainer to move the tooth rather than mutilating it with excessive occlusal grinding. When the tooth-to-tooth relationship is as correct as the orthodontist believes it can be, the occlusion should be refined. The combination of occlusal stability and the stabilizing effect of the retainer allows the entire dentition to become quite stable in a greatly reduced time. The alternative of using a retainer to hold teeth in malocclusion is a poor second choice.

EFFICIENCY IN EQUILIBRATION

An extravagant amount of time can be wasted with inefficient equilibration procedures. With well-trained chairside help and a good procedural approach by the dentist, most patients can be equilibrated initially within an hour's time. This means that all interferences to centric relation can be eliminated and all protrusive and lateral excursions can be harmonized.

This does not mean that the resultant occlusion will require no further adjustments. It would be rare to finalize an occlusion to the point of stability in one appointment because stressed teeth have a tendency to move as excessive occlusal forces are reduced. How long it takes the stressed teeth to regain equilibrium with their periodontal ligaments varies greatly after the stress is removed. The occlusal adjustment must be repeatedly refined as the shifting produces new interferences.

At any one appointment, all the dentist can do is to eliminate occlusal interferences *for the position the teeth are in at that time.* Efficient technique can cut the time required for the initial equilibration and can drastically cut the time required for the subsequent follow-up equilibration appointments.

Role of the chairside assistant

Efficient equilibration is a four-handed endeavor because the manipulation of the mandible requires both hands of the dentist.

The assistant has three responsibilities:

1. Keeping the mouth dry so that the ribbon will mark effectively
2. Holding the marking ribbon in place while the dentist manipulates the jaw
3. Keeping the teeth cool while the selective grinding is being performed

For the assistant to be efficient in accomplishing her responsibilities, she must learn to effectively alternate three implements in concert with the procedures of the dentist: marking ribbon, the evacuator suction tip, and the air syringe.

One of the secrets to rapid equilibration is to work in a dry mouth. Letting the teeth get wet prevents the ribbon from marking adequately. The combined use of vacuum evacuation and a stream of air soon dries up all but the worst salivator. We have found very little need for chemical antisialagogues if we have

efficient assisting. Drying the teeth with a cotton roll leaves a thin film that reduces the effectiveness of the marking ribbon. The continuous stream of air on the occlusal surfaces in combination with the vacuum during grinding procedures keeps the teeth cool and dry. The marking ribbon can then be inserted immediately when the grinding is completed for each previous marking.

All equilibration procedures except the final check for "long centric" interferences can be accomplished with the patient in a supine position. The dentist and the assistant can be seated comfortably. The dentist should have easy access to the handpiece. The assistant holds two implements and lays the third on the patient's chest or on the bracket table (Fig. 24-7). (In the supine position, patients do not object to having instruments laid on the napkin near their left shoulder. It is the most convenient place for the assistant.)

Hand and head signals can be used for rapid communication with the assistant. A nod of the dentist's head means to insert the ribbon. Hand positions can be worked out to show where to place the ribbon. Raising the thumb means to take out all instruments so that the occlusion can be checked. Voiceless communication is not only faster, it is a more relaxing way to work.

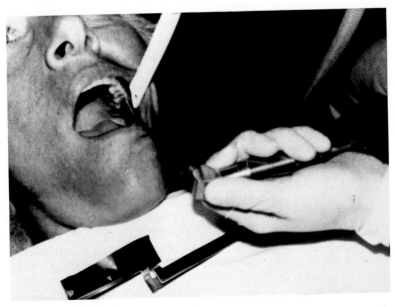

Fig. 24-7. For efficient equilibration procedures, the assistant is responsible for three implements: air syringe, vacuum tip, and marking ribbons. She keeps two of these in her hands at all times while the unused implement rests on the patient's shoulder.

Describing an oft-repeated sequence may provide some insight into efficient equilibration steps:

1. The dentist manipulates the jaw into terminal hinge position and then taps the teeth together (Fig. 24-8). The patient is asked: "Which side contacts first?" Whichever side is indicated by the patient is the side that should be marked. If the patient cannot decide, both sides are marked.

2. Before inserting the ribbon (on a suitable holder such as a Miller ribbon holder), the assistant evacuates all mouth fluids and dries the teeth with the air stream while the dentist resumes the manipulative position with both hands. When the dentist is ready to mark, a slight nod of the head signals the assistant to insert the ribbon. The dentist taps the teeth together, the assistant removes the ribbon, pats it dry on the patient's napkin, and *immediately* returns to the mouth with the vacuum. The vacuum tip keeps the patient from closing and spoiling the marks while it is keeping the mouth dry.

3. The dentist selectively grinds the marked inclines while the assistant directs air on the teeth being ground. With her other hand she keeps the mouth dry with the evacuator tip (Fig. 24-9).

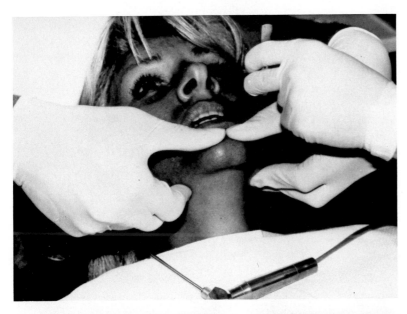

Fig. 24-8. When the mouth is air dried and evacuated of moisture, the air syringe is traded for the ribbon. It is held in place while the dentist manipulates a centric relation closure.

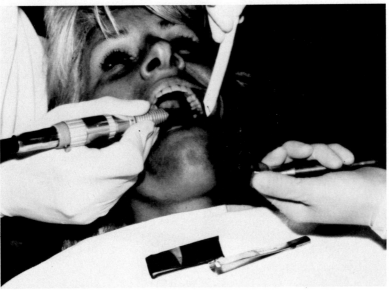

Fig. 24-9. As soon as the interferences have been marked, the ribbon is swapped for the air syringe and the evacuator tip is *immediately* replaced so that the patient cannot close and ruin the marks. The dentist grinds the appropriate interferences while the assistant cools the teeth with air and keeps all saliva evacuated.

4. When the dentist is nearly finished with the grinding of the marked inclines, a nod of the head signals the assistant to lay down the evacuator tip and pick up the ribbon (Fig. 24-10). With the air syringe in the other hand, she continues to keep the occlusal surfaces dry. She immediately inserts the ribbon as the dentist removes the handpiece from the mouth. The teeth are tapped together again to make new marks and the grinding is resumed without a break (Fig. 24-11). The assistant replaces the ribbon with the evacuator tip during grinding.

The sequence depends on the assistant's using three implements with two hands. The air syringe can be kept in one hand while the other hand alternates between the vacuum and the marking ribbons. The vacuum is also used for dust removal during the grinding procedures.

Letting the mouth get wet between grindings slows the procedure greatly because it must be thoroughly dried again before marking. Keeping the mouth dry not only speeds up the procedure, but also has the effect of stopping salivation. The judicious use of smooth-cutting stones need not generate a heat prob-

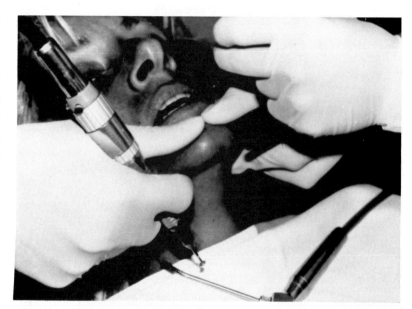

Fig. 24-10. When the dentist nears the end of adjusting a particular mark, a nod of the head signals the assistant to lay down the air syringe and insert the ribbon. Often the mandible can be manipulated into marking the next interference without the handpiece even being laid down.

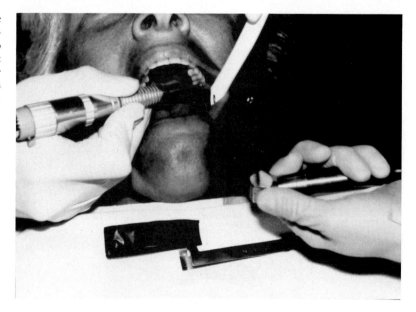

Fig. 24-11. When the mark is made, the handpiece is swung back into position, and the assistant resumes evacuation and air cooling. The sequence is repeated over and over until the equilibration is completed.

lem with a moderate-speed handpiece. High-speed handpieces are more comfortable from a vibration standpoint, but heat production is greater. The use of high speed and water spray is practical for reducing gross interferences, and as better finishing burs have been developed, I have found that the 12-sided football-shaped silicon carbide bur is an excellent choice for the major part of the adjustment. With care, it can be used dry.

Equilibrating with efficiency

Developing a mental visualization of what is to be achieved is essential for efficient equilibration. Possibly the biggest time waste is in the habit of "grinding marks." Just grinding the surface to remove a mark is a slow process. The amount and shape of tooth structure that must be removed to permit nondeviating closure to the most closed position should be visualized. The path of closure and the shape of the interference should be noted and then changed to accept the shape of the cusp that must fit there. The marks should be used as guides, but reshaping need not be confined to the limits of the marks themselves.

Planning the equilibration by adjustment of the occlusion on mounted casts is excellent practice. It is strongly recommended as a routine procedure for all cases. When the dentist is confident of expertise in equilibration, adjustment on casts need be only complete enough to ascertain tooth-to-tooth relationships at the corrected position. In that correct vertical position it is also possible to tell whether the grinding would result in too much loss of enamel. If that is so, alternative treatments, such as orthodontics, can be evaluated. If restorations are to be needed after equilibration, the patient should be told in advance.

Grinding of all nonfunctioning inclines together. If centric relation stops are all established first, the grinding of nonfunctioning inclines can be done with ease. Since most patients should have *no* posterior inclines in any kind of contact, any mark on any incline is indicative of an interference that must be relieved. The only decision that must be made is whether to grind the upper or the lower tooth, or both. The process is greatly simplified by the use of two colors of marking ribbon, a lighter color (red is excellent) to mark all excursions and a black ribbon to mark the centric stops.

The key to the simplicity of this approach is the careful elimination of all centric relation interferences before excursive corrections are made. If all centric stops are well established and correctly contoured, they are preserved. All other posterior contacts are eliminated. The procedure is as follows:

1. In a dry mouth, insert a fresh red ribbon and close the jaw in centric relation. While holding the condyles up with firm pressure, have the patient move forward and back and then left and right. Open and keep the teeth dry while changing ribbons.
2. Immediately insert the black ribbon and tap the teeth lightly together in centric relation. This should produce a small black mark for each centric stop on top of red marks that extend onto inclines.
3. Do not grind any black (centric) marks.
4. Reshape all posterior inclines that have red marks so that they cannot be contacted in *any* excursion. If there is thin enamel on an incline, do the reduction on the opposite arch. The same is true for sensitive tooth surfaces. Convex fossa walls should be reduced in preference over a flatter opposing surface. If fossa walls would be mutilated to receive a wide cusp tip, grind the walls of the cusp to make the cusp narrower. Do not shorten the cusp.

Selective reshaping can be done with complete freedom to reduce any surface of any posterior tooth except centric stops. Such reshaping permits the dentist to improve the shape of any tooth surface with no concern for removing any tooth contacts that are critical to stability or function of the occlusion. Care should always be taken to prevent overgrinding, but this is easily prevented when one pays attention to enamel contours.

5. When the mandible can be firmly guided through all border movements without causing any posterior incline to be marked, eccentric disclusion has been accomplished.

Locating hard-to-find interferences. If an apparently correct equilibration fails to completely eliminate tension or tenderness in either joint musculature or on any tooth or if the patient can detect a prematurity that does not mark, the probable cause is movement of the prematurely contacting tooth. This is particularly common with the most distal molar contacts because those teeth are so frequently depressable. They also often have very smooth facets that do not mark readily. It is, in fact, unusual to find second or third molars that do not have incline interferences still present, even after the most meticulous equilibration because of these factors. A simple procedure can be used to detect such interferences and should be used routinely:

1. After the equilibration has been completed in relation to guided border movements, dry the tooth surfaces with air until they are bone dry. Placement of a cotton roll next to the molars helps to keep the surfaces dry and holds the cheek out of the way.
2. Inserting the ribbon making certain that the entire occlusal surface of the last molar is covered by the ribbon. (It is a common fault to keep the ribbon holder too far to the buccal.) The tip of the ribbon holder must be angled so that it is positioned very close to the buccal of the last molar.
3. While the assistant holds the ribbon, manipulate the mandible bimanually to a confirmed centric relation at the open position. Then ask the patient to chop the teeth together very firmly a few times while firm pressure keeps the condyles loaded up on the centric axis. This firmly loaded chop-chop contact on very dry teeth will mark interfering inclines before the teeth can move. If you have not used this procedure, you will be amazed at the extent of grinding that will commonly be required before all interferences are eliminated.

As a final test, repeat the above procedure with firmly loaded condyles, but also exert firm pressure laterally in both directions when marking.

The reason mobility patterns are so common on the last molars is that they are almost always involved as at least part of the interference whenever there is a discrepancy between CR and CO. Because the last tooth becomes the fulcrum when the condyle is seated up into centric relation, it is easily loosened. Unless a special effort is made to adjust the occlusion to noninterference with the *passive* position of the last molar, it will probably be missed because it is extremely difficult to observe mobility of that nature.

ARMAMENTARIUM FOR EQUILIBRATION
For marking interferences

Ribbons. The most efficient way to mark interferences is to use very thin film impregnated with different colors of ink. The material of choice for me is *AccuFilm*. The thinness of the film prevents it from smudging around the sides of cusps and permits it to mark only surfaces that contact. It must be changed after several markings because the ink is lifted off the film by the pressure of the contacts and transferred to the teeth.

Ribbon holder. AccuFilm and other types of thin marking ribbons are best held in place with a holder. The *Miller ribbon holder* (Fig. 24-12) is excellent. Several holders should be loaded with two colors so that time is not lost at the chair replacing worn ribbons.

Marking paper. Marking paper is not generally the best material for marking interferences because the ink rubs off too easily and smudges. If the paper is not too easily penetrated or torn, it is acceptable as long as it is not too thick. Thick papers do not confine the marks to the first interference. They tend to also mark any inclines that are as close to contact as the thickness of the ribbon. For that reason, I sometimes use a thicker paper for marking balancing inclines that I want more separation for.

Waxes. Thin sheets of dark-colored wax can be placed over the occlusal surface of the teeth in one arch. The opposing teeth are then tapped gently into the wax until it perforates. The perforations represent interfering contacts. They are then marked with a pencil and then reduced with the usual rules for

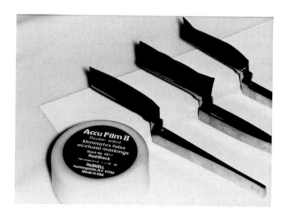

Fig. 24-12. Miller ribbon holders should be set so that articulating ribbon extends 1 to 2 mm past the tip. AccuFilm ribbon is kept sealed in container until needed.

grinding being followed. The procedure is repeated until the perforations are in the right spots.

Wax is an excellent material for finding interferences on sharp-line angles that are often difficult to pick up by other methods. As a routinely used material, though, it is not recommended because it requires an excessively large amount of time, compared with the use of marking ribbons.

Pastes, sprays, and paint-on materials. There is available a variety of materials that can be painted or sprayed onto tooth contact, and then the material is perforated so that the contact areas are made visible. The use of such materials can be extremely accurate because the film thickness is so thin.

METHODS FOR QUANTITATIVE OCCLUSAL ANALYSIS
Photocclusion

For precise determination of occlusal harmony, it is necessary to determine the *sequence* of tooth contacts for any given jaw relationship. the tooth that strikes first must be determined along with identification of subsequent tooth contacts in order of their sequence of contact. Until the photocclusion method was developed by Arcan, only qualitative analysis of occlusal contacts was available. Qualitative analysis can be misleading because the difference is often so minute between the teeth in contact initially and the almost indeterminable space between the teeth that are not in contact. Even the slightest mobility of the first tooth to contact may allow it to be depressed, so that other teeth are permitted to contact, and thus a qualitative marking system would fail to distinguish the critically important first prematurity.

The photocclusion method introduced the first clinical system for quantitative analysis by measurement of the strains induced in a photoplastic wafer, called a "memory sheet." By measuring the birefringence patterns in the memory sheet with a special optical instrument one could determine minute differences in space between the first contact and the teeth that were not yet in contact. The variation in the strains recorded were analyzed by projection of polarized light through the memory wafer onto a screen. The intensity order of the contacts can be distinguished by variations of color that appear on the screen. The black background relates to zero. From that point, a progression of color proceeds through a clearly defined sequence of grey, white, yellow, orange, and red. It then passes through a tint of passage that proceeds with blue, blue-green, green-yellow, orange, and red. Each color represents a step higher on the contact-intensity level.

The strain analysis is made definite for the specific inclines on the occlusal surface when the memory sheet is wiped with a thin layer of silicone impression paste. This gives a clear picture of the occlusal topography with the strain analysis pattern correctly located.

Although the photocclusion method has not achieved the wide usage it deserved, it was a very important stimulus for recognizing the importance of minute occlusal interferences. It was also an inducement for many clinicians to perfect their methods of occlusal equilibration because of the clarity of the recordings that showed that many "perfected" occlusions were not sufficiently equilibrated. The system was too precise to be fooled, and a truly perfected occlusion with equal intensity contacts was necessary for an acceptable recording in the memory sheet.

The method has great value, not only as an aid in diagnosing occlusal disharmony, but also as a record of pre- and posttreatment occlusal relationships.

Computer-assisted dynamic occlusal analysis

One of the most innovative systems for quantitative occlusal analysis was developed by Maness. Through a menu-driven software system, the Tek-scan system (Fig. 24-13) uses a sensor unit that records occlusal contacts on a thin Mylar film and relays the information to a computer. Through analysis of the occlusal contacts it is possible to determine the sequence and timing of which teeth contact and with what degree of comparative force. Comparisons can be made for occlusal contacts in centric relation versus centric occlusion.

The Tek-scan system is practical in that it allows direct real-time recordings of occlusal contacts to be shown on a monitor during any phase of functional jaw movements. It also allows the operator to record contacts at any jaw relationship either on the monitor or on a printout. A special value of the system is that it provides immediate information that is understandable for the patient regarding stressful occlusal contacts. The hard-copy printouts are

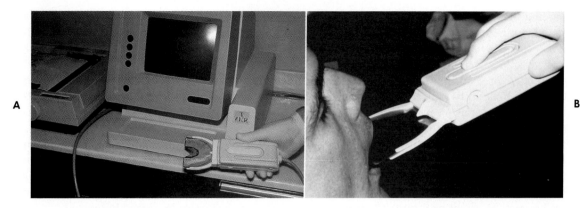

Fig. 24-13. A, Tek-scan unit. Newer models have a built-in printer. **B,** Sensor unit is placed in the mouth to record occlusal contacts.

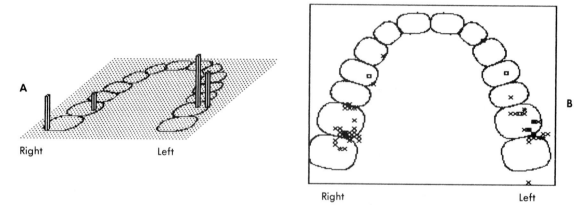

Fig. 24-14. A, Time balance plot showing contacts when the mandible is closed in centric relation. Highest column represents first contact with sequential contacts represented by progressively shorter columns. This occlusion is in need of equilibration. **B,** Time composite display of centric occlusion contacts. Tek-scan analysis permits determination of the sequence of every contact shown from the first contact to the last. This is a function that is shown on the monitor.

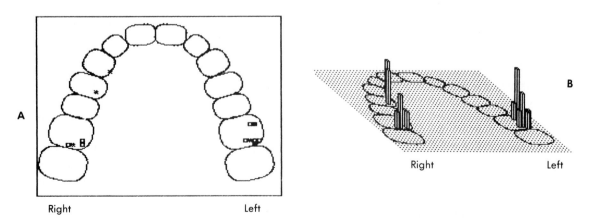

Fig. 24-15. A, Force analysis of contacts in centric relation. Hardest hitting contacts are in molar region with very poor distribution of uneven forces. **B,** Same record showing the forces depicted by columns. The higher the column, the greater is the force.

also valuable as a permanent record. A three-dimensional representation of the occlusal contact data is shown by use of columns that emanate from each contact point. The height of the column indicates relative timing of the contact (Fig. 24-14) or relative force (Fig. 24-15).

The Tek-scan system is so simple to use and provides such clearly defined quantification of both time and force sequence of contacts that it appears to have promise as a practical method for use in routine occlusal analysis and treatment (Fig. 24-16). Posttreatment results

can also be clearly recorded for the patient's permanent record (Fig. 24-17).

With the availability of precise methods for quantifying occlusal contacts, it has become all the more important that dentists understand the importance of multiple equal-intensity contacts and develop the skills for correcting occlusions to such a precise end point. It should be remembered that no instrumentation can take the place of the operator's judgment. Such instruments have little if any value without that judgment and the equilibration skills that go with it.

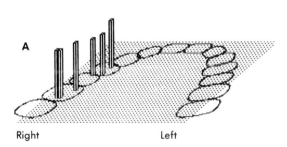

Right   Left

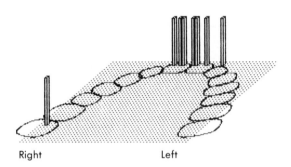

A

Right   Left

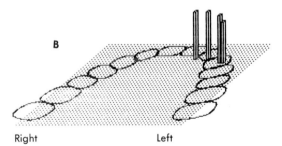

B

Right   Left

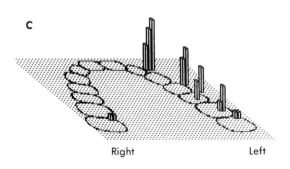

C

Right   Left

Fig. 24-16. Straight protrusive excursion showing even distribution of contacts on anterior teeth but also an unwanted contact on the second molar.

Fig. 24-17. A, Right lateral excursion showing nearly equal group function on the working side with complete disclusion of the nonfunctioning side. This is an acceptable occlusion for patients with anterior open bite. **B,** Left lateral excursion showing ideal anterior guidance disclusion of all posterior teeth. Watching the monitor during excursions enables the dentist to quickly evaluate the disclusive effectiveness of the anterior guidance in all excursions. **C,** Left lateral excursion showing progression of time balance plot as measured from outside in. Notice how the posterior teeth come into contact progressively from the anterior teeth back. This would be considered ideal for group function. Notice the slight nonfunctioning side interference on the right side that comes into contact just before full closure (which was not recorded).

SUMMARY

An understanding of equilibration rationale and procedures is *essential* for complete care of patients in general dentistry practices, as well as most specialty practices. Any dentist who does not develop expertise in equilibration is limited in providing even routine dental services that are nonstressful to the masticatory structures. Failure to understand the principles of equilibration makes even the simplest operative procedure a matter of guesswork.

The effort spent in learning the fine points of equilibration will reap dividends far beyond the ability to adjust occlusions because the knowledge required for equilibration automatically confers an enlightened diagnostic capability.

Remember these important guidelines, and equilibration will be a safe, rewarding experience for both the doctor and the patient.

1. *Diagnose carefully before equilibrating.* Rule out intra-articular problems or pathosis before changing an occlusion. If it must be altered in the presence of joint problems, plan the treatment for specific resolution of specific problems before attempting to finalize the equilibration.
2. *Verify centric relation* before adjusting.
3. *Evaluate on mounted diagnostic casts* before starting equilibration.
4. *Inform* the patient. Be sure the patient agrees to the treatment and understands why it is being done.
5. Don't start an equilibration unless you and the patient are prepared to complete it.
6. *Adjust precisely.* Contacts should all have equal intensity whether the jaw closes firmly or lightly.
7. Prepare the patient for subsequent further adjustments until the occlusion becomes stabilized.

25

Bruxism

The term "bruxism" refers to nonfunctional grinding of the lower teeth against the upper teeth. If uncontrolled, it generally leads to severe abrasive wear of the occlusal surfaces or hypermobility of the teeth and may also contribute to adaptive changes in the temporomandibular joints, resulting in flattening of the condyles and gradual loss of convexity of the eminentiae. In severe bruxers, the masseter muscles are often enlarged, sometimes to the point of noticeable changes in facial contour. Bruxism is associated with muscle spasm, split teeth, and fractured fillings. It is the screeching, grating sound in the night that has kept many spouses awake. One of the most unusual aspects of bruxism is that often the one who does it is not even aware of the habit. Habitual bruxers present some of the most difficult challenges in restorative dentistry, and the difficulty increases with the severity of the wear produced.

The cause of bruxism is not completely clear. Although considerable light has been shed on the problem, there are enough unexplained observations to indicate there is still much to learn. One thing seems certain: there is no single factor that is responsible for all bruxing. It is also rather evident that there is no one single treatment that is effective for eliminating or even reducing all bruxing.

There are, however, reliable methods for reducing the *effects* of bruxing, and in the majority of patients it has been my clinical experience that the signs and symptoms of bruxing

seem to disappear completely with the careful elimination of all occlusal interferences. I am still so confident of this result that I ask every patient to report any sign of bruxism because it may be an indication that the occlusion needs refining.

I have had to moderate my own views, however, regarding the *exclusive* relationship between occlusal interferences and bruxing. In the first edition of this book I stated that bruxing "does not occur without some form of occlusal interference being present." This viewpoint was apparently incorrect though it was also shared by several other clinicians based on the consistent relief of symptoms after meticulous occlusal correction. In a 1961 study, Ramfjord[1] had found that "some kind of occlusal interference will be found in every patient with bruxism." Electromyographic studies done by Ramfjord and Ash showed that "a marked reduction in muscle tonus and harmonious integration of muscle action follows the elimination of occlusal disharmony."

The results of the Ramfjord and Ash research is consistent with many later electromyographic studies that show a direct relationship between occlusal interferences and muscle hyperactivity, including muscle incoordination. Williamson's[2] classic study showing the effect of eccentric posterior tooth contact clearly relates muscle hyperactivity to occlusal interferences. It further documents the reduction in muscle tonus when the eccentric contacts are removed. If study after study confirms the causal relationship between occlusal interferences and muscle hyperactivity, it would be inconsistent to deduct that occlusal factors play no role as a causative factor in bruxing.

It is also obvious that occlusal interferences can trigger parafunctional jaw movements that were not present before the interference was introduced. The consistently observed "erasure mechanism" can be predicted to occur any time the envelope of function is encroached on. Restriction of the anterior guidance, almost without exception will produce excessive abrasive wear on the restricting surfaces. Furthermore, correction of a restricted anterior guidance almost always eliminates the wear problem. Providing a fraction of a millimeter of "long centric" often makes the difference between excessive wear or no observable wear on the anterior contacting surfaces.

Even in patients with no interferences to centric relation, parafunctional pressure against inclines will most likely occur if the inclines interfere with any functional eccentric jaw movements. Pressure against the restrictive inclines usually causes severe wear, but it may also result in hypermobility of the interfering teeth, or the teeth may be forced out of alignment until they no longer interfere.

Severe wear is a common occurrence in postorthodontic patients whose teeth have been held in functional interference for an extended period by a retainer. Even if centric relation harmony is perfected, eccentric wear will most likely occur against inclines of teeth that are prevented by a retainer from moving out of the position of restricted function. When teeth are prevented by the retainer from adaptively moving into a nonrestrictive alignment, the wear occurs rapidly and often causes severe damage in a short time. The severity of wear in such young postorthodontic patients is abnormal for their age and can only be explained as resulting from parafunctional rubbing. Unless the teeth are moved to a noninterfering functional alignment, the wear will continue even if the worn surfaces are restored. However if the functional alignment is corrected, the wear problem can almost always be predictably eliminated. This consistent clinical observation would indicate that bruxism can be caused by occlusal interferences and can be eliminated, at least in some patients, by correction of the occlusion.

Despite the obvious relationship between occlusal interferences and muscle hyperactivity, it appears that occlusal correction alone may not always be a sure cure for habitual bruxing. Rugh[3] showed that habitual nocturnal bruxism continued to occur even after occlusal interferences were removed. By monitoring muscle activity during sleep, electromyographic recordings seemed to indicate about the same amount of masticatory muscle contraction after occlusal correction as there was before. It also showed a direct relationship to emotional stress.

The time of muscle contraction during sleep appears to fluctuate up in direct relationship to stress-causing stimuli such as an argument before bedtime. Periods of emotional peacefulness seem to result in less masticatory muscle activity.

More research is needed, particularly research that distinguishes between the horizontal rubbing patterns found in the habitual bruxer and the stationary clenching action of many people during sleep. Most studies have measured only the duration of elevator muscle contraction, which may be unrelated to horizontal parafunction. Furthermore, the current studies do not explain why masseter muscle hypertrophy is reversed in some patients after occlusal correction, sometimes to such a degree that facial contour is noticeably changed as the muscles become reduced in size.

To be considered valid research, any studies regarding the effect of occlusal interferences on bruxism must compare the time and intensity of parafunctional jaw movement "with" versus "without" occlusal interferences. This requires meticulous occlusal correction as well as verifiable evidence that all occlusal interferences have been completely eliminated. That includes both noninterference to centric relation and disclusion of all posterior teeth during eccentric jaw pathways. Thus proper research protocol would require verification of centric relation as part of the study.

TREATING THE BRUXISM PROBLEM

Despite the controversy that still clouds the cause of bruxism, it is rather clear that habitual elevator muscle hypercontraction has the potential for severe overload on the teeth, the supporting structures, and the temporomandibular joints. In the presence of such an overload, damage to some part of the system is almost inevitable. The destructive effects can be reduced by distributive of the load to the maximum number of equal-intensity tooth contacts during intercuspation. Harmonizing those contacts with centrically related condyles reduces the overload on both the teeth and the joint structures and eliminates the trigger for incoordinated lateral pterygoid contraction. Thus, even if the patient clenches, it need not result in prolonged isometric contraction of opposing muscles.

By perfecting the occlusion for a habitual bruxer, full muscle loading occurs only in centric relation when all parts are aligned. Immediate disclusion of all posterior teeth eliminates any potential overload in eccentric positions and it reduces muscle loading of the joints and the anterior teeth. It is probably this reduction of muscle contraction in eccentric jaw movements that is responsible for the reduction in size of hypertrophic elevator muscles.

To eliminate the signs and symptoms of bruxism, it is particularly critical that centric relation interferences be eliminated with extreme preciseness. This is so because even the slightest premature contact can activate the contraction of the lateral pterygoid muscles and cause incoordinated elevator-muscle hypercontraction. The problem of equilibrating to such preciseness is made more difficult by the slowness of depressed teeth to rebound, and depression or interfering teeth is common in the bruxing patient.

Against teeth that interfere, strong clenching has the effect of compressing the periodontal ligaments. Clinicians now know that rebound from that compressed intrusion can take 30 minutes or longer before the tooth reaches a passive equilibrium in its socket. When a strong clencher or bruxer is being equilibrated, sufficient time for rebound must be provided before the occlusion is finalized or the bruxing trigger may immediately return. Even after careful equilibration, new interferences can easily develop within an hour or less. This may explain why many investigators have reported that their patients continue to grind their teeth even after the occlusion was perfected. The problem of communication that results in this controversy is the same problem that creates such divergent views regarding the causes of temporomandibular disorders. The difficulty of perfecting an occlusion is not always considered by the investigator, and the

so called occlusal perfection may fall far short of complete elimination of interferences.

If the occlusal therapist does not use precise methods for manipulating the mandible into the terminal hinge position, it will be impossible to achieve an interference-free occlusion, even in centric relation. However, perfection in centric relation alone is not enough. Minute interferences in *any* excursion can trigger a bruxism pattern, and so manipulation of the mandible is again essential to find and mark every incline that interferes with any border movement of the mandible within the limits of a correct anterior guidance.

The bruxism habit may actually be a form of a *protective* response to occlusal interferences. It could conceivably be nature's built-in mechanism for self-adjustment of occlusal interferences.

For thousands of years before modern man came along with his soft, refined diet, coarse, abrasive foods were the usual daily fare. As proximal tooth contacts wear and the teeth migrate forward, there is a continual need for occlusal adjustment to compensate for the mesial drift. The coarse foods of premodern man were abrasive enough to wear away interfering cusps and inclines when the bruxism mechanism was stimulated by the pressoreceptors around the roots. In effect, a natural "erasure mechanism" developed as a response to occlusal stress, and the coarse diet supplied the grit to adjust the occlusion to within tolerable limits.

The "erasure mechanism" is still with us, but our modern diet does not supply the grit. So instead of wearing off the interferences, the more frequent tendency is to wiggle the teeth until they become loose.

The excessive wear that occurred from the bruxism patterns of ancient man did not create a severe problem because of the short lifespan. By the time the teeth wore down to the ridges, there was usually little need for them. If the individual lived an unusually long life, the proliferation of the alveolar ridges themselves provided an adequate chewing surface. In modern man, neither loose teeth nor excessively worn teeth are acceptable, and so it is up to the dentist to prevent the results of bruxism.

If we conclude that all bruxism is caused solely by emotional stress, we will have to conclude also that virtually all our ancestors were emotionally unstable! Coarse diets undoubt-edly contributed to a great degree, but it is un-likely that the amount of wear seen on skulls of our early ancestors would have occurred with-out a considerable degree of parafunction also.

No one would deny that emotional stress could be a *contributing* factor in bruxism. If muscle tension is increased by stress, the ten-dency to grind the teeth is also increased, but only if interferences are contactable. A minute interference in a stressed person may trigger bruxism that may cease with either the elimi-nation of the interference or the reduction of muscle tonus when the stressfulness is normal-ized.

The observable results that are attainable with occlusal therapy do not seem to depend on the psychologic state of the patient. We would attempt to adjust the occlusion of a tense person just as quickly as we would treat a relaxed patient. In fact, many patients obvi-ously suffer an increased tension from the mal-occlusion itself. The concurrent muscle spasm that is so often present in the patient with se-vere bruxism, is often responsible for a consid-erable amount of facial tension, discomfort, and even pain.

The discomfort from muscle spasm may in some patients be a causative factor in emo-tional stress rather than vice versa. Results of treatment in a large number of patients seem to indicate that such is the case.

When signs and symptoms of bruxism are observed, a meticulous occlusal examination is in order. Whether occlusal interferences *cause* bruxism has not been clearly established, but it is very clear that occlusal interferences in a bruxing patient can be extremely damaging.

So regardless of whether the cause is emo-tional stress or occlusal triggers, the occlusion should be perfected. In fact, the more likely it is that a patient bruxes, the more important it is to keep the occlusion as perfected as possi-ble. The more perfect the occlusion, the less damage can be done to any of the structures of the masticatory system. In addition, overload-ing individual interfering teeth not only does direct damage to the interfering teeth and their supporting structures, but also the inter-ference causes the additional problem of mus-cle incoordination during the bruxing.

Whether treatment for bruxism is directed at eliminating the cause or the effects of the problem is at this point academic. It appears that regardless of the cause the most effective treatment is perfection of the occlusion. This can be accomplished in two ways:

> *Directly.* By equilibration, occlusal restora-tions, or orthodontics
>
> *Indirectly.* By occlusal splints

Direct occlusal correction

Before alteration of an occlusion is accom-plished directly, a careful analysis should be made on mounted diagnostic casts. If it can be determined that the corrections can be made with selective grinding without mutilation of enamel surfaces, equilibration is most often the method of choice. If restoration of posterior teeth will be needed for other reasons, equili-bration procedures can be used to correct the occlusion directly even if some enamel pene-tration is necessary. Even though restoration of the ground surfaces is planned anyway, the oc-clusion should be stablized as much as possible by equilibation before restoration.

If there is uncertainty about patient accep-tance or operator skill, correction of the occlu-sion should first be done indirectly by use of a removable applicance. At some point, how-ever, it will be in the patient's best interest to eliminate any appliance that is not necessary and correct the problem directly.

Whenever possible, equilibration should re-sult in multiple equal-intensity stops in centric relation with immediate disclusion by the ante-rior guidance in all excursions.

Use of appliances

If occlusal splints are prescribed, complete occlusal coverage should be used to perfect equal-intensity centric stops on all teeth against the splint and immediate disclusion of all posterior teeth the moment the mandible leaves centric relation. Disclusion should be accomplished by an anterior guidance ramp built into the occlusal splint.

The occlusal splint has some possible advan-tages for severe bruxers. Coverage of all the teeth in one arch has the effect of diminishing the proprioceptive response in the individual teeth that are covered by the splint. The splint coverage may also prevent the minute re-bound effect from occurring in teeth that has been intruded. This improvement in stability may better preserve the perfected relationship that is accomplished at equilibration.

A further value of the occlusal splint is to

reduce wear that might otherwise occur during nocturnal bruxing. The acrylic splint may become worn but is more easily replaced than tooth structure.

Even though there are obvious advantages in the use of occlusal splints, they are only advantages if they are needed. If there is no evidence of excessive wear or no signs of hypermobilty after occlusal equilibration or restoration, there is nothing to be gained by routine use of an appliance.

If the occlusion is perfected, I find the need for occlusal splints is very limited, and the need is especially reduced whenever I am able to disclude all posterior teeth in all eccentric excursions. For several years I have almost eliminated the use of nighttime appliances, preferring to keep patients free of any unnecessary prosthesis. I do, however, explain to patients the possibility of needing such an appliance if I notice signs of wear or mobility on routine health maintenance appointments. Up to now, very few patients have showed enough signs to warrant use of an appliance. Thus there is no rationale for prescribing appliances for all patients just because they previously had a wear problem.

Appliances can serve a useful function in some bruxism situations as a temporary adjunct to occlusal correction. Acrylic night guards may help to stabilize hypermobile teeth and reduce tendencies to bruxism during treatment. In unusual situations, they may also serve as compromise substitutes for restorative stabilization or correction when such treatment is impractical for financial or health reasons.

The beneficial effect of acrylic splints or night guards is the result of occlusal correction in the appliances themselves and the stabilizing effect they have on the teeth. The elimination of signs of bruxism will occur with virtually any technique that eliminates occlusal interferences, either on the teeth themselves or on an appliance that fits over the teeth. If there is no deviation of the mandible required, the muscles can relax and either bruxism tendencies disappear or the corrected occlusion prevents bruxism from doing harm.

Soft vinyl mouth guards. One of the more difficult bruxism problems to eliminate is in the patient with chronic sinusitis. An occlusion that is perfected one day is off the next day if pressure in the sinuses moves the upper teeth. It is impossible to keep an occlusion refined to a sufficient degree to keep bruxism patterns eliminated when the positions of the upper teeth are forever changing.

A reasonable solution to the problem is to supply the patient with a well-made soft vinyl mouth guard that can be worn at night to cushion the teeth from the effects of transitory occlusal interferences (Fig. 25-1). When the sinusitis subsides, the appliance is not needed.

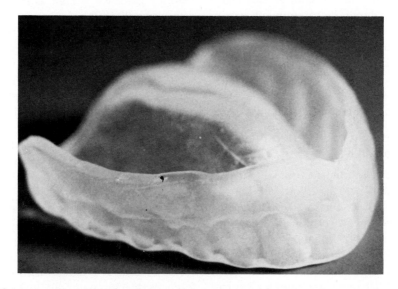

Fig. 25-1. A pliable vinyl mouth guard that can be worn as a temporary "cushion" for teeth that have been moved by sinusitis pressure on upper posterior roots. A soft appliance should not be used as a bite appliance except when there is a problem of sinus pressures. It is not a substitute for a perfected occlusion on a hard occlusal splint.

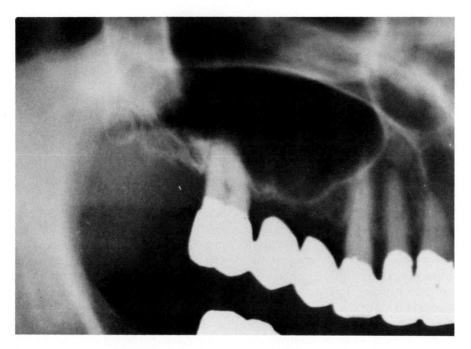

Fig. 25-2. Pressure from sinusitis can actually move teeth with roots that extend into the sinus. The patient should be aware of the difficulty of stabilizing such teeth in the presence of sinusitis pressure against such root surfaces.

Caution should be urged to perfect the occlusion during a time when the sinuses are normal. The appliance should not be a substitute for occlusal harmony.

Questioning the patient regarding sinus headaches, postnasal drips, and nasal stuffiness is an important part of the clinical examination. Radiographs should be carefully observed for the presence of extensive sinuses that extend past the roots of the upper teeth (Fig. 25-2). It is best to advise the patient in advance of the possible need for such an appliance during sinusitis episodes so that he will have an understanding of the limitations of treatment.

Stopping the bruxism habit when the occlusion is worn flat

The most difficult bruxism problem to be faced is the patient who has worn the entire occlusion flat and has shortened the anterior teeth into an end-to-end relationship. The effect of bruxism is easy to eliminate if the flat anterior guidance can be maintained, but often such a patient wishes to have the anterior esthetics improved. There is sometimes no way to improve the esthetics without steepening the anterior guidance. A steepened anterior guidance almost always promotes parafunction.

The solution to the problem is at best a compromise. In order to improve the appearance, I will accept a degree of bruxism. The damage from the bruxism can be minimized if the anterior guidance is perfected to disclude all posterior teeth in all excursions while the anterior guidance is kept as flat as acceptable esthetics will permit.

An increased thickness of metal or porcelain should be used to provide more length of wear on the lingual surfaces of the upper anterior teeth, and the patient should be told in advance of the probable continuation of wear. Some splinting may be required to give added stabilization against stress.

The anterior guidance should be worked out in the most meticulous manner possible.

BRUXISM IN CHILDREN

No one who has ever heard the screeching sounds emanating from a child's bedroom would doubt that children are capable of violent bruxism. Most children grind their teeth at some time or another since occlusal interferences develop naturally during the eruption of teeth. During the mixed-dentition stage, bruxism is common, and some children develop such severe bruxism patterns that they may wear their deciduous teeth flat. There are many old wives' tales for explaining why children grind their teeth. The most popular is probably that the child "has worms."

There may be many different contributing factors that increase the tendency to bruxism, but its effects are negligible in the absence of occlusal interferences. This statement becomes academic because all children have occlusal interferences at some time or other. The problem is not generally serious despite the volume of noise that the bruxism generates. A child's resistance to the stress of bruxism is so high that it does not constitute a threat to the dentition.

If the bruxism becomes so severe that it constitutes an irritant in itself, or if the occlusal wear appears to be more extensive than normal, some occlusal adjustment may be in order. Precise refinement is not necessary when a child's occlusion is adjusted, but it is helpful to polish and round all sharp edges and eliminate any gross interferences if the correction can be done without mutilation of a permanent tooth.

Orthodontic appliances may be in order, or some form of bite plane may be used to disengage an offending tooth until other teeth can erupt into contact or necessary corrections can be made. Gross occlusal adjustment usually reduces the bruxism to tolerable limits.

26

Procedural steps in restoring occlusions

The resolution of any occlusal problem must follow an orderly sequence. When the problem must be solved by restorative means, the sequence followed very often determines the outcome. Restoring posterior teeth before the anterior guidance is finalized is an example of a common error of sequence. The anterior guidance is a determinant of posterior occlusal form, and so its contours must be determined before it can in turn determine its effect on the posterior teeth. Dentists who do not understand how one segment of an occlusion affects another segment very often proceed in wrong directions before realizing it. Steps should always be taken to proceed with any restorative procedure in an orderly fashion to ensure that one sequence will flow smoothly into the next without need for going back to make changes in steps that have already been completed.

Two of the best rules to follow for staying out of trouble with restorative procedures are as follows:

1. Never begin any restorative procedure unless all the procedures that follow are outlined in advance and properly related to one another in correct sequence.
2. Never begin any restorative procedure unless the result is visualized and understood.

PRELIMINARY MOUTH PREPARATION

Restorative procedures are the last step in the treatment plan. All prelminary treatment should be completed before the final preparations are started.

1. *Mouth hygiene instructions* should be given. Patients should demonstrate the ability and interest in proper home care before extensive restorative procedures are started.

2. *Caries control* should be achieved. Deep carious lesions should be corrected and endodontic procedures completed when possible. Pin-retained amalgam techniques are advantageous for large lesions near the gingival margin prior to full coverage preparations.

3. *Periodontal therapy* should be completed. Time should be allowed for tissue maturation before final preparations are completed.

4. *Minor tooth movement* should be completed. Stabilization of the occlusion after any orthodontic procedures should have occurred. When restorative procedures must follow orthodontic movement, temporary bridges can often be used as an esthetic replacement for the usual retainers. When teeth have been moved, ample time should be given for reorganization of the periodontal fibers and bony support before final impressions are made for restorations.

5. *Necessary extractions* should be done and tissues healed before permanent placement of fixed prostheses. Immediate extraction techniques may sometimes be used in carefully selected cases, especially when replacement of the extracted tooth is by removable appliance.

6. *Equilibration* should be completed before preparation of the teeth. *The temporomandibular joints should be comfortable before finalization of any restorative treatment.* Doing restorative procedures before getting the occlusion as static as possible is an invitation to extra work and possible failure. When the occlusion has been harmonized to stability, two advantages are effected:

1. Any occlusal reduction will represent the same amount of thickness for the restoration in any excursion.
2. The teeth will have more of a tendency to stay where they were when the impression was taken.

When unstable teeth are prepared, they may continue to shift even after permanent restorations are placed. Excessive adjustment to stabilize the occlusion then may mutilate the new restorations.

It may be necessary to fabricate provisional bridges or splints in order to optimize the preliminary mouth preparation. The goal of such procedures should be to get the joints comfortable, the teeth stable, and the tissues healthy before final preparation and placement of permanent restorations is considered. Too many occlusal reconstructions fail because of failure to carry out these important preliminary necessities.

SEQUENTIAL STEPS FOR RESTORING DIFFERENT COMBINATIONS

Following is a general list of the variations in restorative needs of different patients. A suggested sequence of restorative procedures is outlined for each type of case. The outline is general, and it may be necessary to vary the procedures or the sequence for particular needs of certain patients.

An understanding of how each sequence affects the next will enable the dentist to vary technique approaches without jeopardizing the result. The sequences are based on the restorative methods outlined in the previous chapters of this book. Other methods may be used to complete many of the steps, but no technique should be considered by any dentist who does not thoroughly understand its rationale. The dentist must know what he or she is trying to accomplish and why; then whatever method is suitable for accomplishing the goal should be selected. This can be done segment by segment or for the entire treatment plan.

RESTORING ALL UPPER POSTERIOR TEETH ONLY

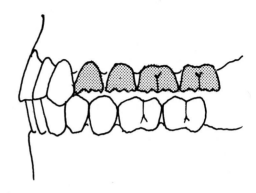

1. All preliminary mouth preparation should be completed.

2. By selective grinding, any deformities of tooth form, marginal ridges, cusp height, and so on, on the lower posterior teeth, should be corrected.

At this time, a decision must be made regarding whether posterior disclusion is the goal. If it is it must be worked out on the lower posterior teeth by equilibration *before* preparation of the upper teeth. This should be verified with marking ribbon to ensure that there are no incline contacts on any lower posterior tooth. Only centric relation stops are permissible.

If group function is to be the choice, there should still be no incline contacts on lower posterior teeth. This will ensure noninterference with centric relation stops but will not prevent group function.

3. All the upper posterior teeth should be prepared.

4. The correctness of the anterior guidance should be verified and modified if necessary. Any modification at this point should be minimal. Equilibration during preliminary mouth preparation should have resulted in good harmonization of the anterior guidance with consideration for the posterior teeth. Flattening out of the lateral anterior guidance must be accompanied by a corresponding opening out of lower fossae contours. This is accomplished more accurately before the upper posterior teeth are prepared, while the upper lingual

cusps are still in place to check lower inclines against them.

5. *If posterior disclusion is the desired result,* it can be achieved in the following ways:

a. By completion of the restorations on a semiadjustable articulator *with the condylar path set flatter than the patient's.* A 20-degree condylar setting will work for most patients. (In all cases the progressive side shift is set to a 15-degree minimum.) See Chapter 12 regarding the rationale for selecting the correct instrument approach. Use of a set-path condylar guidance will be effective in most patients who can be equilibrated to posterior disclusion by the anterior guidance, but there are exceptions that relate particularly to the occlusal plane or unusually flat condylar paths.

b. By completion of the restorations on an articulator that duplicates the condylar path and by carving all inclines out of excursive contact.

If group function is desired, functionally generated path procedures can be used on the upper posterior teeth. Restorations can then be fabricated against the functional core. Contact should be maintained against the core for any incline that must maintain group function contact.

6. Upper posterior restorations are placed and any necessary minor corrections made. All excurrsions should be checked by manipulation of the mandible to border positions.

RESTORING ALL UPPER TEETH BUT NO LOWER TEETH

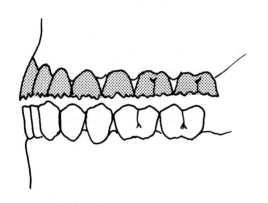

1. Preliminary mouth preparation should be completed.

2. By selective grinding, lower occlusal surfaces should be made as ideal as possible. Any irregularities in marginal ridge contours,

cusp height, and the like should be corrected, with your making sure that lower fossae contours are correct before preparing upper teeth.

Preliminary mouth preparation of the occlusion is the same on the complete upper arch as it is for the posterior upper segment. The decision must be made before tooth preparation regarding whether posterior disclusion or group function is the desired goal.

3. All upper posterior teeth should be prepared. Preparations should be completed in all detail.

4. Correctness of the anterior guidance should be verified and minor modifications made if necessary.

5. One central and the oposite side lateral incisor, or any suitable combination to guide the technician in determining precise incisal edge position and labial contours, should be prepared.

6. An impression of the upper arch should be made. It is not necessary to retract tissue for any of the preparations for this impression. This cast will be used for making the customized anterior guide table and also for waxing up the "throw-away patterns" in the "every-other" cast for duplicating the anterior contours. This cast must be mounted with a facebow.

7. A centric bite record should be made at the correct vertical dimension and anterior teeth put into centric contact.

8. The lower impression should be made and the cast articulated against the first upper cast, with use of the centric bite record.

9. The preparation of the upper anterior teeth should be completed and the impression taken for the master die model. This model will fit into the same bite record made before completion of the anterior preparations.

10. A customized anterior guide table should be made by use of a first model with upper posterior and the two anterior teeth prepared.

11. The upper anterior restorations should be completed using the first model for incisal edge position and labial contour. Those patterns should be transferred to the master cast to serve as guides for contouring the other anterior restorations. The custom anterior guide table will dictate lingual contours.

At this point there are several options regarding how to proceed with treatment.

a. The anterior restorations can be placed and verified for correctness. A new impression can then be made for completing the posterior teeth. If this procedure is followed, the posteriors would be completed later in the same manner prescribed for upper posteriors when the anterior teeth are all right. The options for posterior disclusion or group function would be handled in the routine manner after the anterior teeth are placed.

b. Restorations for the complete upper arch can be completed, and then all upper anterior and posterior restorations can be placed at the same appointment. There are no disadvantages to this as long as the laboratory work is meticulously done on carefully made dies and casts. Bite records and mountings must be precisely monitored for accuracy. The anterior restorations must duplicate the anterior guidance as dictated by the customized anterior guide table before posterior occlusal form can be finalized. After the anterior teeth are completed on the casts, the posterior teeth can be fabricated to relate to them. The options for posterior group function or disclusion can be satisfied on the articulator. If posterior disclusion is desired, the condylar paths should be set flatter on the articulator than they are in the patient. This will automatically result in posterior disclusion without affecting the anterior guidance.

c. The method of choice is up to the operator. As long as the posterior restorations end up in noninterfering harmony with both anterior guidance and condylar guidance, the choice of technique can be made on the basis of personal preference.

12. Balancing-incline contact should be eliminated by "hollow grinding" of the buccal incline of lingual cusps between cusp tips and fossae centric contacts.

13. Working-incline contact should be reduced on any tooth determined to be discluded in lateral function.

14. All upper restorations should be placed. Occlusion should be checked carefully and any necessary corrections (which should be minimal) made.

RESTORING ALL POSTERIOR TEETH BUT NO ANTERIOR TEETH

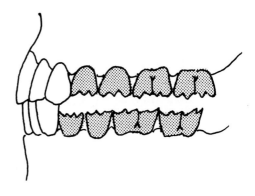

1. Preliminary mouth preparation should be completed.

2. On mounted models the optimum occlusal plane should be determined. When all posterior teeth are to be restored, the Broadrick Occlusal Plane Analyzer is probably the simplest method for determining an acceptable occlusal plane. Preparation plane guides should be made for use when preparing the teeth.

3. All lower posterior teeth should be prepared accordingly.

4. If needed, the anterior guidance should be harmonized by selective grinding. A master impression should be taken and centric bite record made with the anterior teeth in contact.

5. Using the special pin, a fossae-contour guide is made.

6. Lower posterior restorations should be completed following procedures for waxing lower posterior teeth and for carving lower fossae contours (Chapter 21).

7. Lower restorations should be placed.

8. Upper posterior teeth should be prepared.

9. Upper posterior restorations should be completed and occlusal contours finalized.

10. All balancing incline contacts should be eliminated. Working inclines should be refined to desired degree of group function or disclusion.

11. Upper posterior restorations should be placed.

12. Any minor interferences that result from cement thickness hould be corrected. Selective grinding requirements should be minimal.

RESTORING ALL UPPER AND LOWER TEETH

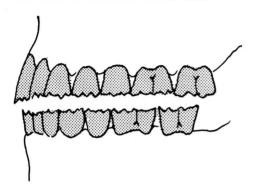

1. Preliminary mouth preparation should be completed.

2. Lower anterior teeth should be prepared. If anterior relationship is acceptable, the lower anterior teeth can be completed against the upper anteriors. If changes are needed in incisal edge position, provisional restorations should be completed on both upper and lower anterior segments before finalization of the lower teeth. When acceptability of contours and function has been verified for both arches, an impression is made of the lower provisionals in place. The temporary splint is then removed, preparations are checked for adequate clearance, and the master impression is made.

3. Lower anterior restorations are completed by use of an index to copy incisal edge position from the cast of the corrected provisionals.

4. Lower anterior restorations are placed after verification that they are correctly related to the corrected upper anterior teeth in centric relation and all excursions.

5. The upper anterior teeth are completed. All guidelines worked out on the teeth directly or on provisional restorations should be copied by the laboratory. These guidelines must be communicated through a centric relation–mounted cast of the corrected anterior segment. A customized anterior guide table and an index for incisal edge position should be made from the cast.

6. Upper anterior restorations are placed and checked for accuracy.

7. Lower posterior teeth are completed. All fosae should be related to the anterior guidance to determine allowable fossa-wall angulations for disclusion.

8. Upper posterior teeth are completed. At placement they should be carefully checked to make certain that each tooth has accceptable holding stops, that all posterior teeth contact simultaneously with equal intensity, and that there are no interferences to either anterior guidance or condylar pathways.

RESTORING ALL LOWER TEETH BUT NO UPPER TEETH

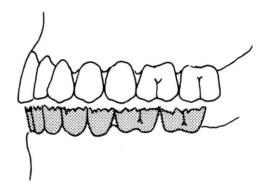

1. Preliminary mouth preparation should be completed.

2. Any imperfections in the upper arch should be refined *before* completion of the lower restorations.

   a. Uneven marginal ridges should be corrected.

   b. Occlusion should be equilibrated to optimum.

   c. Anterior guidance should fulfill its function.

3. Every other lower anterior tooth and all posterior teeth should be prepared and an impression taken. Dies should be made for the prepared anterior teeth.

4. A centric bite record should be taken at the correct vertical dimension. The unprepared anterior teeth should be in contact.

5. The remaining teeth should be prepared and the master impression taken. Dies should be made for all teeth.

6. Both models should be articulated. Anterior patterns should be made on the first model to maintain precise incisal edge position and contour of lower anterior teeth and those patterns transferred to master die model to serve as guide for contouring other patterns. If porcelain jackets are to be made, either they can be made on the first model and transferred to the second or wax patterns can be used

solely as guides on the second model and then discarded. Porcelain veneers can be handled in the same manner.

7. Posterior restorations should be completed with particular care being taken to correctly place all cusp tips.

8. All restorations should be placed and any occlusal discrepancies corrected.

Since all lower cusp inclines are discluded in function, there should be minimal occlusal adjustment required if the models are articulated carefully. The more accurately the instrumentation duplicates jaw movements, the less adjustment will be necessary. However, it should be minor, in any case, if the centric bite record was correct and the arches were properly equilibrated before preparation. Setting the condylar path flatter than the patient's will ensure posterior disclusion.

To prepare fewer teeth at a time, you may complete the lower anterior teeth before starting the preparations on the posterior teeth.

PREPARING ALL UPPER TEETH AND LOWER POSTERIOR TEETH ONLY

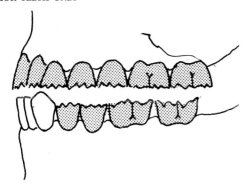

The sequence for this combination would be the same as the outline for preparing all upper and lower teeth, starting with the completion of the lower anterior teeth. There are some modifications, though, that may add practicality to the sequence.

Since the anterior guidance must be finalized before restoration of the lower posterior teeth and since it is easier to harmonize the guidance with the posterior teeth out of contact, it is sometimes easier to go ahead and finish the lower posterior teeth even before restoring the upper anterior teeth. This is a practical sequence *only* if all anterior guidance contours are definite.

If there is no need to modify the anterior guidance further, it is not essential to complete the actual restorations before proceeding with the lower posterior teeth. The fossae contour guide can be made and used on the lower restorations, and they can be completed before any preparation is started on the upper teeth. Then the upper posterior teeth and every other upper incisor are prepared. An impression is made and a centric bite record taken at the correct vertical dimension. This model is used to make the customized anterior guide table, and the sequence is carried out the same as if upper teeth only are being restored.

The practicality of this approach lies in the simpler requirements for temporization. Preparing all upper teeth at the same appointment enables us to make one temporary and one master impression and eliminates any need for having both arches prepared at the same time.

27

Requirements for occlusal stability

Occlusal *stability* is the first goal of occlusal diagnosis and treatment planning. To be maintainably healthy, the teeth must be maintained without excessive wear, hypermobility, or migration out of an acceptable alignment. From the standpoint of occlusion, any dentition can be assumed to be stable if the supporting structures are healthy and there are no problems of wear, mobility, or migration of the teeth, *regardless of what it looks like.*

There are definite criteria for determining whether any occlusal relationship is stable. These criteria are not based on preconceived ideas of what an "ideal" occlusion should look like. Rather they are based on an analysis of whether five specific requirements for occlusal stability are fulfilled. An understanding of these requirements makes it possible not only to determine if an occlusion is stable or unstable but also to select treatment for that instability with logic and in proper sequence.

Stable dentitions that are not in an ideal Class I relationship are often treated erroneously to "correct" the malocclusion, and the corrected occlusion is often more unstable than it was before treatment. An understanding of the requirements for occlusal stability must also include recognition of the *exceptions* to the rules.

There are no occlusal stereotypes that fit all patients. There are no averages that apply to all patients. But there are *principles* of occlusal stability that are reliable guidelines for evaluating any occlusion. They include five requirements and two exceptions. They are so definitive they can be used to evaluate any type of occlusal relationship. If all five requirements are correctly fulfilled, the occlusion will be stable. If any one of the requirements is not fulfilled, the occlusion will be unstable, unless the rules for exceptions are met.

Learning these rules and the exceptions that go with them is the basis for evaluation, diagnosis, and treatment planning of occlusal problems. They should be understood, memorized, and used until they become an automatic part of diagnosis.

The five requirements that must be fulfilled if an occlusion is to function with optimum stability are as follows:

1. Stable stops on all teeth when the condyle-disk assemblies are properly aligned in their most superior position against the eminentiae (centric relation)
2. An anterior guidance that is in harmony with the border movements of the envelope of function
3. Disclusion of all posterior teeth in protrusive movements
4. Disclusion of all posterior teeth on the nonworking side (the side of the orbiting condyle)

5. Noninterference of all posterior teeth on the working side with either the lateral anterior guidance or the border movements of the condyles

The working-side posterior teeth may contact in lateral group function if they are in precise harmony with the anterior guidance *and* condylar border movements, or they may be discluded from working-side contact by the lateral anterior guidance. Determination of the need or amount of group function is dependent on varying requirements of distribution of lateral stress.

It should be obvious that many patients have healthy, maintainable dentitions despite the fact that they fail to fulfill one or more of the stated criteria. It is possible to have a completely healthy, maintainable occlusion without fulfilling a single requirement, but to do so one very important condition must exist: *there must be a substitute for any unfulfilled requirement or else the need for that requirement must be specifically eliminated.*

Before clinical judgment can be developed regarding occlusal stability, there must be a clear understanding of *why* each requirement is important. Then it is essential to learn about the many different ways of effectively substituting for requirements that have not been satisfied. Finally, the diagnostician must be able to recognize when the need for any requirement has been eliminated. Such judgment can be developed, and it is certainly the key to diagnosis of any case presenting a problem related to occlusion.

I will discuss the requirements one by one to give a better insight into how these principles work.

Stable Centric Stops on all Teeth

There are three basic reasons for having stable centric stops on all teeth:
1. The more teeth that are in contact in centric relation, the less stress will be exerted on any contacting tooth. This maximum distribution of stress is most important in centric relation, the position that the mandible physiologically assumes when the muscles close the jaw with the greatest force.
2. The more teeth that contact correctly in centric relation, the less wear will occur on each contacting surface.
3. A correct centric holding contact on

each tooth prevents the supraeruption that results when teeth have no opposing arch contact.

The first reasons are to a degree the "nice-to-have" goals, but the third reason should be our critical concern in diagnosis and treatment.

Although it is possible to minimize problems of stress and wear to a practical degree without having *every* tooth in centric contact, it stands to reason that stress and wear on each contacting tooth will be greater if only four teeth contact their opponents than if the stress and wear can be distributed to eight teeth, or twelve, or on up to sixteen.

Of course, all teeth that are going to contact must contact simultaneously to take advantage of this basic rule of physics because if any tooth strikes prematurely that individual tooth absorbs all the stress at contact instead of allowing it to be distributed to the other teeth.

The most important reason for having contact in centric relation is to prevent unopposed teeth from supraerupting. Unless a tooth is opposed by *something* it will continue to erupt, often taking the alveolar process with it, until it is stopped by some physical obstruction. The obstruction that stops the eruption is normally and ideally an opposing tooth, but eruption may also be stopped by the tongue, the cheeks, the lips, a thumb, or any other force habitually applied to the teeth. Such forces applied to teeth after they have erupted into a correct relationship may even cause those teeth to lose the contact they once had by actually depressing them into the alveolar bone.

To be good diagnosticians of occlusal problems, it is essential that we thoroughly understand these phenomena. Whenever a tooth is not in centric contact with an opposing tooth, we must determine whether the patient has provided a substitute for the missing tooth contact. If he has not, we must provide the contact for him through our plan of treatment. On the other hand, if the patient has substituted for the missing contact, the problem must be handled differently. If lost centric contact is restored without first elimination of a tongue- or cheek-biting habit that caused the separation, the case will fail. The interposed tongue or cheek will force the restored teeth apart by moving them laterally or depressing them even further because of the added thickness of the restorations.

Habit patterns such as biting a pencil or a pipe stem may cause teeth to lose their centric contact. Such lost contact should not be restored while the habit persists. Eliminating the habit allows the teeth to erupt back into contact and then restoration is not necessary.

Although it may appear that tongue- and cheek-biting habits are the cause of many malocclusions, I am convinced that in a large number of cases the opposite is true. To avoid an unpleasant premature contact, many patients learn to hold the tongue between the teeth or suck the cheeks in to cushion the teeth when they swallow. Some patients create a negative pressure in their mouth that sucks part of the lower lip in between the front teeth. Such tongue-lip or cheek positions are more comfortable to the patient than the disagreeable malocclusion and a habit pattern develops. The habit in effect was actually caused by the malocclusion. In many cases adjustment of the occlusion eliminates the need for cushioning the teeth and the habit disappears.

Before attempting to change a habit pattern for any patient, we must first determine whether the habit is harmful. Some habits may actually contribute to the stability of the occlusion. A case in point is the Class II patient with severe upper anterior overjet. A tongue-thrust swallowing pattern may be the only thing that keeps the lower incisors from erupting into the palate. In such a situation, the tongue acts as a substitute for the missing tooth contact in centric relation (Fig. 27-1).

In prognathic arch relationships the upper lip usually serves as an effective stop for the lower incisors. It thereby substitutes for the missing contact with the upper anterior teeth.

Individual teeth will readily supraerupt if they lose centric contact. Lower incisors that have been shortened to improve the esthetics will erupt back into contact unless steps are taken to prevent it. Such steps may include restoring the lost contact on the opposing upper teeth or splinting the noncontacting tooth to one or more teeth that do have centric stops. Before initiating restorative procedures, however, it should be positively established that there is a need for stabilization. Frequently, the cingulum of a lower incisor that is not in cen-

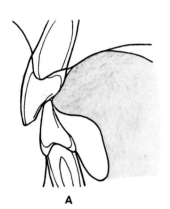
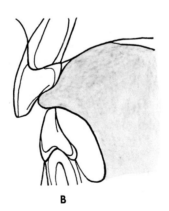
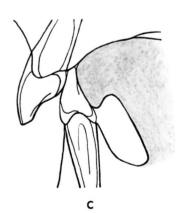

A   B   C

Fig. 27-1. Tongue position and occlusal stability. The position of the tongue during swallowing is an important consideration in the diagnosis of occlusal problems. When there is stable anterior contact in centric relation, **A,** the tongue presses against the lingual surfaces of upper and lower anterior teeth during each swallow. The outward pressure of the tongue is counteracted by the inward pressure of the pursed lips. The net effect has a stabilizing influence on the anterior teeth. In upper anterior overjet relationships, the tongue may serve as a substitute for missing centric contact. If the tongue is thrust between the teeth during deglutition, **B,** and the occlusion is stable, many such arch relationships may be maintained without anterior tooth contact. The tongue thrust may be either the cause of the problem or the solution to an arch malrelationship. It is the diagnostician's job to determine which is the case. In deep overbite problems, **C,** there is no room for the tongue to get over the lower incisors to prevent their supraeruption into the lingual soft tissues. For this reason such occlusal relationships almost always deteriorate in time. Close analysis with correctly mounted models is essential to determine the potential for harm in such relationships. Usually the occlusion must be altered to provide either centric stops or some other substituting stabilization.

tric contact may be locked under the proximal contours of adjacent teeth that are in contact. The *need* for centric contact is thereby eliminated for the locked-in incisor.

Frequent eccentric contact in function may serve as a substitute for centric contacts. A common example of this type of stabilizing contact can be noted in some anterior relationships. Anterior teeth that do not touch in centric relation but do touch at the front end of a "long centric" will usually be quite stable.

Some very capable dentists believe that the anterior teeth should not even touch at all in centric relation. They believe that contact should not occur until the mandible is slightly protruded. However, if concepts of "long centric" are understood, it will be obvious that this horizontal freedom can occur without sacrificing the stress-distributive benefits of centric contact on the anterior teeth.

When centric contacts are lacking and the patient cannot provide a substitute, it is safe to predict that problems will occur. It is certainly better to intercept a predictable problem and correct it before damage has been done than to wait until obvious deterioration has taken place.

One type of occlusal relationship that almost always leads to trouble is the deep overbite with no anterior tooth contact. The lower incisors almost invariably erupt on up into the palatal tissue just lingual to the upper anterior teeth. The reason such problems are so predictable is that it is impossible for the tongue to fit into the space above the lower incisors and provide a substitute for the missing tooth contact. The treatment of such problem cases is discussed in detail in the chapter on solving deep overbite problems.

In analyzing problems that relate to lack of centric contact, two general recommendations could be made:

1. In *normal* arch relationships, when one or more teeth are not in centric contact, corrective procedures should not be initiated until it has been determined *why* the teeth have been held apart.

2. In *abnormal* arch relationships, when any teeth are not in centric contact, corrective procedures will depend on whether the patient has provided an acceptable substitute for the missing contact or the need for such contact has been specifically eliminated.

ANTERIOR GUIDANCE IN HARMONY WITH FUNCTIONAL BORDER MOVEMENTS

There are many factors influencing the position of the anterior teeth. In normal arch relationships, the critical balance between tongue and lips is an important contributor to the eventual positioning of the erupting anterior teeth. Functional demands of sucking, swallowing, and even breathing determine the habitual positions of the tongue and the lips. The teeth are merely guided into position by the repetitious forces of function. As the teeth erupt, movements of incising, chewing, and speaking are influenced by the position of the teeth and habitual patterns of function develop. When the anterior teeth and the envelope of function are in harmony with each other and also with all the other normal relationships of the musculature and the joints, there is a stable anterior relationship.

Anything that adversely affects this harmonious relationship will have a deleterious effect on the long-term stability of the occlusion. Although the proprioceptive sensors around the teeth have the job of programming the muscles to accommodate to the best fit of lower teeth against upper teeth, they can also initiate nonfunctional patterns of erasure as an attempt to eliminate any interference to harmonious muscle activity. Such erasure movements consist in bruxism, clenching, or pushing jaw movements that over the years contribute to premature deterioration of the dentition.

If the anterior guidance is in harmony with the envelope of function, there will not be a tendency for destructive nonfunctional movements.

Very often, disturbances to the anterior guidance are a direct result of mandibular deviations to avoid posterior interferences. Correction of posterior occlusal interferences is *always* a prerequisite of determining the adequacy of the anterior guidance.

An excellent method for evaluating the anterior relationship on centric mounted study models has been suggested by Fillastre. It consists in simply placing a dowel pin or two in each posterior segment of the lower study model. Separator should be painted over each segment and the second half of the model poured. We can then saw down to the separation just distal to the cuspid, and the posterior teeth become removable from the lower model. The anterior relationship can be studied to see whether there is any deviation from first contact in centric relation, and the character of the centric contact can be noted. Lower incisors may hit lingually to the uppers when centric interferences have been removed. This kind of information is certainly critical to any treatment planning. The case is always simplified if anterior contact can be accomplished in centric relation.

Another method of determining this information on mounted study models is to duplicate the models and equilibrate them on the articulator until the anterior relationship can be noted without deviation from posterior teeth.

All that these techniques will establish is whether the anterior relationship is acceptable in centric relation. It will be possible to get a general idea of excursive movements from the articulated models, but we must evaluate in the mouth of each patient to determine how well the myoneural mechanism has adapted to or is capable of adapting to the guidances established by the anterior teeth.

Some patients function comfortably and maintainably with severe restriction by a steep anterior guidance (sometimes even with irregular interlocked anterior teeth). The anterior guidance is thus in harmony with the "chop-chop" envelope of function.

Other patients, because of long-standing habit patterns or because of varying degrees of periodontal destruction, may not be able to cope with the excessive lateral forces that are imposed on steep inclines. The guidance of such patients must be "opened out" or flattened to permit more lateral freedom from restriction by teeth that are too weak to handle the job.

Some patients require the anteroposterior freedom of a "long centric." It is an essential part of their envelope of function. Failure to provide it will produce unnecessary wear and stress on the anterior teeth.

Since the anterior guidance determines how the front end of the mandible is moved, it is referred to as the *anterior determinant of occlusion.* As a determinant of occlusion, it is quite proper that it should be in harmony with functional movements *before* the posterior occlusion is restored. Understanding the clinical aspects of such harmony is the key to the whole occlusal scheme for any patient. The chapters that follow go into detail on solving problems of tooth and arch relationships, and

in each problem that is faced, the envelope of function is an important consideration. The further importance of relating the anterior guidance to the envelope of function cannot be overemphasized.

DISCLUSION OF ALL POSTERIOR TEETH IN PROTRUSIVE MOVEMENTS

When the mandible is protruded, the only teeth in contact should be the anterior teeth. This is so because when the mandible is protruded the condyles are no longer braced. Since the amount of flexing of the mandible depends on varying degrees of contraction of the closing musculature, there is no way to harmonize the posterior teeth to all the different degrees of muscle force. The anterior teeth, being farthest from the fulcrum and not nearly so subject to the flexing, are in the best position to carry the load. Protrusive stresses on posterior teeth are further compounded by the fact that such forces are usually directed toward inclines of the upper cusps as the wider part of the lower arch moves forward into the narrower part of the upper arch.

Because there is no need for posterior teeth to touch during incising, because posterior tooth interferences in protrusion are among the most damaging, and because it is impossible to harmonize the posterior occlusion to all degrees of muscle force in protrusion, the logical approach to minimizing stress on the occlusion is to disclude the posterior teeth completely by letting only the anterior teeth contact in protrusion. It is rather unlikely that a substitute can be provided by the patient for protrusive disclusion of the posterior teeth, but it is possible to eliminate the need for satisfying this criterion. Prognathic patients, as an example, have no anterior guidance and so have no means of discluding the posterior teeth when the mandible is protruded, but prognathic patients have no reason for protrusive movements. Protruding the mandible only makes their arch relationship worse; so almost all patients with prognathism use only vertical, "chop-chop" functional movements, and protrusive disclusion of posterior teeth becomes unnecessary.

On the other hand, patients with Class II occlusions with extreme anterior overjet have no anterior guidance to disclude the posterior teeth, but the need for such protrusive disclusion is rarely eliminated. Class II patients usually do protrude, and unless the stresses can be moved off the back teeth and onto a guidance that is as far forward as possible, the probability of accelerated deterioration of the back teeth is increased.

DISCLUSION OF THE BALANCING SIDE WHEN THE MANDIBLE MOVES LATERALLY

The reason for disclusion of the balancing side when the mandible moves laterally is similar to the one just discussed. As the mandible moves laterally, the orbiting condyle on the balancing side is not braced by ligament, and so it is impossible to harmonize the occlusion to all the varying degrees of muscle contraction against a flexible mandible.

To illustrate the amount of flexing of which the mandible is capable, we may place a paper match between the teeth on the working side. (That would be between the teeth on the left side if the jaw is moved toward the left.) The teeth on the balancing side should be separated (if they are not, there are severe balancing-side interferences). Now the patient squeezes firmly and the separated teeth on the balancing side can probably be made to contact. This is simply because the mandible bends under the contraction of the muscles, and since the unbraced condyle on the balancing side is free to slip up the incline as the mandible bends, the teeth can be brought into contact. More importantly, they can be brought into stressful incline contact. This does not occur on the working side because the rotating condyle is braced against ligament.

It is possible to harmonize the teeth on the working side, but we must beware of falling into the trap of believing that we can accomplish "cross-arch balance." It is possible and even desirable with complete dentures because the resiliency of the denture-bearing tissues allows them to accommodate to any mandibular flexibility. In mouths where opposing natural teeth are present, the stressful, torquing contacts are passed on to the periodontal structures. Balancing-side interferences are considered to be one of the most destructive types of interferences because:

1. The stresses are increased because of the proximity to the condylar fulcrum.
2. The stresses are intensified because they are almost always directed against inclines.

3. Balancing interferences have a tendency to torque or rotate because of the direction of the forces.
4. The unbraced condyle and the flexible mandible enable the patient with bruxism to exert extreme force against even slight interferences.

In light of the preceding, it may seem strange to refer to the side of the orbiting condyle as the "balancing side." This term is apparently a carry-over from reference to the stabilizing effect that cross-arch balance has on complete dentures. When natural teeth are being considered, *nonfunctioning side* would be a more descriptive term for the side of the orbiting condyle, and this term is now preferred.

Regardless of what it is called, the simplified rule to remember is: *When lower posterior teeth move toward the tongue, they should not contact upper teeth.*

NONINTERFERENCE OF ALL POSTERIOR TEETH ON THE WORKING SIDE

If any posterior tooth interferes with the lateral anterior guidance on the same side, it is referred to as a working-side interference. The more distal the working-side interference is found, the more stress will be exerted against the inclines of the interfering tooth.

Ideally, the lateral guiding inclines of the working side should be found on the anterior teeth. The cuspids are usually in the prime position of importance for lateral guidance, but they can be effectively helped in this role by group function with other anterior teeth.

In healthy mouths with good arch relationships, there is rarely a need for the posterior teeth to contact in working excursions. The anterior teeth, by virtue of their distant position from the fulcrum, their usually good crown-root ratios, and their normally dense bone around long roots, are quite capable of guiding the front end of the mandible without help from the posterior teeth.

When arch relationships are not ideal or when anterior teeth have lost a considerable amount of their periodontal support, it is often necessary to allow the posterior teeth to work in group function with the lateral anterior guidance.

When posterior teeth maintain contact in working-side excursions, they must not interfere with *either* the anterior guidance or the condyle border movements. An interference to either places the fulcrum onto the interfering posterior tooth inclines. This is a condition that is extremely stressful to the teeth involved. It is possible and entirely practical for posterior teeth to contact in working excursions without constituting an interference. However, disclusion of all posterior teeth in *all* excursions is the choice whenever practical because of the effect the disclusion has on reducing muscle contraction.

In the examination and evaluation of any occlusion, we must always *manipulate* the mandible into a right and left border excursion. If the anterior teeth are discluded by the posterior teeth, the stress distribution will be unfavorable. We must evaluate what changes are necessary to permit the anterior guidance to do its job.

If the arch relationship does not permit anterior tooth contact in lateral excursion, the anterior guidance cannot disclude the balancing side and the job falls to the posterior teeth on the working side. The front tooth in contact becomes the lateral anterior guidance tooth, but if it is a bicuspid, it is rarely strong enough to carry the load of lateral guidance by itself. It may become necessary to either reinforce the guide tooth by splinting procedures or else distribute the stresses over more teeth by bringing the working side into group function.

Very often the group function approach eliminates the need for splinting in borderline cases. Working-side interferences can be caused by an improper plane of occlusion, faulty occlusal contours, an inadequate anterior guidance, or poor arch relationships. Finding the cause of the problem is the key to correcting it.

USING THE REQUIREMENTS

Proper use of the *requirements for occlusal stability* can greatly simplify and coordinate the diagnosis and treatment planning of occlusal problems.

The following sequence has proved to be a practical system:

1. Determine which requirements have not been fulfilled.
2. Determine *why* any unfulfilled requirements have not been satisfied.
3. Determine whether the patient has either substituted for the unfulfilled requirement or eliminated the need.
4. Determine all the possible methods of providing for the needs that result from failure to fulfill any requirement.
5. Select the *best* method for fulfilling the demands of each unfulfilled requirement.

The preceding sequence is used to determine the treatment for each of the common occlusal problems outlined in the following chapters. A complete understanding of the reasons for each requirement should be developed until it becomes an automatic part of diagnostic thinking.

SUGGESTED READINGS

Fillastre, A.J., Jr.: The restorative practice, seminar manual, Lakeland, Florida, 1987.

Guichet, N.F.: Principles of occlusion, a teaching manual, Anaheim, Calif., 1970, The Dénar Corp.

Kaplan, R.L.: Concepts of occlusion, Dent. Clin. North Am., pp. 557-590, Nov. 1963.

Ramfjord, S.P., and Ash, M.M.: Occlusion, ed. 3, Philadelphia, 1983, W.B. Saunders Co.

Schuyler, C.H.: Occlusal harmony as a basic requisite in orthodontia, N.Y. J. Dent. **24**:174, 386-388, 1954.

Schuyler, C.H.: Factors contributing to traumatic occlusion, J. Prosthet. Dent. **11**:708, 1961.

28

Solving occlusal problems through programmed treatment planning

Some occlusal problems appear almost insurmountable when we see them for the first time. This is especially so when multiple problems of periodontitis and caries are found in combination with arch relationship problems, destructive habit patterns, and drifted or elongated teeth. Problems of excessive wear on some teeth may be found in the same mouth with elongated teeth. Esthetic problems along with a myriad of other demands for correction of stress direction and distribution may appear unsolvable.

There is one basic rule that must be followed in the resolution of any occlusal problem: *Never start any orthodontic or restorative procedure unless the result can be visualized.*

Visualizing the result is in effect the setting of a clearly defined goal. Determining this goal of treatment and being able to conceptualize what it must accomplish is the most important factor in treatment design. It is the essence of good problem-solving technique.

The determination of treatment goals must be specific and well defined. The generalized goal of healthy maintainability must be the major criterion for every treatment plan, but it must be applied specifically to each individual

tooth and each segment of the occlusion. Problems of maintainability should be carefully searched out by systematic tooth-by-tooth exploration.

A treatment plan should consist in an orderly sequence of procedures that are necessary to:

1. Eliminate pain
2. Eliminate infection
3. Restore all supporting tissues to healthy maintainability
4. Reshape, reposition, or restore the dentition when necessary for optimum maintainability, esthetics, comfort, and function

Too often, the treatment plan is determined before the *problems* have been isolated. The first step in setting up a treatment plan is to diagnose the problems. *Every* problem must be clearly defined, and this requires thoroughness in the examination stage.

It is hard to imagine how a thorough evaluation can be made without properly mounted diagnostic casts and a complete radiographic survey. Knowledgeable dentists would not attempt to plan a treatment without such aids. Models that have been mounted with facebow and centric relation bite record show the terminal hinge interocclusal position at the first point of contact. Occlusal interferences can be eliminated on the models to show what the tooth-to-tooth relationships will be *at the correct vertical dimension.*

Once tooth-to-tooth relationships at the correct vertical dimension are known, each segment of the occlusion can be evaluated regarding its potential for long-term maintainability. Teeth that are not in a maintainably stable relationship can be studied to determine whether corrections should involve removal, reshaping, repositioning, or restoring. Such corrections can actually be accomplished on the models, and the projected treatment goal can then be assessed for feasibility and correctness. There can be no better way to visualize the goals of a treatment plan than to have an actual model of the projected result.

PROBLEM SOLVING

Problem cases are more easily solved with a programmed approach. Developing an orderly sequence of procedures to use for each new patient is a must. It simplifies the planning of chair time and eliminates confusion for the office staff. Most importantly, though, it enables the dentist to program his or her thinking into sequential patterns. A multiple-problem case loses most of its complexity when individual problems can be isolated and solved one step at a time. In my office, we have found that two visits are essential for treatment planning.

First appointment

The first appointment with a new patient should be planned to accomplish the following:

1. The patient's complaints must be ascertained. The first part of the appointment is *listening time.* We must find out what the patient's problems are from his or her own point of view. We must get feelings on esthetics, long-term expectations, and present comfort level. We have to ask questions. An assistant should write down all pertinent information so that the dentist can give undivided continuous attention to the discussion with the patient.

2. Present conditions are charted. There should be a convenient place on every patient record for charting present conditions. It should be kept simple so that it will be used. A cursory examination is all that is needed at this time because the detailed examination

will be completed at the second appointment. Information that is needed includes the following:

a. *Present restorations.* The general condition of the present restorations should be noted. Specific problems that will obviously need attention should be charted.

b. *Prosthetic.* Is the patient wearing any prosthetic devices? An appraisal of each appliance should be given and patient's comments regarding same noted.

c. *Occlusion.* The type of arch relationship should be noted. Tooth relationships in a manipulated terminal hinge closure should be examined and first point of contact and direction of slide noted. Any patient comments about the occlusion should be recorded.

d. *Temporomandibular joint.* Have there been symptoms, past or present, that could be related to temporomandibular joint dysfunction? Such a question should be asked. One of the examination forms for diagnosis of temporomandibular joint problems may be used. Palpation for muscle tenderness should be routine.

The joints should be tested to see if a verifiable centric relation can be determined and to rule out any intra-articular problems. If there is a history of any signs or symptoms or the examination reveals any abnormalities, we would routinely use Doppler auscultation at this appointment. If further diagnostic tests are needed, they would be recommended.

e. *Periodontal.* A general appraisal of the periodontal condition should be noted at this time. Each tooth should be checked for hypermobility and any mobility patterns should be noted on the chart at this appointment. Obviously unsavable teeth should be so noted also.

f. *Oral lesions.* The mouth should be carefully examined for any lesions of soft tissues.

g. *Caries.* Carious lesions should be charted at this appointment.

h. *Mouth hygiene.* A general appraisal of the patient's mouth hygiene and attitudes about proper mouth care should be noted.

3. Impressions, bite records, and facebow record for mounted diagnostic models are taken.

4. A radiographic survey is completed. Periapical films of all teeth are essential. Radiographs showing temporomandibular joints should be made for evaluation of any joints suspected of possible problems or pathosis.

Purpose of the first appointment. The first appointment is a *generalized* information-gathering session. Enough information must be gained to permit practical study of the radiographs and mounted models before the second appointment. A tentative treatment plan must be formulated from this information, but the final treatment plan should not be accepted until the detailed examination is completed at the second appointment.

The first appointment can proceed in a very orderly manner if it is organized to do so. Impression materials should be measured out in advance, facebow equipment should be ready, and bite-record materials should be on hand.

This appointment is ideally conducted with the patient's participation. By allowing the patient to observe all aspects of the examination in a large hand mirror, we can explain what we find and describe what we are seeing as we examine. By spending more time at the original examination appointment, we find the treatment explanation is more readily understood and accepted at the second appointment.

Second appointment

After an evaluation of generalized problems has been completed, it is time to get down to specifics. In most cases, the tentative treatment plan that is worked out on the models is generally correct and requires minimal changes and additions at the final examination appointment. In problem cases, however, an acceptable treatment plan may be formulated only by careful examination at the chair using the combination of radiographs, models, and clinical probing.

This is the appointment at which each tooth is meticulously examined for any factors that would cause deterioration or prevent its maintenance. At this appointment, a complete periodontal examination should be completed. Pockets should be charted and each tooth should be evaluated for periodontal maintainability. If the patient is to be referred to a periodontist, the examination does not need to be quite so definitive, but any area of questionable prognosis should be recorded. The effect of periodontal treatment on the restorative treatment plan should be appraised.

When multiple problems exist, the following programmed approach to problem solving may be used:

1. Each tooth should be evaluated individually. Can it be saved and made maintainable by any procedure? Any special requirements for saving, such as endodontics, hemisection, post coping, and the like, should be noted.

2. Teeth that *cannot* be saved or maintained should be indicated on study model and chart.

3. Questionable teeth should be indicated by a question mark being put on the model and chart.

4. The remaining teeth should be evaluated on the basis of stress direction and distribution. It should be determined whether questionable teeth are key teeth in minimizing stress problems. If a questionable tooth offers no advantage for the remaining teeth, it may be a logical decision to extract it. If so, this should be indicated on the model. Questionable teeth should be treated and the results of treatment determined before they are used as key teeth in any restorative plan.

5. Evaluation should be made as to whether remaining teeth would best be served by fixed or by removable prostheses. If removable, should it be tooth bearing or tissue bearing?

6. The problems should be reevaluated. Sometimes the whole complexion of a case changes when unsavable teeth are removed. Actually doing this on mounted models helps to clarify the process of isolating individual problems. Occlusal problems should be attacked first, and then restorative decisions should be tailored both to the needs of individual teeth and to the occlusal requirements.

DESIGNING OCCLUSAL TREATMENT BASED ON THE REQUIREMENTS FOR OCCLUSAL STABILITY

The requirements outlined for occlusal stability serve as the guideline for planning treatment. If any one of the requirements for stability is not fulfilled, it is almost a certainty that one or more teeth will either get loose, wear excessively, or migrate out of proper position *unless:*

1. The patient provides a substitute for the unfulfilled requirement, or
2. Specifically eliminates the need for that particular requirement not fulfilled.

Both exceptions are clinically discernible, and we should always look carefully for either substitutes or factors that eliminate the need for any requirement before we attempt to treat any occlusal problem. We cannot base treatment on appearance of the occlusion alone. We must evaluate every tooth individually to determine if it does or does not have a problem with stability. We must also evaluate the occlusion by segment, looking first at the anterior guidance and then at the posterior segments.

The requirements for occlusal stability should be analyzed and treatment planned *in correct sequence*. The first requirement of stable holding contacts for each tooth must be satisfied in the plan before treatment planning for the next requirement of anterior guidance can be properly thought out.

Primary treatment objective: stable holding contacts

If the first requirement has not been fulfilled, the analysis should be directed at determining the following:

1. Can we *provide* stable holding contacts for each tooth?
2. If we cannot provide holding contacts, can we *substitute* for the missing contact?
3. If we cannot provide or substitute, can we *eliminate the need?*

The ideal treatment objective is to *provide* the holding contacts, and so that is the first priority of our treatment plan. With correctly mounted diagnostic casts we can analyze the effects of various treatment approaches in regard to accomplishing this goal. If we can't logically accomplish it, we proceed to analyze methods for substitution or elimination of the need.

To determine the best method of solving any occlusal problem, we should analyze as many different methods as possible before selecting a treatment plan. The sequence to follow in our analysis is as follows if we apply it to determining the best method for *providing* holding contacts (fulfilling the first requirement for occlusal stability):

1. *Reshaping.* Can equilibration or occlusal recontouring reestablish stable holding contacts on teeth that don't have them? If it can do it satisfactorily without our grinding through enamel, we have solved the problem

in the simplest manner possible. This is always our first choice of treatment if all needs of the patient can be satisfied by this method.

2. *Repositioning.* Can teeth be moved into correct alignment? Moving teeth is almost always preferable over unnecessary restorations.

3. *Restoring.* If teeth can be reshaped into stable holding contacts by restorations, the decision to use or not use this method can be made logically only by comparing it with other treatment plans. If the teeth would benefit from restorations for other purposes, the decision is easy. If the teeth do not need restorations for other reasons, the alternative methods should be evaluated and pros and cons of each explained to the patient. Factors of treatment time, expense, esthetic considerations, and patient health may influence the decision.

4. *Surgery.* If the occlusal problem cannot be resolved by reshaping, repositioning, or restoring the dentition, it may be necessary to reposition parts of the skeletal base to achieve the best overall result.

5. *Combining methods.* Many problem occlusions are best treated by a combined approach to treatment. The sequence is still followed as outlined. Some occlusions can be helped dramatically by judicious reshaping, but optimum occlusal stability cannot be completely achieved without some movement of teeth in combination with the recontoured occlusion. It is not unusual to combine three or even four methods in order to solve some occlusal problems.

Substitution. If stable holding contacts are absent and the patient has not substituted for them by posturing the tongue or lips as a stop for eruption, the *treatment plan* may employ a substitute. An example is an occlusal splint that provides holding contacts when worn at night. The nighttime wear may be all that is needed to prevent eruption of unopposed teeth and may provide a simple alternative to an extensive treatment plan.

Elimination of need. If stable holding contacts are absent and treatment is necessary to stabilize a segment of the occlusion, that stabilization may be accomplished in some instances without either providing contact or providing a substitute. As an example, unopposed teeth can be splinted to teeth that *are* opposed; thus the need for holding contacts is eliminated.

Selecting which treatment approach to

use. For many occlusal problems the stability of the dentition can be accomplished in several ways. Astute treatment planning, however, requires evaluating all the different possible ways to solve the problem by comparing the methods from several standpoints. Just because we *can* stabilize an occlusion by complete arch splinting does not automatically make it the correct treatment. We must weigh each alternative from several perspectives:

1. Is it the best plan for achieving a *maintainably* healthy mouth?
2. Is the *cost* of the plan reasonable or necessary for the results it achieves? This evaluation may be looked at differently from different patient perspectives.
3. Is the *time* required to achieve a result logical in comparison with other plans? Again this decision may be different for different patients.
4. Does the *health* of the patient warrant an extensive treatment plan?
5. Is the prognosis favorable enough to make extensive procedures logical?
6. Is the prognosis, *without* treatment, unfavorable enough to warrant an extensive treatment plan?

All these decisions really boil down to making two honest appraisals regarding the proposed treatment:

1. Is the treatment really optimally beneficial for the patient?
2. Would a simpler plan work?

I have a very reliable way for helping me to make every complex decision regarding recommendations for treatment: Would I want the same treatment plan used on me? Would I treat my wife or children in the same way I'm proposing to treat the patient? If I can't honestly answer yes to each of those questions, I don't suggest such treatment for the patient. If the patient must compromise, I try to approach alternative plans that are in line with the best interests and special considerations of each patient. These decisions require understanding of individual circumstances and an empathetic approach to doing the best service possible within the means of the patient and the patient's emotional and intellectual ability to understand it and maintain it.

The treatment planning procedures outlined above should be applied to analyze each of the five requirements for occlusal stability and strategize the best method for fulfilling each requirement, or substituting for it, or eliminating the need for it.

Analyzing the anterior teeth. Only after decisions have been made regarding the first requirement of stable holding contacts on every tooth do we then determine the method of choice for satisfying the second requirement of an anterior guidance in harmony with the envelope of function. The evaluation of any anterior guidance must be based on an understanding of the factors that determine anterior tooth relationships. In the following chapters on solving the various problems of occlusion, it will be apparent that working out the correct position and contour of each anterior tooth is the key to solving most of the other problems.

Anterior relationship problems must be solved as a separate entity before we proceed with posterior occlusal problems, unless the posterior teeth must be changed to permit an optimum anterior relationship.

Analyzing the occlusal plane. If posterior teeth interfere with the anterior guidance in any mandibular position, the occlusal plane should be carefully evaluated to determine how it can be corrected. Methods for analyzing the occlusal plane are outlined in Chapter 20. Remember that the front of the occlusal plane starts where the incisal plane ends, and so it is essential to have the lower incisal edges correctly aligned with the interpupillary line *before* the occlusal plane can be determined. Many of the problems we see with poor treatment results are obviously the consequence of restoring posterior teeth without first determining the correct anterior relationships. The sequence of analysis and of treatment is a critical factor that is too often ignored.

Analyzing posterior tooth-to-tooth relationships. After the acceptability of the occlusal plane is either confirmed or corrected, the tooth-to-tooth relationships can be established within those acceptable limits. Within the framework of those limits, a variety of tooth-to-tooth relationships are possible. Many factors influence the type of occlusal contours that are suitable. Whether the problem is a crossbite, an end-to-end relationship, or a posterior open bite, cusp position and contour will need to be decided upon before treatment decisions are finalized. Sometimes the final contours are refined in provisional restorations, but there is always a reason for every cusp-tip position and every fossa contour.

Those decisions are more logically made when they are related to the requirements for occlusal stability.

Be certain that whatever occlusal design is used for the posterior teeth, they must not interfere with the disclusive function of the anterior guidance. If occlusal contacts can be positioned in line with the long axes of each tooth so that they meet in simultaneous contact in centric relation with no interference to any anterior tooth contact position, they will probably be at least acceptable. They will, at worst, be adjustable.

Solving restorative problems. Determining the type of restorations to use can be on a tooth-by-tooth basis once the total occlusal scheme has been resolved. The corrected models will show clearly which teeth must be altered by restorations, and the restorative needs of each individual tooth should also be considered. The decision should be made on the basis of what restoration will best serve each tooth and then the choice of restorations evaluated in relation to the combined need of other teeth. The type of restorations selected should fulfill the needs of strength, protection, and esthetics.

When a comprehensive treatment plan has been completed and a careful reevaluation of all factors indicates that the plan will produce optimum oral health for the patient, a sequence of treatment should be outlined in writing. Such an *order of treatment* should be in a prominent place on the patient's record. It has several advantages.

1. It eliminates the need for time-consuming review of treatment every time the patient reports for an appointment. It serves as a ready reference for what has been completed and what is yet to be started.
2. It provides an excellent reference for setting up and reserving appointment times in advance.
3. It aids the staff in preappointment preparations for each office procedure. Auxilia-

ries always know what procedures to prepare for before the patient arrives.

4. It enables the dentist to present an orderly sequence of treatment to the patient. Patients appreciate an explanation of what they can expect in terms of future appointments. We never attempt a consultation with a patient until we have outlined the sequential order of treatment in writing on the chart.
5. It forces the dentist to follow a basic rule of treatment: *Never begin any restorative procedure unless all the procedures that follow are outlined in advance and properly related to one another.*

An understanding of the principles outlined in Chapter 27 is essential if we are to effectively evaluate any treatment plan. It should be reviewed if necessary and every problem case evaluated on the basis of these criteria. Treatment planning can become the most rewarding challenge in dentistry for the dentist who learns how to search out problems and then find solutions to each problem uncovered.

SUMMARY

Solving problems of occlusion is simplified when one follows an orderly sequence in examination and treatment planning. Only problems that are recognized will be solved. A complete mouth survey must include thorough radiographic analysis, periodontal examination, occlusal analysis on correctly mounted casts, and a systematic tooth-by-tooth search for every factor that could cause accelerated deterioration.

Every problem should be listed. *All possible solutions* for each individual problem should be evaluated. The *best* solution for each problem should be determined. The result of treatment should be visualized. Corrected models should be used whenever necessary. A sequential, step-by-step procedure for completing the treatment plan in the most orderly manner should be designed.

Finally the plan should be followed.

29

Splinting

The decision of whether to join teeth together for stabilization can sometimes be perplexing to resolve. For each advantage that splinting may offer, there is at least one disadvantage that must be accepted. The determination to splint should be made only when the benefits clearly outweigh the negative aspect of having the teeth connected to each other.

The disadvantages of permanent fixed splinting are rather obvious:

Splinted teeth are more difficult to clean. The ease of flossing unsplinted teeth verses the difficulty and time consumption of threading floss under each contact is reason enough not to splint unnecessarily.

Permanent splinting requires extensive restorative procedures. Teeth that may not otherwise require restorations must often be restored.

Splinting is costly. It demands meticulous care, skill, and judgment to accomplish it acceptably. A splint, like a chain, is no better than its weakest link. Quality cannot be compromised on any restoration involved in a splint.

Splinted restorations are difficult to repair. Problems that could easily be resolved on an individual tooth may require extensive and expensive procedures when that tooth is part of a splint.

Splinted teeth are difficult to check. Hypermobile teeth may be depressed during cementation, and the marginal seal may be defective. Caries can occur as the cement line washes out, and the tooth can become loose under the splinted crown without showing any signs until the problem is well advanced. Splinted teeth must be checked extra carefully, but even then it is possible to miss problems in their early stages.

It is often difficult to provide optimum crown contours on splinted teeth. Particularly on short teeth or teeth that are close together, the interdental papillae are easily crowded or overprotected.

Splinting (with full coverage) may require more tooth reduction. To achieve a "line of draw" it is often necessary to reduce teeth considerably more than would be required for individual restorations.

When all the disadvantages of permanent fixed splinting are evaluated, it should be apparent that it is a procedure that should not be used unless it is first determined that the benefits of splinting are essential to the preservation of the remaining teeth or it is needed to enable the patient to function comfortably.

The single observation that teeth are hypermobile is not in itself an indication for splinting. Even extremely mobile teeth often respond to occlusal correction and become firm, functional, and maintainably healthy without splinting. Occlusal correction should be completed to the point of achieving as much occlusal stability as possible before a final decision is made regarding permanent fixed splinting. If destructive tendencies can be *reversed* without splinting, the chances are good the teeth can be *maintained* without splinting.

It may seem out of place to enumerate the disadvantages of splinting before even discussing its rationale and indications, but the negative aspects must be considered before a positive decision can be logically made. There are definite indications, and many otherwise unsavable teeth have been made comfortable and maintainable by applying the principles of splinting. This does not alter the fact, however, that splinting should not be used as a "shotgun" security measure for every tooth that has lost some of its periodontal support. Individual teeth have so many advantages over splinted teeth that splinting is definitely contraindicated unless it is necessary for the comfortable maintainability of the teeth. Dentists who understand the principles of stress direction and distribution will have less need for splinting because they will reduce stresses effectively through occlusal contouring.

RATIONALE OF SPLINTING

Splinting refers to any joining together of two or more teeth for the purpose of stabilization. The benefits that can be derived from the effects of splinting are varied and specific. The desired effect should always be tailored according to specific requirements of stabilization. The advantages of splinting are directly related to the following effects that can result from joining teeth together:

Redirection of stresses. Perhaps the most important single benefit of splinting is its effect on the redirection of forces. Notice in Fig. 29-1 how even lateral forces are directed progres-

sively more parallel with the long axes of the teeth as the base is widened by splinting. Splinting around a corner expands the base in two directions and redirects both mesiodistal and buccolingual forces. It is this principle of stress redirection that enables us to effectively save teeth with minimal remaining bone support. Teeth that are not capable of normal function individually can serve as effective abutments for fixed bridges because of this redirection of forces.

Redistribution of forces. When teeth are joined together, any force on an individual tooth is distributed to all of the splinted teeth. Root surfaces that may resist stresses poorly in one direction may provide good resistance in another direction. Thus the combined effect of splinting weak teeth together is to capitalize on whatever strength any tooth can offer to the group.

Prevention of migration. It is sometimes difficult to keep loose teeth from migrating out of correct occlusal relationships. Splinting has the effect of stabilizing the teeth and preventing the constant need for realignment.

Prevention of supraeruption. Teeth with no opposing contact have a tendency to erupt until stopped by the soft tissues. Harmful supraeruption can be stopped by splinting of nonopposed teeth to those having contact.

Stabilization of tipped teeth. Tipped molars with maintainable periodontal tissues can be utilized as effectively as uprighted teeth if the tilted tooth is splinted to the tooth in front of it. When further tipping has been prevented, the stress direction is completely acceptable and there is no need for uprighting procedures before such teeth are restored or used as bridge abutments (Fig. 29-2).

Simply extending the contours of tilted teeth into contact is usually not sufficient to stabilize them because the lateral tilting forces are too great and too far off center from the longitudinal axis.

Elimination of food impaction. Although elimination of food impaction is not in itself a reason for splinting, splinted contacts prevent such impaction into interproximal areas.

Stabilization and strengthening of abutments. Properly made partial dentures with precision attachments have a stabilizing effect themselves on their abutment teeth if the partial denture is completely seated before

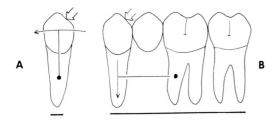

Fig. 29-1. The main value of splinting is its effect on the *direction* of forces. A single tooth is stressed laterally by forces that rotate it around a fulcrum within the root, **A.** The same occlusal force on splinted teeth, **B,** would result in stress directed almost vertically. As the base is widened by splinting, the fulcrum moves over the center of the base and the stress direction changes accordingly.

pressure is applied. Experience has shown, however, that patients do not always make sure of complete seating before biting down with force. A piece of food in the attachment can turn a stabilizing partial denture into a leverage arm that is capable of fracturing the abutment tooth. Double abutting is a form of splinting two teeth together to resist such accidents. It is usually good insurance.

Abutment teeth that have lost alveolar bone support may have to be splinted to provide better resistance to the lateral forces exerted by the partial resting on resilient tissues. Upper abutments with severe bone loss may have to be splinted to provide resistance to the weight of the removable partial denture.

METHODS USED FOR SPLINTING

Teeth may be splinted either permanently or provisionally. *Provisional splinting* may be used for a variety of purposes and may or may not be followed by permanent splinting. The stabilization that can be attained by provisional splinting provides an environment that is conducive to periodontal healing or bone fill-in after orthodontic movement. If the teeth are stable after periodontal treatment or temporary stabilization, it may not be necessary to continue the splinting. In such cases, provisional splinting techniques that are reversible should be used. Reversible splinting techniques include:

1. Use of ligature wire
2. A-splint techniques
3. Removable appliances
   a. Hawley type of retainers
   b. Continuous clasps
   c. Swing-lock partial dentures

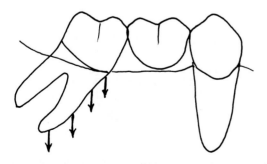

Fig. 29-2. Tilted teeth may serve very well as abutments when splinted. The forces on such a splinted tooth have no tendency to torque the tooth. If there is no unmaintainable crevice on the mesial, tilted molars can serve as abutments without being uprighted.

Provisional splinting techniques that involve irreversible tooth preparation may be used if the involved teeth require restorations for other reasons. The provisional restorations can be splinted, but the option can be left open regarding the necessity or degree of splinting required in the permanent restoration phase. If there is no need for restorations and the necessity of permanent splinting has not been ascertained, reversible techniques should be used whenever possible for the provisional phase.

If it can be predetermined that *permanent splinting* will be necessary, reversible techniques are not necessary for provisional splinting. If full-coverage restorations are to be used for permanent fixed splinting, it is usually also the choice of restoration for any provisional splint that precedes it. Processed full-coverage acrylic splints that effectively stabilize the teeth without being obtrusive esthetically can be made. They can also be shaped to improve occlusal contours and provide adequate cleanability. They can be reinforced with metal copings and strengtheners when needed. They may be constructed to last several months when necessary.

Provisional splinting may be used to determine the feasibility of permanent splinting. In some severely involved periodontal problems, the prognosis is not predictable enough to warrant the time and expense of permanent splints. Provisional splinting provides an opportunity to observe the effects of stabilization before a final commitment to extensive restorative procedures is made.

Splinting with ligature wire

Stainless-steel ligature wire can be used in a variety of ways to stabilize anterior teeth. It is simple to use and quite effective as a reversible method of provisional splinting. It is not a good method for use on posterior teeth because the wire has a tendency to slip into the narrower part of the teeth, although one or two premolars may be included in anterior splints.

Dead-soft 0.010- and 0.007-gage stainless-steel ligature wire should satisfy all requirements for anterior splinting.

There are two techniques of applying the ligature wires that permit the greatest ease of application and yet still provide adequately stability. These are the inverted S tie and the interdental hairpin tie.

A 5- to 6-inch piece of stainless-steel liga-ture wire is bent so that about a third of the wire extends from the starting tooth around the labial surfaces of the teeth to be splinted and extends a few millimeters past the last tooth. The longer portion wraps distally around the starting tooth and is bent to follow the lingual contours of the starting tooth at about contact level. The long end of the wire is poked under the labial wire from the lingual and pulled to firm wrap-around contact with the starting tooth. While the wire is held in po-sition with the fingers, the long end is folded back over the labial wire and pulled through the contact (Fig. 29-3). This procedure is then repeated for each tooth in the splint. The wire should not be pulled too tightly, since some slack is needed to form the labial loops. At the distal of the last tooth, the two ends are twisted together and the excess wire is cut off.

A curved explorer is then inserted in the center labial loop, and the loop is twisted about one turn. This is repeated for the other loops (Fig. 29-4) unless they are tight enough without the procedure. Additional tightening is then performed as needed to assure a firm grip of the ligature wire around each tooth. The twisted loop is then folded over toward the in-cisal edge if the occlusion permits. Otherwise it is folded gingivally, with an attempt made to avoid crowding of the interdental tissue.

The teeth and wire are thoroughly dried and then self-curing acrylic is applied at the contacts. A small amount of acrylic powder is picked up by a brush dampened with mono-mer and carried to each contact area. This serves to lock the ligature wire in position and covers the wire loop to prevent soft-tissue irri-tation.

Some dentists object to the use of acrylic at the contacts, fearing it will promote caries and absorb objectionable odors. This has not been a problem in my clinical experience, and I be-lieve that the advantages of stability outweigh all other disadvantages. Of course the proce-dure should not be used in a highly caries-sus-ceptible person, and in all cases the teeth should be thoroughly clean before the acrylic resin is applied. Only enough acrylic should be used to lock the wire at the correct height. It should never be allowed to fill the interproxi-mal space or interfere with cleanability.

Ligature wire splinting with interdental hairpin ties

This procedure is one of the simplest meth-ods of ligature wire splinting because it does not involve the manipulation of long strands of wire. It is a good procedure when extra strength is required because double strands of wire can be used if desired.

A long U-shaped wire is adapted to the la-bial and lingual surfaces of the teeth to be splinted, and the two loose ends are tied by twisting them around each other (Fig. 29-5). Premade hairpin ties are placed from the lin-gual at each embrasure and tied on the labial side. The splint is secured by tightening the large loop ends and the individual hairpin ties (Fig. 29-6). The ends of the ties are cut about

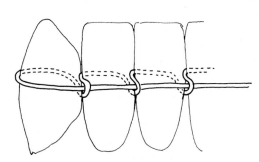

Fig. 29-3. Provisional splinting with the inverted S tie. Stainless steel ligature wire is wrapped around each tooth, through the contact, around the labial wire, and back through the contact. The procedure is repeated for each tooth, and then it is twisted together with the labial wire at the distal of the last tooth to be splinted.

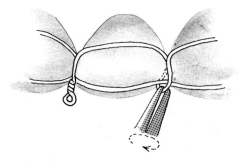

Fig. 29-4. Each loop is then twisted with pliers or an ex-plorer until the wire is pulled tight around each tooth. The loops are then folded over, and the wire can be stabilized at the contacts with self-curing acrylic resin applied by brush.

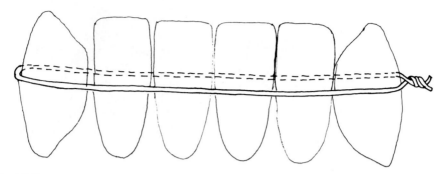

Fig. 29-5. The first step of the hairpin tie. The wire is wrapped around all teeth to be splinted and twisted at the end. A double wire may be used here if more strength is needed.

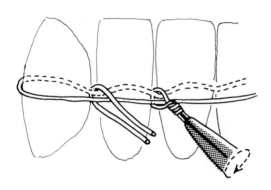

Fig. 29-6. Hairpin-shaped wires are placed at each contact and twisted tight. Contacts may be stabilized with acrylic resin if desired.

2 mm in length and folded back, making sure they do not interfere with either the occlusion or the interdental tissues.

The ligature may be locked in place by application of a small amount of self-curing acrylic resin at the contacts.

A-splint techniques

The A-splint is an intracoronal, provisional, fixed splint that involves minimal tooth reduction. It may be used on either anterior or posterior teeth, and it provides good stability with acceptable esthetics. All the procedures can be accomplished at one appointment. It is an economical way to provide stabilization for fairly long periods of time, and it can even be used to replace missing teeth provisionally.

Although the A-splint is a most practical, conservative approach, it should not be construed as permanent splinting procedure. From a realistic clinical standpoint, it is probably not as consistently dependable as it would appear to be. Even in the hands of careful, experienced dentists, interproximal contours are not always as smooth and cleanable as they should be, and the seal around the reinforcement wire

is not always perfect enough to prevent interproximal caries from starting. It is clearly contraindicated in persons with high caries susceptibility, and anything less than meticulous technique is an invitation to problems. The procedures must be carried out with great care in clean mouths. It does have the definite advantage of easy repairability without disruption of the entire splint.

Anterior A-splint. Using an inverted cone bur or diamond, prepare a channel on the lingual surface of each anterior tooth to be splinted at the height of the contact. The channel is undercut to provide good retention for the filling material. All carious tooth structure is removed, and any loose enamel rods or unsupported filling material is removed.

Braided multiple lengths of 0.010 stainless-steel wire can be cut to size and adapted to the channel cuts. Deeply knurled gold wire may also be used.

After a rubber dam is placed, the teeth are dried and the enamel edges are acid etched in accordance with standard procedures. A composite resin is then placed in the prepared groove, and the wire is seated into the length

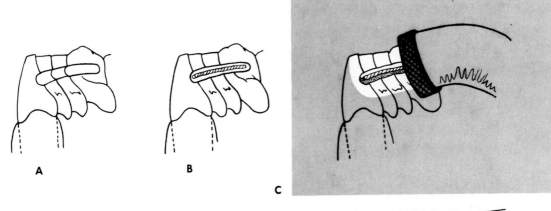

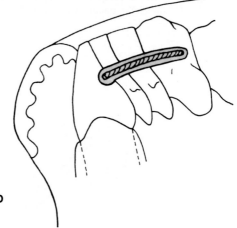

Fig. 29-7. The original A-splint design advocated by Berliner has been made better and stronger by the improved bonding agents. A groove is cut into the lingual surfaces, and a braided length of 0.010-inch stainless steel wire is adapted into the channel, **A** and **B.** Bonding resin is used to cover the wire after all the related enamel edges are acid etched, **C.** Dentin bonding materials are also used. The wire is covered and the surfaces are smoothed, **D.**

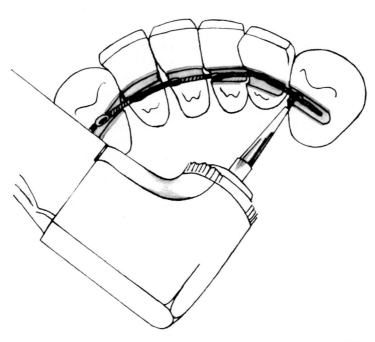

Fig. 29-8. Combination of threaded wire and screws anchors the wire through small loops. After the wire is screwed to the teeth, the groove is filled with a bonded resin. This provides a strong splinting effect with minimum tooth reduction.

of the groove so that it is embedded into the resin (Fig. 29-7). More resin is added over and around the wire to fill the groove. Use of a light-cured composite resin gives ample working time. Curing should be done in small enough increments of resin to ensure complete polymerization.

With care the resin can be applied at the contacts to form fairly acceptable joints. Care must be taken not to infringe on the interdental tissue space, and extreme care is required to prevent rough margins at the interproximal areas. A slight overbuilding is usually helpful on the lingual surfaces so that it can be shaped back to correct contour.

Posterior A-splint. The procedure for A-splinting posterior teeth is essentially the same as for anterior teeth except that it is more difficult to control the interproximal contours. However, the adaptation of interproximal matrices can be done in several ways while room to join the teeth at the contacts is still provided. The reinforcing wire may be used with bonded composite resins or it may be used with amalgam.

The A-splint technique can be greatly strengthened by the use of specially formed wire with loops built in for screw retention (Fig. 29-8). The procedure is the same as for a conventional A-splint, except that the wires are screwed to the teeth before the composite resin material is used to cover it and further strengthen it by the effect of the acid-etch bonding to the enamel.

Various types of metal rods, bars, and meshes are also available for reinforced splinting. They can be used with screw retention or acid-etch composite bonding, or both.

Splinting with removable appliances

Retainers. Orthodontists routinely splint their finished cases with removable retainers until the bone adapts around the repositioned teeth. The same procedure may also be effective as a temporary method of stabilization after periodontal therapy or occlusal correction of hypermobile teeth. It is a very conservative approach for determining the stability of occlusally corrected teeth that had tendencies toward migration before treatment. The patient can be weaned off the appliance for gradually increasing time periods as the teeth become stabilized.

There are many different ways to make stabilizing appliances, but the most commonly used technique is to brace the teeth on the lingual side with the acrylic extension of the palatal coverage or by extension of the lower lingual bar up to contact the teeth. On the labial side, an arch wire is used to hold the teeth in position against the lingual acrylic. These appliances are not practical for stabilizing during periodontal surgery because they interfere with the placement and retention of periodontal dressings.

Continuous clasps. The fabrication of cast continuous clasps can serve as a reversible method of stabilization. They are removable by the patient so that mouth hygiene is made simpler. The difficulty of finding a survey line suitable for an entire arch is sometimes an insurmountable problem, and the esthetic result is so poor that most patients would object to this method of splinting.

Swing lock partial dentures. The stabilization of anterior teeth can be accomplished quite effectively in combination with replacement of posterior teeth through a uniquely designed "swing lock." The teeth are braced from the lingual by an extension of the palatal or lingual bar. A labial brace swings horizontally from a hinge on one side into labial contact with the anterior teeth and is locked into the partial restoration on the other end of the brace.

Swing lock splinting is effective, but it must be remembered that the partial saddle areas are rigidly attached to the anterior teeth and the partial denture is in effect tooth-borne. As such it is essential that the saddles be carefully fitted and the occlusion on the partial restoration be perfected to prevent excessive stress on the abutment teeth. The saddles should be extended distally as far as practical to provide maximum support and should be relined when necessary to maintain perfect ridge adaptation.

The esthetics is generally poor when a swing lock partial denture is used, but we can keep it less obtrusive by masking the labial swing bar with acrylic resin and by keeping it as far as possible away from the incisal edges. In some instances, it may even serve as an artificial gingival cover-up for exposed roots.

The procedure can be used in selected cases for posterior teeth as well as anterior teeth, and it may serve either as an effective method for provisional splinting or a compromise alternative to permanent fixed splinting.

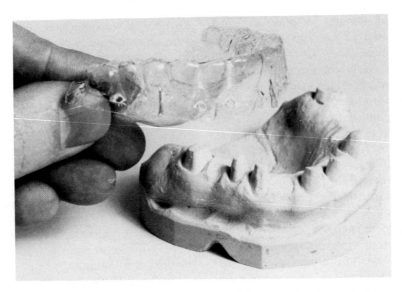

Fig. 29-9. An Omnidental matrix to be used on a model of the prepared teeth for fabricating a temporary acrylic splint (Omnidental Corp., Harrisburg, Pa.). Biostar pressure-molded matrix is also excellent.

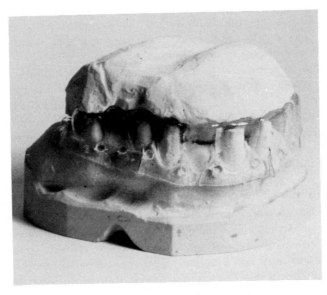

Fig. 29-10. When the matrix is in place, it is reinforced with a mix of stone. Healey's Fast Setting Grey Rock sets very rapidly for this step. This in effect forms two halves of a stone "flask." When the acrylic resin is poured into the matrix and the two halves are squeezed together, firm force can be applied to minimize flash and compress the acrylic. The two parts are held together during setting with heavy rubber bands.

Provisional splinting with full coverage

One of the best methods of provisional splinting is to use acrylic splints with full-coverage abutments. As has already been pointed out, this procedure is only practical in mouths that require permanent splinting or extensive full-coverage restorations. Many periodontal patients are also candidates for extensive restorative dentistry, and so acrylic full-coverage splinting is used quite often.

Attempts at fabricating provisional acrylic splints in the mouth are impractical. It is unnecessarily time consuming, and the results are never as good as a properly processed acrylic splint that is made on a stone model. A simple indirect technique that produces good quality splints with minimum chair time can be used. Auxiliaries may be trained to fabricate the splint from an alginate or hydrocolloid impression of the prepared teeth.

Techniques for making acrylic provisional splint.

1. On a preliminary model that has been corrected for missing teeth or irregular occlusal problems, a matrix is made on an Omnivac or similar vacuum former using Omnidental Temporary Splint Material (0.020-clear).

2. When preparation of the teeth is completed, an impression is taken and poured in hard stone.

3. The matrix is placed on the model of the prepared teeth and adapted correctly to the palate or the retromolar pad area. It should cover some areas that can serve as definite stops or stabilizers when pressure is applied later (Fig. 29-9).

4. With the matrix in place, it is reinforced with a mix of fast-setting stone (Healey's Fast Setting Grey Rock is good). "Stop" areas should be covered completely so that the matrix will not be compressed (Fig. 29-10).

5. The model of prepared teeth should be painted with separator.

6. A mix of self-curing acrylic resin should be poured into the reinforced matrix and compressed against the model. It should be tightly wrapped with heavy rubber bands.

7. The model is immediately placed into a water-pressure manometer flask (Parkell) filled with hot water. (A pressure cooker pot may also be used effectively.) The lid is placed on the flask, and it is compressed to at least 4 atmospheres (Fig. 29-11).

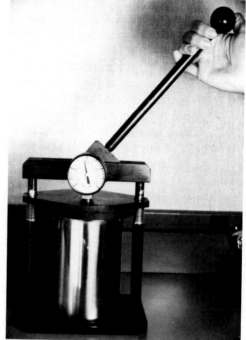

A

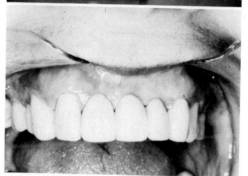

B

Fig. 29-11. A, A water-pressure manometer flask (Parkell). The "flasked" acrylic resin is immediately placed in hot water in the "pot" of the flask, and the lid is placed and closed under pressure. A thick rubber gasket compresses and raises the pressure inside the flask. **B,** Temporary splints processed in this manner cure with no porosity and have a very dense consistency.

8. In 5 to 10 minutes, the model is removed from the flask and the splint is separated from the model. The matrix will peel off easily. Some teeth will probably break off in the splint, but a strong blast of air will usually release them. If not, the stone is divided into two pieces with a round bur and the pieces can then be easily removed.

9. The margins should be trimmed carefully, and additional shaping if necessary is done. Care should be taken not to make interproximal slices too deep because it will weaken the

splint. Any undercuts should be removed, and the inside of the crowns slightly hollowed out to permit a thickness of cement. All external surfaces should be polished.

10. The splint is put into place. Selection of the type of cement will depend on factors of time, tooth preparation, and the like.

If the splint is to be worn for a prolonged period of time or there are long spans that need to be reinforced, cast copings can be fabricated and combined with the preceding technique.

Technique for making acrylic provisional splint with cast copings.

1. A silicone impression of the prepared teeth is made and is poured into one of the strong model or die type of investments. A second model is poured in die stone.

2. Thin copings are waxed directly on the die investment model.

3. The copings are joined together with sprue wax, which will serve as reinforcing rods (Fig. 29-12). They should be placed so that they will not interfere with normal contours.

4. Beads are added to the waxup. They will serve as extra retention for the acrylic resin.

5. The entire waxup is sprued and cast in one piece on the investment model.

6. After pickling and sprue removal, the metal framework is placed on the die stone model.

7. The acrylic provisional splint is then fabricated right over the metal framework in the same manner as it would be done if the metal were not there. The formed Omnidental matrix is placed and then reinforced with stone. The acrylic resin is poured into the matrix, the model is inserted, and pressure is applied. A pressure flask is used to cure the acrylic resin so that it will be dense and nonporous. Margins are trimmed, and the splint is shaped in the usual way.

The procedure is simple, but a warning should be given against making the metal margins too thick. The copings should be kept quite thin to provide room for acrylic resin over the metal. The reinforcing rods should be kept confined within normal contours.

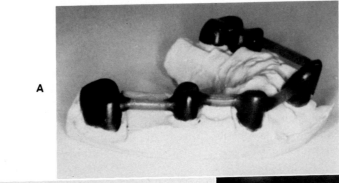

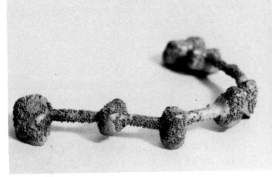

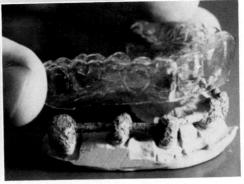

Fig. 29-12. A, Gold reinforced provisional splints can be made rather easily by waxing copings directly on a die investment model and then joining the copings with sprue wax. **B,** The casting made directly on the die investment model. Beads were added to waxup to provide retention for acrylic resin. **C,** A matrix can be adapted to fit directly over the casting, and the acrylic resin can be processed the same as an all-acrylic temporary restoration. After processing, the acrylic is trimmed and polished back to the gold margins. The occlusion is refined either on mounted models or directly in the mouth.

Permanent fixed splinting

Today's dentists have a wide variety of techniques to choose from for permanent fixed splinting. It is no longer necessary to confine all splinting to full-coverage procedures. It is possible to mix techniques so that teeth can be restored in the manner most practical for each individual tooth. This advantage is largely the result of the improvement in techniques of pin retention. The restorative methods that I have found to be most practical for fixed permanent splinting are the following.

Full coverage. Despite its disadvantages, full coverage is still the most practical restoration to use in many splinting situations. It permits recontouring of teeth without loss of esthetics. It can be used to provide protection for sensitive root surfaces. it can be used on severely broken-down teeth, and it can be used to improve appearance while serving as splint abutments.

Parallel pin restorations. Multiple vertical pinholes are drilled parallel to each other in prepared teeth to provide excellent retention for partial coverage restorations. Since the pins provide adequate retention, it is not necessary to wrap the gold around the teeth to retain the restorations. The restorations must still be extended into cleanable areas, and the use of pins does not obviate the need for correct tooth preparation. However, the splinting effect can be achieved with minimal tooth reduction and unobtrusive display of gold (Fig. 29-13).

Although the technique demands extreme preciseness and the use of paralleling devices to assure accuracy, the results are well worth the efforts. Periodontal prosthesis cases that utilized parallel pin retention have been among the most successful long-term splinting results I have seen.

Nonparallel horizontal pin splinting. The nut and bolt retention that is possible with nonparallel horizontal pins (Fig. 29-14) is one of the most reliable techniques for splinting lower anterior teeth. It can be combined with other types of restorations, requires minimal tooth reduction, and is esthetically acceptable.

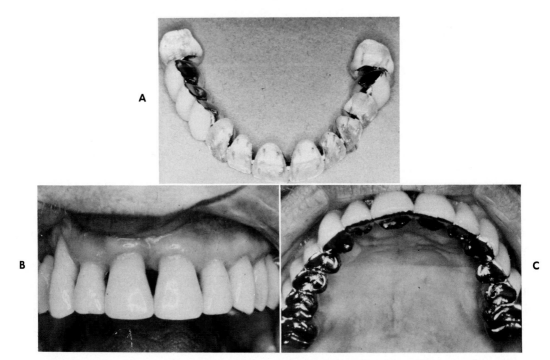

Fig. 29-13. A, Parallel pin retained full arch splint. **B,** Occlusal view of full arch pin splint. **C,** Pin splint in place. There is no gold display, tooth contours are maintained, and labial enamel is preserved. Parallel pin splinting has proved to be an excellent method of stabilizing hypermobile teeth.

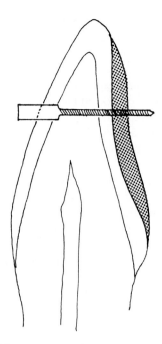

Fig. 29-14. Nonparallel pins (Whaledent) provide nut and bolt retention and minimal tooth preparation. After cementation, both ends of pin are cut flush with the tooth surface. It is one of the best methods that can be used for splinting lower anterior teeth.

It can be used on teeth that would present problems of draw for full-coverage preparations.

Nonparallel vertical pin retention. Teeth that do not require full coverage but that do not lend themselves to parallel pins may be splinted with partial coverage retained by nonparallel threaded pins. The retentive effect of the divergent pins is excellent and the procedure is practical. The same benefits are realized from nonparallel vertical pins as are achieved with parallel pins. However, the laboratory procedures are more complex and placement of the restorations in the mouth is slightly more involved than those for parallel pins.

Splinting with combination fixed-removable restorations

It is often possible to provide an excellent splinting effect for hypermobile teeth while permitting them to serve as abutments for a removable partial denture. Even weak teeth may provide stabilization and retention for the removable appliances, and these appliances in turn provide stabilization for the teeth. To accomplish such reciprocal benefits, there is one cardinal rule that must be followed regarding the partial design: *The removable appliance must be tissue supported simultaneously with tooth support.*

There are several ways to design fixed removable combinations to provide a reciprocal stabilizing effect. Perhaps the method that has been in use the longest is to utilize parallel-walled precision attachments in which the male attachment is fitted into the female slot. This permits the partial denture to rest on soft tissue with simultaneous support from the abutment teeth, even when biting pressure is applied. In fact, the more pressure that is exerted on the removable part, the more firmly it is stabilized by the ridges or the palate. This stability benefits the abutment teeth, which are held in position by the parallel walls of the precision attachment. The application of this principle of design is almost unlimited.

Combination tooth- and tissue-borne removable partial dentures can be designed in a variety of ways to provide reciprocal stabilization for abutment teeth. One of the most dependable combination designs is the *bar partial restoration.* The use of parallel-walled bars attached to restorations on the natural teeth can provide unsurpassed lateral stability. The bar partial denture is held in such perfect opposition to its tissue support that any biting pressure on it is always resisted by an optimum combination of support from the teeth and the ridges or palate. The abutment teeth are held in place by the partial denture during function, thereby minimizing destructive lateral forces even on weak abutment teeth (Fig. 29-15).

My earlier thinking on the use of stress-breaker partials has had to change. I originally followed the popular concept of tissue-supported partials that were stabilized and retained by the abutment teeth but not supported by the teeth. It was believed that if parallel-walled precision attachments were used the male attachment should be shortened so that the slots of the attachments would stabilize but not support the partial. The belief was that the tissue support would prevent any vertical loading on the teeth.

The concept was erroneous because in virtually every instance the teeth would simply erupt until the attachment settled to the bottom of the slot. This left a slight step in the occlusal surfaces where the removable part met

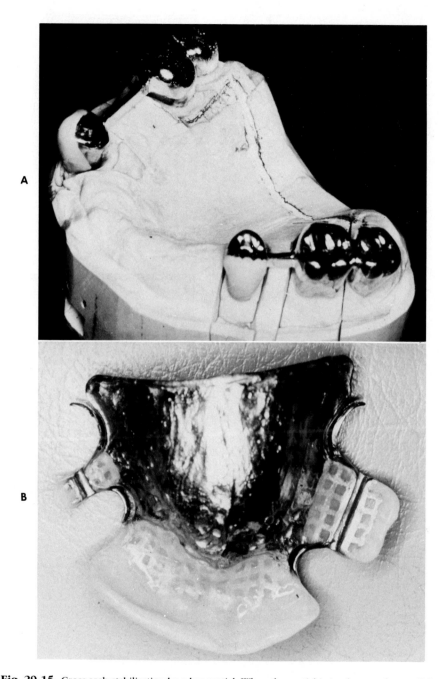

Fig. 29-15. Cross-arch stabilization by a bar partial. When the partial is in place on the parallel-walled bars of the fixed bridge segments, the abutment teeth are prevented from making any lateral movements. The fit of the partial base against the resistive bony palate stabilizes the base during occlusal loading. It in turn stabilizes the abutment teeth while the teeth reciprocally stabilize and retain the partial.

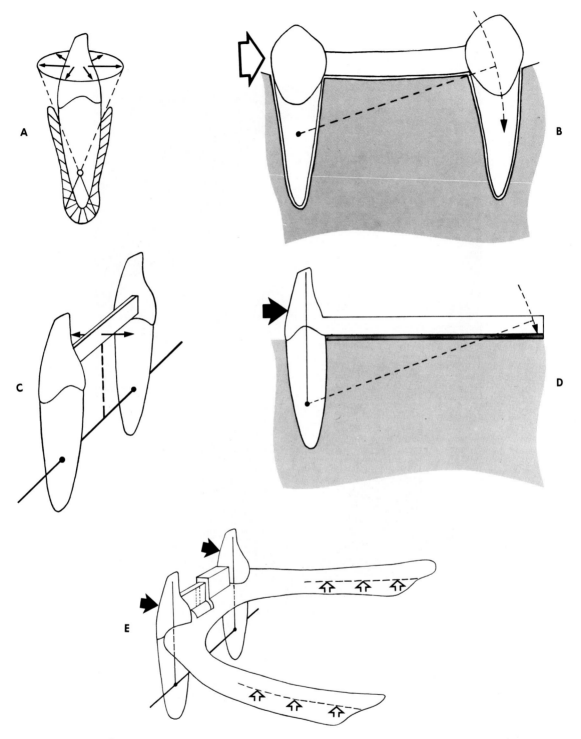

Fig. 29-16. The splinting principle applied to removable appliances. The effect of any parallel-walled attachment is to broaden the base. This has the effect of preventing tooth rotation or lateral movement *if the base fits properly.* This illustration shows the effect achieved with a bar partial, but the effect is identical with any type of parallel-walled precision attachment, guiding plane, or deep-seated rest. **A,** Potential for horizontal movement of a single tooth is in any direction around a rotational point in the root. **B,** Rigid splinting has a redirectional effect that results in near-axial loading. This shows the effect on the fixed segment for a bar partial with a laterally directed stress. **C,** The same segment can be rocked in an anteroposterior direction. **D,** Extension of saddle distally that is fully supported by tissues now resists horizontal pressure. **E,** The effect of a rigidly attached bar partial is to prevent horizontal rocking of the abutment segment. The same effect occurs with properly designed precision attachment partials.

the fixed abutment, but as soon as the abutment teeth and the removable partial were stabilized vertically, stability of both the abutment teeth and the partial were enhanced.

To get the stabilizing effect of fixed removable combinations, the partial should be rigidly attached to the abutment teeth both vertically and horizontally. The saddle areas should fit the tissue with accurate adaptation. This has the effect of one large fixed unit. Because of the broadened base and rigid attachment, lateral movement of the abutments is prevented by the fit of the denture base against the ridge. Even loose teeth with minimal support can often be stabilized by a properly fitted base while serving as a partial abutment (Fig. 29-16).

To accomplish the combination of lateral stabilization, vertical support, and retention in a very small but strong attachment, the precision attachment of choice in my practice is the D2.7 and its more recent modification the D.3 (Fig. 29-17) (Dawson attachment). The reason for these designs is specifically to take advantage of the principles of splinting described in this chapter. By providing the lateral stabilization of parallel walls, the width of the "base" is effectively extended from the abutment teeth to the full dimension of the partial denture base. This has the effect of redirecting almost all forces on the teeth to nearly parallel with their long axes as long as the saddle areas are fitted properly on the ridge and are completely

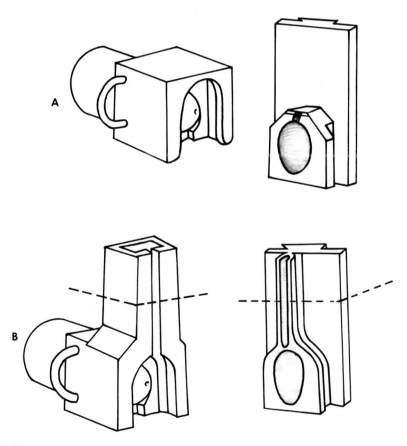

Fig. 29-17. Dawson attachments: The D2.7 attachment, **A,** is designed to provide lateral stabilization, retention, and support in a vertical dimension of only 2.7 mm. The male attachment is attached to the abutment tooth so that less tooth reduction is needed to accommodate it. It is thin enough to eliminate any food trapping under its dimension, and this thinness greatly increases its resistance to fracture. The female portion is attached to the removable partial so that it is replaceable if needed. A spring-loaded plunger engages a dimple for retention. The plunger and spring are both replaceable. The D.3 attachment, **B,** provides a longer male stabilization rod, but it can be shortened as needed. It can also be completely covered over if desired.

seated when the attachment is in place. Teeth that are rigidly attached with parallel-walled attachments are prevented from rocking or moving in any lateral direction while the denture base is seated. Compression of the partial denture base by occlusal forces should actually stabilize the base even more solidly against the ridge, at which point lateral movement of abutment teeth is prevented during periods of greatest force. This stabilization effect can be gained with any parallel-walled attachment or deep-seated rest as long as the saddles are seated completely on the tissues simultaneously with complete, passive alignment of the attachments with the abutment teeth.

Full-coverage splinting of divergent teeth

Teeth that must be splinted using full-coverage abutments do not always permit a line of draw for multiple restorations. To provide enough parallelism of the preparations, it would be necessary to devitalize some teeth unless alternative solutions can be found. There are two good alternatives and usually one or the other is practical for almost all cases:

1. The use of copings to align divergent crown preparations
2. The use of precision slots or interlocks to permit the joining together of divergent segments

Of the two solutions, I much prefer the use of interlocks. Full arch splinting can be effected with multiple segments locked together in the mouth. Interlocks facilitate the repair of a segment without destroying an entire splint, and they permit the preparation of teeth without excessive reduction.

Copings usually require extra reduction of tooth structure to prevent excessive bulk of the finished restoration. It is extremely difficult to provide esthetic contours, especially at the gingival margins, when the added thickness of the coping is present.

Copings do serve a purpose when splinting is required on terminal type of periodontal prostheses. Some patients, because of poor body metabolism and excessive loss of periodontal support, cannot be provided with a

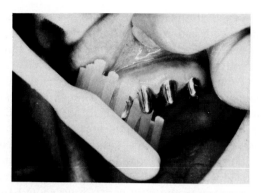

Fig. 29-18. Copings can be used on periodontally involved teeth to simplify cleaning procedures when such teeth must be used as splint abutments. As a *routine* procedure for splinting, however, copings have more disadvantages than advantages. Their use should be reserved for the special, severely involved problem cases that can benefit from easy removal of the splint.

predictably successful result. Such patients can often prolong the maintenance of their natural teeth if they are provided with access for exceptional cleanability. Making the splint fit so that it is removable by the patient facilitates easier maintainability by the patient (Fig. 29-18) and provides a simpler method of making changes in the restorations if there is a further loss of teeth.

The use of copings on vital teeth *as a routine procedure* has little merit. It should be reserved for patients who can derive definite benefits from the added expense, greater tooth reduction, and associated problems of bulky contours and less than ideal esthetics. Fortunately, the need for such procedures is unusual.

Rigid versus nonrigid splinting

Over the years, the controversy of whether splinted teeth should be joined together with rigid or nonrigid joints has been discussed pro and con. There seems to be a feeling by some that the teeth should be allowed to move and "roll with the punches." Such arguments certainly seem to have no validity from either a practical or a clinical standpoint.

The purpose of splinting is to stabilize the teeth against lateral movement. Healthy teeth in good occlusion do not move noticeably in function, and I have never seen a tooth that was harmed by being stable. Clinical experience with hundreds of patients has not turned up any evidence that I can interpret as contraindicating rigid contacts for stabilizing hypermobile teeth.

The use of nonrigid connectors imposes a considerable amount of additional complexity in both laboratory and chair procedures. It greatly increases the cost, and makes it more difficult to fabricate smooth, cleanable, interproximal contours.

Lower full arch splints are subjected to potential stresses as the mandible flexes. For this reason distal abutments should be prepared for the best retention possible. If full arch splinting is not necessary on the lower arch, it is good insurance to restore in segments if multiple restorations are needed. If full arch splinting is required, it can be provided as long as the teeth are prepared with good retentive form. Many long-term clinical results have attested to this.

SUMMARY

Splinting is contraindicated unless it is necessary for the comfortable maintainability of the teeth. Hypermobility in itself is not an indication for splinting. The response to occlusal correction should be noted before any decision is made to splint hypermobile teeth. If teeth can function comfortably and the occlusal relationship can be maintained without splinting, there is no advantage to be gained by joining teeth together. The difficulty of cleaning splinted teeth is reason enough to splint only when it is needed.

Clinical judgment may supersede the preceding comments because of the multiplicity of factors such as root contour, crown-root ratios, bone density, occlusal relationship, and the need for extensive restorative procedures. Splinting may be used as insurance against future problems if the risk of not splinting is determined to be high. However, such a decision should be made only after thorough evaluation of all the factors. It should never be a routine decision.

30

Solving occlusal wear problems

All occlusions wear to some degree. The parabolic contours of the cusps were designed to permit the maximum amount of wear without penetrating into dentin. Even the proximal contact surfaces of teeth wear as the result of rubbing against each other during function. So physiologic wear results in both shortening the vertical length of the teeth and narrowing the horizontal width of the teeth. If the masticatory system is kept in equilibrium, the occlusal wear compensates for the normal proximal wear and the minimal loss of enamel will be of little concern. In a balanced masticatory system with a normal diet, the dentition can stay intact for a long lifetime. The teeth should outlast the body.

To understand problems of occlusal wear, one must understand how the adaptive process compensates for wear. Built into the design of the system, there are two adaptive processes for maintaining the following:

1. Vertical dimension of occlusion
2. Tight proximal contacts

The vertical dimension of occlusion is maintained even when rapid abrasive wear occurs. As the occlusal surfaces of the teeth wear, the dentoalveolar process elongates by progressive remodeling of the alveolar bone. The increase in vertical length of the alveolar process matches the loss of occlusal height, and so the vertical dimension of lower facial height is maintained at a constant dimension throughout adult life unless the teeth are lost.

The horizontal dimension of length around the arch is shortened by several millimeters during life. The proximal wear is compensated by a constant forward pressure that keeps the contacts close together. Not unlike the vertical stabilizing factors, it is part of the adaptive process for maintaining the equilibrium of the parts of the masticatory system.

These adaptive processes continue to function throughout life. They are beneficial if all parts of the system are correctly interrelated. They may contribute to the destruction of the dentition if the interrelating parts get too far out of functional harmony.

Because elongation of alveolar bone matches the amount of occlusal wear, restoration of severely worn teeth is not simply a matter of restoring lost tooth structure. To do such restoration results in an increase of vertical dimension that may in some patients actually intensify the problem. Analysis of a severe wear problem should take into consideration how normal muscle function would move the mandible if there were no barriers from interfering teeth, either vertically or horizontally. In other words, an analysis should be made of mandibular function to determine how and why any part of the dentition is in interference with any jaw movement. The treatment plan should

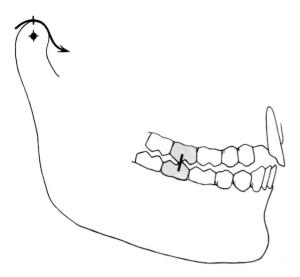 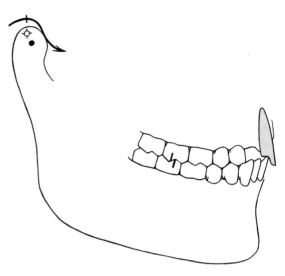

Fig. 30-1. Facets of wear that correspond to the first contact in centric relation can almost always be found. The wear may be severe, or it may just serve as an incline that causes the mandible to shift forward.

Fig. 30-2. If the mandible shifts forward into an opposing incline, the end point of the slide may wear more severely than the site of the interference. This is a common cause of severe anterior wear.

then be directed toward alteration of the dentition so that it is in complete conformity, with no interference to any functional jaw position or excursive movement. Very often the wear patterns themselves are the key to determining the functional pathways of the mandible.

In analyzing any dentition, we should make a distinction between physiologic wear and excessive wear.

Physiologic wear is normal. It results in progressive but very slow loss of convexity on the cusps, accompanied by flattening of cusp tips on the posterior teeth and loss of mamelons on the anterior teeth. Some facets of wear may be found, but they should be minimal in length and depth. Physiologic wear must be evaluated according to age, habit patterns, and history of the wear. It should not result in premature deterioration of the dentition to the extent that it would require correction.

Excessive wear refers to any level of occlusal wear that can be expected to require corrective intervention in order to preserve the dentition. Excessive wear results in unacceptable damage to the occluding surfaces, and it may destroy anterior tooth structure that is necessary for acceptable anterior guidance function or for esthetics.

Excessive abrasive wear is diagnostic. It is dependably related to tooth surfaces that are in direct interference with the functional or

parafunctional movements of the mandible. Tooth structure that is not in the way of jaw movements will not be worn excessively.

Excessive wear can be stimulated either at the site of a direct interference to jaw movement (Fig. 30-1) or at the end point of a slide. Severe anterior wear is often the result of a posterior interference that displaces the mandible forward into a pressured contact of the lower anterior teeth against the upper lingual inclines (Fig. 30-2). Lateral displacement of the mandible may also result in stressful contact against posterior tooth inclines at the end of a slide. The wear problem on the inclines that stop the slide is often more severe than the wear on the inclines that cause the displacement. This will be particularly so if the displacement forces lower teeth into a wedging contact with steep upper inclines.

TREATMENT PLANNING FOR WEAR PROBLEMS

Treatment for any excessive wear problem should be designed to accomplish six things:

1. Equal-intensity contacts on all teeth in a verifiable centric relation.
2. An anterior guidance that is in harmony with the patient's normal functional jaw movements.
3. Immediate disclusion of all posterior contacts the moment the mandible

moves in any direction from centric relation.

4. Restoration of any tooth surfaces that have problem wear through the enamel.
5. Counseling, so that the patient understands that normal jaw posture keeps the teeth apart except during swallowing. ADVICE: "Lips together, teeth apart."
6. Nighttime occlusal splint if habitual nocturnal bruxism persists after occlusal correction.

Determining what treatment is necessary to correct an occlusal wear problem depends directly on what changes are necessary in the dentition to make it conform to the first four goals.

Relating the combination of anterior guidance and condylar guidance to occlusal wear

Because successful reduction of most wear problems requires the separation of all posterior teeth in all jaw positions except centric relation, the analysis of any severe wear problem must focus on how that goal can be achieved best. Thus *both* the anterior guidance and the condylar guidance must be analyzed because posterior disclusion depends on a combination of anterior guidance and condylar guidance, and it is very common to find that either or both guidances have been severely flattened whenever extensive occlusal wear has occurred.

If the anterior guidance is worn flat, the downward path of the condyles must be relied on for separating the posterior teeth in excursions. If the normal convexity of the eminentiae is intact, the condyles *must* travel down when the jaw moves forward, and so posterior disclusion can be worked out even with a flat anterior guidance. But if the condylar guidance has been flattened also, that disclusive effect is not available.

Observation of posterior wear patterns will indicate whether flattening of the eminentiae has occurred because such flattening does not occur without simultaneous wear of the upper lingual cusps. On the other hand, flattening of upper lingual cusps cannot occur with normal condylar paths because lower posterior teeth can move neither forward nor toward the midline without moving downwardly unless the eminence is flattened. This is so even with a zero-degree anterior guidance.

If *only* the anterior teeth are worn flat, it is an indication that acceptable posterior disclusion can be achieved without the anterior guidance being steepened.

If both the anterior and the posterior teeth are worn flat, it is a probable indication that posterior disclusion must be accomplished by steepening of the anterior guidance.

The exception to the above rules may occur when there is a severe curve to the occlusal plane so that the plane slants up in back making it nearly parallel with an undamaged condylar path. When the occlusal plane at the molars parallels the condylar path (Fig. 30-3), the posterior teeth may be worn flat, but that problem can usually be corrected when the occlusal plane is lowered in back without the anterior guidance being steepened.

It is always advantageous to work out the disclusion of the posterior teeth without steepening the anterior guidance if it is possible to accomplish it, because steepening the anterior guidance restricts the existing envelope of function and triggers further parafunctional bruxing. It is my consistent observation that when a patient with a horizontal envelope of function is forced to function more vertically, there is routinely an attempt to regain the more horizontal function by wearing away the steeper anterior inclines, or by loosening the anterior teeth, or by moving them out of the way. The instability of a steepened anterior guidance often goes unnoticed because it does not generally cause any discomfort to the patient.

Regardless of whether a steepened anterior guidance may cause increased wear of the anterior teeth, it may still be the only option for posterior disclusion if the condylar path has been flattened.

The analysis of the condylar path is critically important in severe occlusal wear problems for two reasons.

1. To determine how much help can be expected from the condylar path for discluding the posterior teeth.
2. To determine whether the condylar path will be stable after occlusal correction.

Because the health and alignment of the condyle-disk relationship is so critical to the long-term prognosis for occlusal wear treatment, an analysis of severe occlusal wear should include a determination of whether the disk is intact and aligned during function. Dis-

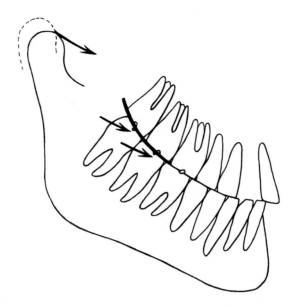

Fig. 30-3. If the occlusal plane at the posterior segment of the occlusion is steeper than the condylar path, it is possible to wear upper teeth (including the lingual cusps) flat.

placement of the disk eventually leads to loss of condylar height by flattening of the condyle and eminence. This, in turn, perpetuates the occlusal wear problem by repetitively recreating an interference with the most posterior teeth on the side of the displacement, which in turn causes muscle incoordination and elevator muscle hyperactivity. For this reason, patients with irreducible disk derangements must expect a continuing need for repeated occlusal corrections, done periodiocally to compensate for the continuing loss of condylar height from progressive breakdown of the articular surfaces.

It appears that the wear problem from a displaced disk can be minimized for both the damaged joint and the occlusal surfaces when a perfected occlusion is provided. Maintaining that perfected occlusion should especially be considered an important follow-up step whenever synovial fluid flow to the articular surfaces is disrupted by a displaced disk. The wear problem is generally manageable but may require replacement of restorations in less time than normal wear would require.

Analysis of the condylar path can be accomplished in the following ways:

1. *Clinical observation.* If the anterior guidance can disclude the posterior teeth in protrusive excursions, there is not a condylar path problem. If the anterior guidance *cannot* disclude the posterior teeth, further analysis of the condy-

lar path should be made by one or more of the following methods.
2. *Protrusive checkbite* at the incisal edge-to-edge position, for setting the condylar path so that its effect can be analyzed on semiadjustable instrumentation.
3. *Pantographic, axiographic, or stereographic recording* of the condylar path for precise analysis. (All methods are described in Chapter 12.)

Analysis of the occlusal plane can be more critical when the condylar path is known. Even a severely flattened condylar path will most often have some angulation downward. As long as the occlusal plane at the molars is flatter than the condylar path, it can be discluded, even by a zero-degree anterior guidance.

Analysis of the occlusal plane is critical when severe posterior wear is being evaluated. There are two ways to increase the eccentric separation of the posterior teeth by alteration of the occlusal plane:

1. By flattening a curved occlusal plane
2. By lowering the occlusal plane in back

Either of the above procedures can increase posterior disclusion without requiring an increase in anterior guidance steepness as long as the posterior half of the occlusal plane is flatter than the condylar path and fossa-wall angulation is flatter than the anterior guidance.

Analysis of the anterior guidance must relate to the existing paths of function *after* wear has occurred. Even though functional movements were originally more vertical, they become more and more horizontal as the teeth are abraded. Once a more horizontal envelope of function has been developed, the flattened anterior guidance cannot be steepened without the probability of triggering more wear against the anterior teeth. Thus a tobacco chewer who has worn the occlusion flat will attempt to regain the flattened pathways if they are restricted by a steepened anterior guidance.

Some parafunctional wear against anterior teeth can be corrected without triggering a recurrence of the wear. If the anterior wear occurred primarily as a result of posterior interferences that are still present, the anterior surfaces can often be restored with a good prognosis after the posterior interferences are eliminated.

Analysis of a worn anterior guidance cannot be made accurately until all posterior interferences have been eliminated. This is best done on mounted diagnostic casts. After the casts have been equilibrated, a diagnostic waxup of the anterior teeth should be done. The waxup should recontour the anterior teeth to the flattest possible guidance consistent with maintaining correct incisal edge position. The first analysis should be at the most closed vertical dimension. Four primary questions should be answered by the diagnostic waxup of the equilibrated casts in the following order:

1. Can the lower incisal edges be correctly contoured?
2. Can a definite holding stop be provided for each lower incisal edge against its upper lingual surface?
3. Can the upper incisal edges be corrected or maintained without interference to the existing neutral zone or lip-closure path?
4. Can an anterior guidance be worked out between the established centric stops and the upper incisal edges?

The above questions should be analyzed first at the most closed vertical of the equilibrated casts. If the anterior relationships can be worked out without increasing vertical dimension, that is ideal. If vertical must be increased to accomplish an acceptable anterior relationship, it should be increased only as much as necessary. A goal of treatment is to reduce requirements for adaptation to the minimum, and this is done best by maintenance of the existing vertical.

The next step in analysis is to determine the effect of the waxed-up anterior teeth on posterior disclusion. The key questions to resolve are as follows:

1. Can the anterior guidance (as waxed) disclude all posterior teeth in all excursions?
2. If the anterior guidance cannot disclude the posterior teeth, can the problem be resolved by changes in the posterior segments?

Failure to answer the above questions early in the diagnostic analysis is probably the major cause of failure in the treatment of wear problems. Disclusion of the posterior teeth in all excursions is an essential element of successful treatment. It must be thought out in advance because if steepening the anterior guidance is the only way to provide posterior disclusion it must be accomplished as the first restorative priority.

Testing the treatment plan with provisional restorations

After an acceptable anterior relationship has been waxed up, it still must be refined in the mouth. The waxup should be duplicated in stone and a matrix made for construction of the provisional restorations in acrylic resin after the teeth are prepared.

When anterior wear is severe, it is best to complete all refinements before either segment is cemented. Upper and lower provisional restorations are usually placed, and all adjustments are made before the lower segment is copied. The lower anterior restorations should be completed in final form, but they should not be cemented until all function excursions have been verified against the upper temporary restorations. The anterior guidance should be checked carefully at this stage to make certain that posterior disclusion is effective and that the upper contours conform with the lip-closure path and phonetic requirements. At that point the lower permanent restorations can be cemented, and the upper anterior restorations can be finalized. Care should be taken in the laboratory to duplicate incisal edge positions and guidance contours that were worked out on the provisional restorations (Fig. 30-4).

If splinting is not required, it may be practical to complete the upper and lower anterior restorations before the posterior teeth are prepared. The posterior teeth will, of course, have to be equilibrated as part of the preliminary mouth preparation before finalization of the anterior guidance either in the provisionals or in the permanent restorations.

If the posterior teeth are prepared at the same time as the anteriors, the provisional restorations can be made for the full arch. The anterior guidance can still be worked out in the normal manner, and the posterior teeth can still be adjusted so that they are discluded by the anterior guidance on the temporary resto-

rations. The entire occlusal scheme can thus be worked out provisionally in this manner before any final restorations are fabricated. It then becomes a matter of reproducing all the guidelines that were determined in the mouth. This can be done in the laboratory with precise accuracy if all the guidelines are communicated.

If the provisional restorations are full arch splints, the posterior segments can be sectioned through the distal canine contact and

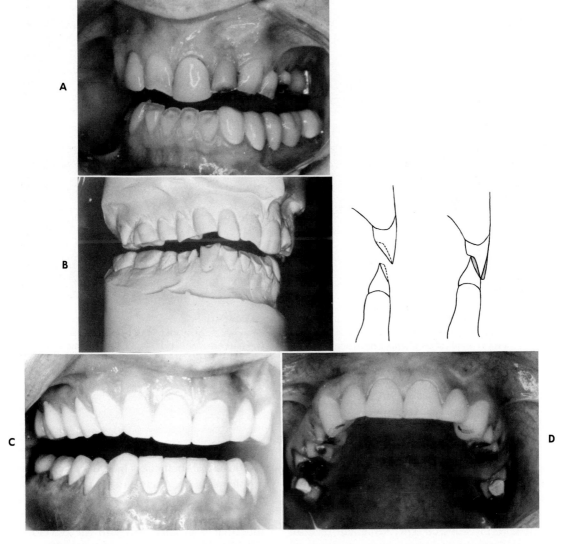

Fig. 30-4. A, Severe wear. **B,** Casts mounted in centric relation are corrected by restoration of lower incisal edges and reshaping of upper lingual contours. Labial surfaces of upper anterior teeth will need to be thickened to provide acceptable incisal edge contour. Diagnostic waxup is then duplicated and is used to fabricate matrixes for provisional splints. **C,** Lower restorations are completed according to plan (see Chapter 17). Upper provisional restorations are then refined against the lower teeth. **D,** Posterior segments of the upper provisional splint are removed. A centric bite record is made for mounting cast of provisionals and the die model.   *Continued.*

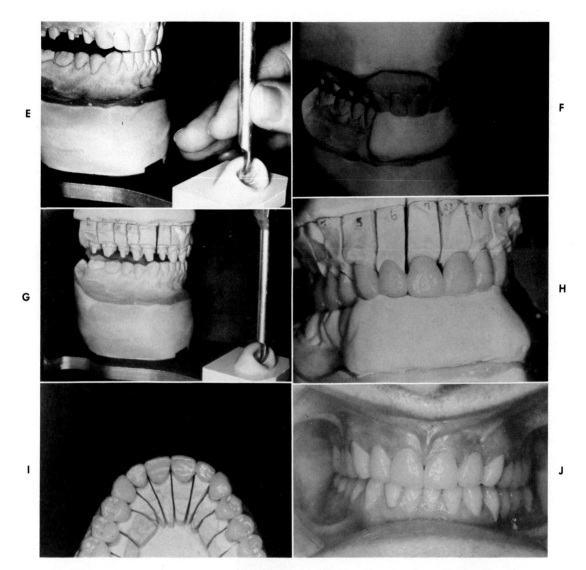

Fig. 30-4, cont'd. **E,** Customized anterior guidance is fabricated by use of cast of the corrected anterior provisional restorations. Notice how pin stops at incisal edge alignment. **F,** Index is made for precise duplication of upper provisional restorations. **G,** Master die model is mounted with same centric bite record that was used to mount provisional restorations. Thus it relates perfectly to the custom anterior guide. **H,** Checking incisal edge position against the index shows up a lab error in contouring left side of incisal edges. Error was corrected. **I,** Notice definite stops for lower incisal contact. **J,** Completed restorations.

removed. An impression of the anterior segment in place can then be made. A centric relation bite record can be made on the posterior teeth at the correct vertical dimension with anterior contact. This same bite record can be used to articulate both the master die model and the cast of the anterior provisionals in place. From these two articulated casts, the customized anterior guide table can be fabricated as well as an index for incisal edge position.

The secret to success in solving severe wear problems is definitely keyed to working out the correct anterior guidance. If posterior disclusion can be achieved with an anterior guidance that is in harmony with the envelope of function, the prognosis will be excellent.

If the anterior guidance must restrict the envelope of function in order to disclude the posterior teeth, the result will still be acceptable and patient comfort can be good, but a

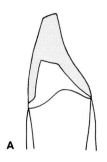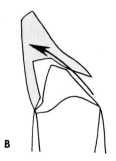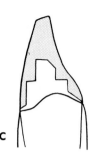

Fig. 30-5. Preparation for retention on short teeth is often inadequate because it provides no resistance to rotation off the prepared tooth, **A** and **B**. Retention can be increased greatly by preparing in steps so that opposing walls are nearly parallel, **C**. This prevents the restoration from being rocked off.

varying degree of progressive wear can be expected on the anterior teeth. A nighttime occlusal splint can be used to reduce wear from nocturnal bruxing.

If it is necessary to steepen the anterior guidance, the posterior teeth should be monitored periodically for any signs of excursive interferences as the anterior guidance is flattened by recurrent wear. The same monitoring is especially important if an irreducible disk derangement is present because of potential loss of condyle height.

Restoring severely worn posterior teeth

Restoration of the posterior occlusion is dependent on determination of the correct anterior guidance first. In the analysis of various types of occlusal wear, the focus should be directed first to the anterior teeth. The posterior teeth must be fitted in between the anterior guidance and the condylar guidance, but they must not interfere with either. Thus the establishment of stable holding contacts is the primary goal of the posterior occlusion.

With long-term wear, the posterior teeth are sometimes abraded nearly to the gum line. There are generally four choices for treatment of such severely worn teeth:

1. *Pin-retained all-gold restorations.* The use of parallel pin retention permits restorations of the exposed dentin without significant increase in vertical dimension. This is not always esthetically acceptable in the anterior segments.

2. *Increase the vertical dimension.* An increase in the vertical dimension may improve the esthetic result but in some patients can lead to excessive stress. Although increasing the vertical may be

the best choice for some patients, it is contraindicated if the alveolar bone is sclerotic and the masticatory muscles are hypertrophied.

3. *Crown-lengthening procedures.* It may be necessary to surgically expose enough tooth structure to provide retention and esthetic contouring.

4. *Pulp extirpation and endodontic post and coping construction.* This choice can provide retentive form when needed. It may also require an increase in vertical dimension. Pulp extirpation may also be combined with crown lengthening to provide improved esthetics and retention without increasing the vertical dimension.

Retentive preparation for severely worn teeth

It is often possible to restore shortened teeth with suprisingly good esthetic results, especially if the lip line covers the cemento-enamel junction. Retention is jeopardized whenever the restoration can rotate off a tooth. Preparing with opposing, near-parallel walls prevents rotation and provides maximum retention (Fig. 30-5).

When should occlusal wear be restored?

All occlusal wear does not need to be restored. Even penetration into dentin may not need treatment. If the cause of the wear can be eliminated through equilibration so that worn surfaces are no longer subjected to parafunctional contact, exposed dentin may remain intact for years. Whether the worn surfaces should be restored depends on the answers to the following questions:

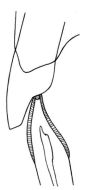

Fig. 30-6. If cupped incisal edges are recontoured with resin bonded to the enamel ring, the resin prevents wear on the dentin but is not subject to occlusal wear because most of the function occurs against the enamel contact. Dentin bonding agents have made this procedure even more practical.

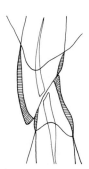

Fig. 30-7. When severe wear occurs on both contacting surfaces, correction sometimes requires a choice of either devitalizing the teeth or increasing the vertical.

1. *Will treatment be complicated by delay in restoring the wear?* Often the same type of restoration would be possible without compromise even if more wear occurs. In such cases there is no need to rush treatment, especially if there is a chance the wear problem has been corrected by the improved occlusion.
2. *Is restoration necessary to control sensitivity?* Exposure of dentin produces different responses in different patients.
3. *Is restoration required to satisfy esthetic desires?* Worn teeth can be unsightly. Matching restorations to look like adjacent worn teeth severely limits the esthetic result that could be achieved. The patient should always be informed of the options.
4. *Is it relatively certain that restorations will eventually be required?* If so, the patient should be fully informed about the probable time frame, and the condition should be monitored on a regular basis if the patient elects to delay.

Conservative correction of incisal wear

When incisal wear penetrates through the enamel, the softer dentin begins to cup, leaving an elevated ring of unsupported enamel rods. This leads to chipping away of the enamel and makes the incisal edges unsightly and rough.

A preventive measure that seems to help considerably in stabilizing the incisal edges while improving the appearance is to bond composite resin into the cupped-out dentin area. If the resin is bonded to the ring of acid-etched enamel, it replaces the dentin bond and prevents the destruction of loose enamel rods.

Dentin bonding agents have further enhanced this procedure, and more wear-resistant resins have also helped though the incisal edges do not function on the composite resin except in end-to-end relationships. Instead, most functional contact occurs against the enamel ring (Fig. 30-6). As long as this procedure is performed before the enamel ring has been destroyed, the prognosis is good enough to make the procedure recommended over the unnecessary use of full coverage.

TYPES OF ANTERIOR WEAR PROBLEMS
Severe wear on labial of lower teeth and lingual of upper teeth

If the contacting surface enamel is worn severely on both the upper and lower anterior teeth, there is sometimes no room to restore the surfaces back without either invading the pulp or increasing the vertical dimension (Fig. 30-7).

This type of problem is usually treated by opening the vertical. As the mandible swings open, the lower anteriors arc away from the worn surface contact (Fig. 30-8) providing room for restorative materials that are necessary regardless of the treatment selected.

Treating the problem in this manner generally has a good prognosis if the increased vertical is kept to a minimum and stable holding contacts are provided for the anterior teeth.

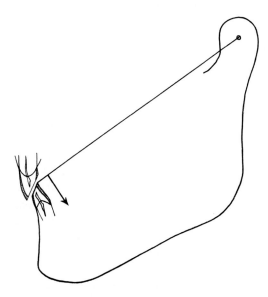

Fig. 30-8. Increasing the vertical on an anterior wear problem does two things: it opens space vertically, and it opens space horizontally because of the opening arc around the condylar axis. This provides room to restore worn surfaces on the labial of the lower or the lingual of the upper incisors.

Care must be taken to reinforce the incisal edges with sufficient thickness to prevent fracturing thin unsupported porcelain. There is generally no problem working out the anterior guidance because in this type of wear the envelope of function is quite steep.

All details of the anterior relationship should be refined in provisional restorations, which are then copied in the laboratory. Care should be taken to avoid interference with a tightly restricted neutral zone and lip-closure path, which usually are present with this type of wear.

All interferences to centric relation should be removed before any details of the anterior relationship are worked out.

Severe labial wear of lower incisors

When lower incisors wear severely on their labioincisal surfaces, it is usually a sign of improperly contoured upper lingual restorations (Fig. 30-9).

It is a classic example of interference to the envelope of function that generally requires a concave upper lingual contour for noninterference. The thick bulbous lingual contours that are so prevalent in upper anterior restorations must be altered if the problem is to be treated successfully.

Sometimes the restorations can be reshaped to provide a stable stop on the cingulum and a

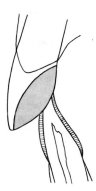

Fig. 30-9. One of the most common wear problems results from improper contouring of upper lingual surfaces. Bulbous, convex contours invariably lead to excessive wear of the lower incisors and instability of the anterior segments. Convex contours usually fail to provide a stable holding contact and also interfere with normal functional jaw movements.

corrected path from the centric stop to the incisal edge. Even if this requires remaking the upper restorations, it should be recommended or restoration of the lower worn surfaces will fail. Wear will continue to be a problem as long as tooth structure interferes with functional jaw pathways.

After reshaping the upper lingual surfaces, the lower incisal and labial contours should be perfected in provisional restorations and then copied in the laboratory.

Severe lingual wear on upper anterior teeth

Excessive wear on upper lingual inclines is most often the result of posterior inclines that deflect the mandible forward. The lower incisal edges are driven forward into the upper lingual surfaces where bruxing patterns may wear the surfaces nearly to the pulp (Fig. 30-10, *A*). If we observe the relationship in centric occlusion, it will appear impossible to restore lost tooth structure without opening the bite. If the mandible is manipulated into centric relation, however, we will find it is often posterior to the acquired worn position.

Elimination of centric relation interferences by selective grinding so that the mandible can fully close without forward deflection will often provide room between the lower incisal edges and the upper lingual inclines without increasing the vertical (Fig. 30-10, *B*).

Severe anterior wear that results in an end-to-end relationship

Badly worn teeth that have drifted into an end-to-end relationship present a real restorative challenge. It is difficult to lengthen the appearance of the upper teeth without severely steepening the anterior guidance. A compromise that permits the lower incisal edges to move forward on a fairly flat guidance and then progress into a steeper incline as gradually as possible by way of a concave pathway is usually called for (Fig. 30-11).

To make the concave contour possible, it is usually necessary to restore the worn lower teeth with full coverage, to narrow the broad incisal edges from the labial, and to position the incisal edge lingually. By moving the incisal edges lingually, we can lengthen the lower incisors to provide some overjet for the upper teeth. With sufficient overjet, the upper incisors can then curve down from the cingulum centric stop, providing more length for the upper anterior teeth. Both esthetics and function are improved by such a procedure.

It should be remembered that even though the esthetics and function are improved by the above process the envelope of function will still be restricted from its flattened pathways. It will usually be necessary to either splint the upper restorations or provide a nighttime retainer to prevent movement. The nighttime

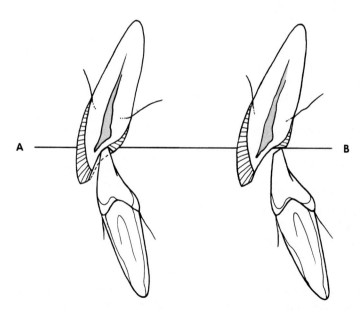

Fig. 30-10. Extreme lingual wear is often the result of posterior deviating interferences that deflect the jaw forward. If the relationship of the teeth is observed in the acquired centric occlusion, **A**, it would appear impossible to restore the worn lingual surfaces without opening the bite. If posterior interferences to a centric relation closure are eliminated, the jaw is often able to close to the original vertical dimension on a more distal arc of closure, **B**. There is then sufficient room to restore the lingual surfaces without increasing the vertical dimension.

retainer can include full occlusal coverage to reduce wear on the steepened anterior inclines.

Uneven wear

Anterior wear is not always equal on both arches. Severe wear may be found on upper teeth with minimal wear on the lower ones. When the enamel is penetrated on one arch, the softer dentin may wear rapidly permitting the teeth with harder enamel surfaces to erupt up into the more rapidly wearing teeth. Such uneven wear patterns can create very difficult occlusal plane problems (Fig. 30-12).

When the upper teeth wear rapidly, the lower anterior segment erupts up to form a severe reverse smile line that is very unattractive (Fig. 30-13). Correction is difficult because the eruption of the lower teeth occurs by elongation of the alveolar bone sometimes making the soft-tissue juncture of the lower teeth too high to correct by restorative procedures alone.

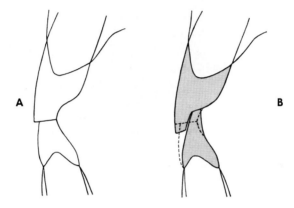

Fig. 30-11. As the anterior teeth wear, the lower teeth migrate forward, eventually wearing to an end-to-end relationship, **A.** They can be restored to more esthetic contour without increasing the vertical by thinning the lower incisal edge back and lengthening it if needed, **B.** The upper incisors can be shortened at the lingual and lengthened at the incisal. This process does restrict a flat anterior guidance and may result in some added horizontal stress to the anterior teeth.

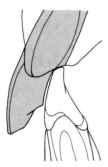

Fig. 30-12. If the lower teeth erupt up far enough into the worn root surfaces of the upper incisors, the lower segment is too high to correct restoratively. The lower incisal plane, being so high, distorts the normal appearance.

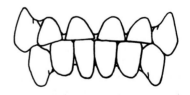

Fig. 30-13. Lower incisors erupt up with their alveolar process when upper teeth wear severely. This creates one of the most difficult problems to solve because the cementoenamel junctions of the lower incisors are often above the level of the occlusal plane. The resultant reverse smile line is also a difficult esthetic challenge.

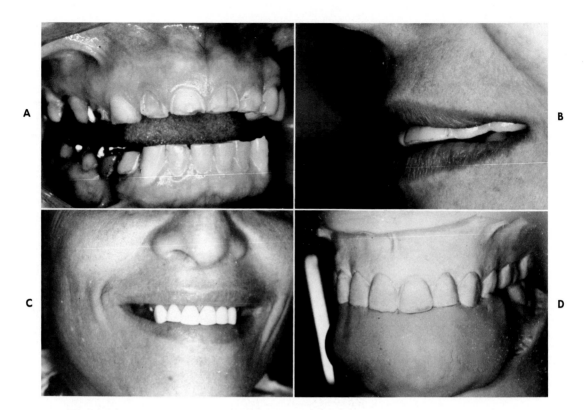

Fig. 30-14. Severe wear of upper anterior teeth, **A.** Provisional anterior restorations, **B,** are used to determine ideal incisal edge position before the anterior guidance can be worked out. An attempt is made in the provisionals to satisfy the esthetic and functional requirements at the most closed vertical possible. Although some increase is necessary, it should be kept as close to the original vertical dimension as possible. Resolving the anterior guidance problems is the key to successful treatment of most wear problems. **C,** Provisonal restorations are contoured within the established incisal plane and labial contour that had been determined from the lip-closure path, smile line, and phonetics. **D,** Index made on cast of corrected provisional splint will be used to guide the technician.

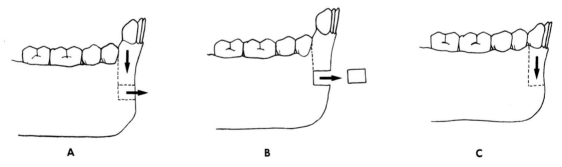

Fig. 30-15. Segmental osteotomy is a practical approach for inferiorly repositioning the lower anterior dentoalveolar segment when the alveolar process has become elongated. The gingival margins of the incisors were too high for restorative correction, **A.** The alternative of pulp extirpation and crown lengthening surgery is often more radical than osteotomy when the elongation has been severe. This procedure permits an esthetically acceptable solution that can also reestablish an effective anterior guidance, **B** and **C.**

The solution requires lowering of the lower incisal edges to permit a more normal upper smile line. The methods for accomplishing this should be evaluated in the same manner as other programmed treatment planning by consideration of all choices in proper sequence:

1. *Reshaping.* Can the lower incisors be shortened by grinding?
2. *Repositioning.* Is it possible to intrude the lower incisors orthodontically?
3. *Restoring.* Can the lower incisors be shortened restoratively? Can the occlusal plane be improved by an increase in the vertical (Fig. 30-14)?
4. *Surgery.* Would a segmental osteotomy be the best way to lower the entire anterior dentoalveolar segment (Fig. 30-15)?

The solution to the problem of uneven wear will be more readily determined if a structured approach to analysis takes into consideration all the possible options, or combination of options. Solutions will be as varied as the problems that are presented, but the answers will be found in this orderly process.

PREVENTING OCCLUSAL WEAR PROBLEMS

Tooth structure that is not in the way of jaw movements will not wear excessively.

There is probably no better reason for advocating functional harmony of the entire masticatory system than for the effect that a peaceful neuromuscular system has on preventing wear problems.

Except for habitual function against abrasive materials, most wear can be prevented. At least it can almost always be reduced to a level whereby the dentition can last a long lifetime. The best way to ensure against an excessive occlusal wear problem is by maintaining the optimum harmony possible between the articulation of the teeth and the articulation of the temporomandibular joints. This is best accomplished by the following:

1. Preserving the best possible alignment of the condyle-disk assemblies
2. Observing and correcting any signs of instability in the dentition.
3. Observing and correcting as much as possible any problems of masticatory muscle hyperactivity.

When a wear problem is noticed, meticulous attention should be given to providing equal-intensity contacts on the maximum number of teeth possible. Occlusal contact should occur in centric relation, and all posterior teeth should disclude the moment the jaw leaves centric relation. The anterior guidance should be nonrestrictive if possible.

Wear problems should be diagnosed early and treated before tooth structure is worn beyond the point of acceptable restoration.

Patients should be advised of the consequences of noxious habits.

31

Solving deep overbite
problems

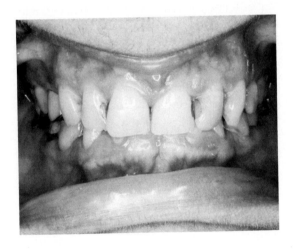

A deep overbite is not itself a problem. Many patients are treated unnecessarily to "correct" a deep overbite that was not a problem at all. Often the "corrected" anterior relationship is less stable than the deep overbite relationship. In deep overbite relationships, the eruption of the anterior teeth was guided by pressures from the lips and the tongue. The teeth are usually positioned quite naturally in their respective arches, and because they were guided into position by lip and tongue pressures, they are usually in harmonious position with them.

There is no problem, or even prospective problem, with teeth in a deep overbite rela-

tionship *if the teeth have stable centric contacts.* The degree of difficulty in treating problem deep overbites is directly related to the problems associated with establishing acceptable centric holding contacts.

Patients with deep overbite relationships that do not provide centric contacts for the anterior teeth are almost always in trouble. Some form of treatment is indicated in most of these patients. Patients with deep overbite relationships that have stable anterior contact in centric relation are almost never in trouble (from the arch relationship). Such patients rarely need corrective treatment.

The key word in the preceding statement is "stable." Just having anterior contact may not be sufficient if the contact does not serve as a *stop* to prevent continuous eruption of the lower anterior teeth. Eruption of the lower anterior teeth into the gingival tissues or into the palate is the number one problem associated with deep overbites. Treatment should always be designed to prevent this from happening or to correct it in a *stable* fashion if it has already occurred.

Sometimes one can correct a deep overbite problem by simply reshaping the upper lingual contours, shortening the lower anterior teeth, and having the patient follow a simple exercise to reposition the lower anterior teeth. The case must be selected carefully, and the patient

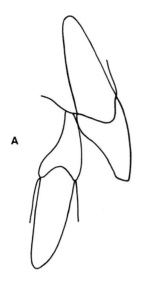

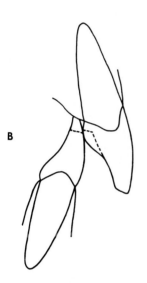

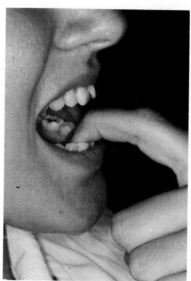

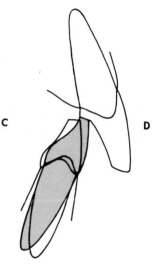

Fig. 31-1. A, Deep overbite problem with unstable contact or near contact at the gingival margin. This relationship is predictably deteriorating because there are no holding contacts to prevent supraeruption into gingival tissue. **B,** To provide stable holding contacts, the lower incisors are shortened and ledge type of stops are ground into the upper lingual surfaces. Lower teeth should be ground to allow for slight eruption during the movement forward. **C,** Some method of moving the lower incisors forward must be used. Sometimes just finger pressure to pull the lower teeth forward is all that is required. Removable orthodontic appliances should be used when necessary. If the teeth are slightly crowded, contact will not be lost as they are moved. If contact is lost, a restoration or two may be necessary to restore it. **D,** Centric contact is established. Once a *stable* stop is provided, there is rarely any tendency toward relapse to the former relationship.

must cooperate, but the procedure works surprisingly well in cases with slight crowding of extruded lower anterior teeth that contact or nearly contact at the lingual gingival margin (Fig. 31-1). Three steps are required:

1. The height of the lower anterior teeth should be reduced so that they do not contact soft tissue.
2. With a sharp-edged stone, a definite centric stop should be cut for each lower anterior tooth into the upper lingual surface. A flat ledge should be formed that will be just above each lower incisal edge position when the jaw is closed.

3. The patient should be taught to exert a forward pressure on the lower anterior teeth using the index finger. The finger should be hooked over the incisal edge and pulled forward for several minutes several times a day.

The pulling pressure moves the teeth forward as they erupt slightly up into contact against the stable stop. There is no further tendency for the teeth to slide up the lingual incline into the soft palatal tissue. Once they are seated into a properly contoured contact, the relationship becomes quite stable.

Often the ledge must be cut almost at the

level of the lingual gingival tissue. This presents no problem to the tissue. If there is any question about the patient's cooperation, a lower removable orthodontic appliance should be used to move the lower teeth forward. This is generally not necessary if the patient cooperates with the finger pressure and if the movement required is minimal.

If the lower anterior teeth are in good alignment and cannot be moved forward without causing a separation at their contacts, the pre-

ceding procedure should not be used. It is sometimes practical to move the upper anterior teeth in slightly after the holding notches are cut.

After the teeth have been positioned into the centric stops, the anterior guidance should be refined to harmonize excursions from the new centric contacts forward and laterally. Minimal adjustment is usually required because patients with deep overbite have naturally steep, near-vertical patterns of function.

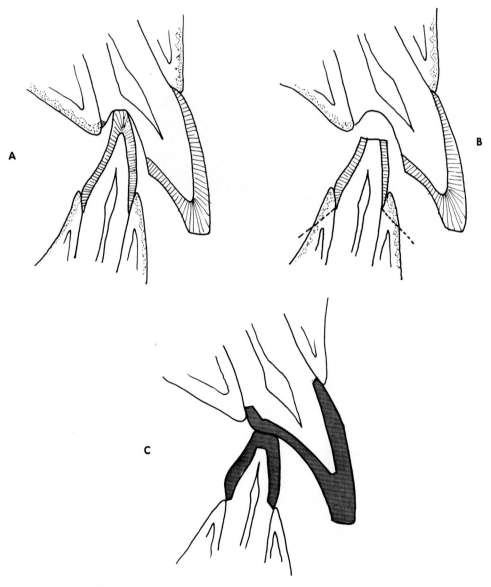

Fig. 31-2. A, Deep overbite with supraeruption of lower incisors into badly worn upper anterior teeth. It is not uncommon for the lower incisal enamel to remain intact while the upper lingual surface wears. When this occurs, the eruption of the lower teeth keeps pace with the wear. **B,** The solution always involves shortening the lower anterior teeth. This must even be done if it requires endodontics and reduction of supporting tissues. **C,** After posterior deflective contacts have been corrected and the reduction of lower anterior teeth is completed, both upper and lower anterior teeth must usually be restored.

DEEP OVERBITE PROBLEMS ASSOCIATED WITH AN ANTERIOR SLIDE

If a deep-overbite problem is complicated by posterior interferences that deflect the mandible forward, there is often a tendency to produce extreme wear on the upper anterior lingual surfaces. Sometimes the bruxism effect of the lower incisors carves out the lingual contours and forms a concavity that extends up above the level of the gingival margin. The eruption of the lower incisors keeps pace with the wear on the upper, and the anterior contact ends up in a hole in the upper teeth (Fig. 31-2, *A*). This type of case sometimes looks unsolvable, but an understanding of what has taken place will serve to simplify the treatment plan.

Such a problem calls for a three-step solution:

1. We must equilibrate to permit the mandible to close without deflection.
2. We must shorten the lower incisors to position the incisal edges in an optimum relationship to previsualized centric stops on the upper incisors (Fig. 31-2, *B*). The lower anterior teeth must always be shortened in such cases, even if it necessitates endodontic treatment. Sometimes periodontal surgery is necessary to lower the gingival margin on the mandibular teeth because of eruption of the teeth and corresponding vertical growth of the alveolar bone.
3. We must restore the upper lingual contours to establish stable centric stops (Fig. 31-2, *C*). We must be certain to harmonize the protrusive and lateral excursions after the centric contacts have been determined.

In some deep overbite cases, the upper lingual surfaces are worn severely and are in contact with the entire labial surface of the lower incisors. In some such cases, elimination of the deflecting posterior interferences is all that is required to provide room for restoring the upper anterior teeth. When they are restored, the centric contact should be moved as much as possible from the labial surface to the lower incisal edge. The labioincisal edge of the lower should normally be the contact in centric relation, but because of the naturally steep inclines, contact in protrusive and lateral excursions may be almost entirely on the labial surface. There is no harm in such an arrangement

as long as the patient is given whatever freedom is needed for "long centric" before the surface-to-surface contact occurs. When needed, even a fraction of a millimeter of "long centric" seems to be the difference of whether patients continue their wear problems or eliminate them.

DEEP OVERBITE PROBLEMS WITH NO DEFLECTIVE INTERFERENCES

Not all deep overbite problems are associated with deflective interferences. One of the most difficult problems to solve is the extremely worn deep overbite that contacts surface to surface in centric relation (Fig. 31-3). Sometimes the upper lingual surfaces have worn almost through the teeth, leaving a sharp, thin incisal edge. If the lower labial surfaces have also worn, the problem is complicated even more.

One may wonder how the problem can be solved without either increasing the vertical or moving teeth. The answer is that it cannot. Unless either the upper anterior teeth are moved labially or the lower teeth are moved lingually, there is insufficient room to restore the lost surface of either. Increasing the vertical dimension will provide room for the restoration, but this necessarily involves the restoration of posterior teeth also.

It is usually difficult to move the lower teeth lingually, and so the orthodontic reposi-

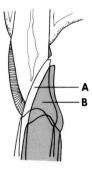

Fig. 31-3. One of the most difficult deep overbite problems to solve. If there is extreme surface-to-surface wear and no deviation into centric relation, there is no way to provide room for the restorations unless teeth are moved or the vertical dimension is increased. *A,* Centric relation surface-to-surface contact. *B,* Position of the teeth at an increased vertical dimension provides the needed room for restoration. The arc of opening directs the teeth back as well as down. If this procedure is used, posterior teeth must also be restored to the new vertical dimension.

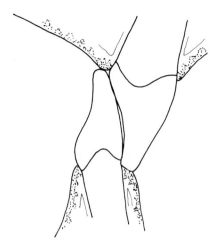

Fig. 31-4. Deep overbite with lingually inclined anterior teeth almost always ends up in trouble because there are no stops for either upper or lower teeth. Notice impingement of gingival tissue by incisal edge.

tioning most often is confined to the upper anterior teeth. It is not difficult to move these teeth with a removable appliance, but patients with deep overbite generally have tight upper lips. The trick is to *keep* the teeth forward after the appliance has been removed.

Since the badly worn upper anterior teeth will need to be restored anyway, we can go ahead and prepare them as soon as they are in the desired position and make a plastic provisional splint to serve as a retainer. The temporary splint stabilizes the teeth very well while the bone fills in and the periodontal fibers become realigned. It also introduces the patient to the new overjet, which has been necessarily increased, gives us plenty of time to work out acceptable esthetics and function, and lets the patient adapt to the slightly changed appearance and phonetics.

Even though the teeth are moved only about a millimeter or so, to the tight-lipped patient with deep overbite it feels like more. It is well to let such a patient get used to it and verify its comfort before proceeding with the permanent restorations.

An important clinical judgment that will have to be made is whether to splint the upper anterior teeth when the labial surface has to be moved forward. An extremely tight lip can force the teeth back to the original lip—labial surface relationship. If the anterior guidance is in good harmony, normal function against the

lingual surfaces will tend to counterbalance lip pressure, but if good bone support has been diminished by periodontal disease, the upper anterior teeth may need the extra stabilization that splinting would provide.

Deep overbite problems that result because of unstable centric contact are generally easier to solve if there has not been a great deal of wear because there is usually room to reshape the teeth to establish stability of the centric stops. A relationship that, given enough time, usually ends up in trouble is the deep overbite with lingually inclined anterior teeth (Fig. 31-4). When the upper anterior teeth tilt back toward the lingual, there is no convenient stop for the lower teeth. The centric contact is usually made against the lower labial surface by the upper incisal edge. The contact in combination with lip position is usually sufficient to stabilize the upper teeth, but there are no stops to prevent the lower incisors from erupting on up into the palate. Sometimes the combination allows the upper anterior teeth to supraerupt also, and so the incisal edges of the upper teeth traumatize the lower labial gingiva while the lower incisal edges injure the palatal side tissues.

The resolution of such problems almost always involves reshaping the upper lingual surfaces and shortening the lower incisors. If the upper teeth impinge on labial tissues, they must be shortened also (Fig. 31-5).

To solve the problem, the lower incisal edges must be moved forward into stable ledge type of centric stops on the upper surfaces, or upper lingual stops must be extended by restoration. The repositioning of the incisal edges may be accomplished either by restoration or by orthodontic movement. If the lower teeth are moved forward, the contour change on the upper surfaces involves selective shaping of the lingual surfaces to provide definite stops. It may or may not require restorative treatment of the ground surfaces, depending on whether the enamel surface is penetrated.

If it is impossible to provide stable centric stops, an alternative may be to do the necessary shortening of supraerupted teeth and then splint the unstable teeth in each direction until we can join to a tooth on each side that has as a stable centric stop. The splinted teeth will be unable to erupt back into tissue contact because they will be held in check by the teeth with the stable stops.

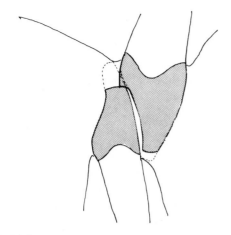

Fig. 31-5. After shortening of both upper and lower anterior teeth, some type of stop must be provided. If the lower teeth can be shortened enough, the stop can usually be added on to the upper lingual surface. Because of intense lip pressure, even orthodontic correction will fail unless stable stops are provided as part of the treatment. If it is possible to move the lower anterior teeth forward, one can often provide the stop by grinding the upper lingual surface to provide a ledge. This does not require movement of the upper teeth and so does not disturb the balance of the teeth with the pressure of the lips.

Complete orthodontic resolution of the problem is always the first choice of treatment if it could provide stability. This is particularly so if it would eliminate the need for extensive restorative procedures that would otherwise be unnecessary. However, if orthodontic movement is contemplated on patients with lingually inclined upper and lower anteriors, the factor of an extremely strong buccinator–orbicularis oris complex must be considered. The lingual inclination is almost surely associated with a very strong lower band in a high position. The surgical release procedure described in Chapter 6 may be considered if anterior tooth angulations are to be changed.

DEEP OVERBITE PROBLEMS WITH NO CENTRIC CONTACT

Of all the occlusal relationships observed, the one that will most predictably lead down the path of eventual destruction is the deep overbite relationship when there are no centric stops to prevent the lower anterior teeth from erupting into the soft tissues.

The proximity of the upper and lower teeth in a deep overbite makes it nearly impossible for the tongue to substitute for the missing centric contact. The tongue can rest against the lingual surfaces, but there is not enough room for it to be interposed between the lower incisal edges and the palate. Thus there is nothing to stop the continual eruptive process of the lower anterior teeth until they meet the soft tissues.

Unfortunately, two of the most common approaches to solving this problem are methods that have absolutely no chance of success. In fact, the procedures are harmful. They are (1) shortening the lower anterior teeth by grinding and (2) depressing the lower anterior teeth with an anterior bite plane that also allows extrusion of the posterior teeth.

Unless the shortened teeth are provided with stable centric stops, they will simply erupt, alveolar process and all, back into the palatal tissue. We have seen lower anterior teeth that have been shortened so many times that they had been ground off to the gum line. The elongated alveolar process was then hitting into the palate.

A basic rule to follow when treating deep overbite problems is: *Never shorten the lower anterior teeth unless stable centric stops are provided* or some means of stabilization is effected.

Another popular treatment for deep overbite is even more detrimental: Increasing the vertical height of the posterior teeth to correct a deep overbite problem is absolutely contraindicated unless stable holding contacts are provided for the anterior teeth. In the absence of anterior contact, the lower incisors will erupt, while simultaneously the upper incisors are usually inclined lingually by the lip pressure. The posterior teeth will not maintain the increased vertical, and they will be intruded by an amount equaling the dimension of the vertical increase. The end point of such treatment almost invariably is a stepped occlusal plane along with a worsened problem of anterior guidance disharmony.

Some patients manage to maintain a stable occlusal relationship despite the lack of centric tooth-to-tooth contacts. Patients with wide, smooth incisal edges in contact with dense resistance palatal tissue may be able to maintain stability if their functional cycle is nearly vertical. Such patients usually have steep cuspid protection and utilize practically no lateral or protrusive excursions. This, in combination with the type of tooth-tissue contact, is within the resistant range of the tissues, and nothing needs to be done.

If restorative treatment is necessary, the same steep cuspid inclines should be maintained. Unless the lower incisors require restorations, they should be left undisturbed. If the anterior teeth require restorations for other reasons, we would then go ahead and correct the relationship at the same time. Otherwise, we do not try to alter an occlusion that is comfortable and being maintained in good health.

Such maintainability with tissue contact is unusual. It can exist, but it would not be wise to count on it unless the patient has been stable with it for several years. As a general rule, deep overbite relationships that do not have definitive means of stabilizing tooth positions should be treated to prevent the problems from occurring. When problems already exist, the immediate effect should not only be relieved, but steps should also be taken to prevent the recurrence of the problem.

There are five basic approaches for solving deep overbite problems when anterior tooth contact is missing:

1. Orthodontic tooth movement
2. Restorative reshaping
3. Splinting
4. Use of bite plane appliances at night
5. Establishment of contact on the palatal bar extension of a removable partial restoration

None of the preceding approaches is applicable for all cases, but the advantages and disadvantages of each should be evaluated before any treatment plan related to a deep overbite problem is determined. Selective grinding and reshaping of the natural teeth must usually be done in combination with any of these procedures, and it is often necessary to combine procedures to achieve the best results.

Correcting deep overbite problems orthodontically

A basic restorative tenet is to avoid unnecessary restorative treatment. If we can avoid restorations by moving the teeth into a correct relationship, orthodontics is the method of choice.

Improved methods of torquing the anterior teeth into stable contact make it possible to correct the unstable deep overbite and improve esthetics at the same time. The key to successful orthodontic treatment is the same

key used for restorative success—stable centric contacts. The ideal relationship is lower incisal contact against the upper cingulum. In accomplishing this, we must take care to avoid moving the upper incisal edges into the lip-closure path (Fig. 31-6). If this cannot be achieved, combining selective grinding with tooth movement is often the practical approach, followed by reshaping the upper lingual surfaces to provide a stable stop and then moving the teeth so that the lower incisal edge fits into the stop. Elongated lower anterior teeth must frequently be shortened to permit correct repositioning.

The orthodontist should be the best judge of the practicality of solving any deep overbite problem by tooth movement. If complex, long-term orthodontic treatment is required, it can be weighed against other methods or combinations of methods. A comparison of advantages and disadvantages can be made, and a logical solution can be determined. In the young patient with healthy virgin teeth, however, all possible steps should be taken to avoid the restorative approach.

It is essential for the treating orthodontist to understand the concepts of anterior guidance. Too many deep overbite problems are actually *caused* by faulty orthodontic procedures, and many orthodontic attempts at solving deep overbite problems fail because of inadequate understanding of anterior guidance. A strong recommendation may be made to review the principles of anterior guidance (as outlined in Chapter 16) before the treatment plan is finalized.

It has been a pleasure to collaborate on numerous cases during the past few years with enlightened orthodontists who understand the problems and know how to solve them. The methods are available, but they will work only in the hands of those who understand the goals of anterior function and long-term stability.

Solving deep overbite problems by restorative reshaping

The preparation of anterior teeth and subsequent reshaping by restorations can accomplish many benefits.

1. Full coverage restorations on shortened lower anterior teeth can be shaped to move the incisal edges forward. Often this is all that is necessary to provide stable contacts.

2. The lingual surface of upper anterior

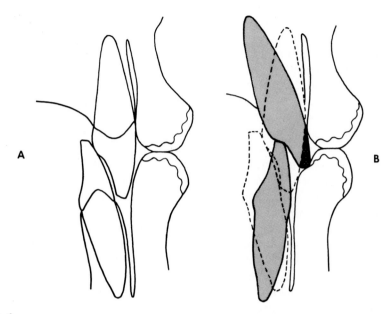

Fig. 31-6. When teeth are moved from an unstable deep overbite relationship, **A,** to a position that has an acceptable stop, **B,** care must be taken not to incline the upper incisors too much and thereby move the incisal edges into an interference with the lip-closure path.

teeth can be contoured additively toward the lingual to provide holding contacts for the lower anterior teeth (Fig. 31-7). The extent of such lingual contouring is strictly limited, however, by the effect that it has on the health of gingival tissues. Under no circumstances should contours that overprotect the gingival margins be permitted. Clinical judgment mixed with common sense must be the deciding factor regarding the limits of the lingual extension.

3. A combination of restoring upper lingual surfaces to provide improved centric stop locations and of restoring lower anterior teeth to provide improved incisal edge location is often a practical approach. It is particularly logical when the anterior teeth require restorations anyway for other reasons.

In a nutshell, restorative procedures can either be used to move lower contacts forward or upper contacts inward. In the process the contacts can be either raised or lowered. The changes must fall within the limits of acceptable stress direction for each tooth and within contour limitations dictated by requirements for maintainable gingival health.

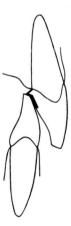

Fig. 31-7. In some instances the upper cingulum can be extended slightly to provide a stop for a lower tooth (usually after the lower tooth has been shortened). Care must be taken not to overprotect the gingival tissue from such extensions.

Solving deep overbite problems by splinting

In some arch relationships, too much stress would be directed off the long axis if teeth are moved or restored to contact. Teeth that have supraerupted into the palatal tissue can be shortened to relieve the pressure against the soft tissues, but unless they are stabilized in some manner, they will reerupt right back up. Splinting is often the most practical method of stabilizing such lower anterior teeth. By joining the teeth with no stops to a tooth on each side that does have a centric contact, one can stop any further eruption.

The splinting can be accomplished in a variety of ways. If incisal edge reduction has been necessary to the extent of exposing dentin, full coverage would be the method of choice. If esthetic improvement is not needed and the incisal edges are intact, nonparallel horizontal pin splinting is an excellent method that is both conservative and effective.

When full coverage is used, acrylic veneers are contraindicated. Centric contact on the "stop" tooth should be in a hard material, preferably porcelain, for its esthetic value as well as its durability. Upper anterior teeth without centric contact are usually kept from supraerupting by the lip contact. They would rarely require splinting for stabilization unless other factors demanded it.

In the absence of posterior teeth, the lower anterior teeth can be stabilized by modifications in partial denture design. Combining continuous clasp splinting of the anterior teeth with replacement of the posterior teeth has the effect of preventing their continuous elongation. Swing lock design partial dentures accomplish the same results. Although such procedures are effective, they must be considered compromise approaches to the problem because of their esthetic shortcomings. When possible, permanent splinting is a more desired solution.

Minimizing operative intervention through the use of bite planes to solve deep overbite problems

For reasons of age, health, economics, or timing, it is not always practical for some patients to undergo optimum orthodontic or restorative treatment. When a deep overbite problem is causing discomfort from tissue impingement or future problems are imminent, something must be done to relieve the pain or prevent the problem from worsening or recurring. The least complicated way of preventing supraeruption of the lower anterior teeth is to provide contacts on a removable bite plane. Just wearing the bite plane at night is sufficient to keep the teeth from erupting back into tissue impingement after they have been shortened.

The night guard can also be used as a preventive measure for young adults who have excessive overbite relationships and no holding contacts to prevent supraeruption. It can serve as an interim measure to keep them out of trouble until more definitive measures can be taken when time, circumstances, or economics permit. Fabrication of the night guard should be carried out on centrically mounted models. Maxillary appliances seem to be more comfortable than those worn on lower teeth because of the stability obtainable from palatal coverage. The appliance is most esthetically acceptable when it is made of clear acrylic resin. It must provide stable centric contacts *for all the lower teeth,* and it should be equilibrated so that there is no interference to any excursive movement.

The thin palatal coverage should extend up and over all the posterior teeth. It should extend to the bucco-occlusal line angle to stop as a continuation of the natural buccal contours (Fig. 31-8). The occlusal table should be extended around to allow the lower anterior teeth to contact on the anterior bite plane simultaneously with posterior centric contact. The acrylic appliance should cover the lingual surfaces of the upper anterior teeth, and a comfortable anterior guidance should be worked out in the appliance.

Wire clasps can extend around the distal of the last molar on each side and engage a slight undercut on the buccal. The clasps are really used more for convenient removal of the appliance than they are for retention. For comfort's sake the appliance should fit precisely without rock. Patients should be instructed to thoroughly clean their mouths every evening before insertion of the appliance. It should be worn every night. The Biostar technique (described in Chapter 11) is another excellent method for constructing a night guard appliance that usually eliminates any need for clasps.

Patient acceptance of the night guard is sur-

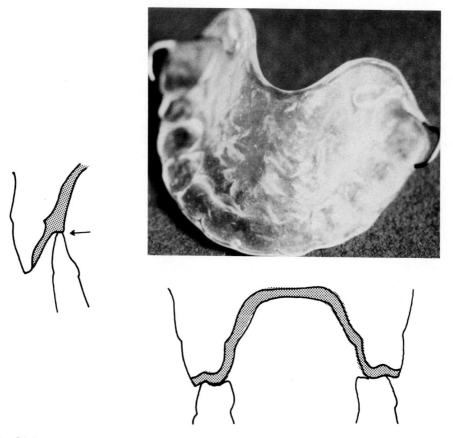

Fig. 31-8. A night guard appliance is very effective as a compromise procedure for preventing the supraeruption of noncontacting anterior teeth. The appliance, *upper right,* is fabricated of clear acrylic resin. Two wrought wire clasps help to stabilize it and provide a simple means of removal. The appliance should be adapted to the palate and should extend to form a continuous smooth contour with the buccal surfaces. A stable centric stop should be provided for the lower anterior teeth, *arrow,* and this stop should be in perfect harmony with the posterior occlusal contacts on the appliance.

prisingly good. Patients report it is comfortable to wear, and some patients have worn such appliances for years rather than undergo orthodontic treatment or resort to splinting procedures for stabilization.

The use of a night guard appliance is a compromise solution for keeping deep overbite patients out of trouble, but it is an acceptable compromise if it is properly made and religiously worn.

Using removable partial dentures to solve deep overbite problems

When an upper partial denture is required, it can sometimes fulfill a double purpose by serving as a contact for the lower anterior teeth. If the palatal bar is designed to cover the tissues behind the upper anterior teeth, the lower anterior teeth may be permitted to con-

tact the palatal bar to prevent supraeruption. The contour of the palatal coverage may be designed to permit protrusive excursions of the lower anterior teeth to slide smoothly from the palatal coverage onto the lingual inclines of the upper anterior teeth.

Although this seems to be the most practical way to solve some unusual deep overbite problems, it should be cautioned that the restorative procedures demand extreme preciseness and perfect occlusal harmony of the removable segment. Too much pressure will cause tissue problems on the lingual gingival area.

Tooth support for the partial, in combination with tissue support, is an absolute requirement.

This procedure is something of a last-resort solution that has its main value in arch relationships that do not have sufficient posterior tooth support. When some tissue support is needed from the upper teeth to enable the lower anterior teeth to actually carry part of the stresses of the lower arch, this procedure has merit. In situations where the lower anterior teeth are not actually needed to lend support, splinting the anterior teeth to prevent supraeruption will suffice. This procedure is not needed.

SUMMARY

A deep overbite is a problem only when the anterior relationship is not stable. All methods of treating deep overbite problems are designed to either provide stable holding contacts to prevent supraeruption of the lower anterior teeth or to stabilize by other means teeth that cannot be positioned or restored to contact sufficiently in function to maintain their position.

32

Solving anterior overjet problems

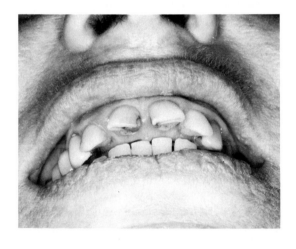

Patients with excessive overjet have two specific problems, each of which may contribute to accelerated deterioration of the teeth and supporting structures.

PROBLEM 1: In excessive anterior overjet relationships, the lower anterior teeth have no stabilizing contact with the upper teeth, either in centric or near centric relation. Hence they have a tendency to supraerupt, drift out of alignment, and frequently impinge on the palatal tissues.

PROBLEM 2: Excessive overjet relationships make it difficult or impossible for the anterior guidance to do its job of posterior disclusion.

A third problem that is often associated with excessive anterior overjet is esthetics. The classic bucktooth appearance has long been used by cartoonists to depict stupidity. It is not a pleasant appearance, and it is often the real reason why patients seek treatment.

The resolution of anterior overjet problems involves four considerations:
1. Stabilization of the lower anterior teeth
2. Providing the best possible anterior guidance for posterior disclusion in protrusion
3. Providing the best possible relationship for disclusion of the balancing inclines
4. Improving the position, alignment, or shape of the upper anterior teeth for better esthetics

Although all four of these requirements are interrelated, they can be considered separately for simplicity. It is helpful to keep in mind that anterior overjet problems may result from either maxillary anterior protrusion or mandibular anterior retrusion. Regardless of the cause of the problem, the requirements for stable occlusion do not change.

SOLVING THE PROBLEM OF STABILIZING THE LOWER ANTERIOR TEETH

It is not always necessary to stabilize lower anterior teeth just because they lack contact in centric relation. If the anterior overjet problem is not too severe, the teeth may contact in protrusive and lateral function enough to stabilize them and prevent their supraeruption.

Even in severe overjet problems, the tongue may position itself between the palate and the lower anterior teeth during each swallow. The tongue thus acts as a substitute for the missing tooth contact and serves to stabilize the position of the teeth. There are many patients with healthy mouths who do not have anterior tooth contact in any functional position. There is no need for operative intervention to stabilize teeth that are already stable.

There are other substitutes for anterior tooth contact. The lips sometimes are positioned in ways that serve to stabilize teeth with an apparent anterior overjet problem. Lip biting, sucking in the lower lip, and other habit patterns are very often beneficial because they serve as substitutes for missing tooth contact. Many times such habit patterns are all that is needed to stabilize the position of the teeth and prevent problems. No treatment plan should ever be initiated that does not consider the effect of habit patterns.

In evaluating habit patterns, we must differentiate between habits that stabilize teeth when there is a true interarch malrelationship and habit patterns that cause problems. Some habit patterns are actually responsible for the overjet problem we are trying to resolve. Harmful habit patterns are those that lead to instability of the occlusion.

A major facet of diagnosis is to determine whether there is occlusal instability. If a habit pattern has substituted for missing tooth contacts, if the teeth are firm, if the patient is comfortable, and if in our clinical judgment the stability is maintainable, there would be no need for operative intervention. However, such a relationship should be kept under careful scrutiny because it takes very little to disturb the delicate balance of an occlusion that depends on a habit pattern for its stability.

If a habit pattern is the primary cause of the overjet problem, elimination of the habit is the major aspect of treatment. Limited success has been reported in correction of such occlusal relationships with myofunctional therapy. However, if the habit can be eliminated by any practical means, it would certainly be the treatment of choice.

Some habits result from attempts to cushion the teeth against striking an occlusal interference. Equilibration sometimes eliminates the

need for such habit patterns, and when there is no reason to bite the lip or hold the tongue between the teeth, the normalized lip pressures return the upper anterior teeth back to their correct relationship with the lower teeth.

When a habit pattern cannot be broken, we have no choice but to work around it. As an example, it would be folly to restore lower anterior teeth to come into contact in the presence of an unbreakable tongue-thrust swallowing pattern.

In the presence of a habit pattern, attempts at stabilization of the lower anterior teeth should follow this sequence:

1. It should be determined whether the anterior relationship is stable because of a beneficial habit pattern.

2. It should be determined whether a harmful habit pattern is contributing to the problem. If it is, we must evaluate the possibilities of either eliminating the habit through myofunctional therapy or eliminating the cause of the habit or a combination of both.

3. If the habit is beneficial or a potentially destructive habit cannot be eliminated, we must design the treatment to cooperate with the habit. In any conflict between the teeth and a habit pattern, the teeth will lose.

Not all overjet problems are related to habit patterns. The majority are interarch relationship problems that require intervention of some type to resolve the instability. Unstable lower anterior teeth can be treated with some of the same options that are used for deep overbite problems. Deep overbite relationships with no anterior contact are also actually problems of overjet. The following five options may be used singly or in combination to solve the problem of supraeruption of the lower anterior teeth in patients with overjet problems.

1. For patients with severe overjet, the *orthodontic approach* often requires some extractions. Orthodontics is usually the first choice of treatment.

2. *Restorative reshaping* to establish holding contacts is usually not possible in patients with severe overjet unless the teeth are repositioned orthodontically first.

3. *Splinting* is often necessary in severe overjet problems to prevent the lower anterior teeth from supraerupting. In very severe overjet problems, it may be necessary to extend the splinting all the way around the arch to stabilize lower posterior teeth that cannot contact ideally. If the contacts cannot be designed

to direct the forces down the long axis, splinting may be necessary to counteract the lateral stress.

4. *Night-guard biting planes* may be used as a compromise treatment. They can be used as a Hawley type of retainer also to stabilize upper anterior teeth that have been repositioned lingually. If nighttime use of the appliance is sufficient to stabilize the occlusion, it may serve as a practical alternative to exten-

sive restorative treatment when circumstances rule out more complex approaches. Details for fabrication are in Chapter 31. It is the same type of appliance that may be used in deep overbite problems.

5. The *use of removable partial dentures* to stabilize the lower anterior teeth may have special adaptation for patients with severe overjet. Sometimes it is the only practical way to achieve stabilizing contact for the lower an-

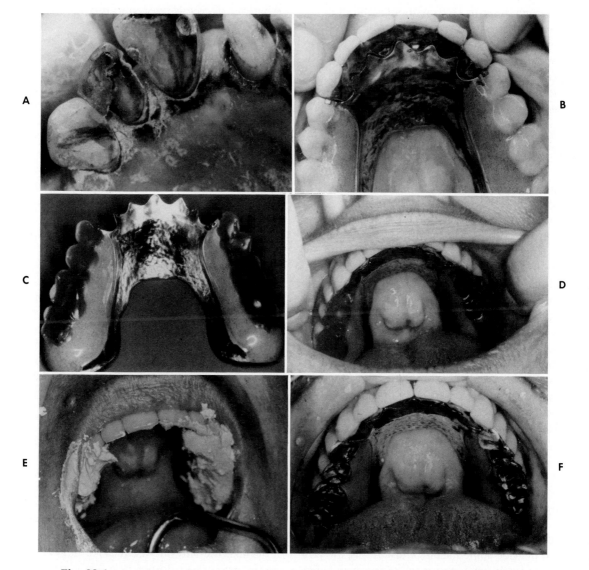

Fig. 32-1. A, Overjet problem. Marks on tissue indicate contact of lower incisors, lingual to upper tooth contact. **B,** Restorations and partial denture in place. Notice that palatal bar extends to form continuous contour with restored lingual tooth surface. Centric contact is on palatal bar. Excursive movements continue on to tooth surfaces. Posterior teeth are plastic. **C,** After anterior guidance is determined to be correct, the posterior plastic teeth are reduced and functional wax is added to the surface. **D,** All border movements are captured for the occlusal surfaces using functionally generated path technique. **E,** The functional core is formed in the mouth before the partial denture is removed. **F,** Gold occlusals are fabricated against the functional core. The result is a very harmonious occlusal relationship between the anterior guidance, the partial dentures, and the condyles.

terior teeth. The lower anterior teeth can contact the upper palatal bar to provide excellent stabilization (Fig. 32-1). In severe arch relationship problems, the saddle area of the partial restoration may also provide contact for lower posterior teeth that are in severe lingual version.

Lower removable appliances may also be used to stabilize teeth. Partial restorations with continuous clasps or swing lock designs, as well as extended overlay partial dentures may sometimes be used as compromise treatments.

Lower anterior teeth without stable holding contacts can be prevented from supraerupting if we provide either something for the teeth to contact or something to hold the teeth in place so that they cannot supraerupt. The five methods of accomplishing this should be reviewed in Chapter 31 for further details.

PROVIDING PROTRUSIVE DISCLUSION OF THE POSTERIOR TEETH

Patients with severe anterior overjet rarely have vertical patterns of function. The vertical "chop-chop" biters are mostly confined to those with steep anterior guidances or those who have no need to protrude the mandible. Patients with end-to-end relationships and anterior crossbites have nothing to gain by mandibular protrusion. However, patients with too much anterior overjet *have* to protrude the mandible to allow the anterior teeth to function. Consequently, their pattern of function is usually quite horizontal. Unless the posterior teeth are discluded in protrusion, they are subjected to excessive stress. Therefore the arch relationship that needs posterior disclusion the most often has no way to provide it because the anterior teeth are not in contact until considerable protrusion has already occurred.

One of the most common problems seen in severe anterior overjet relationships is hypermobility of the posterior teeth with varying degrees of periodontitis. The overjet patient is particularly susceptible to traumatogenic periodontal breakdown unless the treatment plan can provide some means of discluding the posterior teeth when the mandible is protruded. The rule to follow for protrusive disclusion is: *When the anterior teeth cannot provide the guidance to disclude the posterior teeth in protrusion, the job should be assigned to the most anteriorly positioned tooth on each side that can.*

The cuspids can usually be shaped to provide a protrusive guidance, but it is sometimes necessary for the upper first premolars to assume this role. In really severe overjet conditions the job may even be given to the upper second premolars. Which teeth serve as the protrusive guidance is not too important as long as the guiding tooth on each side discludes all the teeth distal to it. If a first premolar is in the best position to serve as the guidance but is not strong enough to assume the role, it should be strengthened by splinting to whatever degree is needed to provide the necessary stabilization.

Even a pontic may serve as the protrusive guidance. It is *position* that is important. The stress diminishes as the distance from the condylar fulcrum increases, and so the farther forward the guidance can be positioned, the less stress is exerted on the guiding tooth (or the bridge abutments if the guide tooth is a pontic). Contouring the guidance tooth for protrusive disclusion is accomplished the same way that the protrusive pathway of any anterior guidance is worked out.

PROVIDING DISCLUSION OF THE NONFUNCTIONING INCLINES

In severe anterior overjet relationships the anterior teeth may not be able to contact in lateral excursions. In such cases, disclusion of the nonfunctioning inclines must be accomplished by posterior teeth on the working side. When only posterior teeth contact in working excursions, the lateral anterior guidance must be established on the contacting tooth that is farthest forward. From that point back, varying degrees of group function can be worked out to distribute the lateral stresses.

It is usually preferable to have all the posterior teeth is group function when they do not get help from the anterior teeth, but this is not an unbreakable rule. The distribution of lateral stresses must always be worked out according to the resistance capabilities of the teeth sharing the occlusal forces.

Unlike the anterior teeth, posterior teeth in eccentric contact do not have the capacity for shutting off elevator muscle contraction, and so premolars are not generally capable of resisting the same forces that the cuspid can. Premolar roots are usually much shorter than the average cuspid root, and premolars do not have the benefit of the dense bone of the cuspid eminence. Deep flutes or bifurcations make the premolars more susceptible to irreversible periodontitis than the single-rooted cuspid. Finally, premolars, being closer to the condylar fulcrum, are in a position of greater stress than the cuspid. For all these reasons, a single premolar should rarely serve as the lateral anterior guidance.

When excessive overjet prohibits the anterior teeth from contact in lateral excursions, the balancing inclines should usually be discluded by group function of all or most of the posterior teeth on the opposite side. When posterior group function must occur without any help from anterior teeth, the working inclines must be perfectly harmonized to make sure the lateral stresses are evenly distributed. Functional inclines should never be steeper than the patient's normal functional pathways. To accomplish this in posterior restorative cases, we should correct the lingual inclines of the most forward guiding tooth, following the same rules that are applicable for harmonizing any lateral guidance. All teeth distal to the guiding teeth should then be harmonized to both the guide tooth and the condylar guidance. Functional path procedures work well to accomplish this harmony. It can also be done with several different instrument approaches. If restorations are not needed, inclines must be corrected by equilibration until group function is achieved.

IMPROVING THE POSITION OR SHAPE OF UPPER ANTERIOR TEETH WITH EXCESSIVE OVERJET

Improving the esthetics of buckteeth is one of the most stimulating challenges a dentist can face. The improvement in appearance is especially gratifying when it also helps to stabilize the occlusion, reverse destructive tendencies, and provide better comfort. These are all achievable goals that can be fulfilled if the treatment plan is carefully designed for optimum results rather than for expediency.

Too often the correction of maxillary anterior protrusion is attempted by simple reshaping of the teeth with full-coverage restorations. Many cases can be solved in this manner, but better results can be achieved for most patients with problem overjet if the upper anterior teeth are moved into better alignment before any restorative reshaping is finalized.

Correcting upper anterior tooth position orthodontically

Circumstances permitting, complete orthodontic treatment is always the method of choice if it eliminates the need for extensive restorative procedures. But if extensive restorative treatment is needed anyway, minor tooth movement procedures are still beneficial in a large percentage of the cases we treat. Furthermore, minor tooth movement is often simplified when it is combined with a restorative approach. Teeth can be narrowed or shortened to provide direct access to their corrected position. Esthetic temporary bridges can sometimes be used to hold teeth in position after they are moved, and provisional restorations can sometimes serve the same purpose as orthodontic bands.

One of the most practical methods for repositioning upper anterior teeth is to use a removable upper appliance with an anterior bite plane to keep the lower anterior teeth from supraerupting during treatment. A rubber band extends around the labial surfaces of the upper anterior teeth to apply pressure lingually. the palatal acrylic appliance contacts the lingual surface of each tooth (Fig. 32-2).

The appliance is activated when the acrylic splint is cut back for whatever amount of movement is desired. Cutting it back a little at a time prevents the movement from occurring too rapidly and serves as the control for the *amount* of movement. Guides can be cut into the acrylic splint to direct teeth laterally or to rotate them. Teeth that are in correct position can be stabilized by the lingual acrylic bite plane while others are selectively moved. The rubber band is not too obtrusive and very few patients ever object to its appearance.

Narrowing the upper anterior teeth is often necessary to permit sufficient lingual movement. The stripping procedures can be accomplished a little at a time as the teeth are moved (Fig. 32-3). Movement can be accomplished by activated wires or by rubber bands.

As the upper anterior teeth are being moved back into a better alignment, their relationship with the lower incisors should be repeatedly checked with the appliance removed. It is usually necessary to reshape the upper lingual surfaces after they are moved to provide stable holding contacts for the lower anterior teeth. The reshaping can wait until the teeth are in their final position, though, because the

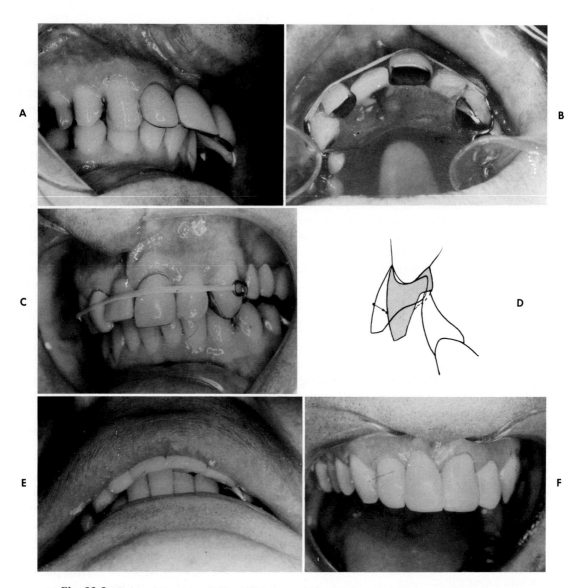

Fig. 32-2. A, Anterior overjet problem. The upper anterior teeth are in complete labial version to the lower anterior teeth. The problem is complicated by a fixed bridge. **B,** The pontic is removed to permit individual movement of the teeth. It is replaced on the appliance. When the appliance is in place, it is stabilized by its approximation to the posterior lingual contours plus a wrought wire clasp on the distal abutment on each side. Pressure is exerted lingually by the rubber band, which can be replaced by the patient. The amount and direction of movement can be controlled by the manner of reducing the acrylic material that is lingual to each tooth. **C,** Compare the position of the left central with its position in **B.** As the upper teeth are moved, their lingual surfaces must be ground to form a centric stop that can be engaged by the incisal edges of the lower teeth. Notice also the comparative incisal edge position. Moving the upper anterior teeth with this type of appliance has the effect of improving the smile line. **D,** This illustration shows why the lingual contours must be ground as the upper anterior teeth are moved in. If the hollow grinding is not done, the lingual movement is stopped by the lower teeth. The hollow ground area becomes the holding contact after the teeth are moved. Excursive function must be adjusted additionally. **E,** After completion of the orthodontic movement, the teeth can be prepared for a provisional acrylic bridge. It serves as an excellent retainer, is esthetic, and enables the patient to evaluate the new anterior guidance. Refinements can be made for function, phonetics, and esthetics, **F,** before fabrication of the permanent restorations. Notice centric relation contact (in **E**) on teeth that originally had a severe overjet problem.

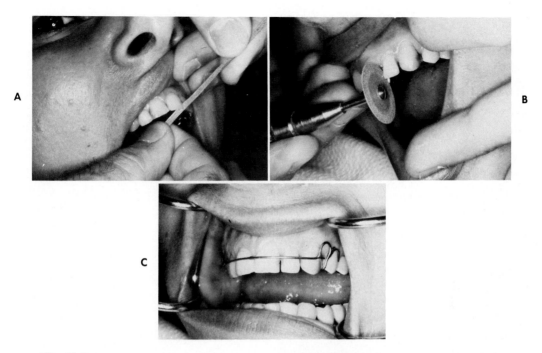

Fig. 32-3. **A,** When posterior occlusal relationships are acceptable, an anterior overjet problem can frequently be resolved when the upper anterior teeth are narrowed and then moved lingually. The narrowing procedure is started with a double-edged lightning strip. **B,** Thin separating disks can be used to narrow teeth. **C,** An activated labial arch wire on a simple removable appliance is used to move the teeth lingually. Lingual contours must be hollow ground as the teeth move.

bite plane prevents the lower teeth from interfering. The shaping should be done immediately after the appliance is removed.

When anterior contact has been established, the appliance can be modified to permit all the teeth to contact. The rubber band should then be replaced by a labial retainer wire to stabilize the teeth in their new position for a few weeks.

If the anterior teeth are to be restored, preparations can be made for making a provisional splint to serve as a retainer. The temporary splint can also be used to refine the anterior guidance and resolve any esthetic problems.

Reshaping the anterior teeth with restorations

Any time a major change is made in the shape of anterior teeth, it should be made first in temporary restorations. The changes should be worked out on mounted study models so that the result can be visualized before treatment is started. When the teeth are prepared and the preplanned temporary restorations are placed, the anterior guidance can be refined for minimal stress and optimum comfort. Modifications can be made to achieve the best esthetics and phonetics. Complete patient approval can be secured before the final restorations are fabricated.

The methods described in Chapter 31 are also applicable for patients with overjet problems. There are some special considerations, though, that should be noted:

1. Malposed teeth should not be restored until they have been moved into the best possible position (Fig. 32-4). "Warping" the labial surface of malposed teeth back into alignment can sometimes produce a round, very unnatural appearance. When the root goes one way and the crown goes another, the appearance is unpleasant and artificial. As far as practical, the root should be aligned to the restored crown. This also produces better stress direction.

2. The restored lingual contours should not be allowed to overprotect the gingival tissues. Sometimes our attempt to achieve centric contact results in too much lingual extension. If the contours are not compatible with main-

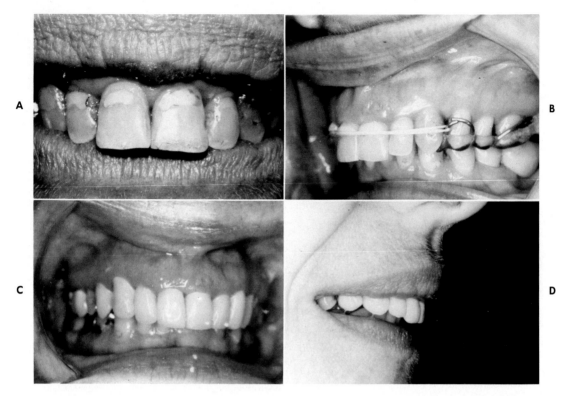

Fig. 32-4. Overjet problem that requires restorations, **A.** Position determines contour. Unless teeth are moved into better alignment first, restorations will be too round on labial surface. Both esthetics and function will be compromised. Movement back is controlled by acrylic stops on the lingual. Rubber band moves teeth to the stops, **B.** After positioning, teeth are stabilized for 3 to 4 months with a provisional splint. **C,** Splint is also used to work out final details of contour. Lip-closure path and esthetics are greatly improved. Permanent restorations copy details from provisionals, **D.**

tainable tissue health, they are not acceptable. Alternatives to centric contact will have to be considered.

3. We must be *certain* to provide sufficient "long centric." Some patients with excessive overjet develop a protruded "jaw set" to compensate for the malrelationship. It becomes such a definite part of their functional movements that any interference to it is annoying. Even though the "new look" is a great esthetic improvement, such patients may complain constantly that the upper anterior teeth have been "pulled in too far." Fortunately, such patients are in the definite minority, but the potential problem should always be considered. If the final restorations are not fabricated until the relationship has been approved in the temporary restoration, it is unlikely that such a problem will occur.

EQUILIBRATING THE OVERJET PROBLEM

Some patients with excessive overjet have anterior contact only in their protruded, acquired occlusal position. The following inquiry is often made: What will happen if I equilibrate such a patient and permit closure back into centric relation? The anterior contact in the acquired position would be lost. Wouldn't equilibration be contraindicated in such cases?

The answer has many facets to it. *Proper* equilibration is rarely contraindicated. If a patient is comfortable and has no sign of any problem or any potential for accelerated deterioration, there would be no reason to equilibrate. But as I have already pointed out, patients with malocclusion and no problems are rare. Patients with excessive overjet with occlusal interferences and no problems are *ex-*

tremely rare. We should correct any problem that has a damaging effect on the long-term health of the teeth and supporting structures. Each case demands clinical judgment in this regard.

Equilibrating such patients does not usually create a problem. Most often, what appears to be a long slide is really a minimal protrusive deviation. The difference between centric relation and centric occlusion is usually a fraction of a millimeter when the interferences are eliminated. If anterior contact occurred in the acquired position before equilibration, it has been my clinical experience that most patients will have enough contact in excursive function to maintain the position of the lower anterior teeth after equilibration.

If there has been any forward movement of the upper anterior teeth as a result of the protrusive deviation, lip pressures will probably bring the upper anterior teeth back in after the interferences are removed and the mandible stops deviating forward. Lower anterior teeth frequently erupt on into contact if arch relationships permit.

If loss of anterior contact does cause a problem as a result of equilibration, the problem is treated the same as any other overjet problem. The options for solving the problem are the same. However, if there was contact in acquired centric occlusion before equilibration, it should take a minimum of minor tooth movement to regain the contact in centric relation. Removable appliances can usually be used most effectively to solve the problem with very little difficulty.

SOLVING OVERJET PROBLEMS WHEN THERE IS INSUFFICIENT POSTERIOR ANCHORAGE

When upper anterior teeth have flared labially because of lost posterior tooth support, a twofold problem is created. There is a loss of vertical stops by the posterior teeth. This loss allows the lower anterior teeth to close too far on a forwardly directed arc; thus the lingual movement of the upper anterior teeth is blocked (Fig. 32-5). The problem is compounded by insufficient posterior anchorage for providing a stable base for moving the anterior teeth. Since movement of the anterior teeth is usually required to reposition them in a more favorable relationship, it is essential to find acceptable anchorage. There are four ways of accomplishing this, as follows.

Extraoral anchorage. The use of headgear provides sufficient anchorage, but for adult patients such headgear is usually unacceptable.

Intraoral tissue-supported base. A tissue-supported base with posterior teeth can provide the increased vertical to unlock the lower anterior teeth from upper lingual contact. But tissue support makes poor anchorage and often results in soft-tissue irritation from moving the base rather than the teeth. This problem can usually be solved by the application of pressure to move only one tooth at a time while the other anterior teeth are used as anchorage for the partial. Movement can be controlled by removal of acrylic material on the lingual of one tooth and waiting until that tooth is moved to contact it. Then some acrylic resin is removed on a different tooth. By alternating with one tooth at a time, we can make the fit of the partial base in the palatal vault serve as resistance without creating too much pressure on the soft tissues (Fig. 32-6). The higher the vault, the better this method works. Very flat ridges do not provide sufficient anchorage to utilize this method.

Implant anchorage. If there is sufficient bone in the posterior ridge areas to get an os-

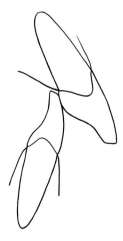

Fig. 32-5. Upper anterior overjet. Anterior teeth are flared out from lower incisor contact against the lingual slope of the cingulum. This problem frequently occurs from loss of posterior support. A special treatment problem is created because of loss of posterior tooth anchorage for moving the incisors back. The upper incisors are also blocked by the lower incisors.

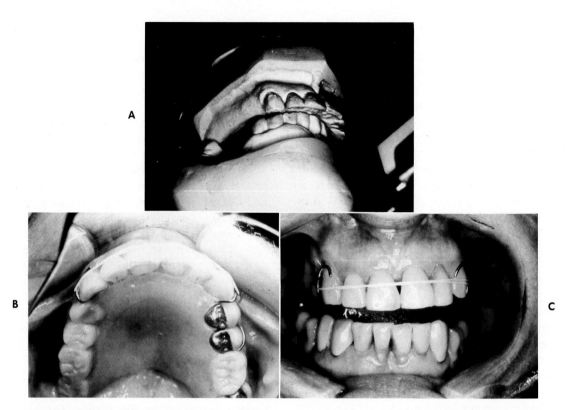

Fig. 32-6. Treatment series showing movement of one tooth at a time using palatal adaptation of partial as resistance in combination with two bicuspids. Anterior teeth that are not being moved also can serve as resistance to the one that is under pressure. By alternating from one tooth to another, one can eventually move all the anteriors back. **A,** Before treatment. **B,** Appliance in place. Only left lateral incisor is being moved during this stage. Notice how acrylic material has been removed on lingual side of that tooth only. **C,** Corrected alignment. Lingual surfaces had to be slightly recontoured to provide acceptable vertical stops for lower anterior teeth.

seointegrated implant on each side, the implants can serve as anchorage for moving the anterior teeth. It will still be necessary to open the vertical enough to disengage the lower anterior teeth from the upper lingual surfaces.

Anchorage from lower arch. If there is a sufficient number of lower posterior teeth, they may be banded for added stabilization and used as anchorage for elastics attached to the upper anterior teeth.

SURGICAL CORRECTION

In severe arch malrelationships, the treatment of choice may be orthognathic surgery. Before any surgical approach is selected, a careful evaluation should determine whether the overjet problem is the result of maxillary protrusion or is from mandibular retrusion, or is a combination of both. The rule to follow always is: Leave what is right; change only what is wrong.

Cephalometric analysis is a helpful diagnostic method, but it must be used in combination with neutral zone analysis and esthetic profile observation. Please read Chapters 38 and 39 for more information regarding cephalometric determinations and surgical methods for correcting severe arch malrelationships.

SUGGESTED READINGS

Burstone, C.J.: Lip posture and its significance in treatment planning, Am. J. Orthodont. **53:**262-284, 1967.

Geiger, A., and Hirschfeld, L.: Minor tooth movement in general practice, ed. 3, St. Louis, 1974, The C.V. Mosby Co.

Goldstein, M.C.: Orthodontics in crown and bridge and periodontal therapy, Dent. Clin. North Am., pp. 449-459, July 1964.

Graber, T.M.: Orthodontics, principles and practice, Philadelphia, 1962, W.B. Saunders Co.

Hinds, E.C., and Kent., J.N.: Surgical treatment of developmental jaw deformities, St. Louis, 1972, The C.V. Mosby Co.

MacIntosh, R.B.: Orthodontic surgery: comments on diagnostic modalities, J. Oral Surg. **28:**149-159, 1970.

Profit, W.R., and White, R.P.: Treatment of severe malocclusion by correlated orthodontic surgical procedures, Angle Orthodont. **40:**1-10, 1970.

Schwartz, A.M., and Gratzinger, M.: Removable orthodontic appliances, Philadelphia, 1966, W.B. Saunders Co.

33

Solving anterior open bite problems

Treatment planning for anterior open bites requires that the *cause* of the open bite be considered. If the cause of the separation is still an active factor, closure of the opening will be unsuccessful unless that factor can be altered along with the changes in occlusion.

An important decision that must be made in solving an anterior open bite problem is to determine whether it is really a problem that needs solving. Since many anterior open bite problems are the result of habit patterns, the habit must be eliminated or treatment must be planned to work with the habit if it is unbreakable.

The major causes of anterior open bite in order of probable frequency are as follows:
1. Forces that result from thumb or finger sucking, use of pacifiers.
2. Crowding. If anterior teeth are rotated forward off their basal bone, the forward inclination causes separation.
3. Airway obstruction:
   a. Inadequate nasal airway creating the need for an oral airway (mouth breather)
   b. Allergies
   c. Septum problems and blockage from turbinates
   d. Enlarged adenoids or tonsils
4. Lip and tongue habits.

5. Neurologic problems (such as cerebral palsy).
6. Skeletal growth abnormalities, probably resulting from the above problems as well as from pure skeletal growth asymmetries.

There are varying degrees of habit-caused anterior open bites. Since the degree of anterior separation is usually a clue to the habit that caused it, this is where the analysis should start. It should be understood that noticing the amount of anterior separation is, at best, empiric. It is not meant to be a precise criterion. Even such generalized evaluations, however, can serve as helpful starting points from which to evaluate the cause of problems and formulate practical treatment approaches.

MINIMAL ANTERIOR OPENING

An anterior separation of approximately 1 mm is usually caused by a lip-sucking habit. The patient develops a negative pressure and sucks the mucosal tissues between the front teeth. The *inner* part of the lower lip at or below the vermilion border is involved, and so the habit is not readily apparent.

This habit is usually developed as a protective device to avoid a posterior interference. Perfecting the posterior occlusion through selective grinding eliminates the *need* for the habit and it usually ceases after equilibration. When the habit is eliminated, the anterior teeth move into contact and no further treatment is needed.

The time required for the teeth to reposition themselves after the cause of the habit is eliminated varies. I have seen complete self-correction of the anterior relationship occur within 2 to 3 weeks, and in other patients it requires months. If the arch relationship permits anterior contact and there is nothing interposed between the teeth to prevent eruption, the lower anterior teeth will erupt and the upper anterior teeth will find their balance with lip pressures.

If the anterior teeth do not require restorations for other reasons, we must not get impatient if we do not see immediate results. We should keep the posterior occlusion refined as perfectly as possible and let nature take its course. Very few patients will fail to respond.

There will be some patients who will not break the lip-sucking habit regardless of how perfect the posterior occlusion is. We have no choice but to work around the habit, and this can be done very effectively.

If anterior teeth must be restored in the presence of an unbreakable habit, the restored surfaces must be positioned the same as the natural surfaces were. Some minor esthetic corrections can usually be made, but the labial and lingual surfaces must be positioned the same.

Preparing every other anterior tooth, as outlined in Chapter 18, is the most practical approach. By doing that, both labial and lingual contours can be duplicated according to the adjacent unprepared teeth. Incisal edge positions can be precisely duplicated, and the restored teeth will fit right into the position that the unbreakable habit pattern dictates.

When the habit prevents the anterior guidance from carrying out its disclusive functions, we must be sure that the working side can effectively disclude the nonfunctioning side and also be sure that protrusive disclusion is taken care of by the most forward teeth that can do it.

Many patients function comfortably with a slight anterior open bite. It is not an esthetic problem, and it usually does not interfere with function. What, if anything, we do about it depends on our appraisal of whether it is contributing to accelerated deterioration. If the mouth is healthy and maintainable, nothing needs to be done.

MODERATE ANTERIOR OPEN BITES (1 TO 5 MM SEPARATION)

If the arch relationship would permit anterior contact but there is a separation of approximately 1 to 5 mm, the cause of the problem is usually a tongue-thrust swallowing pattern, though lip-biting habits may also account for the separation.

It is rather surprising how forcefully the tongue can be thrust against the anterior teeth in swallowing. Some separations of little more than 1 mm may fool us because the separation between the upper and lower anterior teeth does not appear to provide sufficient room for interposing the tongue. However, close examination with the lips separated during a swallow will often demonstrate the tongue pressed so firmly against the lingual surfaces that a thin ridge of blanched tongue tissue can be seen wedged into the separation. Inward lip pressure apparently holds the upper anterior teeth in and prevents the separation from getting any worse.

Lip-biting habits may also produce a smaller separation than might be expected. Patients with very thin lips sometimes interpose the lower one between the teeth without causing the amount of separation that would normally be anticipated. It is usually a "protective" habit. The same habits may produce more severe open bite problems. A tongue thrust may open up the anterior teeth several millimeters and may extend around to include some of the posterior teeth as well. Not only does the character of the tongue thrust determine the extent and the amount of anterior opening, but also the shape and amount of the opening give us a clue to the type of tongue thrust. Purely on the basis of clinical experience, I know that some types of tongue-thrust malrelationships respond to treatment rather predictably whereas other types respond unfavorably. It pays to know the difference.

If habit patterns can be eliminated, separations of up to 5 mm or so can usually be corrected very effectively with minor tooth movement, or restorative procedures, or a combination of both. The prognosis is particularly good if posterior occlusal harmony is established along with the anterior correction. In some cases no treatment is required because the teeth are realigned by the changed lip and tongue posture.

We can easily diagnose separations caused by holding objects between the teeth by asking questions or by observing. Open spaces should not be closed unless the patient is willing to stop the habit. If a pipe stem is the cause of the separation, the separation should be duplicated in any restorations of the area if the patient plans to continue the pipe smoking. Pencil biting, nail holding, or other occupation-related habits should be treated similarly.

It should be determined whether a moderate anterior opening is really a problem. If the cuspid guidance is not disturbed by the separation of the incisors, the potential for stability of the occlusion is good. The occlusion should be checked carefully to make sure that there are no balancing-side interferences, and posterior teeth should be discluded in protrusion by the most forward teeth that can do the job. When posterior occlusal harmony is perfected, it is surprising how often the anterior opening closes down, but even if it does not, there will be no harm caused if the stresses can be distributed over most of the posterior teeth.

SEVERE ANTERIOR OPEN BITES (5 MM OR GREATER SEPARATION)

Although it appears certain that abnormal deglutition and other tongue-thrust patterns play some role in all severe anterior open bites, it is also apparent that in most instances there is a vertical dysplasia within the bone system itself. In many anterior open bites, the anterior teeth are actually supraerupted in their unsuccessful attempt to close the open space. It is doubtful that such supraeruption would result from a depressive type of tongue habit. We must differentiate between such skeletal malrelationships and those that were caused primarily by habits that have depressed the anterior teeth.

Very often, severe open bite problems are the result of habits that were caused by other habits. The anterior open bite that results from a thumb-sucking habit is often perpetuated by a tongue-thrust swallowing habit. The tongue thrust results from an attempt to seal off the anterior opening to develop the negative pressure for the swallow.

Combining occlusal correction with myofunctional therapy has the capability of solving the problem if the patient can cooperate, but it has an uncertain prognosis because it is difficult to predict patient cooperation in changing such a set swallowing pattern. Nevertheless, it should be tried if there is no need for immediacy.

If the problem is habit caused, orthodontic procedures can almost always be used successfully to realign the anterior teeth. The only problem is keeping them there after they are moved.

Solving the problem of achieving a stable anterior relationship may require a three-pronged attack:

1. Orthodontic correction of anterior tooth relationships
2. Myofunctional therapy to eliminate tongue or lip habits
3. Occlusal equilibration to eliminate the need for protective tongue or lip habits

If this combination of procedures does not produce the desired occlusal stability, a fourth procedure may be necessary. Splinting may be required to hold the anterior teeth in their corrected position. Unless anterior restorations are required for other reasons, however, permanent splinting should not be considered until it has been positively determined that it is needed. Stabilization by removable retainers should be tried first. After a suitable time for reorganization of the supporting tissues, the retainer should be removed a day at a time. If no tooth movement occurs, it should be left out for gradually longer periods. Splinting should be considered only as a last resort when maintainable stability cannot be achieved without it. Then it should be used with careful discretion. Even splinted teeth can be moved out of alignment if a strong habit pattern is still present.

If the tongue habit resulted from an initial thumb-sucking habit, the prognosis is better than if the anterior open bite is hereditary. Our success record in correcting anterior tooth position in hereditary skeletal anterior open bites is poor, but the potential for achieving stability of the dentition is good, even without complete correction of the anterior position.

Severe anterior open bite relationships present the following problems:

1. There is poor anterior esthetics. This is often the only reason the patient seeks help.
2. The anterior guidance cannot do its job. Posterior disclusion in protrusive and

balancing excursions cannot be accomplished by the anterior teeth.

3. The posterior teeth are overstressed. The teeth nearest the condylar fulcrum usually receive the greatest stress with no help from the anterior teeth.

With no anterior guidance, elevator muscle hyperactivity is increased, and so the potential for overload on the contacting molars is increased. However, if the teeth that do contact in centric relation can be made to simultaneously contact on both sides with equal intensity, there does not seem to be a problem with maintaining them in a stable relationship. The vertical contracted length of elevator muscles establishes a set dimension between the mandible and the maxilla at the position of the muscle origin or attachment. The teeth erupt into that set space until they meet an opposing force equal to the eruptive force. If the tongue takes up part of that space, it becomes the stop for eruption. It does not appear that the teeth that contact opposing teeth receive any more load than the teeth that contact the tongue.

I have followed several patients with anterior open bite for many years, and if the contacting teeth are adjusted for equal-intensity loading against vertically directed stops, these dentitions stay just as stable as those with full occlusal contact.

Before treatment is initiated, we should determine whether the anterior open bite is the result of a skeletal malrelationship. Cephalometric evaluation can be used to determine whether the problem is skeletal or is the direct result of habit-caused depression of the anterior teeth. If the skeletal relationship is good and the tongue habit is generally limited to protrusive thrusting, the prognosis is good for realigning the anterior teeth.

If a skeletal relationship is the primary cause of the anterior open bite and the skeletal bone is too far separated to permit correction within the dentoalveolar process, the prognosis for realigning the anterior teeth conservatively is poor. But if the tongue thrust is limited to *protrusive* thrusting, the potential for achieving good stability of the entire dentition is excellent. The nonsurgical treatment of choice for this specific problem is to close the vertical dimension by reduction of the height of the posterior teeth. This can be done by selective grinding or by orthodontic intrusion.

The greater the reduction of posterior tooth height, the greater will be the reduction of the anterior opening. In most cases, the posterior teeth can be shortened enough to bring the cuspids into contact. The distribution of stresses on to more teeth can usually be further improved by reshaping of the centric contacts at the closed vertical (Fig. 33-1) and establishment of working-side group function for disclusion of the balancing inclines. If such reshaping exposes dentin, cast restorations should be placed to protect the occlusal surfaces.

The closure of the anterior opening that results from the decreased vertical dimension produces a greatly improved appearance. Even though the space may not be completely closed, any reduction of the anterior opening results in a noticeable esthetic improvement that is gratifying to the patient.

Even though the closed vertical appears stable, there is growing evidence that the actual mandible-to-maxilla relationship does not stay at the new closed dimension. It appears that elongation of the alveolar bone matches the amount of tooth reduction so that the loss of vertical is temporary. Unless, however, the tongue is interposed back between the arches after correction, the corrected occlusal relationship will stay surprisingly stable, and the increased dimension of alveolar bone will go unnoticed.

The preceding results are achievable in skeletal malrelationships if the tongue thrust is primarily a protrusive thrust. The tongue seems to readily adapt to the closed vertical without disrupting the changed alignment. The protrusive thrust in this type of problem was not the cause of the opened bite, and so it can easily conform to a more closed relationship.

If the protrusive tongue habit also includes a *lateral* tongue thrust, however, the prospects for stable correction by closing the vertical are practically nonexistent. This is true regardless of whether the lateral tongue thrust occurs with or without a skeletal malrelationship.

TREATING PROTRUSIVE LATERAL TONGUE THRUST PROBLEMS

In a protrusive lateral tongue thrust, the tongue is spread out and held between all the anterior and posterior teeth except the most distal teeth on each side (Fig. 33-2). Often the only teeth in contact are the second or third molars. Unlike the straight protrusive tongue

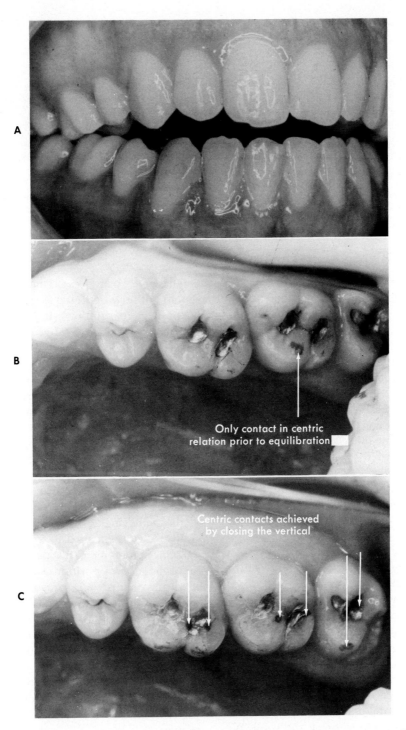

Fig. 33-1. **A,** Anterior open bite. Relationships in which the opening increases progressively toward the anterior teeth can almost always be stabilized when the vertical dimension is closed to bring more posterior teeth into centric contact. **B,** In anterior open bite relationships, it is not uncommon to have centric relation contact on only one tooth on each side. Posterior teeth that are stressed in this manner frequently become hypermobile and develop periodontitis. **C,** Closure of the vertical dimension permits more teeth to come into centric relation contact, the stresses are better distributed, the anterior teeth can come closer together, and the result is routinely quite stable.

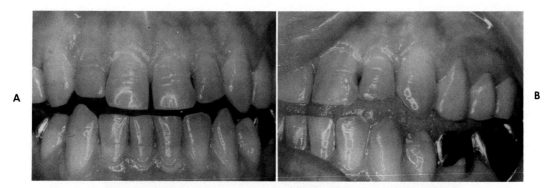

Fig. 33-2. **A,** Anterior open bite that has same amount of separation on posterior teeth as it does on anterior teeth. The only teeth in contact are the last molars on each side. **B,** Tongue position during swallowing. Tongue is thrust laterally as well as protrusively. Closure of the vertical dimension to obtain contact on more teeth usually fails because the tongue habit recurs.

thrust with its progressively much larger anterior opening, the lateral tongue habit usually produces a fairly even separation of all the noncontacting teeth. Although it usually occurs with a slightly prognathic mandible, it can occur with any arch relationship.

Correction of the occlusal separation *appears* very simple. Shortening one or two opposing teeth on each side that have contact usually closes the vertical dimension enough to bring most of the other teeth into contact. If the arch relationship permits, the occlusion may sometimes be corrected by selective grinding at the closed vertical dimension. Most often, though, occlusal reconstruction would be necessary to provide cusp-fossa relationships with stable form.

When full occlusion is restored to a patient with lateral tongue thrust, the patient will be comfortable, will function well, and will generally be pleased with the good result. There is only one big problem: the good occlusal relationship will almost never stay that way. Unless that lateral tongue habit can be broken, the original separation will recur. I have found it virtually impossible to permanently break severe lateral tongue habits if the anterior teeth were included in the open bite separation.

It is not impossible to break the habit. We have actually achieved occlusal contact on previously separated teeth with no treatment other than retraining the patient to swallow properly. Results have been achieved for up to a year and slightly longer. Eventually the pattern returns and the separation recurs without the patient even being aware of it. It should be

emphasized that our clinical experience should not be interpreted as meaning there are no permanent solutions. It is just honest reporting that we have not been able to maintain long-term occlusal contact with any method we have used up to now. Myofunctional techniques have not provided the answer.

Just because we cannot predict long-term maintenance of occlusal contact does not mean we cannot achieve an acceptable degree of occlusal stability. By working with the habit, we can let the tongue stay interposed between the teeth and can improve the occlusion of the teeth that do contact, so that stress direction is made as ideal as possible on the occluding teeth. Achieving a harmony between tooth contact may seem hard to imagine, but it can be achieved rather easily because the tongue serves as its own positioner. The teeth merely adapt to whatever pressures it provides.

It is a mystery how patients with so little occlusal contact can function, but it does not seem to be a problem as far as they are concerned. Patients can maintain comfort, function, and a surprising degree of stability *with* the protrusive lateral tongue-thrust habit. Before attempting to correct such a relationship, we must be certain there is a real need for change.

There is no way for the noncontacting anterior teeth to provide any anterior guidance, but this is not a problem because protrusive lateral tongue thrusters are usually vertical "chop- choppers." They do not as a rule protrude the mandible or use lateral jaw movements.

Lateral stresses on the contacting posterior teeth should be minimized as much as possible by flattening of cusp inclines.

If a patient with protrusive tongue thrust requires extensive restoration of the posterior teeth because of caries or general breakdown of existing restorations, there may be nothing wrong with making an attempt at occlusal correction in the new restoration. A relapse of the corrected occlusion does not seem to cause any discomfort or injury, and so it may be worth the try. I would, however, draw the line at restoring occlusions to contact that had no other reason to be restored, unless there was positive evidence that the habit could be eliminated and that the restorative procedures were needed to preserve the remaining teeth.

The more predictive approach to treatment, however, is to first determine if the occlusion is stable by checking for signs of hypermobility or change of tooth position. If there is no instability problem, we can restore the occlusal surfaces to the same relationship with the tongue by preparing every other posterior tooth and taking an impression before completing the rest of the preparations. The resulting cast can be used to guide the technician to the precisely correct contours, and the stable relationship with the tongue can remain unchanged.

PROGRESSIVE ANTERIOR SEPARATION

Adult patients who develop progressive anterior open bites (Fig. 33-3) should be observed very carefully for indications of rheumatoid arthritis. The diagnosis is easily made because rarely is this systemic disease ever confined to a single joint. Deformity of other joints is usually obvious. The fingers are most often involved (Fig. 33-4).

The deformity of the temporomandibular joints that occurs in rheumatoid arthritis may cause a separation of the anterior teeth, and the separation may continue to enlarge as the deterioration of the joints progresses.

Attempts to restore or reposition the anterior teeth back to contact are contraindicated. The patient should be kept comfortable by maintenance of the best possible occlusal relationship on the teeth that contact. Selective grinding can usually be used to eliminate any deflective contacts and to reshape any interfering inclines.

If a pain-dysfunction syndrome should develop in a patient with rheumatoid arthritis,

the degree of joint deformity will have no effect on the resolution of the pain aspects of the syndrome. with rare exceptions, these patients respond just as quickly and just as predictably to occlusal therapy as patients with normal joints.

Even though the disk is destroyed in the rheumatoid joint, there can still be a bone-to-bone stop for the condyle that does not require lateral pterygoid muscle resistance to the elevator muscles. Although the nature of this uppermost position is tenuous, patients can be kept reasonably free of muscle pain in the joint region by correction of occlusal interferences on the posterior teeth that strike.

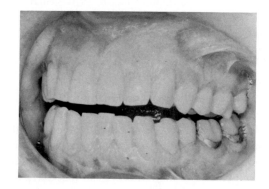

Fig. 33-3. A progressively occurring anterior open bite. Any occlusal relationship that starts to open in front in later years should be evaluated for rheumatoid arthritis. Since the disease rarely affects a single joint, observation of the hands will usually show deformity of the finger joints also. Patients with rheumatoid arthritis can usually be kept fairly comfortable in the temporomandibular joint region by equilibration of the posterior teeth that contact to direct the stresses as favorably as possible. No attempt should be made to close the anterior teeth back to the original relationship.

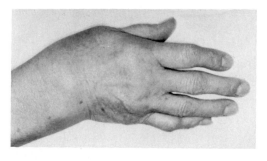

Fig. 33-4. Swollen knuckles typical of rheumatoid arthritis.

ABNORMAL TONGUE SIZES

If an abnormally large tongue is responsible for the open bite, no amount of occlusal reconstruction or myofunctional therapy will be able to achieve maintainable occlusal contact. It should not be attempted. Restoration of the occlusal surfaces, when needed, should follow an occlusal plane that is in harmony with the existing tooth position if that position has achieved stability.

Correction of irregularities in cusp height, marginal ridges, and so on can be accomplished without upsetting the balance between the tongue and the teeth if the overall plane of occlusion is maintained as it was. If any major changes in the occlusal plane should be necessary, tongue position should be evaluated and considered as a definite factor. Provisional restorations should be used to verify comfort and function before the restorations are finalized.

ORTHODONTIC CORRECTION OF ANTERIOR OPEN BITES

It appears that conventional intraoral orthodontic techniques would be successful only in patients who have tooth derangements without a severe skeletal malrelationship. If the morphology of the mandible itself must be changed, it appears rather logical that extraoral orthopedic appliances would be needed. Graber has pointed out that such orthopedic appliances can effect a change in a relatively short period of time *if the treatment is accomplished during a period of fairly rapid growth.*

Dentists have the obligation to their young patients to notice any open bite tendencies because of such skeletal malrelationships. Patients should be referred for orthodontic evaluation early enough for the orthodontists to take advantage of the growth periods.

In adult patients, it is easier to shorten teeth than to depress them. Shortening a second molar 1 mm produces as much as 3 mm of anterior closure; so the best approach for resolving severe anterior open bite problems appears to be a combined effort between the restorative dentist and the orthodontist.

The vertical dimension should be closed as much as possible by reduction of the height of the posterior teeth. Severe shortening will require restoration of the occlusion. There should be orthodontic alignment of the anterior teeth into the best relationship possible after they have been brought as close together as possible by the vertical closure.

Surgical correction of anterior open bite problems has become more and more a logical choice of treatment. Very often the correction can be done better and faster by surgery, and the facial profile may be improved at the same time.

Surgical correction is discussed in more detail in Chapter 39.

34

Treating end-to-end occlusions

An end-to-end occlusion may occur as an *anterior* end-to-end occlusion, a *posterior* end-to-end occlusion, or a combination of both.

An occlusal relationship is end to end if the incisal edges of the lower anterior teeth are aligned with the incisal edges of the upper teeth, or if lower buccal cusps are aligned with upper buccal cusps, when the mandible is in centric relation at the correct occlusal vertical dimension.

In anterior end-to-end relationships the mandible cannot be protruded without loading all the stresses onto the posterior teeth. The anterior guidance is lost as soon as the lower incisors move forward of their upper tooth contacts. *In posterior end-to-end relationships* the normal working inclines do not contact, and so posterior working inclines may not provide the necessary guidance needed to disengage the balancing side.

In the analysis of end-to-end anterior relationships it is important to determine whether the end-to-end alignment is the result of a skeletal relationship or of severe anterior wear. In a *skeletal* end-to-end relationship the usual requirements of posterior disclusion are minimized because most such patients have vertical functional patterns. They rarely use protrusive movements past the point of anterior contact, and their lateral movements are similarly restricted. From the time of tooth eruption,

functional contact of the opposing arches is limited to a narrow range of horizontal movement, and so lateral stresses against posterior teeth are not generally a problem. Furthermore, if all posterior teeth are end to end, the balancing *inclines* cannot come into contact unless the occlusal plane is incorrect.

Severe wear problems must be treated differently from skeletal end-to-end relationships. If the anterior end-to-end relationship is the result of severe wear, the treatment approach must assume that there is a definite horizontal pattern of function, and the occlusion must be altered to provide disclusion of the posterior teeth in all excursive movements whenever possible. If the anterior guidance cannot disclude nonfunctioning side inclines, the posterior teeth on the working side must be designed to accomplish the disclusion.

If a complete end-to-end occlusion is stable and comfortable and if periodontal support is intact, there is no reason to change it. If any occlusal interferences are noted in such an occlusion, they can be corrected by selective grinding without disturbing the envelope of function and without a normal potential for introducing any problems.

In posterior cusp tip–to–cusp tip relationships, centric relation interferences should be relieved by flattening of the upper cusp tip and, if needed, selective shaping of the lower

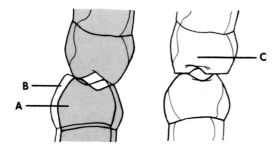

Fig. 34-1. In end-to-end posterior relationships, deviation from a tip-to-tip centric relation contact, *A*, to a more closed deviated centric occlusion, *B*, is equilibrated by flattening the upper cusp tips, *C*. Selective grinding done in this manner eliminates the deviation while providing a more stable centric relation holding contact. Such relationships are usually discluded in all excursions.

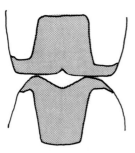

Fig. 34-2. Lower cusp tip to upper flat surface. This type of end-to-end relationship can provide good stability as long as lateral function contact is not needed.

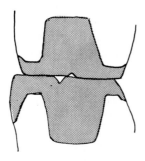

Fig. 34-3. Flat occlusal contours shown diagrammatically. The occlusal contours can be made quite functional and natural appearing by properly placed grooves and ridges carved into the occlusal surfaces.

cusp tip (Fig. 34-1). *The goal is to provide as much stability as possible in centric relation and as much relief as possible in excursions.*

When a lower cusp tip is positioned against an upper surface that is flat, the downward movement of the orbiting condyle is sufficient to disclude the balancing side, even in the presence of a horizontal anterior guidance and a flat working side, if the occlusal plane is correct. Since the teeth in end-to-end relationships are usually in rather good balance with the tongue and cheeks and the direction of force is favorable for both upper and lower teeth, a cusp tip–to–flat surface relationship is quite stable.

If the posterior teeth must be restored, the same decision regarding contour may be made. We have several options for restorative contouring of posterior end-to-end relationships. Which type of occlusal form is selected should depend to a large degree on the answer to the following question: *Can the anterior guidance function as discluder of protrusive and balancing inclines?* In the presence of a functioning anterior guidance, flat occlusal morphology can be used. Stable centric stops can be provided in several ways. Each type should be evaluated from several standpoints.

Lower cusp tip to upper flat surface (Fig. 34-2). This relationship can provide almost normal lower posterior occlusal form, with slight modifications to flatten and broaden upper cusp tips to serve as stops for the more rounded lower cusps. Enough overjet can be provided to hold the cheek away from the contacts. This type of occlusal form is adequate as long as the teeth are positioned in harmony with the checks and tongue and as long as posterior discluion is permissible in all eccentric positions.

Flat occlusal contours (Fig. 34-3). Beautiful occlusal form can be provided that is very stable by use of relative flat occlusal contours. Stresses are reduced by proper contouring of grooves and sluiceways. The surfaces can function as grinders that are capable of mangling the food even though they are discluded in eccentric positions. The lower buccal contours can be recessed enough to provide sufficient overjet to hold the cheeks out of the way. Upper lingual contours can be recessed slightly to avoid pinching of the tongue.

Warped posterior contours. The practice of "warping" posterior contours to move

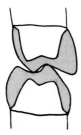

Fig. 34-4. Warped posterior contours. Notice the end-to-end relationship of the preparations. Warping can usually be achieved with this relationship as long as the forces are directed up and down the long axes and as long as the gingival tissues are not overprotected by extreme changes in gingival third contours. Correctly warped contours do permit excursive functional contact.

lower cusps in and upper cusps out (Fig. 34-4) is probably overdone. It often results in stresses that are directed off the long axis. It is done in an attempt to position cusp tips into fossae, but *if stability can be achieved in other ways, there is no need to place cusp tips in fossae if the fossae inclines are not needed in lateral excursive contact.* In normal arch relationships, cusp tip–to–fossa contact is a natural, practical way to achieve stability, but directing the forces off the long axis just to reproduce textbook anatomy is not practical. Rather than thinking in terms of preconceived ideas of *contours,* it is wise to develop concepts of stress *direction* and then locate the directional contacts in a manner that provides the best possibilities for stability. Every occlusal contour should be evaluated in this manner, and this is particularly so when arch relationships are not ideal.

In posterior end-to-end relationships, if it is possible to warp a lower cusp in lingually to an improved fossa location, stress direction can usually be maintained through the long axis of both upper and lower teeth. But warping upper cusps out buccally is usually stress producing. Warping is not practical if it creates buccal or lingual contours that overprotect the gingival margins.

Warping of the buccal or lingual contours may also create a latent problem of stability that is often overlooked in treatment planning. Particularly in patients with strong tongue or buccinator pressures, such contour alterations result in nonconformity to a limited neutral zone. The result is a continuous horizontal migration of the restored teeth until their posi-

tion between the opposing muscular forces is neutralized. For this reason, it is not uncommon for posterior teeth that have been restored with warped contours to require multiple occlusal adjustments after insertion of the restorations. This phenomenon is most noticeable in the molar region where the wider, stronger part of the tongue versus the stronger part of the buccinator muscle creates a firm pressure against any tooth surface that is extended outside its neutral zone position.

Warping cusp tips and repositioning fossae is good restorative technique if it can be accomplished within limits of correct stress directioning, adequate stability, and contouring for tissue maintenance.

UNILATERAL END-TO-END RELATIONSHIPS

If one side of the arch is in an end-to-end relationship but the other side is in a cusp-fossa relationship, there is a definite potential for causing harm to the side that occludes correctly.

The correctly occluding side is capable of discluding the balancing inclines on the end-to-end side, but the end-to-end side has no fossa wall contact to disclude the opposite balancing inclines of the intercuspated teeth. If the anterior teeth are in end-to-end relationships also, they are not capable of providing the lift that is needed to disengage the balancing inclines of the intercuspated side either. There are at least three practical solutions for unilateral end-to-end problems:

Orthodontics. Repositioning the end-to-end side into a correct intercuspation will enable it to assume the job of discluding the opposite-side balancing inclines.

Flattening of the balancing inclines on the intercuspated side. If the balancing inclines are made flat enough, they will be discluded by even a horizontal working-side pathway. The downward path of the orbiting condyle will help in the disclusive effort.

Even an end-to-end relationship of the anterior teeth can serve quite well as a lateral anterior guidance because the lower incisors maintain contact as they pass laterally across the upper incisal edges. The distance traveled in anterior contact is enough to disclude flattened balancing inclines. When end-to-end cuspids disengage laterally, the incisors are still in contact. This is sufficient to protect the posterior teeth from balancing-side interferences if the balancing inclines are made flat enough and the occlusal plane is correct.

Working inclines should normally be flattened also, just to provide symmetry of function. As long as all balancing inclines are discluded, however, it is not imperative that working-side inclines be the same on both sides.

Centralization of the lower cusps. By converging the lower buccal and lingual cusps into single centralized cusps, it is practical to place them in the central fossae of the upper teeth (Fig. 34-5). Stress direction is ideal for both upper and lower teeth and function is excellent. With centralized lower cusps, the upper working inclines can be used to disclude the balancing inclines on the opposite side, and it can be accomplished within the limits of the normal neutral zone.

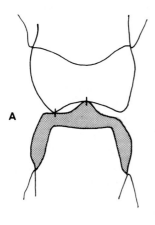

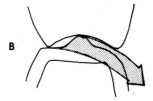

Fig. 34-5. Centralized lower cusps. Posterior end-to-end occlusions that require contact in working excursions can be achieved when the lower occlusal form is contoured into centralized cusps. The direction of force is ideal, and centric contact can even by provided for the upper lingual cusps as shown in **A.** Although the contour is not "normal," it is quite acceptable esthetically if supplemental occlusal anatomy is carved thoughtfully. Patients are routinely quite pleased with the functional efficiency. **B** illustrates the working-side functional contact that can be achieved.

Even though it is a departure from normal occlusal anatomy, lower centralized cusps are an innovative way to solve unilateral end-to-end problems. There are no real disadvantages to the procedure, and even the esthetic difference from normal contours is not noticeable. It permits normal buccal and lingual contours at the gingival level for both upper and lower teeth, and the stress direction can be made so ideal that stability is usually not a problem.

The alternative of warping cusps and relocating fossae works fine if the arch relationship is *slightly* off line, but a true end-to-end occlusion requires too much warping to consider it as a practical approach. The resultant stress directions are too unfavorable.

RESTORING END-TO-END ANTERIOR TEETH

If restorations are a necessity on end-to-end anterior teeth, their anterior guidance function can be improved greatly with subtle changes in contours.

Minimal changes in incisal edge position can effect gross improvements in anterior function. Moving the upper incisal edges forward and the lower incisal edges inward can extend the protrusive contact by a couple of millimeters or more (Fig. 34-6). In combination with the downward movement of the protruding condyles, this 2 to 3 mm of added anterior guidance should be sufficient to disclude the posterior teeth if the posterior occlusal form is correspondingly contoured to be discluded by a flat anterior guidance.

A strong warning should be noted here against steepening end-to-end anterior guidance angles. The guidance should remain nearly flat. Improvement should be made in the form of *extending* anterior guidance contact, not steepening it. Most dentists are surprised to find how effective a perfectly flat anterior guidance can be, but even a horizontal zero-degree guidance can fulfill all the disclusive needs of the posterior teeth if occlusal contours are also kept flat enough and the occlusal plane is correct.

Restorative recontouring of teeth in an end-to-end bite can cause special problems if the stresses are moved off the direction of the long axis. In a long-standing end-to-end relationship, the stresses are so confined to the long axis that the periodontal fibers and the bone trabeculas are not aligned to resist lateral stress. Suddenly changing a tooth's contour to subject it to lateral forces may produce unwanted effects of tenderness or hypermobility until the fibers realign and the bone gets more resistant to the lateral forces. Great care should be taken to avoid contours that will direct the stresses off the long axis. If it is absolutely essential to restore an incisal edge off the long axis too far, it may be necessary to stabilize the tooth in that position by splinting. Fortunately, this is a rare requirement because in most cases it would be better to orthodontically move the tooth rather than restore it to a stressful contour.

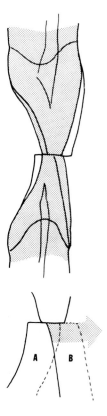

Fig. 34-6. Anterior end-to-end, *shaded,* relationships do not generally present a difficult problem. Notice how little change is needed to provide a flat anterior guidance of several millimeters. In addition to the added protrusive contact *(arrow in lower illustration),* the anterior contact can also be maintained until the lingual incisal line angle of the lower reaches the labioincisal line angle of the upper. Position *A* represents centric relation. Position *B* represents the most protruded relationship possible without los of anterior contact. The changes in incisal edge relationship can be accomplished either restoratively or orthodontically, depending on individual factors in each case.

End-to-end relationships with extreme wear

When anterior teeth have undergone extreme wear, an end-to-end relationship presents a special problem. This is especially true if the wear has penetrated near pulpal exposures on both upper and lower anterior teeth.

The worn incisal edges must be covered with a thickness of restorative metal or porcelain, or both, but the teeth cannot be reduced further without exposure of the pulps. The choice that must be made is between increasing the vertical dimension or endodontically treating the teeth and maintaining the vertical dimension.

Since eruption of the teeth and vertical growth of the alveolar bone do not normally allow loss of vertical dimension, even in extreme wear situations, the addition of restorative materials over the incisal edges must be considered as an *increased* vertical dimension. In end-to-end problems like the preceding, however, increasing the vertical dimension is usually the lesser of evils. When it can be done without too much disruption of muscle balance, it is a better choice of treatment than multiple root canals.

CAUTION: The vertical dimension should be increased no more than is necessary to provide room for the restorative materials on the incisal edges. A 1½ mm increase should usually provide the needed space. As with any increase in vertical dimension, the occlusion should be checked periodically for several months after the restorations are placed.

Special considerations

An end-to-end occlusion is very often treated as a malocclusion simply because it does not conform to the requirements of a Class I relationship. That is not an acceptable reason for altering any occlusion. Instead, the decision to alter the occlusal relationship should be based on a careful evaluation of the following factors.

Stability. Whether an end-to-end occlusion is stable depends principally on two factors:
1. Harmony with the neutral zone
2. Noninterference with the envelope of function

Harmony with the neutral zone can occur with a variety of tooth-to-tooth relationships because strong tongue, cheek, and lip pres-

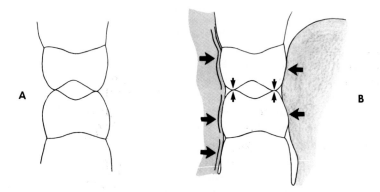

Fig. 34-7. Stability is not totally dependent on cusp-fossa alignment. End-to-end posterior teeth, **A,** may be stable if they have enough stops at the correct vertical dimension to prevent eruption and if they are in horizontal stability with the neutral zone, **B.**

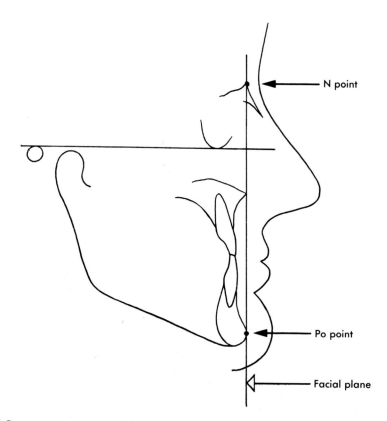

Fig. 34-8. End-to-end relationship of incisors occurs posterior to the facial plane indicating a bimaxillary deficiency. Thicker than normal soft tissue and deep cleft indicate a strong perioral muscle pressure against the anterior teeth. This would normally mean a strong stabilizing influence from the neutral zone where the teeth are now. This type of relationship also occurs with a small orifice.

sures can stabilize teeth just as effectively as perfected intercuspal relationships (Fig. 34-7). In fact, neutral zone conformance is more important to stability than the intercuspal alignment because there is no intercuspal relationship that will remain stable if it is not in harmony with muscular forces.

Occlusal analysis on end-to-end relationships is incomplete unless it includes a careful search for specific signs of instability. If there is no evidence of hypermobility, excessive wear, or migration of teeth, the end-to-end relationship can be considered stable from an occlusal perspective. This stability would not occur with nonconformity to *either* the neutral zone or the envelope of function.

Function. It is rare for a patient with a *stable* end-to-end relationship to complain of inadequate function. I know of almost no instances when such patients even complained of any degree of impairment in function. If there is a sufficient number of stable holding contacts that are coordinated with centric relation, loss of function does not appear to be a problem for the patient with an end-to-end occlusion.

Esthetics. The irony of an anterior end-to-end occlusion is that although many dentists believe it should be "corrected" most patients believe it is the *ideal* relationship. I have had many patients with a normal overbite relationship complain that their teeth were not "correctly" aligned end to end. But I do not remember a single patient with skeletal end-to-end occlusion ever complaining that he wanted his teeth to overlap. In the absence of noxious habit patterns that destroy the incisal plane relationship, an anterior end-to-end occlusion often results in a beautiful smile. It rarely needs to be altered for esthetic reasons.

Skeletofacial profile. There can be several different causes of anterior end-to-end relationships. The effect on facial profile is often a major consideration, and in a notable percentage of patients who seek treatment the chief complaint is more likely to be related to facial profile than it is to the actual occlusal relationship.

Evaluation of skeletofacial profile problems requires cephalometric analysis as well as mounted diagnostic casts. The purpose of the cephalometric evaluation is to determine whether the end-to-end relationship is caused by an underdeveloped maxilla or an overdeveloped mandible, or some combination of both. We can rather easily make this decision by observing the relationship of both arches to one or more of the standard facial planes that can be plotted on a lateral cephalometric radiograph.

The use of McNamara's plane provides an easily used reference for this determination (see Chapter 38).

Neutral zone. If an end-to-end relationship occurs posterior to the facial plane or the McNamara plane, it results in a "pushed-in" appearance as a manifestation of bimaxillary deficiency (Fig. 34-8). This type of occlusal relationship should be treated with caution because it is usually accompanied by a very strong buccinator–orbicularis oris limitation on arch size. If muscular limitation is a factor in restricting arch size, the soft-tissue thickness as shown on the cephalometric radiograph will be greater than normal, especially in the lower lip. If this is observed, any attempts at advancement of maxillary or mandibular segments should be preceded by an analysis of the musculature and possible alteration of the position or length of the muscle itself.

If an end-to-end relationship occurs anterior to the McNamara plane, it indicates a bimaxillary protrusion. In some patients, this procumbency creates a very attractive facial profile, especially when combined with high cheek bones. This relationship probably never occurs in combination with a strong or restrictive buccinator–orbicularis oris complex. Examination of soft-tissue thickness on the lateral cephalometric radiograph will normally reveal a thinner than normal dimension. If surgical correction of either arch length is considered, it should be planned to achieve the best profile. This can normally be accomplished with a predictably good prognosis because there is rarely a conflict with the neutral zone. The exception is evidenced by the finding of an oversized tongue, but this does not usually occur in end-to-end occlusions that have anterior tooth contact in centric relation.

35

Treating splayed anterior teeth

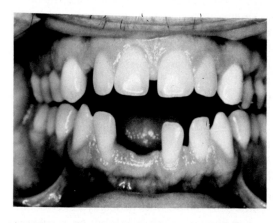

Fig. 35-1. Splayed anterior teeth result from strong pressure from an oversized tongue.

Splayed anterior teeth are those that incline outwardly from strong tongue pressure. The labial inclination results in spaces between the teeth (Fig. 35-1). The condition may or may not be accompanied by a loss of periodontal support. Successful treatment of splayed anterior teeth requires a careful analysis of the relationship of the splayed teeth to the neutral zone.

SPLAYED LOWER ANTERIOR TEETH

It is a relatively simple process to close open spaces by moving lower anterior teeth into a more lingually positioned arch form, but

experience has shown that this too frequently results in an unstable relationship. There are three potential reasons for the instability:

1. Nonconformity with the neutral zone
2. Loss of holding contacts against the upper teeth
3. Loss of anterior guidance for disclusion of the posterior teeth.

Conforming with the neutral zone. It is not uncommon to find lower anterior teeth with no sign of hypermobility even though they are severely splayed and have no proximal contact with adjacent teeth. In the absence of hypermobility or migration, such teeth can be considered to be in perfect conformity with the neutral zone between tongue and lip pressures. Unless there are some overriding reasons for altering the arch form, any restorative or orthodontic treatment should maintain the existing curvature of the arch. It is completely acceptable to close spaces between the teeth either restoratively or by lateral movement within the arch form. The best esthetics is usually achieved by a combination of lateral tooth movement to improve spacing, combined with restorative procedures for reshaping teeth or adding pontics if the space requires (Fig. 35-2). As with any other alteration of anterior teeth, provisional restorations should be used to determine and verify the correct incisal edge positions before comple-

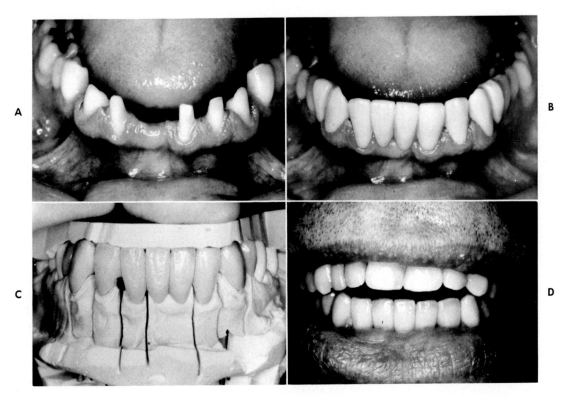

Fig. 35-2. A, Lower teeth are prepared. **B,** Provisional splint is made to copy diagnostic waxup. Waxup maintains the position of all the teeth within the same neutral zone corridor that was established by the strong tongue position. Final adjustments are made in the mouth. **C,** An index is made using firm putty silicone to copy a cast of the corrected provisional splint in the mouth. This shows the relationship of the finished restorations to the index. **D,** Finished restorations. Anterior open bite is maintained along with neutral zone position for all the anterior teeth to conform to strong forward tongue posture.

tion of the final restorative treatment. Spacing requirements should be worked out on mounted casts before we initiate any orthodontic procedures, and a full waxup should be completed. It is often necessary to add an extra incisor to maintain normal tooth size.

Bonding procedures may be suitable for closing spaces between some splayed teeth, but the casts should still be analyzed for proper spacing so that the result produces incisal edges of reasonably consistent widths and normal tooth size.

If the splaying effect has created an unacceptable arch form that must be changed for esthetic or functional reasons, the neutral zone must be changed also. Thus treatment planning must be based on a determination of how the existing neutral zone was established. The same arch configuration may result from different lip or tongue variations, some of which are

easily altered whereas others require more complex solutions.

The most common neutral zone configuration found with splayed lower anterior teeth is illustrated in Fig. 35-3. The effect of a strong forward tongue posture combines with a strong lower band of the buccinator that is positioned low. The tongue pushes the incisal edges forward while the buccinator–orbicularis oris band of muscle holds the roots back lingually. Attempts at changing tooth position by alteration of the arch form in the presence of strong neutral zone confinement will predictably fail. If arch form is to be altered, either the excessive pressure from the tongue, or excessive pressure from the perioral musculature must be reduced, or stabilization must be increased.

Even loose teeth will passively relate to their neutral zone position. If hypermobility

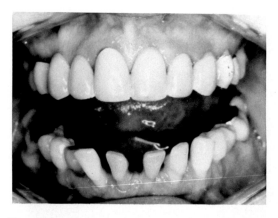

Fig. 35-3. Splaying of lower anterior teeth. Lower band of buccinator holds roots back while strong forward tongue pressure pushes crowns forward. Tongue posture also creates anterior open bite.

occurs coincident with splaying, the hypermobility will almost certainly be related in some way with tooth interference to some functional jaw movements. Varying degrees of periodontal breakdown may be noted, but it may have little relevance to the splaying effect.

Splaying of lower anterior teeth is rarely caused by occlusal interferences. It is almost always a neutral zone phenomenon. An exception to this observation, however, can be noted occasionally in relation to mandibular prognathism. If the upper incisors interfere with the centric relation arc of closure so that the lingual surfaces of the lower incisors strike them, the mandible is forced into a protrusive displacement that also loads the lower incisors in a labial direction. In most cases, the mandible accommodates to the displacement, but in some patients the lower incisors do the accommodating by flaring out labially into a crossbite with splayed incisors.

There are generally no neutral zone problems associated with correction of this type of arch-form problem. It can be treated by use of the same guidelines as are recommended for other anterior crossbite problems.

A method for aligning splayed lower anterior teeth

Lower anterior teeth can sometimes be moved into good alignment without adversely affecting the arch form when elastic ligature is used in combination with a lingual arch bar. The procedure is particularly useful when posterior teeth have been lost.

On corrected diagnostic casts, the arch bar is adapted to the existing curvature of the arch, and a loop is made at each end of the bar. The elastic ligature is then wrapped around each tooth securing it to the bar with a continuous strand of elastic. Fig. 35-4 shows how the ligature is adapted to the teeth and the arch bar to correct the alignment. The pressure from the ligature has the effect of pulling the teeth together while pulling them against the bar. The teeth will even rotate into correct alignment because as soon as one side of the tooth contacts the bar, it is stopped while pressure is still exerted against the other side until the tooth is rotated into full lingual contact with the bar.

After the teeth are moved into correct alignment, they should be held in place with ligature wire or some form of retention until the supporting structures reorganize. They can then be used in whatever capacity is required for the completed restorative plan.

Maintaining holding contacts and anterior guidance

When any changes are made in the position of lower incisal edges, the effect of such changes on the total anterior guidance must be evaluated.

If lower incisal edges are moved or recontoured, each reciprocal holding contact must be reoriented to the new position. The contour and position of each upper tooth stop should be corrected whenever necessary to provide vertical stability to both upper and lower anterior segments. Just having tooth contact may not be enough. Each contact must be properly contoured to prevent eruption and provide axially aligned loading to the best degree possible.

The anterior guidance should always be reevaluated whenever holding contacts are changed on the incisors or canines. The change should not result in restriction of the envelope of function, and it should not result in loss of the disclusive effect on the posterior occlusion.

SPLAYED UPPER ANTERIOR TEETH

If only the upper anterior teeth are splayed, changes in the neutral zone relationship can often be achieved so that lip pressures are reversed. When the lower anterior teeth are upright but the upper teeth are splayed, the lower lip will usually be found substantially

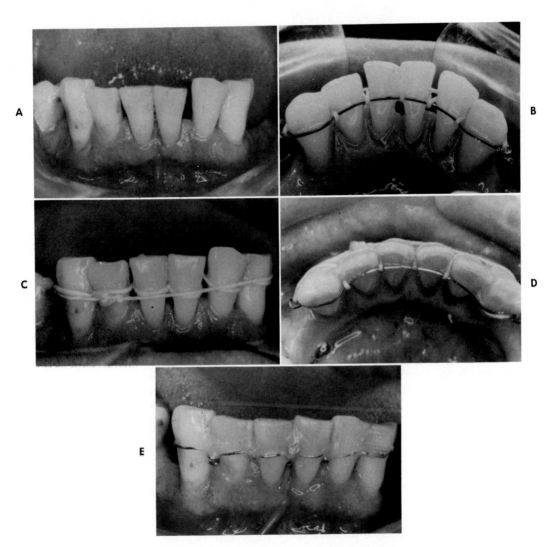

Fig. 35-4. **A,** Splayed lower anterior teeth can be easily realigned without need for bands or removable appliances. **B,** A lingual arch bar is adapted to the corrected study model. Flat 0.01 × 0.02 inch wire is used. A loop is made at the distal of each end tooth. A long strand of medium elastic ligature is held at one end while the other end is run through the loop, around the first tooth, into the interproximal, and then around the arch bar and back out the same interproximal. This is repeated for each tooth while tension is maintained on the ligature. **C,** When the ligature is wrapped around the labial of the last tooth, it is run through the loop at the end and then pulled around and tied to the other end with a double surgeon's knot. **D,** The ligature pulls the teeth together and rotates them, if necessary, against the arch bar. **E,** After the teeth are in position, they should be stabilized with steel ligature wire for at least 2 months. Most such cases require some form of permanent splinting.

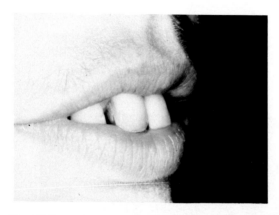

Fig. 35-5. Splayed upper anterior teeth, caused by lower lip pressure, which traps the lip between the lower incisors and the lingual of the upper incisors.

lingual to the upper anterior teeth during swallowing. This lip posture forces the lower anterior teeth lingually and upper anterior teeth labially. The lower teeth have tongue-pressure resistance against the lower lip and so they may actually be stable, but the lower lip is an outward force against the upper anterior teeth that is added to the forward tongue pressure, and this cumulative force easily overpowers the upper lip. The more the upper teeth splay, the less resistance can be applied by the upper lip against the angled labial surfaces (Fig. 35-5).

The treatment approach for splayed upper anterior teeth is often aimed at repositioning of the teeth back into a more upright position. When the incisal edges are moved lingually, the lower lip can slide in front of the upper teeth for a more normal lip seal during swallowing. As soon as the lower lip is postured labially to the upper anterior teeth, the neutral zone is changed. The lower lip assumes an inward resistance role to outward tongue pressure rather than being an additive outward force.

Because the lower incisors generally supraerupt when upper anterior teeth splay, it is often necessary to shorten them to make room for proper upper tooth alignment. It may also

be necessary to alter the shape of the upper lingual surfaces to provide stable holding contacts. Remember that vertical stability of both anterior segments is an essential goal of treatment. It may be provided orthodontically or restoratively if simple reshaping cannot achieve an acceptable result. If holding contacts cannot be provided, the treatment plan should consider whether stabilization with splinting is needed or a bite plane type of substitute is necessary.

Many patients with splayed anterior teeth also have an anterior open bite because of a strong tongue posture, but this would never be the case with supraeruption of lower anterior teeth. When such supraeruption has occurred, stable holding contacts must be provided or the teeth must be vertically stabilized by some other treatment approach.

Severe bone loss in the anterior segments may result in splaying of both upper and lower anterior teeth in the absence of posterior tooth support, but this may still be related to strong tongue pressure. Nevertheless it is often possible to realign the teeth to a more vertical position if stable holding contacts are provided. The prognosis is improved whenever a more normalized lip seal can be facilitated by the better tooth alignment.

SPLAYING AS A RESULT OF AN ENLARGED TONGUE

An oversized tongue may be the sole causative factor in some splayed dentitions. In some patients the tongue force can be overcome by nighttime use of a retainer. If the dentition is healthy and the patient does not object to wearing the retainer, it is a logical treatment approach for some patients. It will not work if the tongue size is too large to be counterresisted.

Surgical techniques for decreasing the size of the tongue have improved and can be considered in selected patients.

Regardless of the treatment approach used for splayed anterior teeth, conformity with the neutral zone should be the first consideration before any treatment plan can be finalized.

36

Treating the crossbite patient

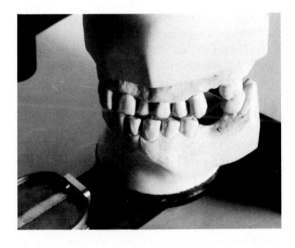

Probably no other type of occlusal problem is treated so improperly so routinely as the crossbite relationship. Far too often, the treatment accomplished to "correct" a crossbite is significantly more harmful than the crossbite itself. This is particularly unfortunate because, when properly treated, crossbite relationships can be among the most stable, most predictably maintainable occlusions.

Crossbite problems should be divided into two categories: anterior crossbite and posterior crossbite. Anterior crossbites present an entirely different set of problems and considerations from posterior crossbites. Although they may or may not occur together, they should

be considered separately because each segment is judged by a different set of criteria.

ANTERIOR CROSSBITE

Mandibular prognathism results from a true basal jaw dysplasia. The horizontal growth of the mandible exceeds the horizontal development of the maxilla, and the lower anterior teeth end up in front of the upper anterior teeth. Anterior crossbite can also result from underdevelopment of the maxilla (maxillary retrognathism).

Because mandibular prognathism is primarily a skeletal malrelationship, it is more practical to prevent it than it is to correct it after it has happened. As with other skeletal deformities, it is amenable to treatment by extraoral orthopedic traction *if treatment is started early enough* to intercept the mandibular growth and manage it through the growth years.

At the first sign of an anterior crossbite, even the youngest patient should be referred to a competent orthodontist. Graber reports successful resolution of anterior crossbites in 3 to 4 months using extraoral appliances worn only at night by children 2 to 6 years of age.

Most orthodontists agree that once an anterior crossbite relation is established, it will get progressively worse with each growth spurt. It makes little difference in the young child

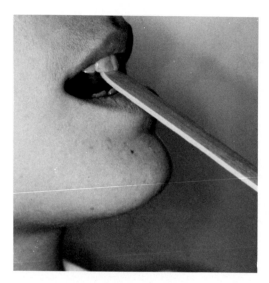

Fig. 36-1. Anterior crossbites in children can often be corrected by pressure from a tongue depressor blade several times a day. A dental nurse illustrates the position of the blade.

whether the crossbite is a true skeletal malrelationship or a pseudocrossbite caused from faulty tooth position; if the lower anterior teeth get in front of the upper anterior teeth before growth has been completed, the tendency will be toward excessive horizontal growth of the mandible. Thus pseudocrossbites in young children usually become true skeletal crossbites in adults.

For early crossbite analysis, computerized cephalometric growth predictions can be useful. Ricketts has set up parameters of comparison regarding growth direction and degree that can guide the diagnostician in selecting the proper course of treatment.

Simple crossbites from tooth malposition can often be corrected in young children by pressure applied several times a day with a tongue blade (Fig. 36-1). As soon as the upper teeth establish an overlap on the lower ones, the exercise can be stopped. They will be guided into position from that point by their own inclines.

After the last of the pubertal growth spurts has finalized the shape of the mandible (about 12 years of age in females and 18 years in males), any treatment of anterior crossbites becomes corrective rather than preventive. What are the problems associated with anterior crossbite that need correction? As with other types of skeletal dysplasias, the "problems" are

often more apparent than real. Patients with anterior crossbite can commonly substitute for unfulfilled occlusal criteria, or they may eliminate the need for some of the usual requirements for stability. Before changes are initiated, each criterion for maintainable occlusion should be carefully analyzed to see whether it is needed.

The problems or potential problems that are commonly associated with anterior crossbites are the following.

Esthetics. The most common reason, by far, that patients seek treatment is to improve their appearance. Elimination of the "bulldog look" of prognathism can be accomplished in several ways, but surgery seems to be the only practical method if the prognathism is severe.

No centric contact on anterior teeth. In many crossbites, the patients do have anterior contact, but it is reversed so that the incisal edges of the upper teeth contact the cingulum of the lower teeth. In more severe malrelationships there is no anterior contact. The usual problem associated with lack of centric contact is supraeruption of the teeth. This is rarely a problem with anterior crossbites because the upper lip substitutes for the contact and holds the lower anterior teeth in place. The tongue prevents the upper teeth from supraerupting. If supraeruption is a problem, it can be solved by provision of centric contact through surgical correction of the arch relationship, by orthodontic repositioning of the teeth, by restorative reshaping, or by splinting to teeth that have centric contact. Combinations of these treatment modes may also be employed.

No anterior guidance. Anterior crossbites cannot provide anterior guidance for either protrusive or lateral excursions. It does not however constitute a problem. Prognathic patients do not use protrusive movements, and so there is no need to provide disclusion of the posterior teeth in protrusion. When a prognathic patient protrudes, it makes the problem worse, and so there is no tendency at all to include such movements in function.

Most prognathic patients limit their function to vertical "chop-chop" movements, but it is wise to provide balancing incline disclusion anyway. The necessary lift can usually always be provided by the working-side inclines. Since there is no anterior guidance to help the posterior teeth, group function of the working inclines is usually the occlusion of choice.

Pseudoprognathism

Some anterior crossbites are not the result of a true mandibular prognathism. The pseudoprognathism results from tooth interferences that force the mandible forward or simply give the appearance of protrusion because of the inverted anterior relationship.

If the upper anterior teeth slant lingually to permit the lower anterior teeth to close in front of them, the prognosis is usually favorable. It is often just a matter of moving the upper anterior teeth forward and jumping them over the lower ones. The rest of the alignment is routine.

It is almost always necessary to open the bite during the correction because the upper teeth must be free to move forward. This can be accomplished with a removable lower appliance that provides a steep incline plane to wedge the upper anterior teeth forward past the lower incisal edges (Fig. 36-2). Such appliances must be worn continuously to be effective and should be removed only for cleaning. They usually accomplish the "crossover" in a matter of weeks. Once the upper anterior teeth are in front of the lower ones, conventional removable appliances may be used to align and refine the anterior relationship if necessary.

Any time the bite must be held open to move teeth, it can take up to several months for the teeth to settle back to their correct vertical dimension. We should not rush any restorative treatment after the use of such appliances. We must make certain the occlusion has stabilized first.

If extensive restoration of all the anterior teeth is required, it may permit a simplified combination approach to correction of the crossbite. By shortening the anterior teeth enough to permit the upper anterior teeth to pass forward of the lower ones, removable appliances that do not require any bite opening can be used. The upper anterior teeth are free to be moved forward, and the lower anterior teeth can be moved inward (Fig. 36-3). As soon as the teeth are in an acceptable relationship, the preparations can be completed and provisional plastic bridges can be made to serve as retainers. Permanent restorations should not be started for a least 2 months after completion of the tooth movement.

Two important considerations should be kept in mind when we are moving linguover-

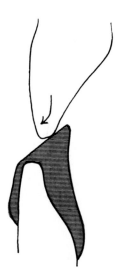

Fig. 36-2. Fabrication of a steep incline plane is often effective in correcting some crossbites. The acrylic appliance must be worn almost continuously until the upper teeth "jump over" the lower ones. The appliance is no longer necessary when the crossover occurs.

sion upper anterior teeth forward. First, we must make sure that there is sufficient alveolar bone labially. Teeth should not be moved so far or so fast that they create dehiscence in the labial plate. Second, when linguoversion upper anterior teeth are moved labial to the lower teeth, the stresses exerted on the teeth are reversed. It takes time for the bone and the periodontal ligaments to realign to these new stresses. The teeth may be tender to function until this realignment takes place.

Some anterior crossbites that appear severe may be false manifestations of occlusal interferences. All such occlusal problems should be evaluated on diagnostic casts *that have been mounted with a facebow record in centric relation.* Without such an analysis, serious mistakes in treatment planning can be made. I have seen patients who were scheduled for surgical reduction to correct a prognathism but who actually required only selective occlusal grinding to permit the mandible to close back in centric relation. Minor orthodontic procedures at the correct jaw position then replaced the "need" for the extensive surgery.

Incorrect analysis more often tends to *oversimplify* anterior crossbite problems, however. Even correctly mounted casts are invitations to trouble if they are not interpreted correctly.

To illustrate the method of analysis, a common anterior crossbite situation can be stud-

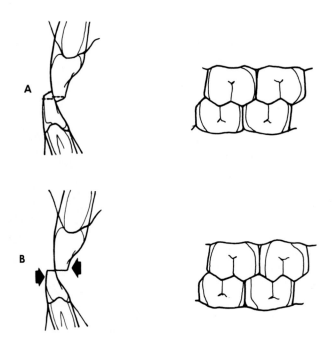

Fig. 36-3. When anterior teeth require extensive restorations, crossbite relationship, **A,** can sometimes be corrected easily when the anterior teeth are shortened. Appliances can then be used to correct the crossbite without even changing the vertical dimension during treatment, **B.**

ied. A 42-year-old male patient presents with a noticeable prognathism when the teeth are closed together (Fig. 36-4). But if the mandible is manipulated into a verified centric relation and held on that axis during closure, the anterior teeth meet end to end (Fig. 36-5). The patient then must slide the mandible forward to get past the upper incisal edges in order to bring the posterior teeth into contact. At that point, the lower anterior teeth are completely in front of the upper anterior teeth and the prognathism is very noticeable. At the end-to-end relationship the facial profile is much improved. The anterior teeth do not need restorations, but the patient is willing to have them restored if it will improve his appearance. There is considerable pulp recession, and so the teeth could be shortened if needed.

What would you do for this problem? The following treatment plan is the approach that many dentists seem to consider. Follow through with it critically to see if it is a practical solution to the above problem.

If we reason that the jaw relationship is a pseudoprognathism that results from tooth interferences, we may wish to take advantage of the receded pulps and might elect to reshape the upper and lower anterior teeth into a nor-

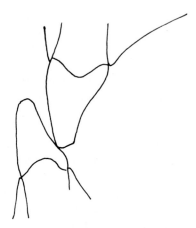

Fig. 36-4. To test understanding of crossbite treatment planning, evaluate this relationship on a 42-year-old patient who wants to look better. His anterior teeth are not in need of restorations, but he is willing to undergo extensive restorative procedures if it will help his appearance.

mal relationship as in Fig. 36-6. None of the posterior teeth need restorations; so we may wish to shorten the anterior teeth at the end-to-end position enough to close the original vertical dimension of posterior tooth contact. Evaluate the process shown in Fig. 36-6, and decide if this is a reasonable approach for correcting the anterior crossbite into a more ac-

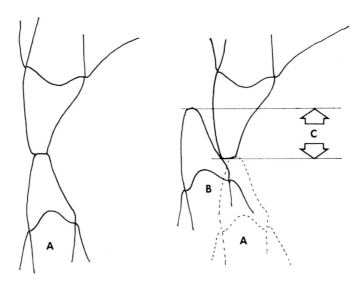

Fig. 36-5. When the mandible is manipulated into the terminal hinge position, the anterior relationship is end to end. From the first contact at centric relation, *A*, he must slide his jaw forward into his acquired position of maximum occlusal contact, *B*. Difference in vertical dimension between first contact and maximum contact, *arrow at C.*

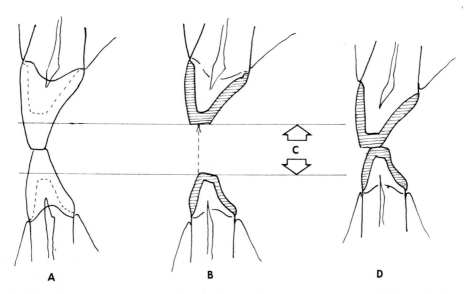

Fig. 36-6. Evaluate this treatment plan, realizing that the end-to-end relationship in centric relation is at an opened vertical dimension. The corrected anterior relationship must be achieved at the correct vertical dimension. The difference between the vertical at first contact and maximum contact is represented by **C.** With this in mind, preparations are done on the upper and lower anterior teeth to shorten them. The tooth preparation is represented by the dotted lines on **A.** Full-coverage restorations are placed that reshape the teeth, **B,** for a better relationship at the correct vertical dimension. **D** represents what many dentists believe will happen when the mandible closes to the correct vertical dimension. Evaluate this treatment plan carefully to see whether you agree. Then compare your decision with Fig. 36-7

ceptable esthetic relationship. Many dentists attempt to follow such reasoning.

An astute diagnostician would have already seen the mistake in the preceding plan. Because such a diagnostician would never plan treatment for a patient with anterior crossbite without *facebow-mounted* diagnostic casts. A common serious error in treatment planning will be made if the casts are mounted on an articulator that does not maintain the correct condylar axis. The above plan may seem feasible if the casts are not related to the condyles, but the arc of closure will be quite different when the mandible closes.

As the anterior teeth are shortened and the mandible arcs are closed, the lower anterior teeth follow an arc around the condylar axis that is in a *forward* direction (Fig. 36-7). The lower anterior teeth *do not follow a vertical upward path of closure.* The only way to know the correct path is by studying diagnostic casts mounted with an open centric relation bite record on an instrument that correctly records the condylar axis. A facebow is essential.

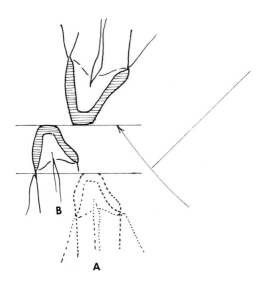

Fig. 36-7. This illustration shows what would really happen if the preceding treatment plan were carried out. *A* to *B*, The arc of closure of the mandible is *not vertical*, as represented in Fig. 36-6. It is *forward.* Many patients undergo extensive restorative procedures because of this error, only to end up worse off after the restorations are completed. This common mistake is the result of trying to plan occlusal treatment on models that are not properly mounted with a facebow. The treatment plan for each case must be evaluated *at the correct vertical dimension in centric relation.* The only way to achieve this is to record the correct arc of closure. A facebow is essential.

Furthermore, it will be necessary to eliminate occlusal interferences on the casts to permit closure of the diagnostic models to the same vertical dimension as the acquired position. This is the only sure way of knowing the correct location of the lower anterior teeth when the mandible is closed to the proper vertical without deviation. We may evaluate various options for improving the anterior relationship only when we know the precise position of the teeth *at the correct vertical dimension.*

Of all the occlusal relationships we may be called on to treat, the necessity for complete preoperative analysis is probably the greatest in anterior crossbite problems. Not only should casts be equilibrated but a complete waxup of all anterior teeth should also be accomplished. The waxup should represent the final contours and tooth position. These finalized goals should then be evaluated to make certain they are attainable, and a step-by-step treatment plan should be outlined to achieve them.

Until an accurate model of the projected result can be fabricated and its practicality verified, it is extremely poor judgment to proceed with any irreversible operative procedures.

It would seem unnecessary to comment any further on the need for correct facebow mountings, but we never cease to be amazed at how often this requirement is ignored. The use of Galetti or Crescent articulators is an open invitation to trouble. The axis of closure is so erroneous on instruments of this type that preplanning is totally inaccurate. It is far too common a mistake to plan a treatment and sell the patient on a beautiful result that cannot be delivered.

Most "hit and slide into" crossbites that appear to be pseudocrossbites are not false at all. They are most often true prognathic skeletal malrelationships. The interfering tooth contacts are usually interferences more to the arcing path of closure than to the final position at full closure.

Many patients who hit end to end in centric relation need only a slight reduction of the upper labial surfaces or a minimal reshaping of the lower lingual surfaces to provide a nondeviating path of closure to the correct vertical dimension (Fig. 36-8). Although the interference may produce an extremely long and devious slide, the length of the slide does not nec-

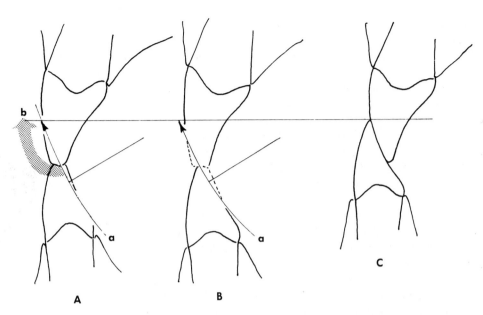

Fig. 36-8. A and **B,** In the correction of anterior crossbite problems, the arc of closure, *a,* is an essential bit of information. Although the slide into the acquired position, *b,* may look severe, the deviation from centric relation is often correctable when the labial surface of the upper teeth and the lingual surface of the lower ones are shaved off. **C** represents the undeviated centric relation position of the teeth after correction. The crossbite is still present, but there is no deviation. This is the treatment of choice for solving temporomandibular joint syndrome problems in many crossbite patients with centric interferences.

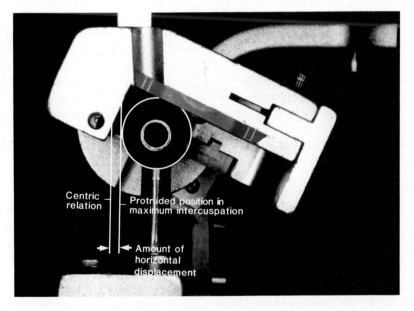

Fig. 36-9. Some occlusal interferences may produce very long "slides" from first point of centric contact to maximum occlusal contact. The slide, however, may closely parallel the normal arc of closure, and the actual horizontal displacement may be minimal. To quickly determine the amount of *horizontal* displacement, one simply notes the difference between the condyle ball when it is in centric relation versus its position when the teeth are maximally occluded. The difference will equal the amount that the lower incisal edges will move back when the occlusion is equilibrated at the correct vertical.

essarily represent the amount of displacement at the closed position. In other words, we may have a long slide with minimal protrusive deviation.

To determine the true horizontal displacement of the mandible at the acquired occlusal position, we note the distance of the articulator condyle from its centric stop position. The distance of the ball from the stop is representative of how far back the lower incisal edges will be moved when centric interferences are eliminated (Fig. 36-9).

If an analysis of the mounted casts indicates that restorative reshaping of the anterior teeth is not feasible, the patient must be told the facts. Temporomandibular joint pain can be relieved by selective elimination of interferences to centric relation closure, but we can make no improvement in the patient's appearance without resorting to more radical methods.

Often, selective shaping of incisal edges improves the appearance noticeably. Orthodontic evaluation would also be in order to see whether tooth position within the skeletal framework can practically be improved.

In a nutshell, the conservative approaches for resolving anterior crossbite problems can be summarized as follows:

1. Selective shaping and occlusal equilibration
2. Orthodontic repositioning of the teeth within present bone framework
3. Restorative reshaping
4. A combination of the above procedures

It is almost always possible to provide comfort, function, and stability to anterior crossbite relations with one or more of the preceding procedures. But it is not always possible to satisfy the esthetic requirements of some patients.

Fortunately one of the most important aspects of an esthetic smile is not related to the upper-to-lower alignment. Rather it is how the upper incisal plane is viewed when the teeth are apart. Normally only the upper anterior teeth show when smiling, and so a pleasant arrangement of the upper incisal edges is not generally affected by the position of the lower teeth except in severe mandibular prognathism. On the other hand, the lower incisal edges show when speaking, and so a nicely ordered lower incisal plane can be attractive, even in crossbite.

A combination of reshaping and restoring is

the method I have found to be preferred for the majority of anterior crossbites that can contact end to end in centric relation. The combination approach usually involves some increase in vertical to hold the posterior contacts at the anterior end-to-end position, and so this method is best reserved for when posterior restorations are needed.

Increasing the vertical dimension causes the lower incisors to arc back more in line with the upper anterior teeth. It also separates the lower teeth from the interfering upper labial inclines that force the mandible forward, and so the occlusion can be reconstructed into a centric relation harmony.

If the increased vertical is established with equal-intensity centric contacts on all the teeth, there will be a favorable prognosis though some occlusal adjustments may be necessary for a period of months while the muscles reorder the vertical dimension to conform to their contracted length.

Despite an increased vertical, many patients I have treated in the above manner have remained completely stable and have required little or no posttreatment equilibration. The probable explanation for this is related to the horizontal displacement of the condyles when the crossbite directed the mandible forward. To displace the mandible forward, the condyles had to move *down* the eminentiae. When the mandible was moved back to centric relation, even though the vertical dimension was increased at the incisors, it was decreased at the angle of the mandible where the elevator muscles attach (Fig. 36-10). This is so because the condyles were allowed to move up as the mandible moved back.

The above option of opening the bite is a logical choice if:

1. An acceptable end-to-end relationship can be achieved at the incisors in harmony with centric relation.
2. The required increase in vertical dimension is acceptable.
3. The posterior segments require restoration for other reasons.

If conservative procedures fall short of optimum esthetics, the patient must make an important decision. There seems to be only two practical choices:

1. Live with the prognathism with fairly good assurances that the dentition can be maintained.
2. Select a surgical correction.

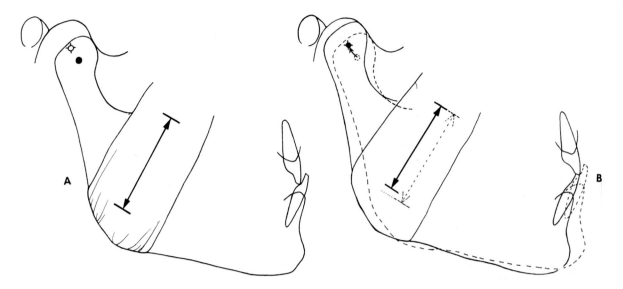

Fig. 36-10. Compare length of elevator muscle when mandible is protruded, **A,** with length of same muscle when condyle moves back *and up* to centric relation, even if the *anterior* vertical is increased, **B.**

Surgical correction of anterior crossbite

There are three methods for correcting an anterior crossbite surgically that seem to be universally accepted as safe, practical solutions:

1. Resection through the ramus so that the body of the mandible can be moved distally into alignment with the maxilla.
2. Horizontal resection of the maxilla so that it can be moved forward into alignment with the mandible.
3. Sectional osteotomies so that an anterior segment can be repositioned. This is not ideal if there is a severe skeletal discrepancy.

At one time, surgical correction was believed to be a radical procedure to be avoided except as a last resort. Advancements in surgical methods have changed this. When indicated, a surgical correction may require far less time and discomfort for the patient than more complex treatments that will not achieve a comparable result.

CAUTION: Before surgery is attempted, the temporomandibular joints must be in optimum position and alignment, and the occlusal relationship must be predetermined in relation to a verifiable centric relation. If the surgical result is to be considered a success, the lower arch must be aligned with the upper arch when the condyles are in centric relation. Fail-

ure to achieve this relationship has been the most common shortcoming of surgical results we have seen. Planning for surgery requires that casts must be mounted with a facebow in centric relation, and any changes in arch position must be related to that three-dimensional alignment.

Surgical methods are described in more detail in Chapter 39.

Temporomandibular joint disorders and anterior crossbite

The resolution of temporomandibular joint pain is accomplished the same for anterior crossbite patients as it is for other arch relationships. Interferences to centric relation must be eliminated to permit the muscles to relax from their state of spasm.

In anterior crossbite relationships, the interfering inclines are usually found on the anterior teeth. Most often, equilibration can be accomplished by shaving off part of the labial surfaces of the upper anterior teeth or the lingual surfaces of the lower anterior teeth, or both surfaces. Some occlusal adjustment may also be needed on the posterior teeth, but selective grinding should follow the usual rules of procedure.

On rare occasions, we may be required to resolve a severely painful occluso-muscle problem on a patient with crossbite who cannot be equilibrated without destruction of the anterior teeth. If the lower teeth are locked forward of the upper teeth and it is not possible to correct the problem with selective grinding, we do have an alternative.

A temporary acrylic bite-raising appliance that provides contact in centric relation can be fabricated for the posterior teeth. The bite must be opened enough for the lower incisors to miss the upper ones so that the condyles are free to go back into their terminal axis.

This procedure is purely a temporary measure to provide relief of severe pain until a logical treatment plan can be designed. Such a treatment plan may consist in any of the usual modes of treating mandibular prognathism, or it may require orthodontics to actually move the upper teeth further lingually to accommodate the lower arch in centric relation. Such a treatment may sound rather extreme, but in some cases it may be the treatment of choice over a surgical approach. It would have the effect of slightly reducing the prognathism by allowing the mandible to retrude back to centric relations. It would not, however, have a noticeable effect on the tooth-to-tooth appearance.

POSTERIOR CROSSBITE

It is difficult to understand why posterior crossbites are so routinely treated as something that must be "corrected." Actually, a posterior crossbite relationship can be every bit as stable, functional, comfortable, and esthetic as its more normal counterpart. Yet how common it is to see such stable relationships warped all out of proportion into contours that overprotect the gingival tissues and invite stresses to be directed off the long axes to a damaging degree, all under the guise of "correcting" a crossbite.

Evaluating posterior crossbites

Most posterior crossbites are the direct result of basal bone relationships. The posterior teeth are usually positioned properly within their own alveolar process, but the width of the mandibular bony arch is proportionately wider than the maxillary bony arch. When the teeth assume the most stable relationship within the bone, the tooth-to-tooth relationship is reversed from what is normally considered "correct." But is such a crossbite relationship *incorrect?* It is not if it fulfills the neces-

sary criteria for maintainable occlusion. Most often this relationship is more correct than it would be if the teeth were changed to the normal form of intercuspation.

In evaluating the acceptability of a posterior crossbite relationship, the following observations should be made.

Tooth-to-bone relationship in the same arch. Are the teeth ideally situated in the alveolar process? Would the tooth-to-bone relationship be improved if the mandibular teeth are moved lingually or the maxillary teeth buccally? If the teeth are properly positioned within their alveolar bone, which in turn is harmoniously aligned with its basal bone, the usual indication would be to maintain this tooth-to-bone balance. There would have to be some very compelling reasons for disturbing such a relationship before any change in tooth position should be considered.

Relationship of the teeth to the tongue and cheeks. Are the teeth in harmony with normal tongue and cheek pressures, or have they been moved into the crossbite relationship by abnormal muscle patterns or habits? If deviate tongue or cheek patterns have moved the teeth into a malrelationship, is it possible to correct the abnormal habit pattern? Would a change in tooth position or contour benefit the tooth-to-muscle harmony or the overall stability?

Occlusal relationship. Upper-to-lower tooth relationships should be evaluated for direction of stresses, distribution of stresses, and stability. If the occlusal relationship causes stresses to be directed favorably up or down the long axes, the first requirement of stability has been fulfilled. If the occlusal contours permit favorable distribution of lateral forces in excursive movements, the second requirement of stability can be fulfilled.

When both of these requirements have been satisfied, neither stability nor function needs to be slighted. Optimum function with excellent stability is just as practically attained in a posterior crossbite relationship as it is with normal intercuspation.

If the posterior teeth are in harmony with their supporting bone, if tooth alignment does not interfere with muscle activity, and if occlusal contours are correctly related to the optimum direction and distribution of stresses, there is no occlusal relationship that is more stable than a posterior crossbite.

Restoring posterior crossbites

One of the most common mistakes we will see is balancing incline interference in posterior crossbites that have been restored. We should take a careful look at the next few crossbite patients who have had occlusal restoration of the posterior teeth. In my experience, most of the patients examined were functioning on the lingual inclines of the lower buccal cusps in mediotrusion (Fig. 36-11). It is a prevalent fallacy that when teeth are in a crossbite relationship the balancing inclines should be reversed from what they normally are. This is a serious error that is extremely stress producing.

Upper inclines that face the cheek or lower inclines that face the tongue should never contact in lateral excursions. This rule should be followed regardless of the arch relationship. A helpful way to remember the preceding rule is to learn another rule: *When the lower posterior teeth move toward the tongue, they must disclude.* The side that moves toward the tongue is always the orbiting, condyle side, and all posterior tooth contact should be eliminated on this side because the condyle is unbraced. There is no way to harmonize the occlusion to all degrees of muscle contraction on the unbraced condyle side. Crossbites are no exception. All inclines should disclude when the lower teeth move toward the tongue.

When posterior crossbites are being restored, the *lower lingual cusps* become the functioning cusps. They fit into the same upper fossae and function against the same inclines as

the lower buccal cusps do in a normal relationship (Fig. 36-12). If posterior group function is desired, the lower lingual cusps contact the lingual inclines of the *upper buccal cusps* in working excursions (laterotrusion). This working incline contact can be used very effectively to disclude the opposite-side balancing inclines.

The *lower buccal cusp* is a nonfunctioning cusp in crossbite relationship, and its lingual inclines should never contact; so it should be shortened slightly from the normal contours so that it does not interfere in balancing excursions (mediotrusion). In patients with a more pronounced curve of Spee, the lower buccal cusps will need to be progressively flatter as we proceed posteriorly.

In establishing the occlusal plane on posterior crossbite relationships, it is best to keep the plane on the low side in back. Nothing is lost if the occlusal plane is lower than necessary on the distal (as long as both upper and lower crown-to-root ratios are considered). However, an occlusal plane that is too high distally could make it impractical to provide centric stops that would be free of protrusive or balancing interferences from the upper lingual cusps and the lower buccal cusp in crossbite.

If the lower teeth are tilted lingually and the upper teeth are fairly vertical, the buccal incline of the lower lingual cusp can serve as the functioning incline for working excursions.

It is difficult to evaluate whether lateral stresses would be resisted any better or worse on the lower lingual cusp incline or the upper

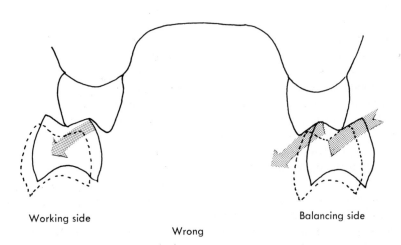

Working side   Balancing side

Wrong

Fig. 36-11. The most common mistake in treating posterior crossbite relationships is to build the balancing inclines into function. This is a very stressful relationship.

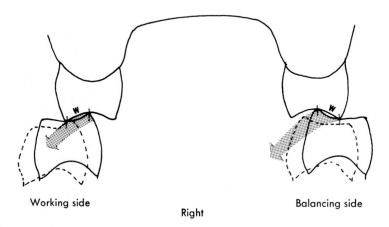

Working side

Right

Balancing side

Fig. 36-12. The correct crossbite relationship. When teeth move toward the tongue, they should never be in contact. The relationship illustrated here is just as functional and just as stable as a normal arch relationship. The working side discludes the balancing side in lateral excursions. The centric stops are stable.

buccal cusp. It is doubtful that it would matter too much whether there is a slight stress difference because whichever incline is used must be in harmony with the lateral anterior guidance and the condylar movements. Furthermore, most crossbite patients do not use lateral functional movements to the usual extent. their function very often follows a more vertical pattern.

If the anterior guidance is capable of resisting all the lateral stresses without help from the posterior teeth, there are no contraindications for posterior disclusion in all eccentric positions.

The *upper lingual cusp* is a nonfunctioning, noncontacting cusp in crossbite relationships. It should be designed to hold the tongue out of the way and to serve as a gripper of fibrous foods without ever coming into contact with the lower tooth. It can come close to contact, but it should never touch.

Fossa contours. There is no difference in the principles of fossa design whether the teeth are in crossbite or not. Lower fossae must be contoured to receive the upper buccal cusps in a stable centric relation contact. Fossae walls must be harmonized so that they are not steeper than the lateral anterior guidance to permit the cusps to pass in and out of the fossae without interference.

The use of the fossa-contour guide as explained in Chapter 21 is just as practical for crossbite relationships as it is for normal occlusions. If the contours of the lower fossae are correctly harmonized, the upper posterior

teeth may be restored by several different approaches, including functionally generated path techniques.

Some dentists believe that in crossbite situations the upper teeth should be restored first and the functionally generated path technique should be used on the lower teeth. This is certainly not necessary if lower cusp tip placement and fossa contours are correct. It is far more practical to restore the lower posterior teeth first and then use the functional path procedures on the upper teeth where it is easier to stabilize the base for the functional wax.

With fully adjustable instrumentation combined with a correct anterior guidance, posterior crossbites can be restored one arch at a time as long as some method of providing correct fossa contours is used, or both arches may be restored together.

Equilibrating posterior crossbites

If the lower lingual cusp is to serve as the functioning cusp, it is treated in the same manner as a lower buccal cusp in normal intercuspation. All upper inclines are treated in the usual way. Upper working inclines are either harmonized to whatever degree of group function is indicated, or they are ground out of contact if disclusion is preferred.

The buccal inclines of the upper lingual cusps are balancing inclines that should always be ground out of all contact in any eccentric jaw position. The only variation in selective grinding of the upper lingual cusp is that the cusp tip can be shortened. It will not be a functioning cusp, and so it can be shaped without regard for maintaining contact of any kind.

In crossbite, the tip of the upper buccal cusp takes on a new importance because, when possible, we want it to serve as a holding contact. Consequently it should never be shortened unless it interfers in both centric and lateral excursions. It is better to shape the upper buccal cusps when necessary to improve the buccolingual position in the lower fossae and then do most of the selective grinding on the lower fossa walls and cusp inclines.

If the lingual inclines of the upper buccal cusps are to serve as the working inclines, the lower fossae can be opened out. There is no need to provide lower working incline contact if it is present on the upper teeth. Conversely, if the buccal inclines of the lower lingual cusps are to serve as the working incline contact, there is no need to provide upper working incline contact. Walls of the upper fossae can be opened out, and all upper inclines become nonfunctional.

There is no harm in providing functional incline contact on both upper and lower teeth

simultaneously, but there does not appear to be any observable benefits from doing it. There would be no reason, however, to grind functioning inclines away if they are already present and functioning correctly.

The equilibration of crossbite relationships, as with other relationships, should provide noninterfering closure into centric relation. Determining which cusps should function against which inclines should be based on a tooth-to-tooth appraisal of what will provide the most stability with the least lateral stress.

SELECTED READINGS

Berliner, A.: Ligatures, splints, bite planes and pyramids, Philadelphia, 1964, J.B. Lippincott Co.

Graber, T.M.: Orthodontics, principles and practice, Philadelphia, 1962, W.B. Saunders Co.

Profit, W.R., and White, R.P.: Treatment of severe malocclusions by correlated orthodontic, surgical procedures, Angle Orthodont. **40**:1-10, 1970.

Schwartz, A.M., and Gratzinger, M.: Removable orthodontic appliances, Philadelphia, 1966, W.B. Saunders Co.

Subtelny, J.D.: Cephalometric diagnosis, growth and treatment: something old, something new? Am. J. Orthodont. **57**:262-286, 1970.

37

Treating the crowded, irregular, or interlocking anterior bite

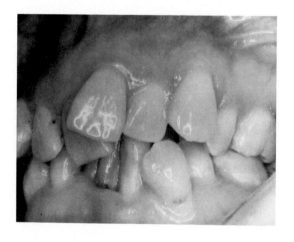

Irregularities in anterior teeth alignment may occur in combination with a variety of other occlusal problems. Crowded incisors may be seen in deep overbites, crossbites, open bites, or almost any other type of arch malrelationship. The anterior misalignment may be the result of an arch malrelationship, or it may be a contributing cause. It may occur in combination with an ideal posterior intercuspation, or the posterior teeth may also be misaligned.

Although anterior teeth must be precisely coordinated with the posterior occlusion, the anterior segments should be evaluated as a separate functional unit. The importance of the anterior guidance as a determinant of posterior occlusion requires that anterior tooth position and alignment have priority over occlusal analysis for the posterior segments. Correction of anterior irregularities must result in a stable relationship that is capable of discluding the posterior teeth in eccentric excursions. At the same time, any changes to anterior alignment must relate to the lip-closure path, phonetic function, and neutral zone harmony.

After a lecture on the importance of anterior guidance, a dentist proceeded to convince one of his 47-year-old patients that she would lose her teeth if she did not have the irregular interlocked anterior bite corrected. Even though the appearance was not particularly noticeable and of no concern to the patient, she agreed to proceed with the extensive plan of orthodontics and restorative reshaping because she did not wish to have her teeth get loose and develop periodontal problems from her malocclusion.

Fortunately, the dentist had second thoughts about his treatment plan when he realized that the lady had no sign of hypermobility, wear facets, or even beginning periodontitis. He reasoned that at 47 years of age she would surely have had *some* signs of deterioration if causative factors of destruction had been present. The patient gratefully accepted his changed diagnosis and continued to live happily with her irregular but healthy dentition.

Unfortunately, all patients are not that lucky because all dentists are not goal oriented to maintainable health. Some are oriented to preconceived ideas of what an occlusion must *look like* rather than how particular occlusal relationships exert their stresses.

Every occlusion must be evaluated on the basis of its potential for destruction, but such an evaluation must consider how the patient functions with a given relationship. An irregular anterior bite is potentially destructive only if:

1. It is uncleanable.
2. It is unstable.
3. It interferes with the patient's functional movements.
4. It fails to provide the necessary disclusive effect for the posterior teeth.

Any one or more of the above problems is reason enough to warrant some type of intervention by the dentist. If none of these problems is being manifested by the irregularity, the only other reason for initiating corrective treatment is *to improve the esthetics.*

Irregular anterior teeth can present a formidable esthetic problem, but in the absence of destructive tendencies it should be the patient's decision to improve the appearance or leave it as it is. However, when the irregularities are definitely contributing to an accelerated deterioration of the teeth or the supporting structures, it is the duty of the dentist to report this to the patient and to suggest ways of solving the problem.

In the absence of any esthetic concern, irregular anterior teeth should be evaluated in each of the potential problem areas.

Cleanability. If the irregularity is great enough, it may be difficult to clean between crowded anterior teeth. Sometimes three teeth may bunch up to form a funnel-like opening between them. If the teeth are not cleanable, they are not maintainable. Lack of cleanability is reason enough to recommend correction of the irregularity.

Stability. Irregular anterior teeth are often unstable because of a lack of centric holding contacts. Teeth that do not have an antagonistic stop will supraerupt unless something substitutes for the missing contact. Cutting off individual elongated teeth to align their incisal edges is a common practice that does not work. Shortened teeth will simply erupt right back out of alignment unless a stop is provided or some form of stabilization is utilized.

Substitutes for centric contact can be provided in several ways. Any noncontacting tooth that does not supraerupt has something that is preventing the eruption. It can always be determined clinically what the substitute is. Some things to look for are as follows.

ECCENTRIC FUNCTION. If the tooth contacts enough in function, it may not need centric contact to keep it from supraerupting.

ANKYLOSIS. Ankylosed roots will keep the tooth from erupting further.

OVERLAPPED CINGULUM. If adjacent contacting teeth lap over the cingulum of a noncontacting tooth, they can lock the tooth into position and prevent any further eruption.

TONGUE OR LIP HABITS. Habitually interposing the tongue or the lips between the teeth will prevent noncontacting teeth from erupting.

If none of the above stabilizers is found, irregular anterior teeth with no contact will supraerupt. This predictable instability is a definite indication for correcting the irregularity, at least to a point of maintainable stability.

Functional interferences. It would appear that the anterior teeth in an interlocking bite would be subjected to abnormal lateral stresses. In most cases, the mandible cannot move forward or laterally without direct interference from some of the malposed anterior teeth. Yet it is common to find patients in their later years with firm, healthy interlocking teeth. The reason is clear. For teeth to be stressed laterally, the mandible must move laterally. Since the interlocking bite restricts lateral movement, the patient develops functional patterns of movement that have no horizontal component. Strictly vertical patterns of movement seem to be the rule in interlocked bite relationships.

If the bite is interlocked in centric relation, there is rarely a problem with lateral stress on either the anterior or posterior teeth. It is not uncommon to find interlocked bites with no deviation from a terminal hinge closure into maximum occlusal contact.

If the bite is interlocked in a *deviated* jaw

position, it would be unusual not to find severe wear facets, some degree of periodontitis, hypermobile teeth, or some related temporomandibular joint symptoms.

Centric interferences can usually be eliminated with selective grinding, but tooth movement may be necessary to resolve other problems. If stable centric relation stops are established, most patients will still maintain the vertical functional stroke in the new occlusal position if the interlocking bite is still present. There is usually no need to provide lateral or protrusive guidances in such cases, but this decision must not be taken lightly. Each case must be carefully evaluated regarding the relationship of the teeth to the envelope of function.

Existing periodontal problems. If periodontal destruction is already noticeable, it is certainly an indication that causative factors are present. A very careful evaluation of the tooth arrangement should be made to determine (1) whether it is contributing to the periodontitis and (2) whether correction of the irregularity is necessary for the resolution of the periodontal problem. If extensive restorative procedures are needed for any reason, it would usually be advantageous to correct the irregularity as a matter of practicality. It depends, however, on the severity of the irregularity and its potential for causing future harm.

METHODS OF CORRECTING ANTERIOR INTERLOCKING BITES

It is very easy to oversimplify the treatment for correction of anterior interlocking bite problems. Some problems are simple to solve. Others may be extremely complex. Cases with interlocked anterior teeth can be divided into two categories:

1. Cases that have sufficient room in the arch to accommodate the anterior teeth when they are properly aligned
2. Cases that have insufficient room for the anterior teeth to be aligned without changing posterior arch form

The first category is easy to solve. It involves primarily the labial or lingual realignment of teeth into spaces that are wide enough to accept them (Fig. 37-1). There is no need for arch expansion in such cases, and excellent results can usually be obtained with removable appliances and minor tooth movement procedures.

When there is insufficient room to align the anterior teeth, the problem becomes more complex. We can no longer simply move the anterior teeth forward or backward into alignment because the teeth are too wide to fit into the space that is available at the position of correct incisal edge alignment (Fig. 37-2).

In general terms, we have at least five possible ways of solving the space problem:

1. We can narrow the teeth so that they will fit into the available space.
2. We can widen the space by reshaping the adjacent teeth.
3. We can reduce the number of teeth that must fit into a given space.
4. We can increase the space by changing the shape of the arch.
5. We can change the axial inclination of the anterior teeth.

The preceding treatment approaches may still be oversimplified because of arch-to-arch relationships. It may be a simple matter to align the teeth in each arch individually, but the resultant arch-to-arch relationship may then be incompatible. It may be necessary to narrow one arch and expand the other.

Orthodontists have excellent methods for evaluating such problems, and any patient who cannot be successfully treated with a simplified approach should be referred to a competent orthodontist.

It should be obvious that properly mounted study models are a necessary part of any treatment planning. No corrective procedures should be started unless the finished result can be clearly visualized and the corrections worked out in detail on the casts.

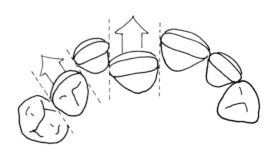

Fig. 37-1. Irregularly arranged anterior teeth that have room in the anterior segment to accommodate the teeth if they are realigned. This is the simplest alignment to correct.

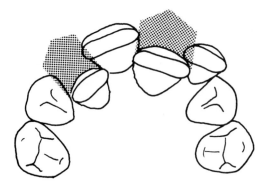

Fig. 37-2. Irregularly arranged anterior teeth with insufficient room for realignment. Teeth cannot be moved into correct alignment without altering either the width of the space or the width of the teeth.

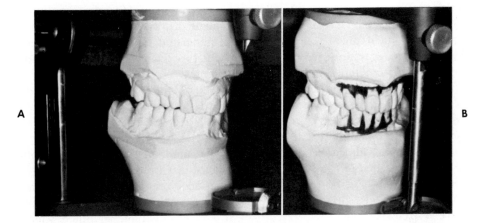

A   B

Fig. 37-3. A, Analysis of crowded anterior teeth can best be accomplished on facebow-mounted models in centric relation. **B,** Equilibration of the models enables us to evaluate the potential stability of the posterior occlusion and at the same time permits a careful study of the anterior relationship at the *correct vertical dimension in centric relation*. It was determined in this case that slight narrowing of the anterior teeth would permit them to be aligned without changing the posterior teeth. Each tooth can be individually separated from the model and measured to determine how much narrowing is required. The teeth should then be repositioned back on the cast in the desired alignment and held in place with wax. This procedure fulfills the prime requirement of proper treatment planning: "Visualize the goal before determining the mode of treatment."

Narrowing crowded teeth to permit alignment

If, on mounted models, the crowded anterior teeth are individually separated and removed from the model, they can then be repositioned back on the cast and tacked with wax in the corrected alignment (Fig. 37-3). Since the space will not be sufficient to accommodate all the teeth in the new alignment, the last tooth is left off. The space that is left is measured and subtracted from the width of the unplaced tooth. The difference will be the total reduction in width that must be distributed over all the anterior teeth in that arch. By dividing that figure by the number of anterior teeth involved, we will know how much each

tooth must be reduced in width to fit into the correct alignment.

Teeth in the anterior segment can be narrowed up to a combined total of 6 mm without the enamel being penetrated. Radiographs of each tooth should be studied to determine the thickness of the enamel before any width reduction is started. The enamel is usually thickest on the distal of the central and lateral incisors, and considerable reduction can be done on either the mesial or distal of the cuspids. If necessary, the mesial of the first premolars can be reduced.

Width reduction is commonly referred to as "stripping." It is accomplished with thin separating disks and abrasive strips, or a mechanical stripper. Ground surfaces should be rounded and polished with sandpaper strips and disks.

After the teeth have been narrowed to the proper width, there are several technique options that can be used for moving them into their predetermined correct position in the arch.

Finger pressure. It is surprising how quickly some teeth can be moved into alignment by having the patient exert finger pressure several times a day in the right direction, once room has been provided.

Ligatures and rubber bands. Elastic ligature material or rubber bands can often be used to align anterior teeth. It can be used alone in some cases but frequently should be combined with arch wires to preserve the arch form. Arch wires can sometimes be incorporated into cemented temporary restorations (Fig. 37-4).

Removable appliances. Very often the simplest approach is to use a removable appliance. The methods of providing directed pressure to the teeth are limited only by the imagination. Tooth movement can be effected by finger springs, rubber bands, spring-loaded devices, and pressurized arch bars.

Bands. Uncontrolled tipping forces against an incisor crown have the tendency to torque the tooth around a rotational axis located near the center of the root. Removable appliances that are designed to move the crown lingually usually produce a concurrent labial movement of the root. Conversely, labial crown movement produces lingual root movement. It is frequently necessary to exert greater control over the axial inclination of anterior teeth than is practical with removable appliances. When teeth are banded, brackets that permit controlled movement of both the crown and the root may be used. There are several methods for exerting the torque effect on the bracket. Square-edged wire that is twisted and then seated into the bracket slot may be used to apply continuous torquing force on the bracket walls as it tries to untwist itself. Twin wires may also be used to accomplish the torquing effect, or light wires may be bent to serve as springs that attach to the brackets. There are many variations in how the force is applied, but the net effect is accomplished through controlling the force through the bracket. The arch wire may exert direct pressure and

torque at the same time, and so the control over specific tooth movement can be very precise.

Although almost any desired tooth movement may be possible with innovative removable appliances, the use of bands is very often the most practical and expeditious method when control of torque is critical.

Cemented brackets

The advantages of bracket control can now be achieved without the disadvantages of bands. New methods of directly cementing the brackets on a lightly etched enamel surface have greatly simplified their use. With directly cemented brackets the thickness of the bands is eliminated between the teeth and the esthetic problems associated with bands are minimized.

The potential variations in using directly cemented brackets are exciting.

Vinyl repositioners

For minor tooth movement, a soft vinyl appliance may be worn. Teeth are cut off and repositioned on a stone model, and the vinyl appliance is fabricated over the corrected model. It is worn much like an athlete's mouth guard, and it has the effect of exerting gentle pressure on selected teeth until they are moved into the predetermined position. It then serves to hold them in place as long as the appliance is worn.

If tooth repositioning is followed by occlusal correction to harmonize the teeth to the new position, stabilization is enhanced, but some form of retention is also necessary until the bone and ligaments realign to the new position.

CORRECTING ANTERIOR IRREGULARITY WITH SELECTIVE EXTRACTION

In the presence of a stable posterior occlusion, the selective extraction of a single lower incisor is sometimes a practical step in resolving the problem of crowded lower anterior teeth. If the combined width of the remaining three incisors equals the space available in the arch and if stable centric holding contacts can be provided for each tooth, there are no real contraindications for the extraction approach.

The fact that there are only three teeth occupying the space that normally has four is not noticeable. It creates no problems of esthetics,

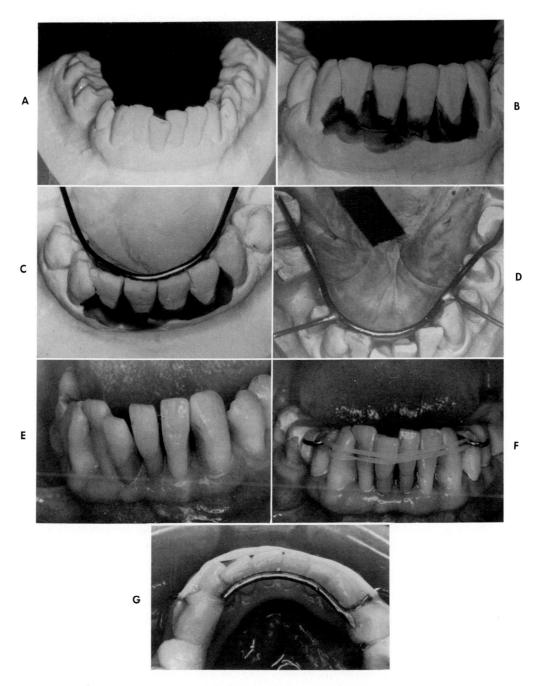

Fig. 37-4. A, Crowded lower anterior teeth. **B.** Analysis of tooth width and position is achieved by separation from the model and repositioning (in harmony with a centrically related upper model). **C,** A lingual arch bar is adapted to the repositioned teeth. It should contact the lingual surface of each tooth. **D,** After necessary preparations are completed on the posterior teeth, a model is made, the arch bar is positioned, and temporary acrylic restorations are fabricated to hold the bar in its correct relationship. A wire is soldered on each side to serve later as a hook for the rubber band. **E,** The anterior teeth are narrowed to their predetermined width. **F,** The appliance is cemented. It serves the dual function of temporization and orthodontic appliance. The rubber band is placed. **G,** The rubber band pulls the teeth into their correctly predetermined positions against the arch bar. Teeth may even by rotated by this method because pressure is exerted on each tooth until the full width of its lingual surface is in contact with the bar.

function, or stability as long as the teeth that remain can be brought into correct anterior function.

If there is a slight size variation between the three remaining teeth and the available space in the arch, one can usually resolve the problem by either stripping the contact area to narrow tooth width further, or selected teeth can be crowned or bonded if more width is needed.

Bands or directly cemented brackets should usually be used if much repositioning of lower incisors is required after a selected tooth is extracted. The brackets permit lateral movement of the root along with the crown so that the teeth may maintain a stable upright position rather than merely tilting them into contact. If the lower incisors are to be included in a restorative splint, the axial relationship of the root is less important. Stabilization will be achieved by the splint.

Extracting all lower incisors

There are circumstances that justify the extraction of all lower incisors when they are crowded. Lower incisors can be replaced with a fixed bridge about as successfully as they can be restored. If periodontitis has resulted in considerable bone loss around the lower incisors, it is difficult to restore the long-exposed root surfaces with full coverage restorations unless the axial alignment is near perfect. Maintenance of gingival health is sometimes complicated by the retention of such teeth, especially if root surfaces are close together or the level of alveolar bone is irregular.

Extraction of crowded lower incisors is indicated under the following conditions:
1. If extensive restorative procedures are indicated that necessarily include the lower incisors whether they are retained or not, and if retention of the lower incisors would not lend any advantage to the remaining teeth
2. If retention of the lower incisors would create problems of maintenance
3. If retention of the lower incisors would require unnecessary complication of the treatment plan without yielding a commensurate value to the plan

Much time, effort, and expense can be wasted trying to save lower incisors that could be restored more effectively with a fixed bridge. The difficulty of cleaning between splinted lower incisors is almost reason enough to recommend it when extensive periodontitis is a problem. If the realigned lower incisors would be cleanable and would have the potential for lending support to other teeth, they should be saved.

Extracting upper anterior teeth

Selective extraction of upper anterior teeth is rarely indicated because of the problems it creates esthetically. However, each case must be evaluated individually. It is sometimes possible to extract both lateral teeth to provide a good alignment, but if extractions are necessary, it is almost always better to extract the first bicuspids to provide room for the correct alignment of all six upper anterior teeth.

Combining selective extraction with restorative reshaping may have great merit for severely crowded anterior teeth if the posterior occlusion is stable (Fig. 37-5). Sometimes the extractions permit narrower restorations than could be achieved otherwise. As an example, extremely wide lateral incisors could be replaced with narrower pontics. Additional room can be gained when the central incisors are narrowed and the mesial of the cuspids is reduced.

Such measures should be used only when complete orthodontic correction must be ruled out for good reason. Combined extraction and restorative techniques should almost never be used on very young patients. They should be reserved for mouths that can benefit in other ways from the restorative procedures. The decision to extract any tooth is a major one that should be made only when the benefits outweigh the disadvantages.

Combining restorative procedures with orthodontics

Restorative reshaping of any tooth should not be considered if the restoration can be avoided by moving the tooth into a better alignment. However, when the need for restoration is evident, the combination of restorative reshaping and orthodontics can often be used to great advantage.

Being able to narrow teeth or shorten them often facilitates their movement through or into spaces that would otherwise not accommodate them (Fig. 37-6). Once in position, they can be restored back to proper contact and occlusion. I believe that the combination

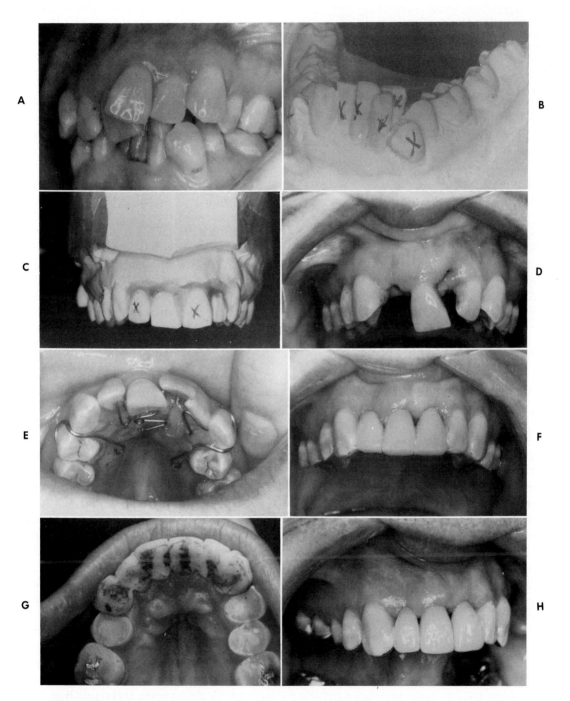

Fig. 37-5. A, Severely crowded anterior relationship with advanced periodontitis around several anterior teeth. The posterior occlusion is stable. **B,** Analysis of the lower arch indicates the necessity of several extractions. **C,** Extraction of the upper left central and right lateral incisor is necessary for periodontal reasons. Teeth are narrowed and repositioned on the model. (Lower arch is of course worked out simultaneously with upper anterior relationship.) **D,** Indicated extractions are completed. **E,** Removable appliance is used to move teeth into their *predetermined* position. **F,** After repositioning, temporary splints are fabricated. They serve as an excellent retainer and also enable the dentist to refine the esthetic contours. The patient has the opportunity to approve the esthetics, phonetics, and function before fabrication of the permanent restorations. **G,** The anterior guidance can be perfected in the temporary restorations. **H,** The finished upper anterior restoration. Posterior arch form has not been disturbed.

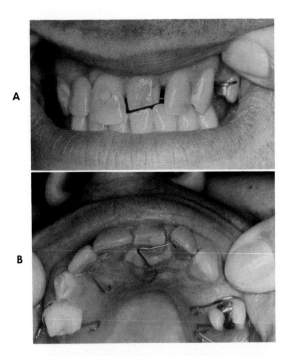

Fig. 37-6. A, A tooth in lingual version that requires (for other reasons) a full crown can be shortened to permit its repositioning without opening the bite or disturbing the rest of the teeth. **B,** Appliance in place. As soon as the tooth reaches its predetermined position, it should be restored back to correct shape with a stabilized temporary restoration.

of restorative reshaping and orthodontics is not generally used to advantage as often as it could be, especially in adult orthodontics.

The advantages do not stop with easier movement of teeth. Temporary acrylic restorations can be fabricated to serve as orthodontic appliances to take the place of bands. They may serve as anchorage, as guides to direct teeth into better position, and finally as extremely good retainers to hold the teeth in place while the supporting tissues reorganize.

RELATIONSHIP OF ANTERIOR TEETH TO POSTERIOR TEETH

I frequently see patients undergo extensive orthodontic treatment involving bicuspid extractions when a more esthetic result could be achieved without extractions, in a fraction of the treatment time and frequently without even using bands or brackets. This should not be misinterpreted as a blanket condemnation of bicuspid extraction. There are arch relationships that are served best by selective extractions (as has already been pointed out). There

are some cases, however, that might be treated differently.

If the posterior occlusion is stable but the anterior teeth are crowded, it should not be considered an *automatic* extraction case. If stripping procedures or restorative reshaping can provide the room for aligning the anterior teeth into an acceptable anterior guidance relationship, there is often no reason to involve the posterior teeth, even when they are not in a Class I relationship.

There are two technique-oriented concepts of orthodontic treatment that might make the above suggestion hard to accept. These concepts are (1) that certain posterior cusps *must* fit in certain corresponding fossae and (2) that a deep overbite relationship is always bad.

Neither concept is valid. Posterior teeth can be maintainably stable in dozens of different relationships from the classic Class I cusp-fossa relationship to an end-to-end bite or even a crossbite. Stability depends on the direction of stress and the distribution of centric holding contacts, not on specific cusp-fossa relationships. The Class I relationship is ideal, but it is not necessary for stability.

In regard to the anterior relationship, there is absolutely nothing wrong with a deep overbite, provided that there are stable centric contacts and the inclines can be harmonized to function. (See Chapter 31.) Given stable centric contacts and functional inclines, deep overbites are just as maintainable as any other anterior relationship, *and the esthetic result is often far superior to the "pushed-in" face of the incorrectly diagnosed extraction case.*

Many patients are far more handsome or beautiful with prominent anterior teeth and a smile line that complements their lip line. Although this may still be accomplished in selected cases with extractions, such a decision should be made on the basis of treating the *face* instead of merely letting the anterior teeth fall victim to some technique concept of cusp tip location and incisal edge relationship.

If the anterior alignment can be corrected without involvement of the posterior teeth —fine! If arch expansion will improve the relationship—that is fine too. If the problem cannot be solved without extractions, we must take out teeth. But we must not get out the forceps until it has been positively determined that:

1. The facial contours, lip support, smile line, and general esthetics will be better with extractions than without
2. The occlusion cannot be stabilized for the long term without extractions
3. The posterior relationship must be changed to correct the anterior relationship; simple expansion of the arch will not suffice or is not practical
4. The above decisions are based on a tooth-by-tooth determination of stress direction and stability of existing centric contacts or potential contacts that might be achieved through reshaping or needed restorations

It is probably worth repeating that it is easy to oversimplify the correction of irregular anterior teeth. Mounted diagnostic models enable the treatment decisions to be tested on the models before any conclusion is finalized. This is a highly recommended procedure.

GROWTH PROBLEMS AND CROWDED LOWER ANTERIOR TEETH

In young patients who have completed successful orthodontic alignment of the anterior teeth, the result is often spoiled later by a delayed crowding of the lower anterior teeth. The same crowding effect may be seen in youngsters who have had naturally well-arranged teeth until their middle or late teens.

Some orthodontic authorities believe that the crowding results from civilized man's failure to wear the anterior teeth into a edge-to-edge relationship. Because of this failure, the anterior teeth supposedly continue to erupt while the posterior teeth do not. The continued eruption is said to cause crowding of the lower anterior teeth as the overbite deepens. This concept is based on studies of Stone Age man's dentition. Some orthodontists still attempt to produce the edge-to-edge bite of severely worn Stone Age dentitions, even in young adults. Hopefully such a stereotyped "orthodontic look" will become a thing of the past as more orthodontists are learning that moderate procumbency is often a desired esthetic trait and that anterior teeth need not be edge to edge to be stable. Even deep overbites can be stable if adequate centric stops are provided.

The problem results from a growth spurt during which the mandible grows faster than the maxilla. The lower anterior teeth are simply caught in the squeeze and crowd up behind the upper anterior teeth, which are held in place by pressure from the lip.

A careful analysis of growth patterns through cephalometrics may enable the astute orthodontists to predict the problem in some cases, but all growing children should be continuously observed for any beginning sign of lower anterior crowding, since it is not uncommon for mandibular growth to continue after maxillary growth has ceased.

The problem is sometimes preventable by use of a simple lingual arch bar bonded or joined to bands on each lower cuspid. The bar prevents the lower incisors from collapsing inward and forces the upper anterior teeth to keep pace with the lower growth spurt. It may have some effect on limiting the growth spurt also, but regardless of how it works, the net effect is to hold the lower anterior teeth in good alignment during the period when mandibular growth occurs at a faster rate than maxillary growth.

Other than minor occlusal adjustment by selective grinding, no other treatment is required except in unusual cases of excessive mandibular development. Once the growth of the mandible has ceased, there is no further need for the appliance. If proper centric contacts are provided and the anterior guidance is in harmony with the envelope of function, there will be no problem of maintaining the relationship indefinitely.

If lower anterior crowding develops *after* the growth years, it is virtually always caused either by a posterior occlusal interference that drives the mandible forward into the upper anterior teeth or by failure to provide adequate centric contact for the lower incisors. Supraeruption and subsequent crowding can occur easily if stable centric stops are not present.

SELECTED READINGS

Altemus, L.A.: Mechanotherapy for minor orthodontic problems, Dent. Clin. North Am., pp. 303-312, July 1968.

Geiger, A., and Hirschfeld, L.: Minor tooth movement in general practice, ed. 3, St. Louis, 1974, The C.V. Mosby Co.

Goldstein, M.C.: Adult orthodontics and the general practitioner, J. Can. Dent. Assoc. **24**:261, 1958.

Goldstein, M.C.: Orthodontics in crown and bridge and periodontal therapy, Dent. Clin. North Am., pp. 449-459, July 1964.

Goldstein, M.C.: Seminar at L.D. Pankey Institute, Miami, Florida, October 1973.

Graber, T.M.: Orthodontics, Philadelphia, 1962, W.B. Saunders Co.

McCreary, C.F.: Personal communication, St. Petersburg, Florida, 1973.

Schlossberg, A.: The removable orthodontic appliance, Dent. Clin. North Am., pp. 487-495, July 1972.

Schwartz, A.M., and Gratzinger, M.: Removable orthodontic appliances, Philadelphia, 1966, W.B. Saunders Co.

Wank, G.S.: The use of grassline ligature in periodontal therapy, Dent. Clin. North Am., pp. 473-486, July 1972.

38

Using cephalometrics for occlusal analysis

Because cephalometrics has been so closely related to predicting growth in children, it has not received the attention it deserves as an aid to treatment planning for adult occlusal problems. Furthermore, the complexity of growth analysis has unnecessarily complicated attempts to simplify cephalometrics for use by general and restorative dentists. It does, however, have great value in occlusal problem analysis for adults, and because growth analysis is unnecessary for mature patients, the use of cephalometrics can be simplified.

Total adherence to cephalometric "norms" does not provide enough information for making a final treatment judgment. Its use must be combined with an analysis of neutral zone factors and established patterns of function. The goal of treatment should be anatomic and functional harmony for individuals that do not always fit cephalometric averages, but the averages can be used as guidelines in combination with other relevant information to tip off the examiner to which segments are in normal relationships and which ones are not. If a dentoalveolar segment that appears normal cephalometrically also appears normal to profile analysis and functional relationships, it should not be changed to conform to a malrelated part. A basic rule in treatment planning is to preserve what is right and change what is wrong.

Cephalometric analysis is an aid to making that decision.

ELEMENTS OF CEPHALOMETRICS

There are two basic elements forming the entire system that must be learned to make cephalometric analysis understandable.

1. Points
2. Planes

Points are precisely located spots that relate to specific bony landmarks. They are the first thing that is located on a tracing of a cephalometric radiograph. Points can also be recorded on soft-tissue landmarks and as intersecting points where two planes cross.

Planes are determined by joining two points with a straight line.

Points

Bony landmarks (on lateral cephalometric analysis, Fig. 38-1). There are 11 bony landmarks that can be easily learned as a beginning foundation for occlusal analysis.

1 *P point* (portion) is located at the most *superior* convexity of the external auditory meatus.

2 *O point* (orbital) is located at the most *inferior* convexity of the external border of the orbital cavity. It is the anterior landmark for determining the Frankfort plane.

3 *Na point* (nasion) is located at the most forward point of the nasofrontal suture. It is the upper

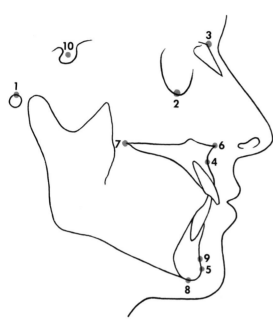

Fig. 38-1. Bony landmarks on lateral cephalogram.

point for determining the facial plane.

4 *A point* (subspinale) is located at the deepest point of concavity on the labial surface of the maxilla between the anterior nasal spine and the alveolus. It is the upper landmark for the A-Po plane. It also signifies the juncture of the basal bone with the alveolar process.

5 *Po point* (pogonion) is the most anterior point on the symphysis. It is the lower landmark for both the facial plane and the A-Po plane.

6 *ANS point* is the anterior tip of the nasal spine.

7 *PNS point* is the posterior tip of the nasal spine.

8 *M point* (menton) is the most inferior point on the symphysis of the mandible.

9 *PM point* (protuberantia mentalis) is a point above the pogonion where the profile changes from convex to concave.

10 *S point* (sella turcica) is the center of the sella turcica.

× *Xi point* is the geometric center of the mandibular ramus (Fig. 38-2).

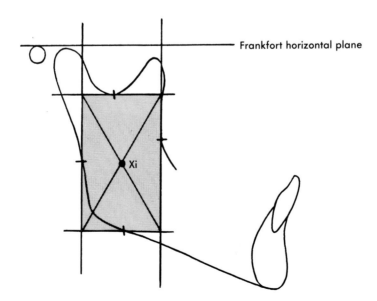

Fig. 38-2. Xi point. A rectangle is formed with the top and bottom parallel to the Frankfort horizontal plane and the sides perpendicular. Each line is drawn to tangent to points on the borders of the ramus to form the rectangle. Xi point is located at the intersection of diagonals and represents the geometric center of the ramus.

Soft-tissue landmarks (Fig. 38-3)

1. *Pn point* (pronasale) is the most anterior point of the nose.
2. *Po' point* (soft-tissue pogonion) is the most anterior point on the soft tissue of the chin.

Planes (related to lateral cephalometric analysis)

For a general appraisal of skeletal, occlusal, and profile relationships we can generate a considerable amount of helpful information by observing two sets of five planes on a lateral cephalometric analysis:

1. Horizontal planes (Fig. 38-4)
   a. Sella nasion plane (S Na)
   b. Frankfort horizontal plane (FH)
   c. Palatal plane (ANS to PNS)
   d. Occlusal plane (OP)
   e. Mandibular plane (MP)
2. Vertical planes
   a. N-A line (connecting nasion with A point)
   b. Facial plane (Na to Po)
   c. A-Po plane
   d. Esthetic plane (Pn to Po')
   e. McNamara line (nasion perpendicular)

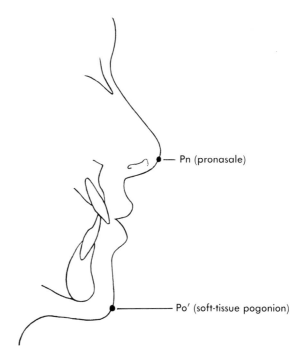

Fig. 38-3. Soft-tissue landmarks.

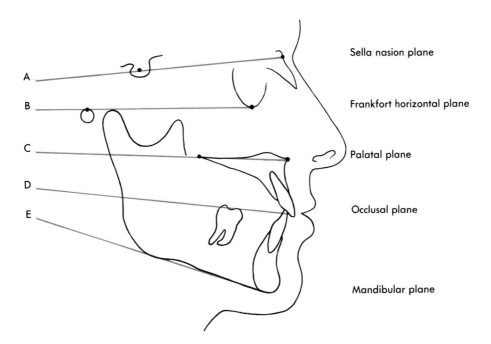

Fig. 38-4. The horizontal planes.

HOW THE PLANES ARE USED FOR OCCLUSAL PROBLEM ANALYSIS

From a lateral viewpoint, the cephalometric planes are an aid for determining five essential relationships that are keys to diagnosis and treatment planning.

1. Anteroposterior relationship of maxilla to cranial base.
2. Anteroposterior relationship of mandible to cranial base.
3. Relationship of upper teeth to maxilla.
4. Relationship of lower teeth to mandible.
5. Vertical relationship of mandible and maxilla to cranial base and to each other.

As stated, a cephalometric analysis is never relied on as the sole determinant of treatment. Rather it is one part of a diagnostic triad that includes the following:

1. Cephalometric analysis
2. Mounted diagnostic casts
3. Clinical examination and evaluation

If all three parts of the analysis are in agreement, the diagnosis can be made with assurance. If any one of the above evaluations does not agree with the others, it should be considered a red flag. Blind dependence on certain cephalometric norms can destroy an attractive facial profile, but this can be avoided when the analysis is combined with clinical observation that includes evaluation of every patient for occlusal stability as part of a total examination. Regardless of the relationship to the norms, a dentition is stable if there are no signs of tooth hypermobility, excessive wear, or migration.

When a stable occlusion is found in combination with an abnormal cephalometric analysis, the reasons for the stability should be determined before any changes are contemplated. The dentition may be stabilized by unbreakable habit patterns or strong neutral zone relationships. Similarly, a unique profile may be attractive and stable, even though it is not "normal."

The significance of skeletal norms must be adjusted for age, sex, and race, but the following makes the most usable analysis as applied to adult white males.

EVALUATING HORIZONTAL POSITION OF MAXILLA

Maxillary depth refers to the anteroposterior relationship of the maxilla to the cranial base. It is determined by the degree of angulation of the N-A line in relation to the Frankfort horizontal plane (FH plane) (Fig. 38-5). This reference determines whether a Class II or Class III malocclusion is attributable to the maxilla.

Norm. A 90-degree angulation indicates that the maxilla is in a normal relationship.

Maxillary protrusion. Maxillary protrusion is indicated by an angulation greater than 90 degrees. The higher the angle, the greater is the horizontal excess of the maxilla.

Maxillary retrusion. Inadequate growth of the maxilla in an anterior direction is indicated by an angulation less than 90 degrees. The lower the value, the greater is the deficiency.

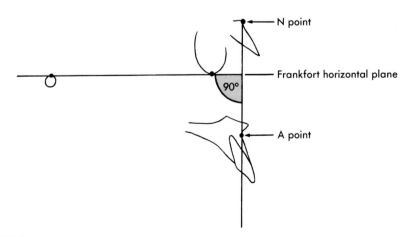

Fig. 38-5. *Maxillary depth analysis* for "normal" anteroposterior relationship of the maxilla to the cranial base. Angle greater than 90 degrees indicates maxillary protrusion. Angle less than 90 degrees indicates retrusion. This analysis indicates whether the maxilla is responsible for a Class II or Class III malocclusion.

EVALUATING HORIZONTAL POSITION OF MANDIBLE

Mandibular depth refers to the anteroposterior position of the mandible to the cranial base. It is determined by the degree of angulation of the N-Po line in relation to the Frankfort horizontal plane (FH plane) (Fig. 38-6). This reference determines whether a Class II or Class III malocclusion is attributable to the mandible.

Norm. A 90-degree angulation indicates that the mandible is in a normal relationship horizontally.

Mandibular prognathism. Mandibular prognathism is indicated by an angulation greater than 90 degrees. The higher the angle, the greater is the mandibular excess in an anterior direction.

Retrognathic mandible. A retrognathic mandible is indicated by an angulation of less than 90 degrees. The lower the angle value, the greater is the mandibular deficiency. A severe deficiency produces an "Andy Gump" type of deformity.

EVALUATING A-P RELATIONSHIP OF MAXILLA TO MANDIBLE

In a normal patient with a straight profile, the A point falls on the facial plane. This indicates a harmonious relationship between the maxilla and the mandible. This relationship is the easiest to treat and is consistent with a pleasant profile.

The relationship of the A point to the facial plane determines the amount of *convexity* of the profile. If the A point is anterior to the facial plane, the patient's profile will be convex (Fig. 38-7).

If the A point is posterior to the facial plane, the profile will be concave (Fig. 38-8).

The convexity analysis relates the maxilla to the mandible. It indicates a retrognathic relationship with a plus dimension of the A point and indicates a prognathic relationship when the A point is posterior to the facial plane. The convexity analysis, however, does not specify which jaw is at fault. Thus convexity analysis should be used with individual analysis of mandibular depth and maxillary depth to deter-

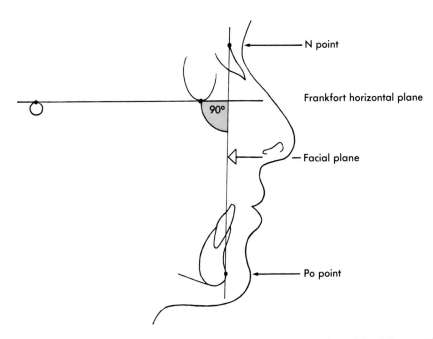

Fig. 38-6. *Mandibular depth analysis* for "normal" anteroposterior relationship of the mandible to the cranial base. Angle greater than 90 degrees indicates mandibular protrusion. Angle less than 90 degrees indicates retrusion, though a slight reduction in value is considered acceptable.

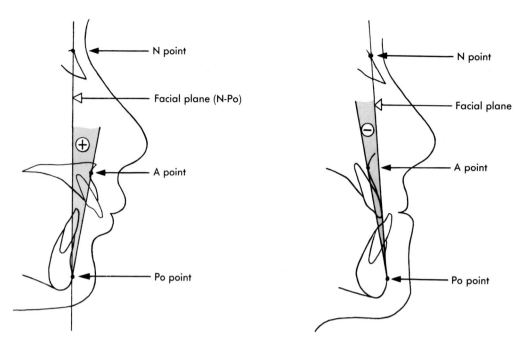

Fig. 38-7. *Convexity analysis.* The A point is anterior to facial plane, an indication of a convex facial profile. This analysis by itself does not show which jaw is at fault because a convex profile can result from either a protruded maxilla or a retruded mandible.

Fig. 38-8. *Concave profile* is indicated by convexity analysis because A point is posterior to facial plane. In this patient, the Class II occlusion is caused by a protruded mandible, but that conclusion is not determinable by this analysis alone. This analysis relates one jaw to the other but does not relate either jaw to the cranial base to determine which jaw is at fault.

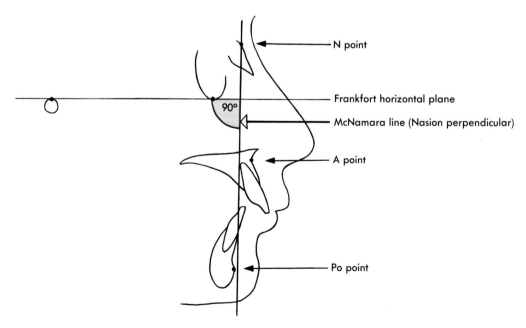

Fig. 38-9. *McNamara line (nasion perpendicular)* is drawn from N-point perpendicular to Frankfort horizontal plane. With this analysis, both the maxilla and mandible can be related to a "true" vertical expression of the anterior facial plane. Both jaws can thus be related to the cranial base in one analysis. In the analysis above, it is obvious that the cause of Class II relationship is a protruded maxilla because the A point is in front of the nasion perpendicular whereas the mandible is slightly behind the line and within a normal distance.

mine where corrections should be made. A quick reference relationship of either or both arches can be analyzed in relation to the McNamara line.

The McNamara line is a reference plane that relates the anteroposterior positioning of both jaws to each other as well as to cranial components. The McNamara line is also referred to as a "nasion perpendicular" because it is constructed by extending a vertical line downward from the nasion, which is perpendicular to the Frankfort horizontal plane (Fig. 38-9).

The construction of a true vertical facial line provides a simple, quick assessment for identification of discrepancies in the horizontal plane that more clearly defines the problem, such as mandibular skeletal protrusion or a maxillary skeletal retrusion (Fig. 38-10) instead of a simplistic diagnosis of Class II malocclusion. It will also indicate when both arches are either protruded or retruded.

The analysis relates the maxilla and mandible to the nasion perpendicular in linear (millimeter) rather than angular (degree) measurements. So the position of the maxilla in relation to the "true" vertical plane is measured in millimeters. In a normal, attractive profile, point A lies on or slightly ahead of the McNamara line.

The relationship of the mandible to the cranial base is also measured in millimeters from the nasion perpendicular, and so it is not influenced by any maxillary reference points. Thus it is a true representation of the chin position in relation to the cranial base. In a growing child with a mixed dentition, the Po point lies normally 8 to 6 mm posterior to the nasion perpendicular. Mandibular growth increases the value approximately 0.5 mm per year until it reaches a normal relationship range of -4 to -2 mm posterior to the McNamara line.

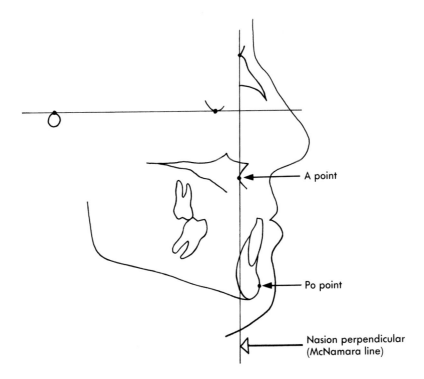

A point

Po point

Nasion perpendicular
(McNamara line)

Fig. 38-10. Clinical example of how cephalometric analysis can aid a prosthodontic treatment plan: This patient was treated unsuccessfully by four different dentists with attempts to prosthetically build out an upper edentulous area to align upper teeth with the lower incisors. This is an example of changing what is right to fit what is wrong. Analysis shows that the maxilla is in correct anteroposterior relationship (A point is on the line). The mandible, however, is severely prognathic (Po point is far anterior to the line). An acceptable result in this patient is not possible without surgical reduction of mandibular length.

RELATING TEETH TO SKELETAL BASES

One of the advantages of using the A point is that it is a *skeletal* relationship that can be evaluated whether or not teeth are present. Thus it can be a helpful determination to make in the analysis of where to relate teeth on a denture.

A-Po plane is the reference plane that relates the denture bases (Fig. 38-11). The A-Po plane is also referred to as the *maxillomandibular line,* and it is an easy reference to which both upper and lower teeth can be related to the maxilla and the mandible. That reference, in turn, can be related to the facial plane.

Upper incisor protrusion is measured in millimeters from the A-Po line. The norm is +3.5 mm, with a deviation of ±2.3 mm.

Upper incisor inclination is measured by degrees of angulation with the A-Po line. The norm is 28 degrees, with a deviation of ±4 degrees.

Lower incisor protrusion has a norm of +1 mm from the A-Po line, with a deviation of ±2.3 mm.

Lower incisor inclination has a norm of 22 degrees, with a deviation of ±4 degrees.

The interincisal angle relates the long axis of the incisors to each other (Fig. 38-12). The norm is 130 degrees. Clinical deviation is 6 degrees. Lower angles indicate protrusion. Higher angles tend toward a deep overbite.

The relationship of the teeth to the skeletal bases is far more dependent on neutral zone factors than on any form of arbitrary positioning based on averages. There is probably no other part of the dentition that is so critically dependent on being in harmony with the musculature. And any malalignment of the teeth with the muscular forces of the tongue or the lips and the perioral musculature will lead to instability. Furthermore it is not necessary to have the anterior teeth conform to any set angulation or even range of angulations. As long as the anterior teeth are in harmony with jaw function and have definite holding contacts to stop their eruption, they can be stable regardless of their interincisal angle.

Many patients with deep overbites and even some lingual inclination (greater than 180 degrees) can be kept completely stable if definite holding contacts are in place (Fig. 38-13).

Lingual inclination of anterior teeth is not uncommon in patients with short upper lips because during swallowing the lower lip must stretch to seal with the upper lip. This creates greater lower lip pressure against the upper labial surfaces, moving the incisal edge toward the lingual. In severely tight-lipped patients it may be necessary to add holding contacts on the upper teeth to prevent supraeruption, but with stable centric stops even lingually inclined anterior teeth can be vertically and horizontally stable. When teeth are related to a naturally tight neutral zone, the lip-closure path is not interfered with, and phonetic relationships are preserved between the lips and the incisal edges. Even though the incisor incli-

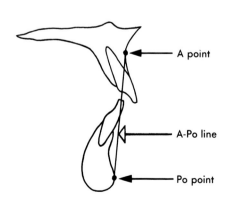

Fig. 38-11. *A-Po line* is the reference plane for the denture bases. It does not relate to the cranial base, but with the addition of the facial plane or the nasion perpendicular the maxillomandibular relationship can be put into perspective with total facial profile. Inclination or protrusion of the anterior teeth relates to this line.

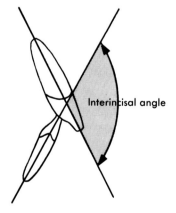

Fig. 38-12. *Interincisal angle* relates the long axis of upper and lower incisors to each other. The norm is 130 degrees, but we put very little importance on this angulation, preferring instead to establish the interincisor angle from functional relationships that vary considerably, even among "normal" dentitions.

nations do not fall within normal values, both esthetics and function may be better served.

Cephalometric norms do not necessarily relate to these important factors, and so the clinical evaluation should have primary importance in diagnosis and treatment planning for anterior tooth inclinations. There seems to be a growing consensus among top orthodontists that cephalometric norms can be used as a quick reference for average anterior tooth inclinations, but clinical evaluation is far more reliable for this particular relationship.

EVALUATING VERTICAL SKELETAL RELATIONSHIPS

Evaluation of the *mandibular plane angle* is one of the most effective ways of determining if an anterior open bite is a skeletal malrelationship. This is an important determination because the treatment of a skeletal open bite is often quite different from an open bite caused by a habit pattern.

The mandibular plane angle relates the mandibular plane to the Frankfort horizontal plane (Fig. 38-14).

Norm is 25 degrees.

Anterior skeletal open bite. A high angulation indicates that the open bite is a skeletal malrelationship caused by the mandible.

Deep overbite. A low angulation indicates that the deep bite is skeletal and is caused by the mandible.

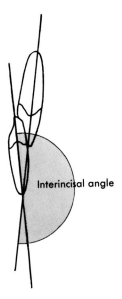

Fig. 38-13. *Lingually inclined anteriors* with an interincisal angle greater than 180 degrees may be completely stable if they have stable holding stops and if they are in harmony with neutral zone factors and functional jaw movements. If a change in inclination is contemplated for teeth in this relationship, care should be taken to maintain the upper incisal edge position in harmony with the lip closure path and a very tight lip relationship.

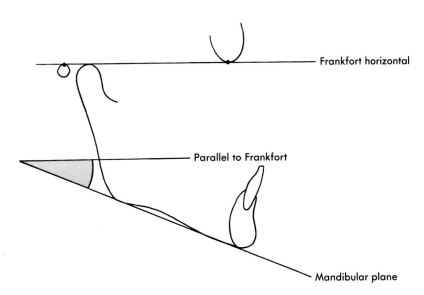

Fig. 38-14. Mandibular plane angle.

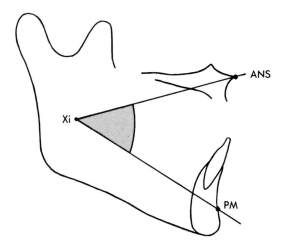

Fig. 38-15. Lower facial height.

Lower facial height is another measurement that relates to the divergence of the maxillomandibular angulation. Ricketts has shown that in normal growth this angle stays constant with age. The measurement is made at the intersection of lines from ANS (anterior nasal spine) to Xi and from PM (protuberantia mentalis) to Xi (Fig. 38-15).

Norm is 47 degrees, with a clinical deviation of 4 degrees.

The higher the angle, the more likely there is a skeletal open bite. The lower the angle, the more there is a tendency for deep overbite.

EVALUATING THE OCCLUSAL PLANE

The *functional occlusal plane* is a plane that relates to the occlusal surfaces of the molars and premolars (Fig. 38-16).

The purpose of analyzing the occlusal plane cephalometrically is to determine its correct vertical position in both the anterior and posterior segments. An esthetically pleasing occlusal plane is close to the center of the ramus (Xi point) at the posterior and slightly below the lip embrasure at the anterior. The lower incisal edges are normally slightly above the level of the functional occlusal plane.

Vertical maxillary excess. If the occlusal plane is too far below the lip embrasure, it indicates a vertical maxillary excess. This refers to the typical "gummy smile." The occlusion may appear normal in every other respect, but when the lips are at rest, the entire labial surface and part of the gingival tissues may be exposed. Periodontal health may be affected because of continuous exposure of the gingival

tissues to the air. The patient may show lip strain from trying to keep the teeth covered.

On treatment of a vertical excess problem in the maxilla it is important to consider the full occlusal plane and the importance of maintaining a correct anterior guidance. The problem is usually solved surgically.

Vertical maxillary deficiency. A high occlusal plane anteriorly may indicate hidden upper incisors and an excessive visibility of the lower anterior teeth. This creates a "bulldog" appearance to the smile, which is unesthetic. With age and a loss of tissue resiliency, the upper lip elongates to a lower level at rest, and so it is a normal occurrence for older patients to expose less of the upper teeth when smiling.

Although cephalometric analysis may relate the level of the anterior occlusal plane to the lip line, it should be remembered that variations in lip length and phonetic function may be more critical determinants. The relationship of the upper incisal edges to the lower-lip smile line can be determined clinically, and the precise incisal edge position can be determined from observation during lip-closure path and lip contact at the *f* and *v* position. In edentulous patients, these guidelines can be determined from wax esthetic controls, and then the denture teeth can be set to those guidelines. My experience would indicate that

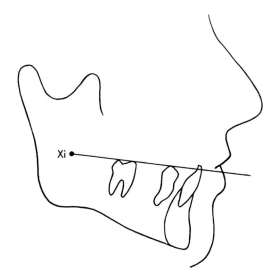

Fig. 38-16. *Functional occlusal plane* relates to the occlusal surfaces of the molars and premolars. It does not bisect the incisors. It is close to the Xi point in the back and aligns slightly below the lip embrasure in the front.

both esthetics and function can be adversely affected by variations in incisal edge position that are so minute that it requires careful clinical observation and testing to determine these guidelines accurately. Cephalometrics can be helpful as a reference, but it is doubtful that it should ever override decisions based on clinical analysis of functional relationships, at least as far as the anterior teeth are concerned.

The posterior level of the occlusal plane should approach the level of Xi point. Problems occur particularly when the posterior occlusal plane is too high because it interferes with protrusive disclusion. The level of the posterior occlusal plane can be so effectively determined on mounted diagnostic casts that it is doubtful that cephalometric analysis is necessary from an occlusal analysis viewpoint. The advantage of mounted casts is that the posterior occlusion can be related to the disclusive effect of the condylar path and the anterior guidance, two very critical factors in determining the acceptability of any occlusal plane.

The use of a Broadrick flag as advocated in the PM technique effectively relates the posterior occlusal plane to the Xi point on mounted diagnostic casts. This is the result achieved, however, only if the *condyle* is used as the posterior survey point in determining the occlusal plane. The use of the Broadrick flag is not applicable for nonrestorative cases though, and so occlusal plane analysis cephalometrically does have real value for orthodontic and surgical analysis if it is used with clinical evaluation.

The superior surface of the retromolar pad is also an effective clinical landmark for locating the posterior level of the occlusal plane. It is especially useful when the posterior ridges are edentulous.

EVALUATING THE SOFT-TISSUE PROFILE

The relationship of the lips to the nose and the chin can be evaluated by analysis of the *esthetic plane* (Fig. 38-17). This plane connects the tip of the nose (Pn point) with the soft-tissue pogonion (Po').

For the most pleasing appearance, the ideal position of the lower lip is close to the esthetic plane. In edentulous patients, the resorption of alveolar ridges allows the lips to sink back. If denture teeth can be positioned to support the lips closer to the esthetic plane, the appearance will be improved.

There are three considerations related to the esthetic plane, as follows.

Size of the nose or prominence of the chin. Excess of either nose or chin may cause the upper and lower lips and teeth to appear retruded. Evaluating the position of the teeth in relation to the nasion perpendicular will give a different perspective in determining whether a profile problem is caused by a normal relationship of the teeth to an abnormal esthetic plane, or vice versa.

Inclination of upper incisors. Protrusion of the upper incisors has a tendency to fold the lower lip and push it forward, creating an unpleasant profile. Changing the neutral zone by inclining the upper incisors back not only improves the esthetics, but also allows the lip to seal more effectively and helps to stabilize the teeth in the more upright position.

Strength and position of perioral musculature. A protruded, button chin with a deep cleft above it forms a very characteristic

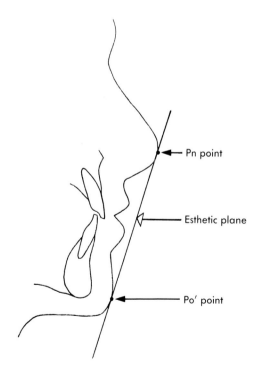

Fig. 38-17. *Esthetic plane.* There are no standards for lip position that are applicable for all patients. However the generally accepted norm is for the lower lip to be within approximately 2 mm from the esthetic plane. This is quite variable in different races and is affected by nose and chin prominence. One can make this analysis clinically by laying a flat ruler against the nose and chin.

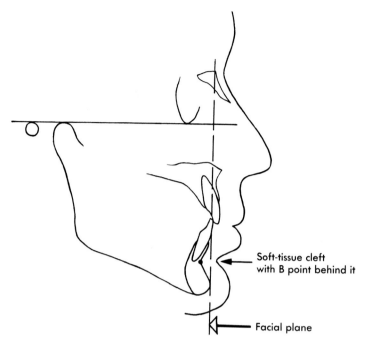

Fig. 38-18. The *B point* is the mandibular counterpart to the A point in the maxilla. It is the deepest part of the concavity between the lower incisor and the bony chin. When it is located too posterior to the facial plane, it indicates the probability of a strong buccinator band limitation on the growth of the dentoalveolar process at the level of the roots. A soft-tissue cleft and button chin are classic profile evidence of this restriction. It may be in combination with normal anteroposterior growth of the skeletal chin.

profile that may be an indication of a strong lower band of the buccinator compressing the underling mentalis muscle. It is often associated with vertical or even lingually inclined incisors because of an exceptionally strong neutral zone effect. The upper band of the buccinator may also be restrictive, creating a retrusion of the upper dentoalveolar process in relation to a normal chin and nose. The restrictive effect of the musculature may also be predominantly directed at the roots and the alveolar process while the tongue exerts a strong forward pressure to incline the crowns forward. The skeletal base may continue to grow while forward growth of the alveolar processes is limited by the tight band of muscle. Cephalometric evidence that this has occurred may be found in a soft-tissue profile with a cleft and a button chin and possibly a B point (supramentale) that is considerably behind the facial plane (Fig. 38-18).

CONCERNS ABOUT THE USE OF CEPHALOMETRICS

One of the most important benefits of cephalometric analysis is the information it provides for determining the anteroposterior relationship of the mandible to the cranial base. This is determined angularly by the relationship of the facial plane (N-Po) to the Frankfort horizontal plane, or it may be determined linearly by relating the Po point to the nasion perpendicular (McNamara line). Either method provides valuable information in determining whether or not the mandible is at fault in a Class II or Class III malocclusion.

The accuracy of the above determinations is totally dependent on the condyles being in centric relation when the lateral cephalogram is made. A significant error is possible if the cephalogram is made in the maximum intercuspal relationship because the mandible can be displaced several millimeters forward of centric relation. This would completely invalidate the relationship of the Po point to the facial plane or the accuracy of the angle formed with the FH plane. Despite this obvious error, there seems to be very limited willingness to change the practice. The errors in diagnosis are very real and are common. In my own practice I have seen numerous patients who have been treatment planned for major corrections that were not needed, including recommendations for surgery where only minimal occlusal correction was required, and the errors in diagnosis were made from inaccurate cephalograms.

Two simple procedures can eliminate the mistakes in diagnosis from cephalometric analysis of displaced mandibles:

1. The use of centrically mounted diagnostic casts as an essential part of occlusal diagnosis.
2. The use of centric relation bite record to hold the mandible at the seated position of the condyles during the radiographic procedure. From that position, the mandible can be closed on the tracing when the condylar axis is maintained near the center of the condyle.

Slavicek has developed a method for correcting the position of the mandible when the cephalometric tracings are made so that the mandible is correctly related to the cranial base in centric relation. These corrections are made by transferal of information from centrically mounted casts so that the position of the mandible on the tracing is correct.

Williamson has consistently emphasized the importance of seated condyles to an accurate cephalometric analysis and utilizes mounted diagnostic casts as an important part of orthodontic treatment planning. Numerous other orthodontists are in agreement and are now including *mounted* diagnostic casts as an essential part of diagnosis.

It is true that an astute diagnostician and master dentist could correct most occlusions without using either mounted casts or cephalometrics just as a master builder could build a house without plans. The question is, "Why would one want to?" Planning from an accurate base of information eliminates trial-and-error treatment and prevents mistakes. Cephalometric analysis can be used to improve the odds. Mounted diagnostic casts and clinical observation, however, are a necessary part of a reasonable occlusal diagnosis.

The second major concern about too much dependence on cephalometric analysis is related to the inclination of the anterior teeth. The success or failure of the anterior relationship depends so much on harmony with the musculature and the surrounding soft tissues, it is not a reliable practice to position these teeth arbitrarily according to averages. It is probable that most postorthodontic instability problems are caused by failure to position the anterior teeth precisely enough in the neutral zone, which is not determinable from cephalometric analysis. Furthermore, the ranges of lip movement *during function* vary so much, even among "normal" faces, that it would seem unlikely that the static analysis of centric relation would be accurate enough to use exclusively, as a definite guideline.

Just as we are unable to precisely determine anterior relationships from mounted diagnostic casts, which are three dimensional, it would be impossible to determine those relationships from two-dimensional cephalograms. Both however provide helpful information, but the final "fine tuning" of anterior teeth inclinations, anterior guidance, and functional relationships can be made accurately only by clinical observation of the dynamic relationship of the soft tissues with the teeth during function.

SELECTED READINGS

Chaconas, S.J., and Gonidis, D.: A cephalometric technique for prosthodontic diagnosis and treatment planning, J. Prosthet. Dent. **56**:567, 1986.

Di Pietro, G.J., and Moergeli, J.R.: Significance of the Frankfort mandibular plane angle to prosthodontics, J. Prosthet. Dent. **36**:624, 1976.

Ricketts, R.M.: Role of cephalometrics in prosthetic diagnosis, J. Prosthet. Dent. **6**:488, 1956.

Skafidas, T.M.: Cephalometric analysis manual, Department of Orthodontics, Emory University School of Dentistry, Atlanta, Ga., 1987.

Wallen, T., and Bloomquist, D.: The clinical examination: is it more important than cephalometric analysis in surgical orthodontics? Int. J. Adult Orthodon. Orthognath. Surg. **1**(3):179, 1986.

39

Solving severe arch malrelationship problems

Arch malrelationship problems fall into two general categories:

1. Those that result from malposition of the teeth in relation to an acceptably aligned skeletal base
2. Those that result from a malrelationship of the skeletal base

Although many arch relationships can be corrected by orthodontic treatment alone, some occlusal problems are too severe to be treated successfully without a combined approach that may involve the expertise of several different specialists. The prosthodontist, the maxillofacial surgeon, and the orthodontist may need to work as a team to solve certain severe malrelationships. When this is necessary, the treatment must be coordinated so that each specialist can perform without constraints that result from lack of understanding by the other specialists regarding the final goals of treatment. Unfortunately even a team approach can fall short of an optimum result if some member of the team does not *direct* the treatment toward a final goal of harmonious occlusion.

For an ideal goal-oriented result, the logical specialist to coordinate the direction of treatment should be the specialist who has the final responsibility for the completion of treatment.

If the orthodontist will have the final responsibility, the orthodontist should direct the surgeon or the prosthodontist regarding the preparation for a finished orthodontic result. If the prosthodontist has the ultimate responsibility for a complete prosthetic result, input from that specialist should clearly outline what is needed from the surgeon or orthodontist. It is terribly discouraging to attempt an acceptable prosthetic treatment plan *after* surgical or orthodontic treatment has been completed with no consideration for the result. This can be avoided if the last person to be responsible for the result is involved in treatment decisions related to preparing the patient for the final treatment result.

Just as with other types of occlusal problems, the treatment of complex arch malrelationships cannot be *solely* directed toward a single textbook version of Class I occlusion, not because it isn't a worthwhile goal in some or even most patients, but rather because it is not a necessary or even acceptable goal in *some* patients. There are many options for treating arch malrelationships, and the prudent diagnostician will evaluate *all* options before recommending treatment. There are many considerations that only the patient can evaluate, and the patient is entitled to know if there is more than one way to achieve a result that would be acceptable. As long as the inviolate goal of optimum oral health is not compromised, the treatment approach that best suits the patient's total needs is the one that should be considered.

The analysis of severe arch malrelationships should result in a treatment plan that accomplishes four specific goals:

1. Optimum oral health
2. Occlusal stability
3. Comfortable function
4. An esthetic result that is acceptable to the patient

Because it may be possible to accomplish the first three goals without satisfying the fourth, severe arch malrelationships should always be analyzed to determine which segments, if any, are properly related to the cranial base and the skeletofacial profile. With improved surgical techniques, realignment of the skeletal base can be accomplished with such predictive results that it should at least be considered as an option to be evaluated before a final treatment plan is determined. Regardless of the mode of treatment selected, the segments of the occlusion that are correctly related should not be altered to conform to the segments that are malpositioned. Thus a careful analysis is in order so that treatment is directed to maintain what is correct and change only what needs to be changed. The process for making such decisions requires an orderly sequence.

The first step in planning treatment for complex arch malrelationships is an interview with the patient to find out from these basic questions what his condition is:

1. Are you uncomfortable?
2. Can you function satisfactorily?
3. How do you feel about your appearance?

There are many arch malrelationships that do not need treatment. If there are no signs of instability, no discomfort, and no complaint about function or appearance, there is no need for intervention. A personal example may help to illustrate this point: A 72-year-old surgeon in excellent health was referred for correction of a severe arch malrelationship. His entire lower arch was completely buccal to his upper arch. He did not have holding contacts on any teeth. There was no anterior guidance, and only the balancing side came into contact in lateral excursion. Upon questioning, he reported no discomfort and no problems of any kind with mastication, and he had 32 firm teeth with no excessive wear. His supporting tissues were completely healthy. When asked about his appearance, he laughed that his prominent lower jaw had never been any concern to him. In fact, he considered it one of his strong features and wouldn't change it, even if he could. No treatment was needed, and none was wanted.

The above patient had a stable occlusion. The tongue and the cheeks *substituted for* the missing holding contacts, and a vertical pattern of function *eliminated the need* for anterior guidance or lateral disclusion. The lack of any sign of instability confirmed that diagnosis.

But would the same conclusion be drawn if the patient had been 32 years of age instead of 72?

The answer is yes. The diagnosis would be the same because regardless of the age of a mature adult the complete lack of any signs of instability *along with an explanation of why the occlusion is stable* is proof enough that treatment is not needed at that time.

The critical element in diagnosis however is the thorough examination. The decision that no treatment is needed can only be made after a careful determination that there are no causes or effects of instability. If tooth positions are changing or teeth are loose or are wearing excessively, some interception of causative factors should be delineated and explained to the patient regardless of how comfortable or how functional the occlusion feels. Patients cannot make an informed decision unless they are aware of all the facts. Patients cannot know the facts unless a thorough examination determines them.

The value of cephalometrics in restorative dentistry has not been well understood, and consequently it has not been used to full advantage. In determining any treatment plan, all practical methods of treatment should be evaluated and compared. The patient should be made aware of the various options and should have a reasonable explanation of why a particular treatment approach is favored. When there are obvious facial profile problems related to the arch malrelationship, cephalometric radiographs are very helpful in the initial stage of diagnosis because an analysis of those films helps us to determine which segments are correct and which segments need to be altered. This is valuable information for determining treatment approaches because each treatment potential can then be analyzed in relation to a correct goal.

With background information from the patient interview, a sequence of analyses can be used to develop all viable options for treatment. Thoroughness requires the following:

1. A complete intraoral examination, including periodontal examination
2. Screening examination and history to determine the condition of the temporomandibular joints; a more intensive TMJ exam when indicated
3. Correctly mounted diagnostic casts in centric relation
4. Complete radiographic series of the teeth and jaws; panoramic films routinely included
5. Cephalometric radiographs if facial profile is a problem or any alteration of the skeletal base is contemplated
6. Completed medical history

Special tests or speciality examination information may also be required for specific problems, and a conference with other specialists who have treated the patient may be in order.

DESIGNING TREATMENT WHEN THE SKELETAL BASE IS ACCEPTABLY ALIGNED

In severe arch malrelationships, the skeletal base is rarely in perfect alignment, but if the skeletal profile appears acceptable and careful interviewing of the patient determines that it is not an esthetic concern, a treatment plan approach is initiated for the purpose of correcting tooth relationships without altering the existing skeletal base. Since the alveolar bone can be made to move with the teeth, it may be effectively altered orthodontically within the context of this approach.

If the skeletal base is not to be changed, diagnostic procedures are aimed at determining where the teeth must be positioned for a stable occlusal relationship. This determination is best organized by use of correctly mounted diagnostic casts. Correct mounting requires verified centric relation bite records and the use of a facebow.

Analysis of the mounted casts must be related to the requirements for stability described in Chapter 27. Each requirement for stability is analyzed *in sequence,* starting with the first requirement of stable holding contacts for each tooth. If we divide our analysis into separate treatment objectives, it greatly simplifies the treatment planning.

FIRST TREATMENT OBJECTIVE—STABLE HOLDING CONTACTS

There are four treatment options that should be analyzed in sequence to determine which option, or combination of options, would best fulfill this objective. The option choices are as follows:

1. Selective grinding—reshaping
2. Orthodontics—repositioning
3. Restoration
4. Surgery

Analysis of first treatment option—selective grinding

On duplicated casts that are also mounted, the first step is to determine how much correction can be accomplished with selective grinding. When all interferences are eliminated so that the casts can close to maximum occlusal contact in centric relation, the results are sometimes surprising. What appears to be a severe occlusal problem may not be severe at all when the occlusal relationship is evaluated in centric relation *at the correct vertical dimension.*

It is amazing how far out of alignment the mandible can be driven by occlusal interferences. Severe facial asymmetries can result from deviation around malposed teeth. Pseudoprognathism can result to a degree that surgical correction might be contemplated if centrically mounted casts were not studied first at the correct vertical dimension. The only effective way to determine the true tooth-to-tooth relationship at the correct vertical is to equilibrate the casts until the articulator can close to the same vertical as maximum occlusal contact. The closure must be confined to the centric relation axis.

The casts can be poured with dowel pins so that the posterior segments can be removed. This permits a quick analysis of the anterior relationship on a centric relation arc. But it does not permit analysis of the tooth-to-tooth relationships of the posterior teeth.

In my practice I have seen several patients with apparent severe arch malrelationships who were scheduled for corrective surgery. But when casts were mounted in centric relation with an open bite record and the interferences to the centric relation arc of closure were cleared, the severe deviation of the mandible was eliminated. Even apparently severe prognathic patients may have acceptable profiles if the mandible is not forced into protrusion by occlusal interferences.

There is no acceptable substitute for centrically mounted diagnostic casts in the diagnosis of arch malrelationships. The casts should be equilibrated to the patient's most closed vertical dimension in centric relation before any further decisions regarding treatment selection are made. A second set of casts should be preserved in their original relationship so that a comparison can be made at any point of treatment.

The decision to use selective grinding should be based on three factors:
1. Amount of tooth reshaping needed
2. Condition of teeth to be reshaped
3. Comparative analysis with other methods of treatment

If gross reshaping is needed on teeth that require restorative procedures for other reasons, even severe reshaping can often be used to advantage. If alternative treatments would be severely complicated or prohibitive for one reason or another from the patient's standpoint, reshaping, even extensive reshaping in some cases, may be the treatment option of choice.

If only minor reshaping is required to achieve an acceptable result, equilibration would generally be the option of choice.

If the problem cannot be resolved by selective grinding, the second step in the sequence should be pursued—orthodontic evaluation.

Analysis of second treatment option—orthodontics

The purpose of this analysis is to determine how much can be accomplished by orthodontics toward moving the teeth into an acceptable relationship. By working with both the original casts and the equilibrated casts, the orthodontist can determine whether it is possible to move teeth within the existing skeletal base into an acceptable alignment or whether it is possible to alter the skeletal framework orthopedically to resolve the malrelationship without surgery. A cephalometric evaluation is an important part of this diagnostic procedure.

By working with both the equilibrated casts and the unchanged casts we can also comparatively evaluate a combination approach whereby reshaping and repositioning procedures are both utilized.

If the problem is too severe to be solved with orthodontics or a combination of orthodontics and selective grinding, the third step in the sequence should be followed—restorative evaluation.

Analysis of third treatment option—restoration

Restorative procedures can be used in a variety of ways to resolve arch malrelationship problems. Restorative options include the following:
1. Restorative reshaping to *eliminate the need* for some holding contacts.
2. Fixed/removable prostheses for *substituting* for missing occlusal contacts.

It is possible to recontour teeth restoratively into unlimited shapes, but unless the recontoured crown form complies with factors of stress direction and tissue health, it may create a bigger problem than it solves. Restorative reshaping should be limited to crown contours that result in axially aligned loading in centric relation. The health of the supporting tissues should never be compromised by overprotection of the gingival tissue regardless of what other advantages may be gained from it. In the evaluation of restorative solutions to arch-relationship problems, periodontal considerations are often the limiting factor that determines the logical extent of the reshaping.

If holding contacts cannot be provided by restorative recontouring, or some combination of restoring, reshaping, and repositioning, the next treatment approach to consider is to see if the need for holding contacts can be eliminated by splinting. If teeth without contact can be joined to teeth that have good occlusal stops, their vertical position in the arch can be stabilized. The decision to splint is sometimes the logical treatment of choice when the teeth to be splinted are also useful as abutments for fixed replacement of missing teeth, or when restorations are needed for other reasons.

But the disadvantages of splinting make its use a secondary choice if it is practical to provide holding contacts by other means.

Fixed/removable prostheses are often an excellent treatment choice when there are edentulous segments that require removable appliances. The combination of tooth and tissue support can often be used effectively to substitute holding contacts on the removable

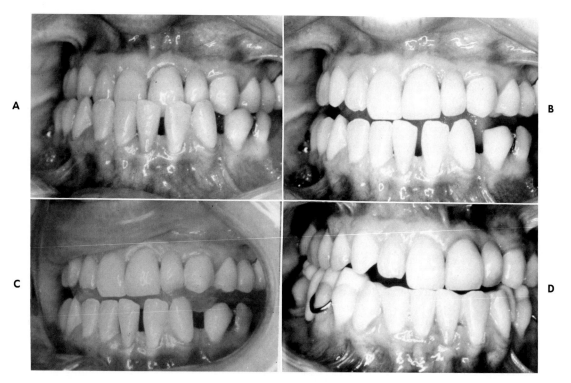

Fig. 39-1. Compromise treatment for a severe arch malrelationship, **A.** Patient had intolerable discomfort, which was diagnosed as occluso-muscle pain resulting from severe displacement of the mandible. **B,** Jaw-to-jaw alignment in centric relation. At this position, joints could accept loading with no discomfort. **C,** Hard Delar wax record in place at centric relation. Patient is comfortable. **D,** Removable splint to coordinate occlusal contact with centric relation resulted in complete comfort for patient.

appliance when stable stops cannot be provided on the teeth themselves. As a compromise treatment, a well-made bite plane can often provide stable holding contacts around an arch that would otherwise require major, complex treatment approaches. I have maintained numerous patients for many years with such appliances who could not afford the more costly surgical and restorative treatment (Fig. 39-1).

Analysis of fourth treatment option—surgery

If the arch malrelationship problem cannot be solved satisfactorily by some combination of reshaping, repositioning, and restorative procedures, it will be apparent on the mounted diagnostic casts. When tooth movement alone, even with recontoured teeth, cannot provide an acceptable occlusal relationship, consideration should be given to surgical repositioning of segments of the dentoalveolar structures on an unchanged skeletal base.

If skeletal base relationships are acceptable and facial profile is not a problem, we can often correct the occlusal malrelationship by shifting a section of the dentition on an un-

changed skeletal base. There are many ways in which sectional osteotomy methods can be used to great advantage. As better surgical techniques have been developed, this procedure has become more useful. Several basic types of sectional osteotomy procedures are illustrated at the end of this chapter along with other surgical methods to show some of the basic methods for surgically correcting each type of arch malrelationship.

The surgical method selected depends on a sequence of diagnostic analyses to determine first the best method, or combination of methods, for establishing stable holding contacts on all the teeth. From that point on, determination of the correct anterior guidance can proceed. The sequence of analysis and subsequent treatment using a combination of specialists is illustrated in Figs. 39-2 to 39-11. In this arch malrelationship the restorative dentist was the coordinator of treatment because he had the final responsibility for an extensive restorative result. In other cases the oral surgeon or the orthodontist may determine the goals of treatment. Regardless of who leads the team approach, it is essential that a very clear model of

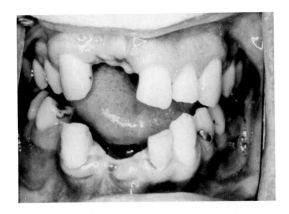

Fig. 39-2. Severe arch malrelationship that resulted from multiple fractures of the maxilla and mandible. The skeletal *base* is acceptable. The dentoalveolar process is misaligned.

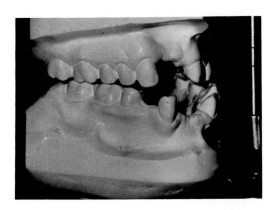

Fig. 39-3. Mounted diagnostic casts at centric relation indicate an anterior open bite and a Class III anterior relationship.

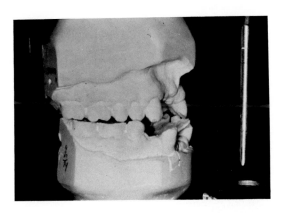

Fig. 39-4. Analysis on cast to see how much correction can be accomplished by reshaping. Some improvement can be made for posterior teeth. Because of multiple fracture lines, onlays are indicated for all posterior teeth regardless of reshaping needs, and so gross reshaping is a logical step to improve the arch relationship.

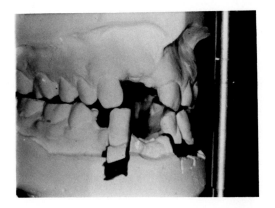

Fig. 39-5. Model of what is needed. A diagnostic waxup will be completed after the teeth have been moved on the second set of casts. This shows a need for more tooth movement than can be accomplished by orthodontics.

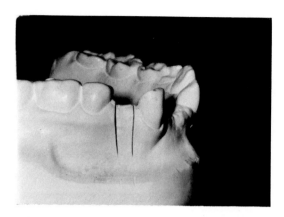

Fig. 39-6. Surgical evaluation shows that an acceptable alignment can be achieved by a segmental osteotomy with a sectional ostectomy.

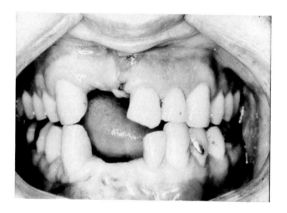

Fig. 39-7. Surgical decision requires movement of lower dentoalveolar segment into better alignment. Removal of a section of bone permits alignment to an acceptable relationship for restoring back to contour. A diagnostic waxup is done again to evaluate acceptability of the alignment so that the result can be visualized.

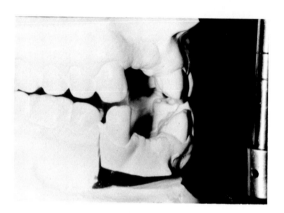

Fig. 39-8. Patient after surgery. Segment in correct position.

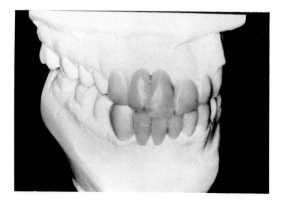

Fig. 39-9. Diagnostic waxup done on postsurgical model to reevaluate planned restorative treatment. This waxup will be duplicated for fabrication of provisional restorations.

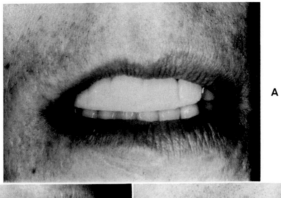

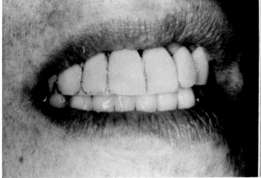

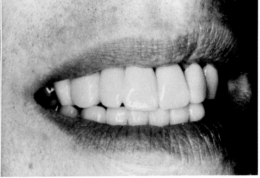

Fig. 39-10. A, Provisional restorations in place after shaping to conform to correct lip-closure path, smile line, and phonetics. Anterior guidance is also worked out on the provisional restorations after incisal edge positions have been determined. No attempt is made to contour individual teeth until position and contour of the incisal plane and the labial surfaces have been determined. **B,** Outline of the individual teeth is drawn on corrected surface contour of the provisional splint. **C,** Provisional restorations after completion of refinement of all contours.

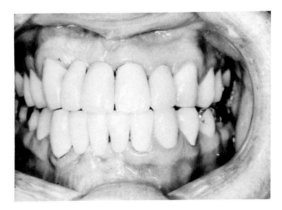

Fig. 39-11. Completed restorations.

the finished result should be constructed in advance of treatment.

No irreversible treatment (other than for an emergency) should be started until the finished result can be clearly visualized and all steps are outlined for the complete treatment.

DESIGNING TREATMENT WHEN THE SKELETAL BASE IS NOT ACCEPTABLY ALIGNED

It is not the purpose of this text to outline all the details of surgical treatment for orthognathic deformities. There are however some underlying principles of treatment planning that relate to what constitutes an acceptable occlusal relationship. And there are some basic surgical objectives that must relate to those goals for good occlusion. By comparing some of the methods with the objectives, we can develop a frame of reference as a basis for communication between the specialties involved.

Starting point for analysis

The starting point for analysis of any severe arch malrelationship must be a determination of the arch relationship when both condyles are in centric relation. If there are any problems of health, position, or alignment of the condyle-disk assemblies, they should be resolved to an acceptable level *before* orthog-

nathic surgery is attempted. Unless the condyle-disk assemblies are in a healthy, physiologically correct relationship, any surgical alignment of the dentition will be misaligned in relation to correct joint position. For that reason, mounted diagnostic casts articulated in a verified centric relation are essential.

Cephalometric analysis should be used with diagnostic casts and a clinical examination to determine the specific parts that need alteration. A review of Chapter 38 is useful to explain some of the ways in which cephalometric analysis is used to guide the determinations.

General practitioners as well as prosthodontists and orthodontists should familiarize themselves with the following basic methods for correcting severe arch malrelationships. In many instances a surgical correction is less traumatic and more readily tolerated than long and extensive orthodontic or prosthodontic treatment, and the results of treatment may be superior. It is an important tenet of restorative dentistry that contour depends on position. Even when extensive restorative treatment is needed, we can often greatly improve it by first correcting the alignment of malrelated arches.

The following surgical methods are illustrated to show how some of the most common arch malrelationships can be corrected (Figs. 39-12 to 39-18).

Text continued on p. 605.

Fig. 39-12. Sagittal split osteotomy *for advancement of the mandible.* This procedure results in a stable forward repositioning, **A,** with little or no relapse because the entire lower band of the buccinator is moved forward with the segment, thus eliminating abnormal pullback from a stretched muscle. Notice how the cut is positioned to avoid the origin of the buccinator. *Heavy dotted line* on **B** shows origin of muscle.

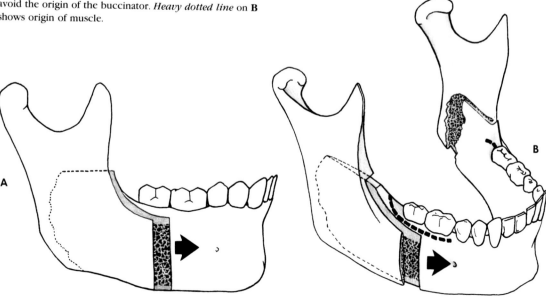

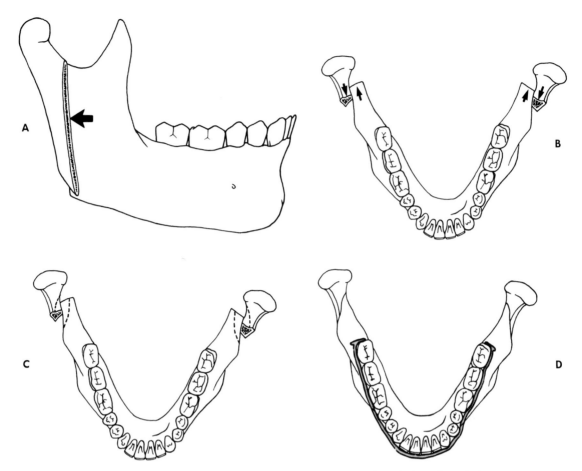

Fig. 39-13. Vertical ramus osteotomy *for mandibular retraction.* A vertical cut through the ramus, **A,** permits the anterior segment to be moved back. The overlap that results, **B,** is reduced to effect a better juncture of the segments, **C.** Notice that the buccinator muscle is unaffected by the repositioning because it is moved in its entirety with the retracted segment, **D.**

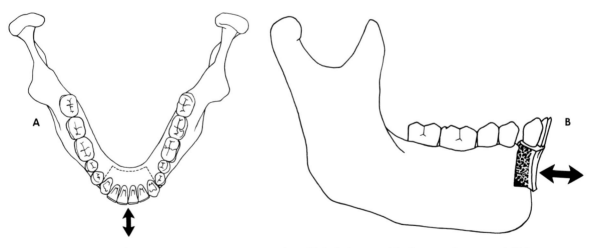

Fig. 39-14. Anterior segmental osteotomy (mandibular) *for repositioning anterior segment.* This procedure is used to reposition the anterior dentoalveolar segment without altering the skeletal base. It can be employed to (1) change the inclination of the anterior segment or (2) level the occlusal plane. **A,** Normal pattern of the cut. **B,** Potential for repositioning. If the section is to be lowered, its height is reduced on the lower border.

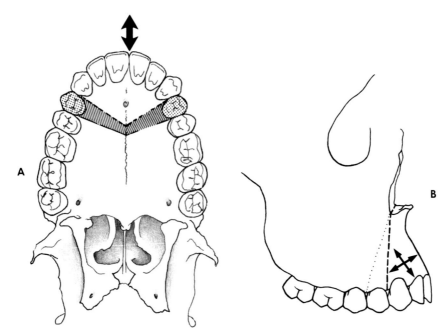

Fig. 39-15. Segmental osteotomy (maxillary) *for repositioning anterior segment.* The anterior segment can be sectioned and repositioned to (1) move the maxillary anterior dentoalveolar segment horizontally or (2) change the inclination of the entire segment or (3) alter the segment's vertical position. It can be combined with removal of a segment, **A. B** shows how the inclination can be altered.

Fig. 39-16. Full maxillary osteotomy *for maxillary advancement.* The maxilla can be sectioned above the roots and the entire dentition advanced forward to correct a skeletal maxillary retrusion.

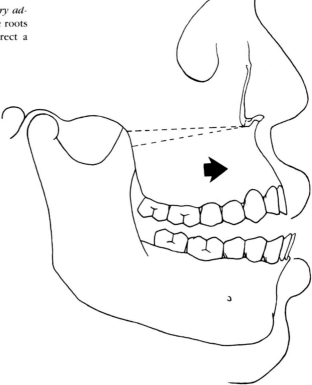

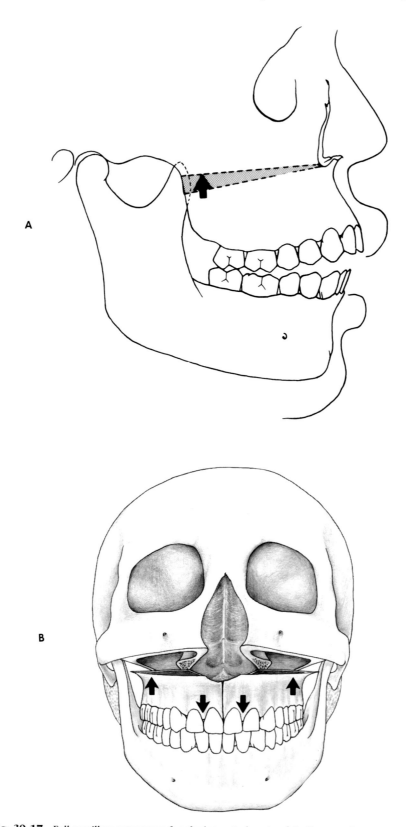

Fig. 39-17. Full maxillary osteotomy *for closing anterior open bite.* By removing a segment from the posterior maxilla, one can elevate the posterior dentoalveolar segment to permit the anterior open bite to be closed, **A.** This up-fracture procedure does not interfere with contracted elevator muscle lengths, and so it provides a very stable result with little or no relapse. A full osteotomy permits a repositioning of the maxilla from several dimensions, **B.**

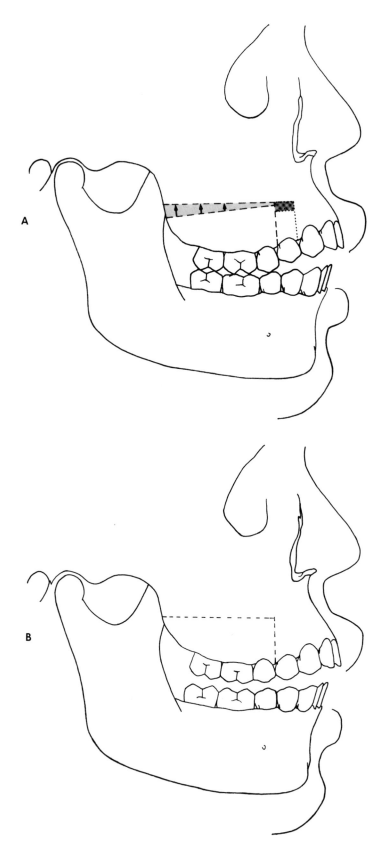

Fig. 39-18. Segmental osteotomy with ostectomy *to level occlusal plane in posterior segments.* By removing a section of bone, one can elevate a segment of the maxillary dentoalveolar process without moving the anterior segment, **A** and **B.** This procedure could be combined with removal of first premolar for horizontal repositioning if needed in addition to the change of vertical. This procedure does not interfere with elevator muscle contraction lengths, and so it results in good stability.

NONSURGICAL TECHNIQUES FOR STABILIZING SKELETAL MALRELATIONSHIPS

Despite advances in surgical technique, a large percentage of arch malrelationships will still be treated by nonsurgical methods. It is possible to stabilize some arch-size discrepancies simply by providing stable holding contacts to prevent supraeruption.

Treating the complete lingual-version lower arch

When all lower teeth are completely lingual to the teeth in the upper arch, there will almost invariably be a skeletal mismatch that is not correctable by orthodontics because there are no occlusal stops—both arches erupt into a side-by-side relationship (Fig. 39-19). Such relationships may be stable if tongue and cheeks substitute for the missing occlusal

stops. If continued eruption is a problem, it can be corrected when holding contacts on the lingual surfaces of the upper teeth are provided and the cusp height on the lower teeth is shortened (Fig. 39-19, *B* and *C*).

If the lower arch can be expanded even slightly to engage the new stops, that is all that will be required to establish stability. There are no concerns about anterior guidance or balancing-side interferences because such patients have vertical patterns of function and have a strong neutral zone horizontally because of the added width between the outward and inward muscle action. In some patients it may be possible to establish stops by simply reshaping tooth surfaces, but it will more often require restorations to provide the holding contacts (Fig. 39-20). There are many configurations that can benefit from this treatment approach, including unilateral arch discrepancies.

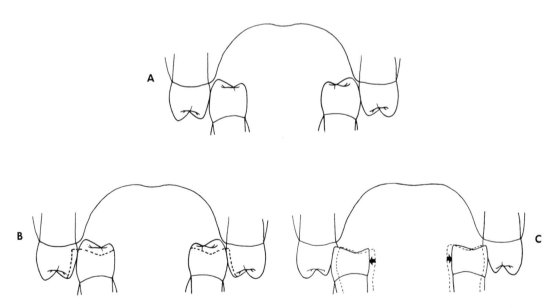

Fig. 39-19. A, When the lower arch is in complete lingual version to the upper arch, supraeruption of the unopposed lower teeth is a potential problem. If the tongue does not substitute for the missing contact, centric holding contacts must be provided. This involves shortening of the lower supraerupted teeth and contouring of the upper lingual surfaces to provide holding contacts. **B,** After contouring is completed, the lower arch is expanded into position for contact in centric relation. This relationship is usually all that is necessary for maintenance of the occlusion. Splinting may be required in some cases. Functional working excursions can be worked out on the upper inclines. **C,** If lower teeth in a lingual-version relationship have supraerupted all the way to tissue contact, the correction is accomplished in the same manner except that the centric stop on the upper teeth may be right at or near the gingival margin. A shallow notch may be all that is necessary to provide a stable centric holding contact. The working excursion in this type of problem is extremely steep, but it does not present a problem because functional movements are almost always vertical.

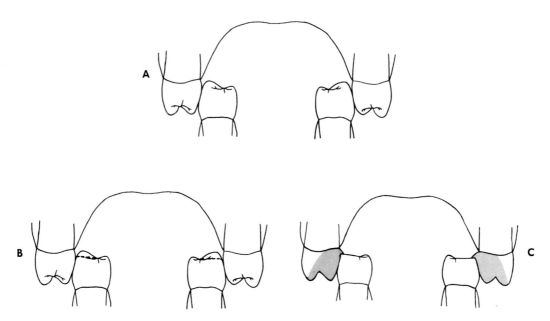

Fig. 39-20. Because of a strong horizontal neutral zone (because of the double thickness of teeth), stability problems are often limited to vertical control of eruption, **A.** Shortening the contact cusp, **B,** and providing a restored stop close to the gum line, **C,** is often all that is needed. Functional movements are limited to vertical, and so excursive pathways are of no concern.

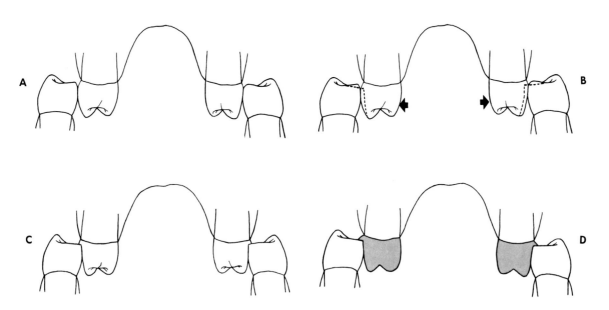

Fig. 39-21. When the mandibular teeth are in complete buccal version to uppers, **A,** the supraeruption of both arches is the principle problem to solve. Stable stops can be established when the lower lingual cusps are shortened and the upper buccal surfaces are reshaped to establish a stop, **B.** The upper arch is then expanded enough to engage the stops, **C. D,** An alternative method is to provide a stop near the gingival margin by restoration.

Treatment choices when lower arch is too wide for upper arch

If the lower teeth are completely buccal to the upper arch, the nonsurgical approach is the same as the treatment for lingual- version lower arches, except that the position of the holding contacts is reversed (Fig. 39-21). There is still no concern about lateral excursions because the steep locked-in occlusion produces a vertical envelope of function.

The decision of how to treat locked in occlusions depends on how the occlusion got that way. If the malrelationship occurred as a result of a congenital arch-size discrepancy, problems with stability will generally be solved when we merely provide centric holding contacts. But if the arch discrepancy resulted from an accidental injury or a poor prosthetic or surgical correction, the locked-in occlusion may not conform with a preestablished pattern of function and stress may result. If any signs of instability are present or masticatory dysfunction is causing discomfort or breakdown, a conservative treatment approach may not be acceptable.

If the occlusion appears stable and the patient is not bothered by esthetics or lack of function, it would generally be in order leaving it as it is. I have observed patients who have relationships like the ones just described who have maintained stable, healthy dentitions for many years with no sign of accelerated deterioration.

40

Transcranial radiography

Transcranial radiography is the method most often used for imaging the temporomandibular joints. The reason transcranial films are so popular is that consistently readable images can be achieved economically and with minimum complexity by use of a standard dental x-ray machine.

With the availability of magnetic resonance imaging (MRI), computerized axial tomography (CT scan) and the wide range of variable techniques for creating images of the joints in any perspective, there is almost no structural problem of the temporomandibular joint that can hide from a persistent diagnostician. Because of these advanced technologies, the use of simple transcranial films may seem to be outdated. There are limitations for transcranial radiography, for sure, but at this writing, it is still the most practical method for assessing the majority of temporomandibular joints radiographically. It should be remembered, however, that transcranial films cannot be used to determine centric relation, and although they may be suggestive of certain disk derangements, neither a positive nor a negative diagnosis of disk displacement should be determined solely from transcranial films.

Even an image of a perfectly centered, normal-appearing joint is not, by itself, assurance of either alignment or health of the temporomandibular joint. Disk displacement can occur without a noticeable displacement of the condyle, and pathologic changes can occur on joint surfaces that are not clearly imaged on transcranial films. Thus a clinical evaluation is an essential preliminary step that must be combined with the radiographic analysis. In fact, the need or purpose of a radiographic examination of the TMJ can be determined only by clinical examination and history.

INDICATIONS FOR TRANSCRANIAL RADIOGRAPHS

Because transcranial films can be made so conveniently and economically, they serve as a practical *first step* for imaging the temporomandibular joints when a potential problem is suspected. Even though the image is predominantly of the lateral aspect of the joint, there will be very few structural problems missed, because most of the pathologic changes that occur on the articulating surfaces start at the lateral half of the joint and are visible on a transcranial view.

If definite clinical signs or symptoms cannot be explained by transcranial radiographs, more specific imaging methods that will more clearly assess the suspected problem area can then be selected. If the lateral view shows no recognizable pathosis, it is a logical second step to view the medial aspect of the joint tomographically. Clinical experience has made us aware that this is rarely necessary.

In some joint problems, the added use of tomography may also fail to clarify the cause of the pathofunction or pain. In such cases, the CT scan may locate the cause of the problem because it can produce a clear definition of the

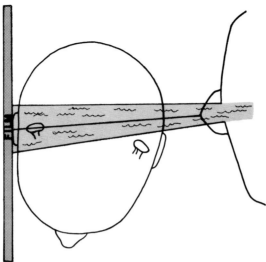

Fig. 40-1. *Individualized* TMJ radiographic technique. Beam is directed through long axis of condyle at 90-degree angle to the film. In this illustration there are no controls for accurate repeatability of head position.

disk and allows visualization of the surfaces and relative positions of the various components of the temporomandibular articulation in both axial and sagittal planes. However, the CT scan has definite disadvantages in addition to its high cost. First, it does not permit observation of the dynamic function, which is necessary for analysis of disk derangements, and, second, it does not show diskal perforations.

At this writing, the only sure method for viewing the *dynamic* function of the disk is through fluoroscopic examination during arthrography. Since this is an invasive procedure, it is reserved for those problems that cannot be diagnosed with simpler procedures. But without an analysis of the joint during function, it is too easy to misinterpret the findings of a static relationship.

The basic purpose of TMJ radiography is to help determine whether we are dealing with an intra-articular problem or with a purely muscular problem related to spasm or incoordination of the masticatory muscles. If we can ascertain that an intra-articular problem does exist, then whatever method is needed should be used to determine the exact nature of the problem so that treatment can be designed that is specific for the pathologic condition. If simple transcranial films can answer the questions that must be answered, there is no reason to put the patient to added expense, inconvenience, or unnecessary radiation.

With above considerations in mind, transcranial radiography is indicated:

1. When there is a history of joint sounds or unexplained discomfort in the joint region
2. Whenever load testing of the joints produces discomfort
3. Whenever any pathologic or structural changes are suspected

If a screening history is negative and a screening examination produces no evidence of intracapsular problems, there is no need for transcranial radiographs, and they are contraindicated. The use of such films must be triggered by clinical evidence.

COMPARISON OF TECHNIQUES

There are several different techniques using different types of positioners for relating the head and the film to the direction of the beam. To simplify a comparison, the differences can be confined to the following:

1. How the head is positioned in relation to the film
2. What direction the beam is in relation to the following:
   a. The long axis of the condyles
   b. The film

The most accurate lateral radiographic image of the condyle is produced when the beam is aimed through the long axis of the condyle, perpendicular to the plane of the film (Fig. 40-1). Updegrave[7] refers to this as *individualized* transcranial radiography, as compared to *standardized* or *fixed-angle* techniques. Although variations in the direction of the beam can oc-

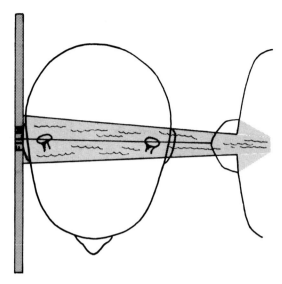

Fig. 40-2. *Standard (fixed-angle)* radiographic technique. Beam is directed at 90 degrees to film but diagonally across condyle. This creates distortion of joint spaces on image.

cur either in the vertical or the horizontal angulations, the major difference between individualized versus standardized techniques is the difference in horizontal angulation of the central ray (Fig. 40-2).

Omnell and Petersson[4] showed that 47 structural changes could be observed in individualized radiographs, whereas only 19 changes could be seen with a standardized technique. If the wide variety of anatomic differences among individuals is considered, it will be obvious why a standardized fixed-angle technique is unacceptable. Therefore the method selected should permit alignment of the beam so that it is as parallel as possible to the long axis of the condyle. With head-holding devices, this beam alignment is usually accomplished by the use of movable ear rods that position the head in relation to the beam.

VERTICAL ANGULATION ALIGNMENT

Vertical angulation of the electron beam is changed when the head is tilted laterally. The degree of angulation is controlled when the height of the ear rods is changed (Fig. 40-3).

According to research and clinical findings by Buhner,[1] setting the vertical angulation of the central beam at 25 degrees will serve as a fairly consistent average for correct imaging of the superior wall, or roof of the glenoid fossa in relation to the Frankfort plane. This angulation is related to the roof of the fossa (not to the condylar head). The space between the condylar head and the roof of the fossa is established by the disk.

According to Farrar and McCarty,[3] a vertical beam angulation of 25 degrees will also minimize superimposition of the petrous portion of the temporal and sphenoid bones over the joint, but this angle will vary to some degree in relation to different head shapes and widths. By moving the ear rod next to the cassette up, the vertical angulation can be increased. Moving the ear rod down decreases the angulation. The vertical angulation on the Acurad head positioner is changed by raising or lowering of the ear plug on the side opposite to the cassette, a range from 21 to 30 degrees, and this range can accommodate almost any patient.

To evaluate the correctness of vertical angulation, the petrous line should be observed on the film. It should intersect the condyle midway between the medial and lateral poles, which should place it slightly above the level of the auditory meatus (Fig. 40-4).

The posterior clinoid process should be positioned slightly anterior to the eminentia, level with the superior outline of the fossa. In many transcranial films the posterior clinoid process is not clearly visible, and so it is not always usable as a landmark.

By analyzing a test radiograph, we can determine if a change in vertical angulation is needed. Increasing the vertical angle will posi-

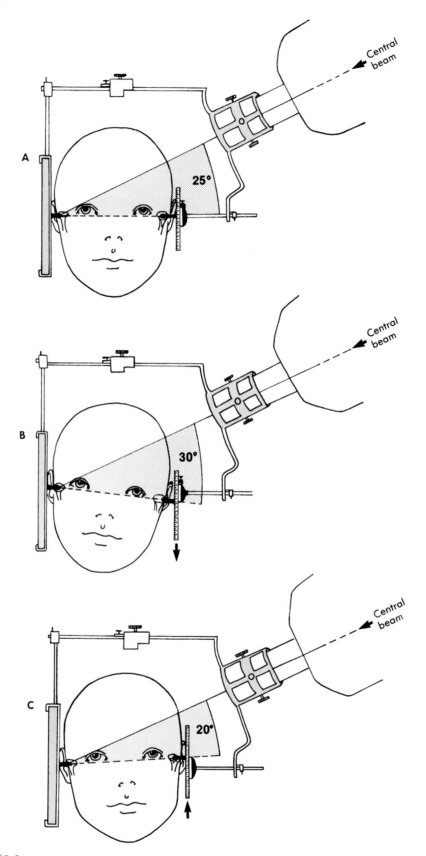

Fig. 40-3. A, Vertical angulation of the beam is altered when the head is tilted laterally. Notice the beam angle when the head is straight. **B,** When the ear rod opposite the cassette is lowered, the chin moves toward the film, tilting the head. This increases the angulation of the central beam. **C,** When the ear rod is raised, opposite the cassette, the chin moves away from the film causing the beam angle to decrease.

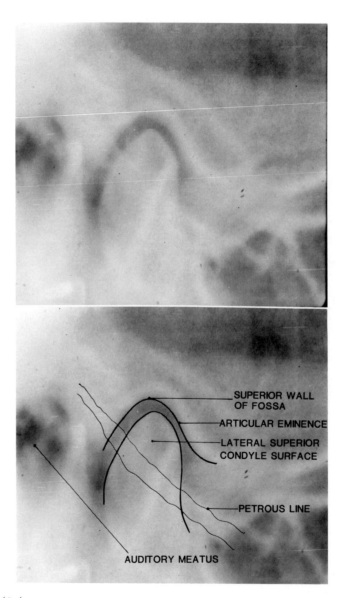

Fig. 40-4. Proper position of petrous line indicates correctness of vertical angulation.

Effect of changing vertical angulation of beam

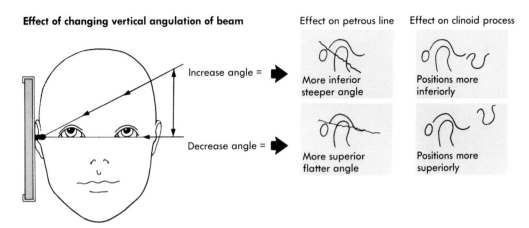

Increase angle =

Decrease angle =

Effect on petrous line

More inferior
steeper angle

More superior
flatter angle

Effect on clinoid process

Positions more
inferiorly

Positions more
superiorly

Fig. 40-5. Effects on petrous line and clinoid process of changing the vertical angulation of beam.

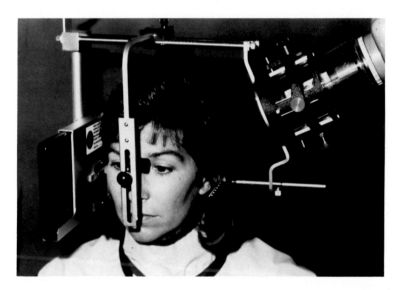

Fig. 40-6. Accurad 200 (Dénar) Head position is controlled by position of ear plugs and nasion positioner. Head does not move during exposure of three different views. Film only is moved after each exposure. The mandible can move in relation to the fixed cranial base for comparative views of joint.

tion the petrous line more inferiorly. The clinoid process is also lowered. Decreasing the vertical angulation raises the petrous line as well as the clinoid process (Fig. 40-5).

All vertical alignments should be made with the Frankfort horizontal plane parallel to the floor. A nasion positioner is used in combination with the ear rods to stabilize the head in that position (Fig. 40-6).

This results in an occlusal plane that is slightly lower in front. This relationship must be maintained when the mouth is opened. The normal tendency to tip the head back during

opening must be prevented. The use of the nasion positioner combined with two ear rods for positioning the head permits reasonable duplication of head position for comparative radiographs. Thus a comparison can be made regarding the position of the condyle in a comfortable centric relation alignment versus its position during maximum intercuspation. A stable head position also permits accurate reproduction of radiographic records for later evaluation of the joint. The use of reproducible reference points is also essential for making corrections in the angulation of the beam.

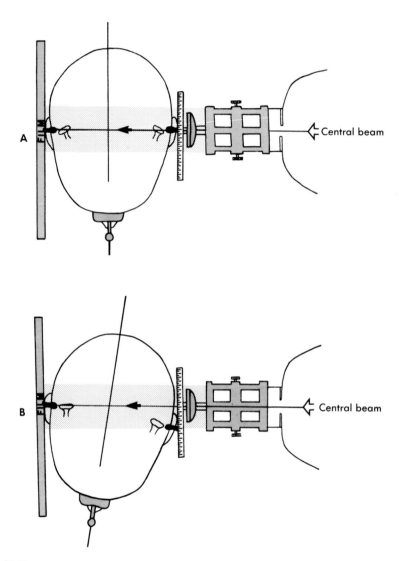

Fig. 40-7. A, Path of central beam when the film is positioned parallel to the midsagittal plane and the beam is directed at 90-degree angle to the film. The image results from the beam crossing diagonally across the condyle. **B,** By moving the ear plug opposite the cassette forward, the head turns toward the cassette. This directs the beam through the long axis of the condyle at 90 degrees to the film. The combination of the two ear rods and the nasion positioner provide three points of reference for ease of duplication.

Effect of changing horizontal angulation of beam

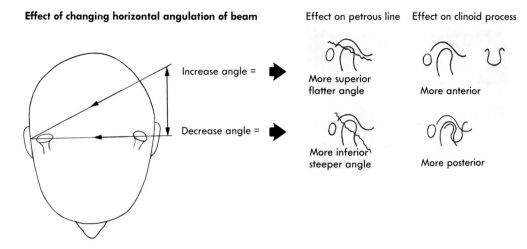

Effect on petrous line   Effect on clinoid process

Increase angle =   ➡   More superior
flatter angle   More anterior

Decrease angle =   ➡   More inferior
steeper angle   More posterior

Fig. 40-8. Effects on movement of petrous line and clinoid process when horizontal angulation of beam is changed.

HORIZONTAL ANGULATION ALIGNMENT

To alter the horizontal angulation of the electron beam, move the ear rod on the opposite side from the cassette holder horizontally. By sliding the ear rod left or right, the head must turn, causing the horizontal angulation of the beam to either increase or decrease (Fig. 40-7).

When the ear plug is moved forward, the head must turn toward the film. This has the effect of aligning the long axis of the condyle with the central beam. It also keeps the film aligned to a 90-degree angle to the rays to provide the least distortion of the image.

The alignment of the head can also be achieved by a combination of horizontal movements of *both* ear plugs. The important consideration is that the long axis of the condyle should parallel the beam, which is, in turn, at 90 degrees to the film. As long as that is accomplished, the image will have diagnostic value. Simple adjustments to the ear plug positions make this a practical procedure.

The location of the petrous line and the clinoid process are also affected by variations of the horizontal angle. The incorrect horizontal angle can result in superimposition of the clinoid process over the fossa and condyle, or the medial pole of the condyle may be projected into the anterior joint space, and such projection could be misinterpreted as an anterior displacement of the condyle.[6]

The petrous line moves superiorly and its angle becomes less steep as the horizontal angle is increased. The clinoid process moves more anteriorly as the head turns toward the film and the horizontal angle is increased (Fig. 40-8).

By relating the relative position of the petrous line and the clinoid process in a trial exposure, compensation can be made in both vertical and horizontal beam angulations by alteration of the position of the ear plugs.

If the horizontal alignment of the long axes of condyles is compared with the transmeatal line (frontal plane), the average angular deviance is approximately 13 degrees according to Yale[8] who studied over 2900 mandibular condyles. He also reported that variations from the frontal plane ranged from 0 to 30 degrees.

The long axis of the condyle generally relates to the ramus at approximately a right angle. In devising a method for taking advantage of that relationship, Schier[5] found that if a flat plane is pressed against the side of the face so that it contacts the high point of the zygomas, the gonion, and the lower border of the mandible next to the molars, the long axis of the condyle would be 90 degrees to that plane. Updegrave takes advantage of this relationship by aligning the cassette with that planar base and directs the ray directly through the condyle at the film. A single ear plug is used on the cassette side to position the film.

OTHER CONSIDERATIONS

The shorter the film distance from the radiation source, the more the distortion occurs in the image. Using a collimated, long cone to lengthen the source-film distance minimizes enlargement of the image of the joint and produces a more readable film.

The use of high-speed intensifying screens permits reduced exposure time and reduced radiation dosage.

Transcranial radiography has definite limitations. It has, however, stood the test of time as a very logical adjunct to a careful clinical examination. Its limitations are more a matter of interpretation than of the radiograph itself and relate to how you plan to use the radiograph. If a transcranial film does not show us what we need to complete a diagnosis, we must proceed to whatever imaging method must be used to provide the needed information.

Cole[2] has suggested three steps in learning to better interpret transcranial radiographs:

1. First, become intimately familiar with the anatomy of the hard and soft tissues of the TMJ.
2. Next, examine the angle of projection of the electron beam and the image it forms, and be sure you understand them.
3. Finally, practice visualizing the TMJ in three dimensions by studying the radiographic image and remembering that the tissue is "translucent" to an electron.

If these three steps are understood, the interpretation of transcranial films can be achieved to a practical advantage.

REFERENCES

1. Buhner, W.A.: A headholder for oriented temporomandibular joint radiographs, J. Prosthet. Dent. **29**:113, 1973.
2. Cole, S.V.: Transcranial radiography: Correlation between actual and radiographic joint spaces, J. Craniomandibular Practice **2**(2):153, 1984.
3. Farrar, W.B., and McCarty, W.L., Jr.: Clinical outline of temporomandibular joint diagnosis and treatment, ed. 7, Montgomery, Ala., 1982, Normandie Publication, pp. 90-100.
4. Omnell, K., and Petersson, A.: Radiography of the temporomandibular joints utilizing oblique lateral transcranial projections, Odontol. Revy **27**(2):77, 1976.
5. Schier, M.B.A.: Temporomandibular joint roentgenography: controlled erect technique, J. Am. Dent. Assoc. **65**:456, Oct. 1962.
6. Tucker, T.N.: Head position for transcranial temporomandibular joint radiographs, J. Prosthet. Dent. **52**:426, 1984.
7. Updegrave, W.J.: Radiography of the temporomandibular joints, individualized and simplified, Compendium of Continuing Education **4**(1):23, 1983.
8. Yale, S.H.: Radiographic evaluation of the temporomandibular joints, J. Am. Dent. Assoc. **79**:102, July 1969.

SUGGESTED READINGS

Craddock, F.W.: Radiography of the temporomandibular joints, J. Dent. Res. **32**:302, 1953.
Weinberg, L.A.: What we really see in a TMJ radiograph, J. Prosthet. Dent. **30**:898, 1973.

41

Postoperative care of occlusal therapy patients

When the active treatment phase has been completed for a patient with an occlusally related problem, a program of postoperative care should be planned that gives the patient the best long-term prognosis.

That plan must be related to the condition of the various parts of the masticatory system after occlusal therapy has been completed. There are seven major considerations that should influence the program of postoperative care:

1. Condition of the connective tissue of the TMJ
2. Presence or absence of an acceptable disk
3. Condition of supporting structures of teeth
4. Degree of fulfillment of all requirements for occlusal stability
5. Presence of habit patterns or nocturnal bruxism
6. Ability or willingness to follow a meticulous oral hygiene program
7. Dietary patterns or general health problems

Abnormalities in any of the above factors may be a reason for special postoperative counseling. If damage to the connective tissues of the joint has weakened the ligaments or surgery has been used to correct such problems, it may be necessary to follow up with physical therapy or a soft diet for a period of months. An excellent help for patients during this reparative stage is *The No-Chew Cookbook*[1] by Randy Wilson. Connective tissue heals slowly, and patients must be educated regarding what they must do or not do to prevent damage.

If the disk is absent or irreparably displaced, patients should be counseled about the importance of maintaining a perfected occlusion. Especially important is the need to correct any posterior occlusal interferences as they may occur because of their trigger effect on muscle hyperactivity. It is also important to advise patients that there is a probability of gradual loss of height of the condyle when the disk is not in place. The occlusion must be checked at each recall appointment to see if the last molar is hitting prematurely, since this is the obvious result of the degenerative joint disease that routinely occurs on the surface of a diskless condyle.

Patients with compromised support for the teeth should be advised of any special requirements for maintenance and may require a closer recall schedule. Mobility patterns should be monitored and recorded for comparison at subsequent appointments. Recordings of sulcular depth should be compared at reasonable intervals.

When any compromise has been made with fulfilling all requirements for occlusal stability, the dentition will be in jeopardy. It should be specifically monitored to make sure that signs of instability are not allowed to reach an irreversible level without the patient being advised of what should be done. It should be noted in the patient's record that the problem was explained and treatment recommended. If patients choose not to follow the advice, they should be told what special measures they should take in home care to at least slow down the expected damage.

Habit patterns can be destructive, or they may have a stabilizing effect on a malrelated occlusion. Any habit pattern should be noted, and effects of such habits monitored for any changes. If the effects of bruxism are progressive, steps should be recommended for reducing the damage. At each recall appointment patients should be informed about the status of any effects resulting from habit patterns.

Different patients respond in different ways to attempts at getting them to follow proper home care procedures. Patients with poor hygiene should be constantly encouraged in a helpful way. Stern lectures and criticism rarely if ever work, and so they may as well be avoided. A record should, however, be kept of each patient's personal oral hygiene, and the patient should always be informed of the effects he or she can expect if procedures are not followed.

Patients who are unable or unwilling to follow hygiene recommendations should be encouraged to come in for more frequent recalls.

Dietary counseling should be a part of any recall appointment if effects that customarily result from an inadequate or imbalanced diet are noted.

The recall appointment for patients with special problems should not be treated in a perfunctory manner as if the problems were normal. That appointment should always be used to help the patient overcome whatever special problems are present so that the destructive effects can be prevented or at least reduced.

Fortunately, most of my patients who accept complete treatment end up with maintainably healthy masticatory systems. The postoperative care for noncompromise patients who have been effectively treated to fulfill all the requirements for occlusal stability must

still be tailored to suit each patient, but I have found great benefit in a technique I refer to as "prodding." Patients are asked to find any disharmonies in a completed occlusal restoration.

In my office, it has been the standard policy for years to *encourage* patients to try to find fault with their occlusal result. It is a policy that eventually leads to excellence in patient comfort because it forces the dentist to accept nothing short of an optimum occlusal result.

Telling patients to critically evaluate their occlusions, to "be fussy about how it feels," is the opposite of what is often implied at the completion of treatment: "This is it. Now you must learn to live with it." Many dental patients end up stressed emotionally because they believe that they have no recourse but to live with their uncomfortable dentistry. Patients truly appreciate the opportunity to point out areas of discomfort. It has been my experience that when given this opportunity they will rarely abuse it. Patients almost always try to be fair to any dentist who is obviously committed to their best interests. Just letting patients know they have the right to expect comfort takes away almost all the urgency and fearfulness about the completed treatment. The dentist can and should systematically evaluate any problem and try to find a solution for it. Such an approach may sound impractical, but it will pay unexpected dividends for both the patient and the dentist (if the dentist is competent enough to correct the problems).

For best long-term maintainability, patients should be instructed in how to evaluate occlusal problems. Early correction of a newly developed interference is usually simple and not very time consuming. Patients should be told to report any of the following indications of occlusal disharmony:

1. Any discomfort in the teeth when chewing
2. Any indication of a "high" tooth or any sign that one or more teeth contact before the rest when closing; any tooth that can be made to hurt by biting on it
3. Any sign of tooth hypermobility
4. Any discomfort in the temporomandibular joint area
5. Any limitation of function

Any one of these signs or symptoms is an indication that the occlusal relationship is producing excessive stress. Each problem is correctable and should be resolved to prevent accelerated deterioration.

Signs of bruxism should also be observed to see if they are related to occlusal interferences. If the bruxing cannot be stopped, it is all the more important to maintain occlusal harmony or to take steps to reduce the damage.

Since there is no restorative technique that can guarantee 100% permanent occlusal harmony, the logical approach to long-term maintainability is to correct occlusal discrepancies whenever they occur and whenever they have the potential for causing breakdown. Enlisting patients' aid in reporting such problems is just as practical as asking them to report bleeding gums or hypersensitivity.

Unless instructions are given regarding what to look for and unless patients are encouraged to be critical about their occlusions, they tend to accept discomfort as part of the normal "breaking-in" experience. Unfortunately, such self-adjustment of an incorrect occlusion usually occurs by getting the stressed teeth loose enough to accommodate to the interfering inclines.

In the absence of an injury, abscess, or severe bone loss, hypermobility is almost always a sign of excessive occlusal stress. It is one of the first detectable signs of periodontal breakdown, and it is almost always completely reversible if corrected early enough. For that reason, no postoperative follow-up appointment is complete without each tooth being checked for hypermobility. Dental hygienists should be trained to examine for hypermobility just as thoroughly as they examine for caries. All postoperative checkups should include such an examination. If any hypermobility is noticed, the occlusal cause of the problem should be located and corrected without delay.

POSTOPERATIVE PERIODONTAL MAINTENANCE

Although there is much evidence that occlusal trauma contributes to many aspects of periodontal breakdown, it is a bad mistake to believe it is the only factor. Until scientific research can provide conclusive proof of singular causes for specific effects, occlusal therapy must be considered as only part of any treatment plan. It should also be regarded as only part of any postoperative follow-up observation.

Even though certain clinical observations may be suggestive of occlusal trauma as the probable cause, all other possible causes should also be considered in a multitreatment approach toward the restoration of optimum health.

An illustrative example is the postoperative formation of gingival clefts. Although there is clinical evidence to associate gingival clefts with occlusal trauma, we know they can also be caused by improper tooth brushing or by improperly contoured restorations, or by postorthodontic pressure from the buccinator—orbicularis oris muscle. Each of these causative factors should be evaluated along with the occlusal factors, and each should be corrected when it is found to be a contributing irritant.

Inadequate or improper oral hygiene is a factor that must be considered in every patient we treat. For the occlusal therapist it is just as important to evaluate, educate, and postoperatively appraise each patient's mouth hygiene as it is to check the occlusion. One of the saddest situations I see is the completely restored patient who has never been taught how to care for his or her investment in extensive dentistry.

Each postoperative checkup appointment should include a careful examination of the periodontal tissues. Either substantial problems should be corrected or the patient should be referred to a competent periodontal specialist.

THE HEALTHY MOUTH—DENTISTRY'S GOAL

Modern dental treatment is designed to focus on one predominant goal: *optimally maintainable oral health.* Any factor that lessens the maintainability of any oral tissue is a factor that must be isolated and corrected. To do less is to fail the task entrusted to us. Dentists who are dedicated to the concept of optimum oral health will not be able to treat one problem while ignoring others. They will search out and correct all factors that contribute to accelerated deterioration.

The role of occlusal stress will never be ignored by any dentist who believes his or her patients are entitled to a healthy mouth. But such a goal-oriented dentist will not be guilty of tunnel vision either. Analysis and correction of occlusal problems will fit in perspective into a total plan of treatment designed to provide and maintain the healthiest mouth possible for each patient treated. The competent dentist of today must be the physician of the masticatory system. There is no other speciality of medicine in which one is adequately trained to assume that role. The modern standard of dental practice should reflect that obligation.

REFERENCE

1. Wilson, J.R.: The no-chew cookbook, ed. 2, 1986, Wilson Publishing Co., P.O. Box 2190, Glenwood Springs, CO 81602.

Index

Page numbers in *italics* indicate illustrations.